Proceedings of the
International Dermatology Symposion (IDS)
Berlin, October 13–15, 1980

Retinoids

Advances in Basic Research and Therapy

Edited by C.E. Orfanos and
O. Braun-Falco · E.M. Farber · Ch. Grupper
M.K. Polano · R. Schuppli

With 215 Figures and 143 Tables

Springer-Verlag
Berlin Heidelberg New York 1981

Prof. Dr. C.E. Orfanos
Director
Department of Dermatology
University Medical Center Steglitz
The Free University of Berlin
Hindenburgdamm 30
1000 Berlin 45, West Germany

ISBN-13:978-3-642-68025-0 e-ISBN-13:978-3-642-68023-6
DOI: 10.1007/978-3-642-68023-6

Library of Congress Cataloging in Publication Data
International Dermatology Symposium (1980 : Berlin, Germany) Retinoids, advances in basic research and therapy.
"Proceedings of the International Dermatology Symposium, Berlin, October 13–15, 1980."
Bibliography: p. Includes index.
1. Psoriasis--Chemotherapy--Congresses. 2. Vitamin A--Testing--Congresses. 3. Acne--Chemotherapy--Congresses. 4. Vitamin A--Physiological effect--Congresses. I. Orfanos, Constantin E. II. Title. [DNLM: 1. Tretinoin--Therapeutic use. 2. Skin diseases--Drug therapy. QU 167 R438]
RL321.I56 1980 616.5' 26061 81-5769
ISBN-13:978-3-642-68025-0 (U.S.) AACR2

Softcover reprint of the hardcover 1st edition 1981

Composition: Fotosatz Service Weihrauch, Würzburg

2127/3321 543210

Contents

Application of Oral Retinoids in Psoriasis

Application of Oral Retinoids in Acne

Oral Retinoid Therapy of Miscellaneous Disorders of Skin and Oral Mucosa

Clinical and Laboratory Monitoring of Oral Retinoid Therapy

Short Clinical and Experimental Reports

Present Status and Perspectives

List of Contributors

Allen, H.B., M.D., Department of Dermatology, University Hospital University of Pennsylvania School of Medicine, Philadelphia, Pennsylvania 19104, U.S.A.

Allevato, M.A., M.D., 1. Cátedra de Dermatologia, Hospital de Clínicas José San Martin, Universidad de Buenos Aires, Buenos Aires, Argentine

Bauer, R., Ass. Prof., M.D., Department of Dermatology, University Medical Center Steglitz, The Free University of Berlin, Hindenburgdamm 30, D-1000 Berlin 45, West Germany

Berecz, M., M.D., Clinic of Dermatology, Semmelweis Medical School, Maria-Straße 41, H-1085 Budapest, Hungary

Berger, H., Prof., M.D., Universitäts-Hautklinik, Von-Siebold-Straße 3, D-3400 Göttingen, West Germany

Bermejo, D., M.D., Department of Dermatology, Polyclinique d'Aubervilliers, F-93300 Aubervilliers, France

Berretti, B., M.D., Department of Dermatology, Polyclinique d'Aubervilliers, F-93300 Aubervilliers, France

Berti, E., M.D., Clinica Dermatologica, Università di Milano, Via Pace 9, I-20122 Milano, Italy

Bialasiewicz, A.A., M.D., Hautklinik Linden, Medizinische Hochschule, Ricklinger Straße 5, D-3000 Hannover 91, West Germany

Binazzi, M., Prof., Chairman, M.D., Istituto di Clinica Dermosifilopatica dell'Università di Perugia, Policlinico Monteluce, I-06100 Perugia, Italy

Blanc, D., M.D., The General Infirmary at Leeds, Department of Dermatology, Great George Street, GB-Leeds LS1 3EX, Great Britain

Blanchet-Bardon, C., M.D., Clinique Dermatologique, Hôpital Saint-Louis 38 à 42, Rue Bichat, F-75010 Paris, France

Boer, J., M.D., Afdeling Dermatologie, Academisch Ziekenhuis-Leiden, Rijnsburgerweg 10, NL-Leiden, Netherlands

Bollag, W., M.D., Pharma Forschung 2, F. Hoffmann-La Roche & Co. AG, Grenzacherstrasse 124, CH-4002 Basel, Switzerland

Bonafé, J.L., M.D., Service de Dermatologie, Hôpital de La Grave, F-31052 Toulouse Cedex, France

Bonnot, G., M.D., Service de Biologie, INSA, F-69621 Villeurbanne, France

Born, W., M.D., Universitäts-Hautklinik, Hauptstraße 7, D-7800 Freiburg, West Germany

Braun-Falco, O., Prof., Chairman, M.D., Universitäts-Hautklinik, Frauenlobstraße 9, D-8000 München 2, West Germany

Bruley-Rosset, M., M.D., Institut de Cancérologie et d'Immunogénétique, Hôpital Paul-Brousse, F-94800 Villejuif, France

Brun, R., M.D. Clinique Universitaire de Dermatologie, Hôpital Cantonal, 1211 Génève 4, Switzerland

Carbrera, H., M.D., Cátedra de Dermatología, Hospital Muniz, Buenos Aires, Argentine

Cardama, J.E., M.D., Cátedra de Dermatología, Hospital Muniz, Buenos Aires, Argentine

Caputo, R., Prof., M.D., Clinica Dermatologica, Università di Milano, Via Pace 9, I-20122 Milano, Italy

Caruso, A., M.D., University of Catania, Department of Experimental Dermatology, Catania, Italy

Christiansen, J.V., M.D., Department of Dermatology, Marselisborg Hospital, University of Aarhus, DK-8000 Aarhus, Denmark

Christophers, E., Prof., Chairman, M.D., Universitäts-Hautklinik, Schittenhelmstraße 7, D-2300 Kiel, West Germany

Contini, D., M.D., Clinica Dermatologica, Università di Milano, Via Pace 9, I-20122 Milano, Italy

Cordero, A.A., Prof., Chairman, M.D., 1.ª Cátedra de Dermatologica, Hospital de Clinicas José San Martin, Universidad de Buenos Aires, Buenos Aires, Argentine

Cunliffe, W.J., M.D., F.R.C.P., The General Infirmary at Leeds, Department of Dermatology, Great George Street, GB-Leeds LS1 3EX, Great Britain

Dabrowski, J., M.D., Klinika Dermatologiczna, A.M. UI. Koszykowa 82a, 02-0088 Warszawa, Poland

Devaux, J., M.D., Service de Dermatologie, Hôtel-Dieu, Place Daviel, F-13002 Marseille, France

Dick, D.C., M.D., Department of Dermatology, University of Glasgow, GB-Glasgow, Great Britain

Dominguez-Soto, L., Prof., M.D., Av. Santiago No. 420, San Jeronimo Lidice, Mexico 20 D.F., Mexico

Donatti, L., M.D., 1. Cátedra de Dermatologia, Hospital de Clínicas José San Martin, Universidad de Buenos Aires, Buenos Aires, Argentine

Dupré, A., Prof., M.D., Service de Dermatologie, Hôpital de La Grave, F-31052 Toulouse Cedex, France

Edelson, Y., M.D., Department of Dermatology, Polyclinique d'Aubervilliers, F-93300 Aubervilliers, France

Farber, E.M., Prof., Chairman, M.D., Department of Dermatology, Stanford University School of Medicine, Stanford, California 94305, U.S.A.

Fischer-Hoinkes, H., M.D., Klinik für Rheumakranke, Dr.-Alfons-Gamp-Straße 1, D-6550 Bad Kreuznach, West Germany

Florentin, I., M.D., Institut de Cancérologie et d'Immunogénétique, Hôpital Paul-Brousse, F-94800 Villejuif, France

Foged, E., M.D., Department of Dermatology, Odense University Hospital, DK-5000 Odense, Denmark

Fredriksson, T., Prof., M.D., Department of Dermatology, Central Hospital, S-72189 Västerås, Sweden

Fulton, R., M.D., Clinique Dermatologique, Hôpital E. Herriot, F-69374 Lyon Cedex 2, France

Gabrielli, M., M.D., Cátedra de Dermatologia, Hospital Muniz, Buenos Aires, Argentine

Gamby, T., M.D., Service de Dermatologie, Hôtel-Dieu, Place Daviel, F-13002 Marseille, France

Gasparini, G., M.D., Clinica Dermatologica, Università di Milano, Via Pace 9, I-20122 Milano, Italy

Gatti, J.C., Prof., M.D., Virrey del Pino 2689, 5° Piso, 1426 Buenos Aires, Argentine

Glazer, S., M.D., Department of Dermatology, Northwestern University Medical School, Ward Memorial Building, Chicago, Illinois 60611, U.S.A.

Gollnick, H., M.D., Department of Dermatology, University Medical Center Steglitz, The Free University of Berlin, Hindenburgdamm 30, D-1000 Berlin 45, West Germany

Gomez, E.C., Prof., M.D., Ph.D., Department of Dermatology, University of California, Sacramento, California 95187, U.S.A.

Gómez, S., M.D., Servicio de Dermatologia, Hospital General "Dr. Manuel Gea Gonzalez", Mexico City 22 D.F., Mexico

Goodman, D.S., Prof., M.D., College of Physicians and Surgeons, Columbia University 630 West, 168th Street, New York, New York 10032, U.S.A.

Gross, P.R., M.D., Department of Dermatology, University Hospital, University of Pennsylvania School of Medicine, Philadelphia, Pennsylvania 19104, U.S.A.

Grupper, Ch., M.D., 38, Rue de Courcelles, F-75008 Paris, France

Guilhou, J.J., M.D., Department of Dermatology, F-34000 Montpellier, France

Haftek, M., M.D., Klinika Dermatologiczna A.M., Ul. Koszykowa 82a, 02-0088 Warszawa, Poland

Happle, R., Prof., M.D., Universitäts-Hautklinik, Von-Esmarch-Straße 56, D-4400 Münster, West Germany

Hartmann, H.R., M.D., Pharma Forschung 2, F. Hoffmann-La Roche & Co. AG, Grenzacherstraße 124, CH-4002 Basel, Switzerland

Hercend, Th., M.D., Institut de Cancérologie et d'Immunogénétique, Hôpital Paul-Brousse, F-94800 Villejuif, France

Hino, H., M.D., Department of Dermatology, Rigshospitalet, University of Copenhagen, Blegdamsvej 9, DK-2100 Copenhagen, Denmark

Hojyo-Tomoka, M.T., M.D., Servicio de Dermatología, Hospital General "Dr. Manuel Gea Gonzalez", Mexico City, Mexico

Hummler, H., M.D., Biologisch-Pharmazeutische Forschung, F. Hoffmann-La Roche & Co. AG, Grenzacherstraße 124, CH-4002 Basel, Switzerland

Hunziker, N., Ass. Prof., M.D., Clinique de Dermatologie, Hôpital Cantonal, Universitaire de Genève, CH-1200 Genève, Switzerland

Imregh, E., Clinic of Dermatology, Semmelweis Medical School, Maria-Straße 41, H-1085 Budapest, Hungary

Jablonska, S., Prof., Chairman, Klinika Dermatologiczna A.M. Ul. Koszykowa 82a, 02-0088 Warszawa, Poland

Jansén, C.T., Ass. Prof., M.D., Department of Dermatology, University of Turku, SF-20520 Turku 52, Finland

Jarząbek-Chorzelska, M.; M.D., Klinika Dermatologiczna A.M. Ul. Koszykowa 82a, 02-0088 Warszawa, Poland

Jeanneret, J.-P., M.D., Clinique Universitaire de Dermatologie, 3, Place Pury, CH-2000 Neuchâtel, Switzerland

Jones, D.H., M.D., The General Infirmary at Leeds, Department of Dermatology, Great George Street, GB-Leeds LS1 3EX, Great Britain

Jorgensen, H., M.D., Department of Dermatology, The Washington Hospital Center, 110 Irving Street, NW, Washington, DC 20010, U.S.A.

Juvakoski, T., M.D., Department of Dermatology, Helsinki University Central Hospital, Snellmaninkatu 14, SF-00170 Helsinki 17, Finland

Kamino, H., M.D., Servicio de Dermatologia, Hospital General "Dr. Manuel Gea Gonzalez", Mexico City 22 D.F., Mexico

Kanerva, L., M.D., Department of Dermatology, Helsinki University Central Hospital, Snellmaninkatu 14, SF-00170 Helsinki 17, Finland

Katz, R.A., M.D., Department of Dermatology, The Washington Hospital Center, 110 Irving Street, NW, Washington, DC 20010, U.S.A.

King, I.A., M.D., MRC Unit on the Experimental Pathology of the Skin, The Medical School, GB-Birmingham B15 2TJ, Great Britain

Kligman, A.M., Prof., Chairman, M.D., Ph.D., Department of Dermatology, University Hospital, University of Pennsylvania School of Medicine, Philadelphia, Pennsylvania 19104, U.S.A.

Kligman, L.H., Ph.D., Department of Dermatology, University Hospital, University of Pennsylvania School of Medicine, Philadelphia, Pennsylvania 19104, U.S.A.

Kober, A., M.D., Department of Pharmaceutical Biochemistry, University of Uppsala S-751 01 Uppsala, Sweden

Koch, H.F., Prof., M.D., Universitätsklinik für Kiefer- und Plastische Gesichtschirurgie, Westdeutsche Kieferklinik, Moorenstraße 5, D-4000 Düsseldorf, West Germany

Komenda, K., M.D., Röntgenabteilung des Krankenhauses St. Marienwörth, Mühlenstraße 39, D-6550 Bad Kreuznach, West Germany

Konstantinović, S., Prof., M.D., Stjepana Radića 19, YU-11040 Beograd, Jugoslavia

Kraińska, T., M.D., Klinika Dermatologiczna A.M., Ul. Koszykowa 82a, 02-0088 Warszawa, Poland

Kummermehr, J., M.D., Strahlenbiologisches Institut der Universität München, Frauenlobstraße 9, D-8000 München 2, West Germany

Landthaler, M., M.D., Universitäts-Hautklinik, Frauenlobstraße 9, D-8000 München 2, West Germany

Lassus, A., Prof., M.D., Department of Dermatology, Helsinki University Central Hospital, Snellmaninkatu 14, SF-00170 Helsinki 17, Finland

Lauharanta, J., M.D., Department of Dermatology, Helsinki University Central Hospital, Snellmaninkatu 14, SF-00170 Helsinki 17, Finland

Leyden, J.J., M.D., Department of Dermatology, University Hospital, University of Pennsylvania School of Medicine, Philadelphia, Pennsylvania 19104, U.S.A.

Litoux, P., M.D., Service de Dermatologie, Hôtel-Dieu, F-44035 Nantes Cedex, France

Lopes, C.F., M.D., II Clinica Dermatologica, Santa Casa de Belo Horizonte, 30000 Belo Horizonte, Brazil

Lubach, D., M.D., Hautklinik Linden, Medizinische Hochschule, Ricklinger Straße 5, D-3000 Hannover 91, West Germany

Lutzner, M.A., M.D., Institut Pasteur, F-75015 Paris, France

MacKie, R.M., M.D., Department of Dermatology, University of Glasgow, GB-Glasgow, Great Britain

Madison, K., M.D., Department of Dermatology, University of Michigan Medical School Outpt. Bldg. C-2064, Ann Arbor, Michigan 48109, U.S.A.

Mahrle, G., Prof., M.D., Universitäts-Hautklinik, Von-Siebold-Straße 3, D-3400 Göttingen, West Germany

Marcelo, C.L., Department of Dermatology, University of Michigan Medical School, Outpt. Bldg. C-2064, Ann Arbor, Michigan 48109, U.S.A.

Marghescu, S., Prof., Chairman, M.D., Hautklinik Linden, Medizinische Hochschule, Ricklinger Straße 5, D-3000 Hannover 91, West Germany

Marks, R., M.D., Department of Dermatology, Welsh National School of Medicine, University of Wales, Heath Park, South Wales, GB-Cardiff CF4 4XN, Great Britain

Massaro, P., M.D., Radioisotopes Unit, Università Cattolica del Sacro Cuore, I-00168 Roma, Italy

Mathé, G., Prof., Chairman, M.D., Institut de Cancérologie et d'Immunogénétique, Hôpital Paul-Brousse, F-94800 Villejuif, France

Meynadier, J., M.D., Department of Dermatology, F-34000 Montpellier, France

Michaëlsson, G., M.D., Department of Dermatology, University Hospital, S-750 14 Uppsala 14, Sweden

Michel, B., M.D., Department of Dermatology, F-34000 Montpellier, France

Mills, O.H., Jr., Ph.D., Department of Dermatology, University Hospital, University of Pennsylvania School of Medicine, Philadelphia, Pennsylvania 19104, U.S.A.

Møller, R., M.D., Department of Dermatology, Rigshospitalet, University of Copenhagen, Blegdamsvej 9, DK-2100 Copenhagen, Denmark

Nall, L., M.A., Department of Dermatology, Stanford University School of Medicine, Stanford, California 94305, U.S.A.

Niedworok, A., M.D., Universitäts-Hautklinik, Von-Esmarch-Straße 56, D-4400 Münster, West Germany

Niemi, K.-M., M.D., Department of Dermatology, Helsinki University Central Hospital, Snellmaninkatu 14, SF-00170 Helsinki 17, Finland

Nigra, Th.P., Department of Dermatology, The Washington Hospital Center, 110 Irving Street, NW, Washington, DC 20010

Nikolowski, J., M.D., Department of Dermatology, Ludwig-Maximilians-Universität München, Frauenlobstr. 9–11, D-8000 München 2, West Germany

Obalek, S., M.D., Klinika Dermatologiczna A.M., Ul. Koszykowa 82a, 02-0088 Warszawa, Poland

Obe, G., Prof. M.D., Institut für Allgemeine Genetik, Arnimallee 5–7, D-1000 Berlin 33, West Germany

Orfanos, C.E., Prof., Chairman, M.D., Department of Dermatology, University Medical Center Steglitz, The Free University of Berlin, Hindenburgdamm 30, D-1000 Berlin 45, West Germany

Orlando, P., M.D., Radioisotopes Unit, Università Cattolica de Sacro Cuore, I-00168 Roma, Italy

Ortonne, J.P., M.D., Service de Dermatologie, Faculté de Médecine, Hôpital Pasteur, F-06000 Nice, France

Ostrow, D., M.D., Department of Dermatology, Northwestern University Medical School, Ward Memorial Building, Chicago, Illinois 60611, U.S.A.

Ott, F., Prof. M.D., Sonneggstraße 55, CH-8006 Zürich, Switzerland

Palmskog, G., M.D., Department of Clinical Research, Roche Produkter AB, Box 250, S-127 25 Skärholmen 1, Sweden

Papini, M., M.D., Istituto di Clinica Dermosifilopatica dell'Università di Perugia, Policlinico Monteluce, I-06100 Perugia, Italy

Paravicini, U., M.D., Biologisch-Pharmazeutische Forschung, F. Hoffmann-La Roche & Co. AG, Grenzacherstraße 124, CH-4002 Basel, Switzerland

Peck, G.L., M.D., Dermatology Branch, National Cancer Institute, Department of Health, Education and Welfare, Bethesda, Maryland 20205, U.S.A.

Pettersson, U., M.D., Department of Clinical Research, Roche Produkter AB, Box 250, S-127 25 Skärholmen 1, Sweden

Pizzi, M., M.D., Service de Dermatologie, Hôtel-Dieu, Place Daviel, F-13002 Marseille, France

Plewig, G., Prof., M.D., Universitäts-Hautklinik, Frauenlobstraße 9, D-8000 München 2, West Germany

Pohl, J., M.D., Universitäts-Hautklinik, Schittenhelmstraße 7, D-2300 Kiel, West Germany

Polano, M.K., Prof., M.D., Postdam 7, NL-2361 BV Warmond, Netherlands

Presti, V. Lo, M.D., University of Catania, Department of Experimental Dermatology, Catania, Italy

Privat, Y., Prof., M.D., Service de Dermatologie, Hôtel-Dieu, Place Daviel, F-13002 Marseille, France

Puissant, A., Prof., Chairman, M.D., Clinique Dermatologique, Hôpital Saint-Louis, 38 à 42, Rue Bichat, F-75010 Paris, France

Rácz, I., Prof., Chairman, M.D., Clinic of Dermatology, Semmelweis Medical School, Maria-Straße 41, H-1085 Budapest, Hungary

Randazzo, S.D., M.D., University of Catania, Department of Experimental Dermatology, Catania, Italy

Reymann, F., M.D., Department of Dermatology, Finsen Institute, DK-2100 Copenhagen, Denmark

van der Rhee, H.J., Afdeling Dermatologie, Academisch Ziekenhuis-Leiden, Rijnsburgerweg 10, NL-Leiden, Netherlands

Rodriques, B.A., M.D., II Clinica Dermatologica, Santa Casa de Belo Horizonte, 3000 Belo Horizonte, Brazil

Roenigk, H.H. Jr., Prof. Chairman, M.D., Department of Dermatology, Northwestern University Medical School, Ward Memorial Building, Chicago, Illinois 60611, U.S.A.

Rufli, Th., M.D., Dermatologische Universitätsklinik, Kantonsspital Basel, Petersgraben 4, CH-4031 Basel, Switzerland

Ruiz-Maldonado, R., Prof., M.D., Dermatology Service, Instituto Nacional de Pediatria DIF, Insurgentes Sur 3700, Mexico 22 D.F., Mexico

Rusciani, L., M.D., Facoltà di Medicina e Chirurgia, Policlinica "A. Gemelli", Università Cattolica del Sacro Cuore, Largo Agostino Gemelli 8, I-00168 Roma, Italy

Schill, W.B., Prof., M.D., Universitäts-Hautklinik, Frauenlobstr. 9, D-8000 München 2, West Germany

Schilling, F., Prof., M.D., Klinik für Rheumakranke, Dr.-Alfons-Gamp-Straße 1, D-6650 Bad Kreuznach, West Germany

Schmidt, H., M.D., Department of Dermatology, Odense University Hospital DK-5000 Odense, Denmark

Schmitt, D., M.D., FRA 11 INSERM, Clinique Dermatologique, Hopital E. Herriot, F-69374 Lyon Cédex 2

Schnitzler, L., M.D., Service de Dermatologie, F-49036 Angers Cedex, France

Schöpf, E., Prof., Chairman, M.D., Universitäts-Hautklinik, Hauptstraße 7, D-7800 Freiburg, West Germany

Van der Schroeff, J., M.D., Afdeling Dermatologie, Academisch Ziekenhuis-Leiden, Rijnsburgerweg 10, NL-Leiden, Netherlands

Schüpbach, M., M.D., Biologisch-Pharmazeutische Forschung, F. Hoffmann-La Roche & Co. AG, Grenzacherstraße 124, CH4002 Basel, Switzerland

Schultz-Ehrenburg, U., Ass. Prof., M.D., Department of Dermatology, University Medical Center Steglitz, The Free University of Berlin, Hindenburgdamm 30, D-1000 Berlin 45, West Germany

Schuppli R., Prof., Chairman, M.D., Dermatologische Universitätsklinik, Kantonsspital Basel, Petersgraben 4, CH-4031 Basel, Switzerland

Schwarz, E., Prof., M.D., Department of Dermatology, University Medical Center Steglitz, The Free University of Berlin, Hindenburgdamm 30, D-1000 Berlin 45, West Germany

Serri, F., Prof., Chairman, M.D., Facoltà di Medicina e Chirurgia, Policlinica "A. Gemelli", Università Cattolica del Sacro Cuore Largo Agostino Gemelli 8, I-00168 Roma, Italy

Sjöholm, I., M.D., Department of Pharmaceutical Biochemistry, University of Uppsala, S-751 01 Uppsala, Sweden

Soós, Gy., M.D., Clinic of Dermatology, Semmelweis Medical School, Budapest, Hungary

Soppi, A.M., Prof., M.D., Department of Dermatology, University of Turku, SF-20520 Turku 52, Finland

Soppi, E., M.D., Department of Dermatology, University of Turku, SF-20520 Turku 52 Finland

Souteyrand, P., M.D., Clinique Dermatologique, Hôpital E. Herriot, F-69374 Lyon Cedex 2, France

Sparberg, M., M.D., Department of Dermatology, Northwestern University, Medical School, Ward Memorial Building, Chicago, Illinois 60611, U.S.A.

Spinnato, F., M.D., Facoltà di Medicina e Chirurgia, Policlinica "A. Gemelli", Università Cattolica del Sacro Cuore, Largo Agostino Gemelli 8, I-00168 Roma, Italy

Sporn, M.B., M.D., Laboratory of Chemoprevention, Divison of Cancer Cause and Prevention, National Institute Cancer Institute, Department of Health, Education and Welfare, Bethesda, Maryland 20205, U.S.A.

Suurmond, D., M.D., Afdeling Dermatologie, Academisch Ziekenhuis-Leiden, Rijnsburgerweg 10, NL-Leiden, Netherlands

Stalder, J.F., M.D., Service de Dermatologie, Hôtel-Dieu, F-44035 Nantes Cedex, France

Stollenwerk, R., M.D., Klinik für Rheumakranke, Dr.-Alfons-Gamp-Straße 1, D-6550 Bad Kreuznach, West Germany

Strauss, J.S., Prof., Chairman, M.D., Department of Dermatology, University of Iowa Hospitals and Clinics, Iowa City 52242, Iowa, U.S.A.

Stüttgen, G., Hautklinik und Poliklinik der Freien Universität im Rudolf-Virchow-Krankenhaus, Augustenburger Allee 1, D-1000 Berlin 65, West Germany

Tabiowo, A., MRC Unit on the Experimental Pathology of the Skin, The Medical School, GB-Birmingham B15 2TJ, Great Britain

Tamayo, L., M.D., Dermatology Service, Instituto Nacional de Pediatria DIF Insurgentes Sur 3700, Mexico 22 D.F., Mexico

Teelmann, K., M.D., Biologisch-Pharmazeutische Forschung, F. Hoffmann-La Roche & Co. AG, Grenzacherstraße 124, CH-4002 Basel, Switzerland

Thivolet, J., Prof., Chairman, M.D., Clinique Dermatologique, Hôpital E. Herriot, F-69374 Lyon Cedex 2, France

Tong, P.S., M.D., Department of Dermatology, University of Michigan Medical School, Outpt. Bldg. C-2064, Ann Arbor, Michigan 48109, U.S.A.

Touron, P., M.D., Service de Dermatologie, Hôpital de La Grave, F-31052 Toulouse Cedex, France

Tsambaos, D., Ass. Prof., M.D., Department of Dermatology, University Medical Center Steglitz, The Free University of Berlin, Hindenburgdamm 30, D-1000 Berlin 45, West Germany

Tsutsumi, V., M.D., Servicio de Dermatologia, Hospital General "Dr. Manuel Gea Gonzalez", Mexico City 22 D.F., Mexico

Urbach, F., Prof., M.D., The Center of Photobiology, Temple University School of Medicine, Philadelphia, Pennsylvania 19140, U.S.A.

Vahlquist, A., M.D., Department of Dermatology, University Hospital, S-750 14 Uppsala 14, Sweden

Venier, A., M.D., Facoltà di Medicina e Chirurgia, Policlinia "A. Gemelli", Università Cattolica del Sacro Cuore, Largo Agostino Gemelli 8, I-00168 Roma, Italy

Verma, A.K., M.D., McArdle Laboratory for Cancer Research, University of Wisconsin, Medical Center Madison, Wisconsin 53706, U.S.A.

Verret, J-L., M.D., Service de Dermatologie, F-49036 Angers Cedex, France

Voorhees, J.J., Prof., Chairman, M.D., Department of Dermatology, University of Michigan Medical School, Outpt. Bldg. C-2064, Ann Arbor, Michigan 48109, U.S.A.

Wagner, G., M.D., Universitäts-Hautklinik, Frauenlobstraße 9, D-8000 München 2, West Germany

Weissmann, I., M.D., Universitäts-Hautklinik, Frauenlobstraße 9, D-8000 München 2, West Germany

Wilkinson, D.I., M.D., Department of Dermatology, Stanford University School of Medicine Stanford, California 94305, U.S.A.

Wokalek, H., M.D., Universitäts-Hautklinik, Hauptstraße 7, D-7800 Freiburg, West Germany

Wolska, H., M.D., Klinika Dermatologiczna A.M., Ul. Koszykowa 82a, 02-0088 Warszawa, Poland

Yokoo, H., M.D., Department of Dermatology, Northwestern University Medical School, Ward Memorial Building Chicago, Illinois 60611, U.S.A.

C.E. Orfanos et al. (eds.)
Retinoids

Introduction

For the first time after the 2nd World War an International Dermatological Symposium (IDS) has taken place in Berlin the former German capital, on October 13–15th, 1980.

Under the auspices of The Free University of Berlin Vicepresident Professor Dr. F. Bschor opened the Symposion addressing nearly 400 dermatologists and basic research scientists from 33 countries all over the world. The meeting, dealing with one of the most fascinating new topics in modern Dermatology was organized by an International Scientific Committee - Professor Dr. O. Braun-Falco, Germany, Professor Dr. E.M. Farber, USA, Dr. Ch. Grupper, France, Professor Dr. M. Polano, Netherlands, Professor Dr. R. Schuppli, Switzerland and myself - and was presented by the Department of Dermatology, University Medical Center Steglitz, Berlin.

The development of Dermatology during the last decades has been influenced to a great extent by the development of new drugs. The introduction of penicillin into therapy in the late 40's has changed the face of modern Venerology; local and systemic application of corticosteroids were an epic development in treating allergic skin reactions and severe bullous diseases, p.e. pemphigus. Synthetic retinoids are extremely effective drugs in various types of keratinization disorders. In addition, they also exert antiinflammatory effects and seem to possess immunomodulatory properties, influencing dermal components such as lymphocytes and macrophages. They seem, therefore, to reestablish normal keratinization and to modulate the general response of the dermal tissue under pathological conditions.

Another interesting aspect to contemplate is the fact that skin research laboratories and dermatologists have contributed significantly in the early stages of the development of retinoids. In Switzerland Bollag and his coworkers, in Germany Stüttgen and our group in Cologne were involved in collecting laboratory and clinical experiences with systemic retinoids since the late 60's. The first publications on both the 13-cis-retinoic acid and the aromatic retinoid etretinate appeared in Europe in 1972/1973 and 1975/1976 respectively. Dermatologists all over the world have now achieved a high level of knowledge on a new group of drugs which may be of significant value in general medicine. The present volume should help to maintain this high level.

The development of this new group of drugs acting primarily on the skin and other ectodermal tissues opened new horizons in systemic dermatotherapy which may lead to a better understanding of the pathogenesis of several skin diseases. Keratotic genodermatoses including psoriasis respond reasonably well to systemic treatment with these compounds. Thus, local therapy with traditional remedies may become less and less important. The management of severe pustular and erythrodermic psoriasis appears now feasible, ichthyotic conditions may be compatible with social life. Also, if some of the presented data will be confirmed in the future, retinoids may definitely enrich therapeutic modalities in oncology, p.e. by inhibiting tumorigenesis. Chemoprevention of skin cancer seems to be a new area of research in which systemic administration of retinoids may play a significant role. Some other reports indicate that retinoids may interfere with the growth of oncogenic virus and virus-induced cancer. It is a unique experience that a great part of the diseases in which synthetic retinoids exert a beneficial effect have been totally resistant to any type of other treatment in the past.

Finally, an important field of common concern are the chemical and laboratory monitoring and long-term side effects of retinoids, particularly in view of their accumulation in the body over several months and their well known teratogenicity in animals. Some significant new information on this particular topic has been delivered during the symposion.

This volume includes nearly all papers presented at the Berlin meeting on the advances on basic research and therapy with retinoids. In the additional closing session some highlights of these reports were summarized presenting our state of knowledge on three main points, (a) the biological effects of the main retinoids, (b) their application in psoriasis and (c) their application in severe acne. There are certainly a few other points which should be discussed thoroughly, however, the main interests were focused on these three at this particular occasion.

The Organizing Scientific Committee of the IDS Berlin also decided to announce and award two prices during the meeting. The price for the best investigational work presented as a poster has been awarded to Dr. I.A. King, Unit in Experimental Pathology of Skin, The Medical School, Birmingham/Great Britain, for his investigation on "Retinoid acid and epidermal cell surface associated carbohydrates". The price for the best clinical work has been given in part to H. Gollnick, Department of Dermatology, University Medical Center Steglitz, The Free University of Berlin, Germany and to Drs. Ch. Grupper and B. Berretti, Polyclinique d'Aubervilliers, France. H. Gollnick won the price for his poster presentation on the "Elevation of triglycerides after oral therapy with aromatic retinoids" in patients with various skin diseases pointing out the significance of additional risk factors for such elevations; Drs. Grupper and Berretti, finally, presented a superb collection of clinical cases treated with the drug showing its clinical efficacy in various skin diseases.

The IDS Organizing Scientific Committee has to mention the Hoffmann-La Roche Company, Grenzach and Basel, for its generous financial support. We highly appreciate in particular the contribution and the personal engagement of Dr. Hennes and Dr. Lefrancq in supporting our efforts for an adequate organization. Finally, we are grateful indeed to Springer-Verlag, Heidelberg, for preparing an appropriate volume of proceedings.

March 1981

C.E. Orfanos, M.D.
Professor and Chairman
Department of Dermatology
University Medical Center Steglitz
The Free University of Berlin

Pharmacology and Toxicology of Retinoids

C.E. Orfanos et al. (eds.)
Retinoids

From Vitamin A to Retinoids: Chemical and Pharmacological Aspects

W. Bollag

Historical Background

Vitamin A is necessary for the development and maintenance of human life. It cannot be synthesized by the body and must therefore be taken in with the food. Either vitamin A alcohol (retinol) and its esters or β-carotene, a provitamin which is split in the intestine to vitamin A, serve as sources. The most important metabolic products are vitamin A esters, which are stored in the liver, vitamin A aldehyde (retinal), which is necessary in its 11-cis isomer form for visual function and vitamin A acid (retinoic acid).

Vitamin A has long been known for its importance in promoting general growth, in regulating proliferation and differentiation of epithelial tissues and in maintaining visual function and reproduction. In particular, the effect of vitamin A on epithelial tissues has attracted much attention, because it had been demonstrated that vitamin A deficiency led to hyperkeratosis of the skin and to squamous metaplasia of mucous membranes. Such alterations not only are observed in various diseases of the skin connected with disorders of keratinization but also in certain precancerous conditions. This link provided the basis for research on the role of vitamin A in dermatology and oncology (2, 6–8, 12, 19). In this article we will be dealing mainly with the dermatological aspects. However, the intimate relationship to oncology will be readily apparent in many instances.

Many dermatological diseases manifest themselves by pathological changes of keratinization such as acne, psoriasis, ichthyoses, lichen ruber planus, Darier's disease, pityriasis rubra pilaris among many other skin diseases. In view of the antikeratinizing properties of vitamin A clinical research focused on this latter group of diseases, in which the occasional benefit of high doses of vitamin A was found. The success rate was, however, too low to recommend this therapy in practical dermatology. Furthermore, the doses needed for therapeutic success were accompanied by unacceptable side effects. These side effects consisted of changes of the skin and mucous membranes, bone, liver and of neurological complications. The next step in the development of a therapeutic agent was the introduction of all-trans-retinoic acid. This compound brought some progress particularly in the systemic or topical treatment of acne, psoriasis, ichthyoses, actinic keratoses and basal cell carcinomas (1, 3, 9, 10, 16, 18, 20). From the scientific, and to some extent from the practical point of view, the clinical results appeared encouraging. However, systemic use of all-trans-retinoic acid, too, was hampered by severe toxic side effects, known as the hypervitaminosis A syndrome and topical use was handicapped by marked skin irritation. It was, therefore, the purpose of our efforts to find new natural or synthetic analogs of vitamin A (retinoids) which would combine better therapeutic activities with less side effects.

The Search for New Retinoids for Use in Dermatology and Oncology

More than a thousand compounds were synthesized by chemical manipulation of the vitamin A molecule at the ring, the side chain and the polar end group, and tested in various biological systems. For oncological screening, animal tumor models could be used for demonstrating preventive or therapeutic antitumor activity. Screening for dermatological applications was, however, more difficult, as only few and rather unreliable animal models exist for testing the antipsoriatic or antikeratinizing property of a compound. To this end a new screening model was developed which made it possible to detect compounds not only with antineoplastic but also antipsoriatic and antikeratinizing properties (4).

The Mouse Papilloma as a Test Model

The following test model was chosen: Skin papillomas of the mouse were induced by using 7,12-dimethylbenz(a)anthracene (DMBA) as an initiating agent painted on the back skin of female Swiss albino mice (2 × 150 µg) on days 1 and 15 and croton oil (500 µg, 2 × weekly) as a promoting agent from day 28 onwards. Papillomas usually appeared after 3–8 months. The papilloma of the mouse is a benign tumor. The question arises whether this model is representative for human diseases such as psoriasis or other keratinizing dermatoses. In both instances increased epidermal proliferation and increased keratinization are typical features. This analogy – to our mind – justifies the use of the papilloma model in screening not only for antineoplastic but also for antipsoriatic and antikeratinizing activities.

Chemically induced papillomas show a marked regression under the influence of retinoids. In a typical therapeutic experiment carried out with well established papillomas the control animals showed an increase in the mean papilloma diameter per animal of 22.7% within 14 days, whereas in the animals treated with all-trans-retinoic acid a dose-dependent regression of up to 51.4% was observed. Clinically, all-trans-retinoic acid used topically or systemically had a more or less satisfying effect in certain oncological diseases as well as in dermatological diseases such as acne, psoriasis, Darier's disease, ichthyoses, lichen ruber planus, actinic keratoses and also in leukoplakias of mucous membranes. These results appeared to validate the use of the papilloma model in the search for drugs in dermatotherapy.

Therapeutic Index

It was our aim to find compounds with a marked dissociation between antipapilloma effect and the toxic hypervitaminosis A syndrome. The therapeutic index was calculated as the ratio between the lowest daily dose causing in a 14 days' study a defined degree of hypervitaminosis A and the dose given once a week for 2 weeks causing 50% regression of papillomas. Thus the therapeutic index enabled us to compare retinoids with each other and to choose the compounds with the most favorable indices for clinical trials. For topical use it was important to know in addition whether the retinoids had an irritating effect on the skin. This was tested on guinea pig skin by topical application for a period of 14 days.

New Compounds

Starting from all-trans-retinoic acid, a large series of esters and amides were synthesized and tested biologically and clinically to some extent, but no significant results were obtained. From many isomers, 13-cis-retinoic acid was chosen for clinical trials because of its low toxicity in mice. It was found to have a marked effect on acne vulgaris and an even more spectacular one on cystic acne (15) when given orally. The aromatic retinoids etretinate (Ro 10-9359) and motretinid (Ro 11-1430) were selected for clinical trials since both compounds showed a therapeutic index ten times more favorable than that of all-trans-retinoic acid. Etretinate (Ro 10-9359) was demonstrated to be of great value in the oral treatment of severe psoriasis and various keratinizing dermatoses (13, 14), whereas motretinid (Ro 11-1430) has a place in the topical treatment of acne vulgaris (17) and is also being tried in the topical treatment of various diseases with pathological keratinization. In Table 1 a series of retinoids are

Table 1. List of a series of retinoids with different chemical structures. The therapeutic index, as well as the dose necessary for an antipapilloma effect, varies markedly between the various retinoids*

Therapeutic Indices of some Retinoids.

	Chemical structure	Hypervitaminosis A (mg/kg)	Antipapilloma Effect (mg/kg)	Therapeutic Index
all-trans-Retinoic acid (Tretinoin)	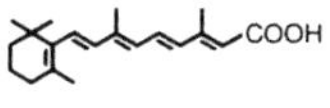	80	400	$\frac{80}{400} = 0.2$
13-cis-Retinoic acid (Isotretinoin) Ro 4-3780	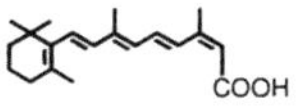	400	800	$\frac{400}{800} = 0.5$
Trimethylmethoxyphenyl (TMMP) analog of retinoic acid ethyl amide (Motretinid) Ro 11-1430	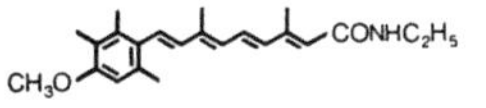	100	50	$\frac{100}{50} = 2.0$
Trimethylmethoxyphenyl (TMMP) analog of retinoic acid ethyl ester (Etretinate) Ro 10-9359	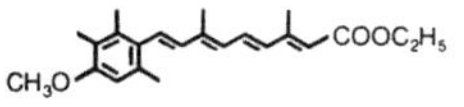	50	25	$\frac{50}{25} = 2.0$
Dichloromethylmethoxyphenyl (DCMMP) analog of retinoic acid ethyl ester Ro 12-7554	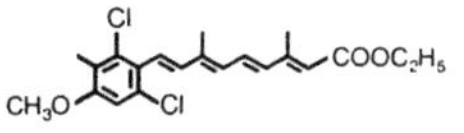	12	6	$\frac{12}{6} = 2.0$
Arotinoid ethyl ester Ro 13-6298	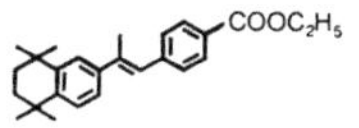	0.1	0.05	$\frac{0.1}{0.05} = 2.0$

* The therapeutic index was defined as the ratio between the lowest daily i.p. dose causing, in a 14 days' study, a defined degree of hypervitaminosis A and the dose given i.p. once a week for 2 weeks causing 50% regression of papillomas.

listed in which the ring, the side chain and the polar end group of the vitamin A molecule have been modified. It can be seen that these compounds which were, or are being, tried clinically, are active at very different doses and possess widely different therapeutic indices. Thus, the dose necessary to induce a 50% regression of the papilloma was 400 mg/kg for all-trans-retinoic acid, but only 0.05 mg/kg for the arotinoid. On the other hand, the therapeutic index of the aromatic retinoids etretinate and motretinid (2.0) was 10 times more favorable than that of all-trans-retinoic acid (0.2).

Other Activities and Mechanism of Action of Retinoids

In addition to the above described activities retinoids show many more interesting properties, which were demonstrated in a series of investigations carried out by many different research workers (7, 8, 11). We will limit ourselves to some investigations in the field of oncology, though other qualities of retinoids, such as their influence on sebum production, on inflammatory phenomena and on immune reactions etc. are, of course, also of utmost importance. Retinoids have been reported to inhibit the growth of certain cell lines in cell cultures. Melanoma cells in particular and preneoplastic and neoplastic mammary cells responded with a marked diminution of growth. In organ cultures hyperplasia and metaplasia of various organs such as trachea, prostate and mammary gland induced by vitamin A deficiency, carcinogenic substances or hormones could be prevented or even reversed by the addition of retinoids. Certain transplantable tumors, particularly chondrosarcoma respond very dramatically to retinoids. A great deal of research has been carried out to ascertain whether retinoids prevent chemically induced tumors. Positive results have been obtained in the prophylaxis of chemically induced tumors of skin, oral cavity, stomach, intestine, trachea-bronchus, urinary bladder, cervix and mammary gland. All the above-mentioned data have given rise to a still increasing effort to study the underlying mechanism of action in vitro and in vivo. The inhibiting effect of retinoids on the proliferation of certain transformed and tumor cells is probably mediated by restoration of density-dependent growth inhibition or of anchorage-dependent growth control. In some instances a direct antiproliferative effect caused by inhibition of DNA synthesis was observed. A further interesting phenomenon being studied intensively is the prevention and reversion of malignant transformation by retinoids in vitro. During the transformation process the cells change the pattern of various properties. Under the influence of retinoids, some of the properties of a transformed malignant cell revert to those of a normal cell. Thus, the restoration of contact inhibition, saturation density, cell adhesiveness, chemical composition of membranes etc. was found. Very recently it was discovered that malignant cells could be induced to regain differentiation by retinoids. Thus, the rapidly proliferating and dedifferentiated malignant cells could reacquire properties of a differentiated cell. Another exciting property of the retinoids is their ability to bind to specific binding proteins, acting as receptors for their action within the cell. Furthermore, the stimulating effect of retinoids on the synthesis of various glycoproteins and glycosaminoglycans may play a decisive role as these components of the cell membrane may determine whether a cell has characteristics of a normal or a transformed neoplastic cell.

All this information was obtained mainly by experiments carried out in vitro. A few examples will now be mentioned to demonstrate that, in vivo also, prevention of the process leading to neoplastic transformation can be achieved by the use of retinoids and that a transition from a proliferative to a differentiated state seems to be attainable. The examples cited below will concern prophylactic and therapeutic treatments with etretinate (Ro 10-9359) in the field of experimental onco-dermatology.

Table 2. Therapy of chemically induced papillomas. Results of treatment of established skin papillomas during 2 weeks with different dosage schedules of the retinoid etretinate (Ro 10-9359)

Dose (mg/kg)		Average sum of the papilloma diameter/animal (mm) Day 0	Day 14	Percent change in the average sum of the papilloma diameter/animal
Controls		21.1	26.0	+ 23.2%
Etretinate				
200	1 x weekly i.p.	25.5	6.6	− 74.1%
100		28.0	8.5	− 69.6%
50		20.4	9.1	− 55.4%
25		24.4	12.5	− 48.8%
12.5		24.8	17.3	− 30.2%
400	1 x weekly p.o.	22.0	4.8	− 78.2%
200		23.7	9.8	− 58.6%
100		21.5	14.3	− 33.5%
50		21.0	16.5	− 21.4%
25		16.0	14.2	− 11.3%
40	daily p.o.	19.5	4.6	− 76.4%
20		16.6	7.4	− 55.4%
10		18.4	9.8	− 46.7%
5		16.5	13.7	− 17.0%

From Bollag (4). By permission of Eur J Cancer

Table 3. Prevention of chemically induced papillomas and carcinomas. Results of treatment with the retinoid etretinate (Ro 10–9359) during the promotion phase of carcinogenesis

			Papillomas		Carcinomas
	Day	Survivors/total number of mice	Mean No. of papillomas per mouse	Mean volume of papillomas per mouse (mm^3)	No. of carcinomas (cumulative number)
Controls	293	47/66	12.4	426.3	46
Ro 10–9359 30 mg/kg orally daily	293	56/66	1.1	6.8	4

From Bollag (5). By permission of Eur J Cancer

Etretinate has a marked *therapeutic* effect on the chemically induced papilloma. From Table 2 it can be seen that even a low dose of 25 mg/kg once a week i.p. leads to a 48.8% regression of the papillomas within 14 days. Not only chemically induced papillomas but also chemically induced squamous cell carcinomas of the mouse skin can be influenced. But for that purpose rather high doses of 200 mg/kg daily i.p. are necessary to achieve a reduction of volume of 53.4%. However, these doses provoke toxic side effects. Etretinate is also highly active in *preventing* induction of skin papillomas and carcinomas by DMBA and croton oil (Table 3). A dose of 30 mg/kg daily orally given during the promotion phase prevented almost completely the appearance and growth of papillomas and carcinomas of mouse skin (5). DMBA-induced keratoacanthoma of the rabbit's ear could also be completely prevented by administering etretinate during the induction phase. Virus-induced skin tumors, too, respond to etretinate. In rabbits inoculated with Shope papilloma virus the appearance of papillomas could be completely prevented by treatment of the animals with etretinate. In established papillomas, etretinate produced therapeutic regression, and, moreover, in squamous cell carcinomas arising from Shope papillomas the growth of the primary tumor and of metastases was inhibited.

Conclusions and Outlook

In this article we have reviewed early and recent investigations with retinoids in the field of experimental and clinical dermatology and oncology. The retinoids, including natural vitamin A compounds and synthetic structural analogs, represent a class of compounds with remarkable therapeutic activity in various dermatological diseases such as acne, psoriasis and many other keratinizing dermatoses. Preneoplastic and neoplastic lesions are also affected by retinoids. In various in vitro and in vivo models the ability of retinoids to prevent or reverse the transformation of a normal to a neoplastic cell could be demonstrated. Mainly by the aid of one particular model (chemically induced skin papilloma of mice) we succeeded in testing a large series of retinoids for their potential ability to influence favorably dermatological as well as oncological diseases. In spite of many therapeutic achievements we are still far from having reached a point where we can be fully satisfied with the practical clinical progress. The main handicap for the practical use of retinoids is their toxicity, manifested by the hypervitaminosis A syndrome. New synthetic retinoids have been shown to possess better therapeutic activity, particularly in the treatment of dermatological diseases. We still hope that further chemical manipulations of the vitamin A molecule will lead to compounds with a wider therapeutic margin both in the fields of dermatology and oncology. Much more work has to be carried out to elucidate the mechanism of action. It is, however, becoming more and more evident that the retinoids possess a large variety of different properties and that every retinoid has its own spectrum of properties. We are at the moment probably only at the beginning of a development which will show that the retinoids indeed represent a new approach to many problems of experimental and clinical dermatology and oncology.

Summary

Vitamin A possesses a regulatory effect on growth and differentiation of epithelial tissues. Vitamin A deficiency leads to hyperkeratosis of the skin and to squamous metaplasia of mucous membranes. Therefore, vitamin A was tried therapeutically for various skin diseases with disorders of keratinization, as well as for prevention and therapy of precancerous and cancerous conditions. The success rate in the treatment of acne, psoriasis and other keratinizing dermatoses was rather low. Retinoic acid was a further step in the treatment of these skin diseases. Systemic use was, however, handicapped by toxic side-effects - the so-called hypervitaminosis A syndrome - and topical use by skin irritation. Our goal was to find retinoids with better therapeutic activity and less side-effects. By varying the vitamin A molecule at the ring, side chain and polar end group many compounds were synthesized and tested in various biological systems. Particular emphasis was put on the following model: Chemically induced papilloma of mouse skin is a benign tumor, on which antineoplastic activity can be tested. Moreover, its increased epidermal proliferation rate with increased keratinization makes it a potential model for screening antipsoriatic and antikeratinizing properties. Thus, the test is useful in both oncology and dermatology. Chemically induced skin papillomas regress under the influence of retinoids. The dose leading to 50% regression of the papilloma was related to the dose provoking hypervitaminosis A syndrome. The calculated index of a compound served as indicator for its more or less favorable therapeutic margin. By means of this test, in conjunction with other model systems a series of compounds useful in dermatology and oncology were discovered. The most important are: 13-cis retinoic acid (isotretinoin), the aromatic retinoids Ro 10-9359 (etretinate) and Ro 11-1430 (motretinid) and the arotinoids.

References

1. Beer P (1962) Untersuchungen über die Wirkung der Vitamin A-Säure. Dermatologica 124:192–195
2. Bollag W (1970) Vitamin A and vitamin A acid in the prophylaxis and therapy of epithelial tumours. Int J Vitam Nutr Res 40:299–314
3. Bollag W, Ótt F (1971) Therapy of actinic keratoses and basal cell carcinomas with local application of vitamin A acid. Cancer Chemother Rep 55:59–60
4. Bollag W (1974) Therapeutic effects of an aromatic retinoic acid analog on chemically induced skin papillomas and carcinomas of mice. Eur J Cancer 10:731–737
5. Bollag W (1975) Prophylaxis of chemically induced epithelial tumors with an aromatic retinoic acid analog (Ro 10-9359). Eur J Cancer 11:721–724
6. Bollag W, Hanck A (1977) From vitamin A to retinoids. Modern trends in the field of oncology and dermatology. Acta Vitamin Enzymol (Milano) 31:113–123
7. Bollag W (1979) Retinoids and cancer. Cancer Chemother Pharmacol 3:207–215
8. Bollag W, Matter A From vitamin A to retinoids in experimental and clinical oncology: Achievements, failures and outlook. Ann NY Acad Sci (in press)
9. Frost P, Weinstein GD (1969) Topical administration of vitamin A acid for ichthyosiform dermatoses and psoriasis. J Amer Med Assoc 207:1863–1868

10. Kligman AM, Fulton JE, Plewig G (1969) Topical vitamin A acid in acne vulgaris. Arch Dermatol 99:469–476
11. Lotan R (1980) Effects of vitamin A and its analogs (retinoids) on normal and neoplastic cells. Biochim Biophys Acta 605:33–91
12. Mayer H, Bollag W, Hänni R, Rüegg R (1978) Retinoids, a new class of compounds with prophylactic and therapeutic activities in oncology and dermatology. Experientia 34:1105–1119
13. Orfanos C, Schuppli R (1978) Workshop "Oral retinoids in dermatology". Dermatologica 157 (Suppl. I): 1–64
14. Ott F, Bollag W (1975) Therapie der Psoriasis mit einem oral wirksamen neuen Vitamin A-Säure-Derivat. Schweiz med Wochenschr 105:439–441
15. Peck GL, Olsen TG, Yoder FW, Strauss JS, Downing DT, Pandya M, Butkus D, Arnaud-Battandier J (1979) Prolonged remissions of cystic and conglobate acne with 13-cis retinoic acid. N Engl J Med 300:329–333
16. Plewig G, Wolff HH, Braun-Falco O (1971) Lokalbehandlung normaler und pathologischer menschlicher Haut mit Vitamin A-Säure. Arch Klin Exp Derm 239:1547–1551
17. Scherrer A, Ótt F (1976) Die Lokaltherapie der Akne vulgaris mit einem aromatischen Retinoid. Praxis 65:453–455
18. Schumacher A, Stüttgen G (1971) Vitamin A-Säure bei Hyperkeratosen, epithelialen Tumoren und Akne. Dtsch med Wochenschr 96:1547–1551
19. Sporn MB, Newton DL (1979) Chemoprevention of cancer with retinoids. Fed Proc 38:2528–2534
20. Stüttgen G (1962) Zur Lokalbehandlung von Keratosen mit Vitamin A-Säure. Dermatologica 124:65–80

C.E. Orfanos et al. (eds.)
Retinoids

Pharmacokinetics and Metabolism of Oral Aromatic Retinoids

U. Paravicini

The preventive effect of Vitamin A and several of its analogs (retinoids) and the induction of precancerous conditions (2) as well as the therapeutic effects on certain hyperkeratotic skin disorders and on chemically induced skin papillomas and squamous cell carcinomas are well known (1).

The present view deals with metabolism and pharmacokinetics of Tigason (etretinate, Ro 10-9359) (Fig. 1), one of the most potent retinoids in terms of its therapeutic ratio in the antipapilloma activity (3).

Metabolism of Tigason

It was the aim of the metabolic investigations, which are briefly summarized, to see whether there are any similarities to retinol and retinoic acid in the metabolic fate of etretinate (6, 7, 15).

On administering a single oral dose of 100 mg radioactively labelled Ro 10-9359 to psoriatic patients, Hänni et al. (8) isolated and identified the parent drug as well as biotransformation products in blood, urine and feces. The question, whether Tigason undergoes enterohepatic circulation, as has been established for retinoic acid (7, 18), has been answered by experiments with bile duct-cannulated rats.

When comparing the *input-output balance* of *total radioactivity* 5 days after single oral doses of [^{3}H]-etretinate in rats as well as in humans, 70 to 80% of totally administered

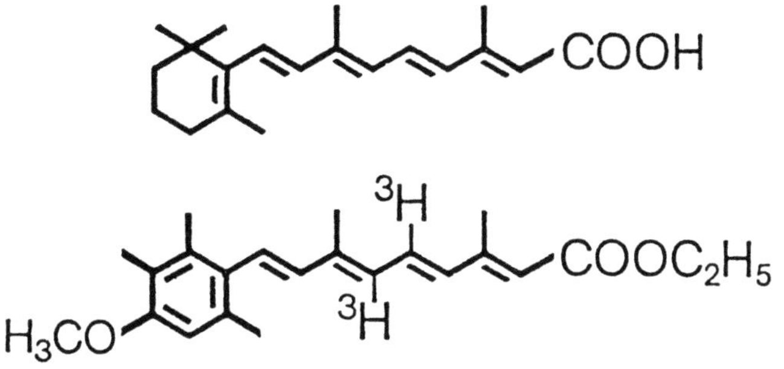

Fig. 1. Chemical structure of the retinoic acid compared with that of the aromatic analog Tigason in its labelled form, which has mainly been used in the experiments discussed

radioactivity appears in the feces, and 10 to 20% in the urine. To what extent this high fecal radioactivity consisted in unabsorbed drug will be discussed later.

In the *rat bile*, which was collected during 48 hours after i.v. bolus, 70% of the administered radioactivity was recovered, whereas after an oral dose, the [^{3}H]-recovery during the same time interval was only 10%. Forty-eight hours after intraduodenal administration of this bile to an untreated rat, 17% of the administered radioactivity was found in the animal's bile.

In *human plasma*, only the *parent drug* and its *main metabolite*, the hydrolysis product (corresponding carboxylic acid), could be isolated after a single oral dose. In the plasma of repeatedly dosed patients, the 13-cis isomer of the main metabolite was identified in addition.

In *human feces* 80% of the radioactivity (60% of the oral dose) was unchanged drug. If the finding from rat experiments, that virtually no drug is excreted unchanged via bile, also holds for humans, then most of the parent drug found in feces must be unabsorbed material.

The pattern of *metabolites*, isolated from *human urine*, looked quite different. Though only a relatively small part of the absorbed material was renally excreted, a large number of different biotransformation products could be isolated (Fig. 2).

The *metabolic pattern in rats* looked much the same as the one in humans, except for *bile*, which was only investigated in rats so far. In rat bile, the majority of metabolites is represented by the glucuronide of the main metabolite. Neither unchanged drug nor compounds with shortened tetraen side chain were detected.

Human urine			
Compounds collected during 5 days after single oral dose			
11% of oral dose		**73**% of total urine radioactivity	
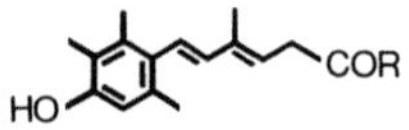	R=OH R=OH conjugate R=NH-CH_2-COOH	10%	**17**%
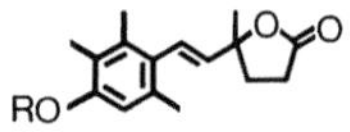 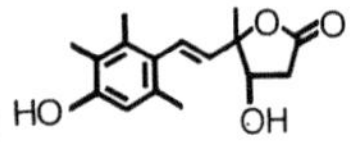	R=CH_3 R=H R=H conjugate	10%	**20**%
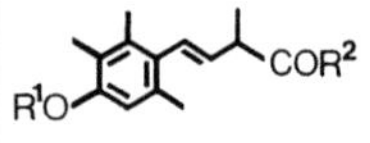	R^1=CH_3 R^2=OH R^1=H R^2=OH R^1=H R^2=OH conjugate R^1=H R^2=NH-CH_2-COOH	10%	**20**%
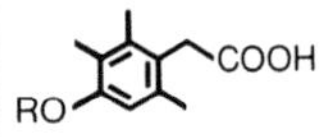	R=CH_3 conjugate R=H R=H conjugate	10%	**16**%

Fig. 2. Structure of compounds, which could be identified in *human urine* after single oral administration of Ro 10-9359

The studies have shown that etretinate undergoes essentially the same metabolic degradation both in humans and in rats. In a first step, part of the absorbed material is hydrolysed. The thus formed carboxylic acid is then biotransformed into three different kinds of metabolic reactions: (1). Formation of the beta glucuronide, leaving the side chain intact, with subsequent excretion exclusively in the bile, (2) cleavage of the side chain, most probably by beta oxidative decarboxylation (4, 8), and (3) demethylation of the methoxy group at the aromatic ring. Metabolites with shortened side chain seem exclusively to be eliminated renally.

Comparisons between retinol and Tigason may lead to the conclusion that the metabolic fate of both essentially resembles one to another. However, it has also to be taken into consideration that there are important questions which remain to be elucidated, namely the transport of Ro 10-9359 at different body sites, and the storage of this drug in the organism.

Pharmacokinetics of Ro 10-9359

Identifying the metabolic fate of a compound yields no information concerning the time course of distribution and elimination of the parent drug and its metabolites. Hence it becomes necessary to investigate the pharmacokinetics of Tigason. Pharmacokinetical analysis is usually accomplished by developing a mathematical model based on the drug concentration versus time profile of a single i.v. bolus administration.

Such an approach is valid provided sufficient data are available for a complete mathematical model description of the single-dose concentration time curve. Moreover, the prediction of other concentration time profiles of different dosing regimens (e.g. higher or multiple doses) by this model assumes that all processes governing the distribution and elimination of the drug are independent of drug concentration and time. Substantial amounts of analytical data from volunteer and patient studies are available for mathematical description of time-dependent concentration changes of etretinate and its main metabolite in the plasma.

The following *dosing regimen* (Fig. 3) was used in a *study with 5 volunteers:*

1. The 5 volunteers initially received an i.v. bolus of 10 mg [^{3}H]-Ro 10-9359. Venous blood samples were collected at appropriate time intervals through 96 hours. Urine and feces were quantitatively collected up to 10 days.
2. Two weeks following the i.v. bolus the volunteers received a single oral dose of 100 mg non-radioactive Tigason. Venous blood samples were collected through 32 hours.
3. Three weeks following the i.v. bolus the subjects received a multiple oral dosing regimen which consisted of 25 mg etretinate administered every 12 hours, except for the first three doses (τ = 8 hours). Blood samples were collected every other day, prior to and three hours after the morning dose.
4. Twelve hours following the last oral dose another i.v. bolus of 10 mg [^{3}H]-Ro 10-9359 was administered and blood samples were collected through 246 hours.

The plasma samples were assayed for the unchanged drug (ester) and its main metabolite (corresponding acid) by using a slight modification of the HPLC method described by Hänni (10). In addition, the plasma samples and excreta obtained from the first i.v. bolus were assayed for total radioactivity.

Results and Discussion

According to the protocol, Fig. 3 shows three different data sets of concentration time profiles of unchanged drug (etretinate) and its main metabolite (corresponding acid) in the plasma of one volunteer. Using the graphical method of residuals, three phases of decline of the drug concentrations following the single i.v. dose were apparent (half-life of the phases:

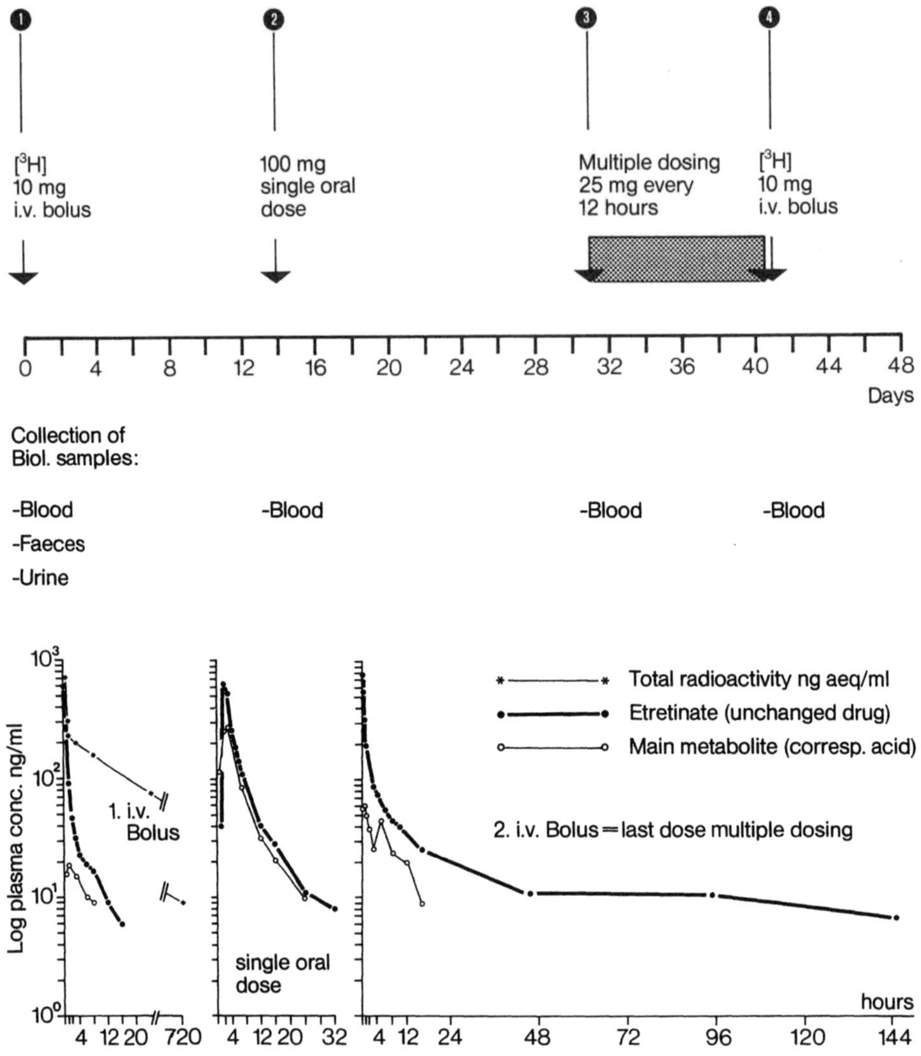

Fig. 3. Protocol for pharmacokinetic studies with healthy male volunteers. Concentration versus time profiles of etretinate and main metabolite (corresponding acid) in plasma of volunteers to whom Tigason was administered according to the protocol. The scale for all 3 graphs is identical

5–10 minutes, 30–60 minutes, 6–12 hours). Although there were indications of at least one other longer phase, the sensitivity limit of the assay did not allow to visualize it. However, fitting the data of four volunteers was performed with a three-compartment model using a non-linear regression analysis program (Nonlin (14)). The goodness of fit as established by the correlation coefficient and visual assessment was good for all subjects.

Although there was erratic absorption in one subject, the oral data could be adequately described using Nonlin (14) with the parameters describing the time lag of one hour as well as the extent of absorption equal to 40% were acceptable since similar values were obtained by alternate methods such as visual assessment and comparisons of area under the concentration time curves (AUC).

Through 24 hours, the time course of concentrations in plasma following the i.v. bolus

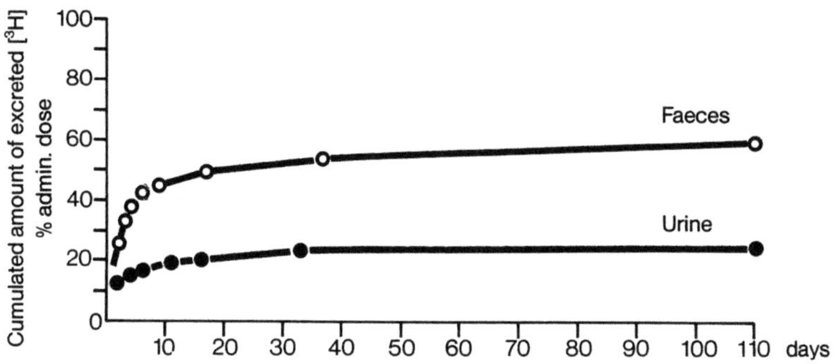

Fig. 4. Cumulated amounts of totally excreted radioactivity as a function of time following an i.v. bolus (Protocol) of [^{3}H]-etretinate to a healthy volunteer

after the ten-day oral multiple dose regimen has the same general shape as after single i.v. bolus. The profile after 24 hours differs in that another pronounced elimination phase with a half-life of 4–8 days is observed. This is suggestive of the existence of another compartment which is "filled up" after multiple dosing to such an extent that analytically detectable concentrations are built up in the plasma.

The cumulated amounts of excreted radioactivity as a function of time after administering the i.v. bolus to a volunteer are shown in Fig. 4. The extremely slow elimination of the compound is obvious, which speaks in addition for a deep compartment.

Further evidence for an existing deep compartment derives from a trial study in psoriatic patients undergoing chronic therapy with 10–25 mg/day Tigason for more than a year. The protocol called for the measurement of 3 trough levels during the last week of therapy and the collection of venous blood samples up to 140 days. The parent drug was measured by the same analytical method (HPLC) as mentioned above. As seen in Fig. 5, the minimum concentrations of unchanged drug at steady state were between 100 and 500 ng/ml plasma which is roughly an order of magnitude higher than that which is observed 24 hours following a single oral dose of 100 mg. Concentration values of 20–50 ng/ml were still observed even 140 days after cessation of the therapy. The persistence

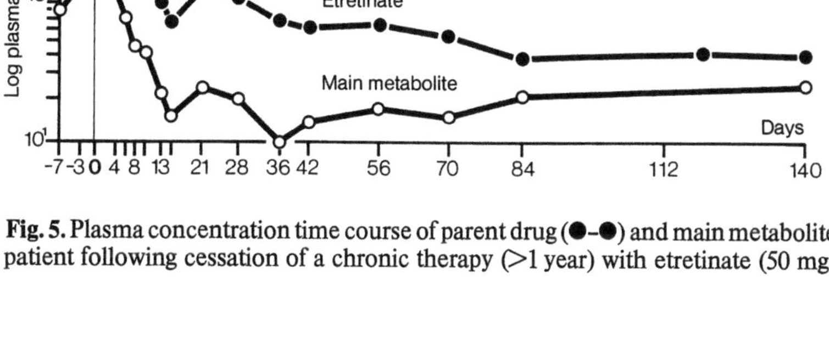

Fig. 5. Plasma concentration time course of parent drug (●–●) and main metabolite (O–O) in a psoriatic patient following cessation of a chronic therapy (>1 year) with etretinate (50 mg/kg)

of elevated Ro 10-9359 levels was associated with a *very* long elimination half-life of about 100 days.

Plasma Levels of the Main Metabolite

Significant plasma levels of the main metabolite (corresponding acid) are observed after oral administration of etretinate, whereas metabolite concentrations after an i.v. bolus are relatively low. Following oral administration the metabolite rapidly appears in the plasma in parallel with the parent drug and subsequently declines in parallel as well.

This kind of behaviour is suggestive of substantial presystemic hydrolysis of Tigason.

Based on the human pharmacokinetic data the following conclusions are reached:

1. The single dose data (i.v. and oral) can be described by a three-compartment model.
2. Prolonged multiple dosing yields a drug concentration-time profile that is significantly different from that which is predicted from the single dose data.
3. The discrepancy encountered with the compartmental analysis could also not be overcome by a non-compartmental approach because of the large errors in the AUC calculations, hence large differences in the clearance values.
4. The non-predictability might either be a result of the limits of the analytical method used or a result of a non-linear process involved in the distribution or elimination of Tigason.
5. Substantial plasma levels of the main metabolite (acid) are observed after oral administration, which is suggestive of presystemic hydrolysis of Ro 10-9359.

The presence of significant plasma levels of etretinate 140 days after the cessation of chronic therapy demands special attention. The extremely slow "elimination" is characteristic of the transfer rate back into the sampling (plasma) compartment from some deep storage compartment. Whether or not the long elimination phase as defined in these studies ($t_{1/2}$ = 100 days) is representative of the final phase in the decline of Tigason concentrations in the plasma cannot be established at present.

This transfer back into the plasma is analogous to an infusion input process and therefore yields sustained levels of Ro 10-9359 (and its main metabolite) long after dosing has ceased. This storage compartment plays such an important role in determining the fate of etretinate in the body, that speculation concerning the identity and characteristics of this storage site seems justifiable.

Although to date little experimental information is available about the type of tissue able to store large amounts of Tigason, one is compelled to compare Ro 10-9359 with vitamin A and its storage site, the liver. Many studies have been carried out in order to determine normal vitamin A liver contents in humans (11, 16), liver storage capacities (13) and storage sites in the liver tissue (12).

Some hints in this direction can be drawn from preliminary experiments with radioactive etretinate in rats.

The primary outcome of these pilot studies indicated that the liver was indeed the tissue, which accumulated Tigason. Briefly the liver took up about 50% of an i.v. dose 10 minutes after administration (unpublished data) and at 6 hours after the drug was administered, the highest tissue to blood concentration ratio was determined for the liver (r = 30.8 (9)). An additional analogy derives from the work of Sauberlich et al. (17), which has shown that the depletion of vitamin A reservoirs take years dependent on the tremendous storage capacity of the liver.

Whether the liver is the preferential storage site of the human organism (vitamin A!) or if Ro 10-9359 is unspecifically bound to various tissues remains to be investigated. Experiments which should answer specific questions related to this problem are presently under way.

Summary

With the aromatic retinoic acid analog Tigason oral and intravenous pharmacokinetic studies have been performed in 5 normal volunteers. Simultaneous fitting of single i.v. and oral data to a three-compartment model assuming first-order absorption was possible. Using Nonlin parameter estimates of the single-dose data, one is able to predict the decline in plasma levels of parent drug following cessation of a 10 days multiple dosing regimen up to 24 hours. The model is however unable to predict a phase of prolonged elimination observed beyond 24 hours. Moreover in 5 patients, who underwent chronic therapy (8–15 months), substantial plasma levels of both unchanged drug and main metabolite (corresponding carboxylic acid) were observed up to 140 days after cessation of the therapy. An apparent half-life of elimination of 80–100 days can be calculated. The drug appears to be stored at some yet unknown storage site.

Investigation of metabolism of Tigason in rats and humans revealed 19 different biotransformation products thus far, most of them appearing in the urine in low amounts (20% of dose). A few of them (mainly the acid Ro 10-1670) after conjugation to glucuronic acid are excreted in the bile in high amounts (60–80% of dose). No drug appeared unchanged in the excreta after i.v. administration to rats.

References

1. Bollag W (1971) Effects of vitamin A acid (NSC-122758) on transplantable and chemically-induced tumors. Cancer Chemother Rep 55:53–58
2. Bollag W (1972) Prophylaxis of chemically-induced benign and malignant epithelial tumors by vitamin A acid (retinoic acid). Eur J Cancer 8:689–693
3. Bollag W (1975) Prophylaxis of chemically-induced epithelial tumors with an aromatic retinoic acid analog (Ro 10-9359). Eur J Cancer 11:721–724
4. De Luca HF, Zile M (1975) Aspects of teratology of vitamin A acid (β-all-trans retinoic acid). Acta Derm Venerol (Stockh) 55 (Suppl. 74):13–20
5. Dunagin PE jr, Zachman RD, Olson JA (1964) Identification of free and conjugated retinoic acid as a product of retinal (vitamin A aldehyde) metabolism in the rat in vivo. Biochim Biophys Acta 90:432–434
6. Hänni R, Bigler F, Meister W, Englert G (1976) Isolation and identification of three urinary metabolites of retinoic acid in the rat. Helv Chim Acta 59:2221–2227
7. Hänni R, Bigler F (1977) Isolation and identification of three major metabolites of retinoic acid from rat feces. Helv Chim Acta 60:881–887
8. Hänni R, Bigler F, Vetter W, Englert G, Loeliger P (1977) Der Metabolismus des Retinoids Ro 10-9359. Isolierung und Identifizierung der Hauptmetaboliten aus Plasma, Urin und Faeces des Menschen sowie aus Galle der Ratte. Synthese von drei Urinmetaboliten. Helv Chim Acta 60: 2309–2325
9. Hänni R (1978) Pharmacokinetic and metabolic pathways of systemically applied retinoids. Dermatologica 157 (Suppl. 1):5–10
10. Hänni R, Hervouet D, Busslinger A (1979) Determination of an aromatic retinoid and its main metabolite by high-performance liquid chromatography. J Chromatogr 162:615–621
11. Hoppner J, Phillips WEJ, Murray TK, Campbell JS (1968) Survey of liver vitamin A stores of Canadians. Can Med Assoc J 99:983–986
12. Inouye T, Minick O, Grubbs C, Moon R, Kent G (1978) Hepatic lipocytes and storages of vitamin A analogues. Fed Proc 37:299
13. Körner WF, Völlm J (1975) New aspects of the tolerance of retinol in humans. Int J Vitam Nutr Res 45:363–372
14. Metzler CM, Elfring GL, McEwen AJ (1974) A user's manual for NONLIN and associated programs. Upjohn Company, Kalamazoo
15. Ott DB, Lachance PA, Lachance MS (1979) Retinoic acid – a review. Am J Clin Nutr 32:2522–2531
16. Raica N jr, Scott J, Lowry L, Sauberlich HE (1972) Vitamin A concentration in human tissues collected from five areas in the United States. Am J Clin Nutr 25:291–296

17. Sauberlich HE, Hodges RE, Wallace DL, Kolder H, Canham JE, Hood H, Raica N jr, Lowry LK (1975) Vitamin A metabolism and requirements in the human studied with the use of labeled retinol. Vitam Horm 32:251–275
18. Zachman RD, Dunagin PE jr, Olson JA (1966) Formation and enterohepatic circulation of metabolites of retinol and retinoic acid in bile duct-cannulated rats. J Lipid Res 7:3–9

C.E. Orfanos et al. (eds.)
Retinoids

In Vivo Immunostimulating Properties of Two Retinoids: Ro 10-9359 and Ro 13-6298

Th. Hercend, M. Bruley-Rosset, I. Florentin and G. Mathé

Vitamin A and some synthetic derivatives exhibit numerous activities; they have been recognized as an important factor in the differentiation of epithelial tissues (12, 13); they possess an antiproliferative effect caused by a reduction of DNA synthesis (9); they can also prevent the development of tumors induced in vivo by chemical carcinogen or even reverse the malignant transformation (1, 10, 15). Many mechanisms could be involved in the antitumor activity of retinoids (2). Stimulation of the host immune system has been considered since retinoids are known to possess adjuvant-like properties (3, 6). However, it is not clear if immunological effect of retinoids play a role in the inhibition of tumor growth.

The first part of this paper is devoted to the analyse of the effect of two synthetic derivatives on the different cell populations of the immune system defined by their functions.

In the second part the capacity of one derivative given repeatedly to restore the immune system of mice depressed by aging, is tested. These aged mice have an increased frequency of spontaneous tumor growth.

The model of aged mice allows to examine at the same time the modifications of immune responses and of tumor incidence caused by a long term treatment with the retinoid and to analyse the relation between host immunity and tumor development.

Two synthetic analogues of the retinoic acid, Ro 10-9359 and Ro 13-6298, differing by the chemical structure, the therapeutic ratio and the toxicity, were chosen for this study.

Material and Methods

I. *Mice:* Eight- to ten-week-old female (C57BL/6 × DBA/2) F1 mice from Roche Laboratories (Switzerland) were used for the study of the effect of two retinoids on immune responses of young mice.

For immunorestoration studies C57BL/6 female retired breeders were purchased at the age of 6 months from BOM Laboratories (Denmark).

II. *Retinoids and treatments*: Two synthetic analogs of retinoic acid, Ro 10-9359 and Ro 13-6298 (chemical formula on Fig. 1) were prepared by Hoffmann-La Roche and administered to young mice i.v. at the dose of 75 mg/kg and 1.5 mg/kg respectively at various days before testing. Ro 10-9359 was administered weekly i.p. to 12-month-old mice during a period of six months at the dose of 1.5 mg/mouse. They were then tested for their immunological reactivity at the age of 18 months.

III. *Immunological tests:*

1. *Assay for macrophage-mediated cytostasis:* The *in vitro* cytostatic activity of peritoneal macrophages was determined by using the tritiated thymidine (^{3}H-TdR) incorporation test. Briefly, $5 \cdot 10^4$ P815 tumor cells/well were cultivated on macrophage monolayers at an effector to target cell ratio of 10 macrophages for 1 tumor cell. Tumor cells, after 18 hours of incubation in the presence of macrophages, were harvested, washed, diluted in fresh medium (RPMI 1640) and redistributed in a

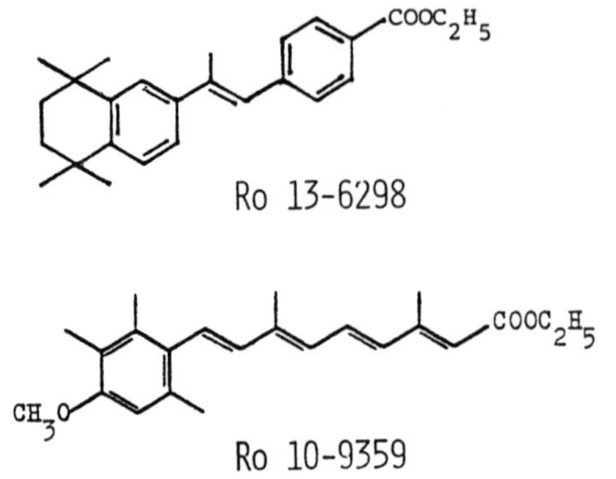

Fig. 1. Chemical structure of two retinoids, Ro 10-9359 and Ro 13-6298

new microplate II. 1 µCi/well of ^{3}H-TdR was then added for the last 4 hours of culture and thymidine incorporated into tumor cells was measured in a β counter. Results are expressed as mean cpm of ^{3}H-TdR incorporation ± standard error of six cultures and as percent inhibition of tumor cell proliferation.

2. *Test for natural killer (NK) cell activity:* Various numbers of spleen cells were incubated for 4 hours at 37 °C with 10^4 ^{51}Cr labelled YAC-1 lymphoma cells into u-shaped microplates. The effector to target cell ratio varied from 200:1 to 50:1. The amount of ^{51}Cr released in the supernatants was measured in a gamma counter. Cultures were done in triplicate and the percentage of specific lysis was calculated as follows:

$$\% \text{ lysis} = \frac{\text{experimental release} - \text{spontaneous release}}{\text{maximal release} - \text{spontaneous release}} \times 100$$

In this test, spontaneous release was obtained by the mean of lysis in six cultures containing 10^4 ^{51}Cr labelled YAC-1 cells as targets and 10^6 thymus cells as negative effectors.

3. *Antibody-dependent cell-mediated cytotoxicity* (ADCC): Various numbers of spleen cells were incubated for 18 hours at 37 °C with 10^4 ^{51}Cr labelled chick red blood cells (CRBC) into u-shaped microplates in the presence of a 1:20,000 final dilution of rabbit anti-CRBC serum. The effector to target cell ratio varied from 100:1 to 6:1. The amount of chromium released in the supernatants was measured in a gamma counter. Cultures were done in triplicate and the percentage of specific lysis was calculated as for NK cell activity but spontaneous release was obtained by the mean lysis in the cultures containing target and effector cells without antiserum.

4. *Cytolytic T cell activity:* $5 \cdot 10^7$ spleen cells were incubated at 37 °C in Falcon flasks in the presence or in the absence of mytomycin-treated P815 tumor cells during four days. The RPMI 1640 culture medium contained antibiotics, glutamine and $5 \cdot 10^{-5}$ mercaptoethanol (ME). After four days of culture, the suspensions were centrifuged and the number of viable cells was enumerated. Various numbers of spleen cells were incubated into u-shaped microplates 4 hours at 37 °C in the presence of 10^4 ^{51}Cr labelled P815 tumor cells, the effector to target cells ratio varying from 30:1 to 3:1. The amount of chromium released in the supernatants was measured in a gamma counter. Cultures were done in triplicate and the percentage of specific lysis was calculated as for NK activity but spontaneous release was obtained by the mean of lysis of cultures containing 10^4 ^{51}Cr labelled P815 as target and varying number of spleen cells cultivated in the absence of P815 tumor cells.

5. *Mortality and pathologic examination:* During the period of treatment, most dead mice or mice killed in poor conditions were necropsied and all surviving mice were killed after the age of 19 months. An autopsy was not performed on mice whose bodies had deteriorated because of cannibalism or because of the length of time elapsed since death. A macroscopic examination of major tissues was performed and all tumors and abnormal tissues were taken for microscopic examination. Tissues were fixed in neutral formalin (10%), embedded in paraplast, sectioned (4 µ) and stained with hematoxylin eosin. The percentage of tumor-bearing mice was evaluated in relation to the total number of mice in the groups at the beginning of the assay.

Results

I. *Effect of two retinoids, Ro 10-9359 and Ro 13-6298 on immune responses of young mice:*

1. *Effect of Ro 10-9359:*

Table 1. Immunological responses not modified by Ro 10-9359

Cell type involved	Cell functions tested	Tests on spleen cells
B cells	B cell activation	LPS, DS responsiveness
	Antibody synthesis	PFC response to TNP-LPS
T cells	T cell helper function	PFC response to TNP-KLH
	T cell mediated cytotoxicity	Mixed allogeneic tumor cell (P815) cultures
	T cell activation	PHA, ConA responsiveness
	Nonspecific suppressor function	Inhibition of normal spleen cell response to mitogens
NK cells	Natural killer cell cytotoxicity	Cytotoxicity against YAC-1

a) *Immunological responses not modified by Ro 10-9359:* Table 1 presents the functions of different cell populations which were not modified at any time by the treatment with Ro 10-9359. No change was observed in the T cell population (helper, killer or suppressor) neither in the B cell (antibody production), nor NK cell population.

b) *Effect on macrophage activation:* Peritoneal macrophages were highly cytostatic at any time after the injection of Ro 10-9359 from day 1 to day 14 (Fig. 2). An inhibition of tumor cell proliferation of 90% was observed at the maximum of the response on day 3.

c) *Effect on ADCC activity:* The ADCC assay was performed at the same days as for the macrophage cytostatic test but the results obtained with mice treated on day 7 are only presented (Fig. 3). At this time the maximum increase of the cytotoxic activity of spleen cells for chicken erythrocytes coated with rabbit antibodies is observed. This activity is low in day 3, high on days 7 and 10, and then decreases on day 14.

2. *Effect of Ro 13-6298:*

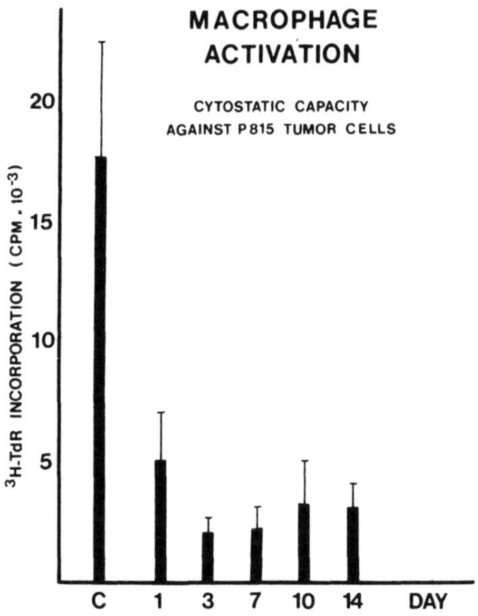

Fig. 2. Macrophage activation in 2-month-old mice treated with Ro 10-9359 at various days

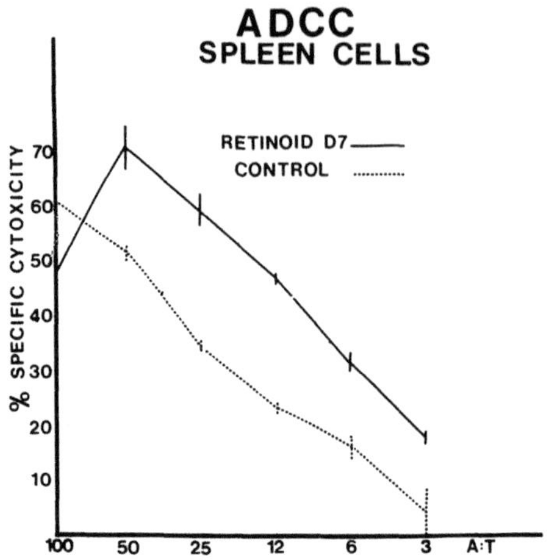

Fig. 3. Antibody-dependent cell-mediated cytotoxicity in 2-month-old mice treated with Ro 10-9359 on day 7

a) *Effect on macrophage activation:* A similar protocol of administration was applied for this derivative but the dose given is much smaller. In this experiment no sign of activation was detected before day 7 after the injection of Ro 13-6298. The maximum of the inhibition of tumor cell proliferation was observed on days 7 and 10 and this activity decreased on day 14 (Fig. 4).

b) *Effect on ADCC activity:* ADCC activity was also highly stimulated by Ro 13-6298 but this effect was maximum three days after its administration (Fig. 5).

The results evidenced that the two derivatives Ro 10-9359 and Ro 13-6298 have a similar pattern of activity. However, the second derivative Ro 13-6298, more toxic for the mice, was also able to induce suppressor cells: the addition of spleen cells coming from Ro 13-6298-

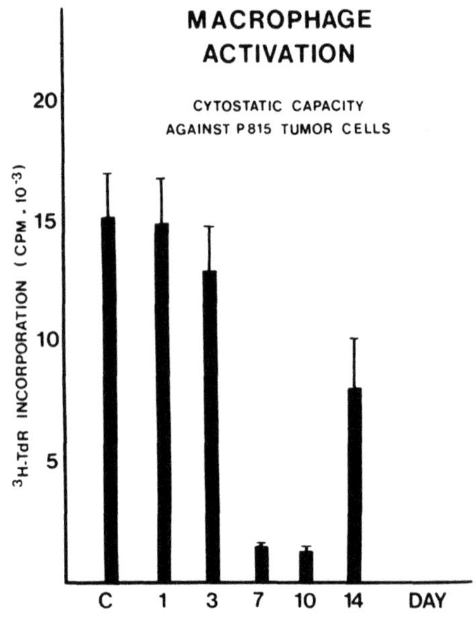

Fig. 4. Macrophage activation in 2-month-old mice treated with Ro 13-6298 at various days

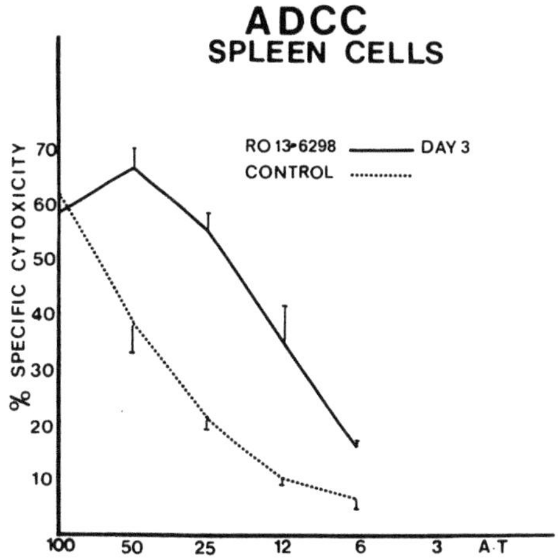

Fig. 5. Antibody-dependent cell-mediated cytotoxicity in 2-month-old mice treated with Ro 13-6298 on day 3

treated mice decreased the response of normal spleen cells to PHA and LPS when they are cocultivated.

II. *Effect of the chronic administration of Ro 10-9359 on immune responses of aged mice:*

1. *Modification of the immune parameters:* After six months of treatment with Ro 10-9359 the mice which at that time were between the age of 18 and 19 months were killed and their spleen cells were tested for immune antitumor activity.

a) *Peritoneal macrophage cytostatic activity:* The effect of the treatment on the capacity of macrophages to inhibit tumor cell proliferation was measured by the inhibition of thymidine incorporation. Tumor cells were cultivated in the presence of macrophages originating from treated or non-treated animals and the results are presented in Table 2. They show that a decrease in the cytostatic capacity of macrophages is associated with aging. Ro 10-9359 is able to stimulate the inhibitory effects of macrophages significantly, but to a low degree.

b) *Natural killer cell activity:* In our experiment, age reduces considerably the natural killer activity of splenic cells from 18% specific lysis at an effector to target cell ratio of 200:1 for young mice to 4.7% for 18-month-old mice and Ro 10-9359 further impairs this activity (Fig. 6).

c) *Antibody-dependent cell-mediated cytotoxicity:* ADCC activity for CRBC coated with

Table 2. Peritoneal macrophage cytostatic activity against tumor cells of young untreated or aged untreated mice, or mice treated by Ro 10–9359

Age of mice Mice treated with:	2 months untreated	18 months untreated	18 months Ro 13–9359
^{3}H-TdR incorporation into tumor cells (in cpm ± SE)	8660 ± 685	28664 ± 1061	23992 ± 846
% inhibition[1] of tumor cell proliferation	70% $p < 0.01$	-	17% $p < 0.05$

[1] % inhibition = $\frac{\text{mean number of } ^{3}\text{H-TdR cpm incorporated into tumor cells in presence of macrophages from young untreated or aged treated mice}}{\text{mean number of } ^{3}\text{H-TdR cpm incorporated into tumor cells in presence of macrophages from untreated aged mice}}$

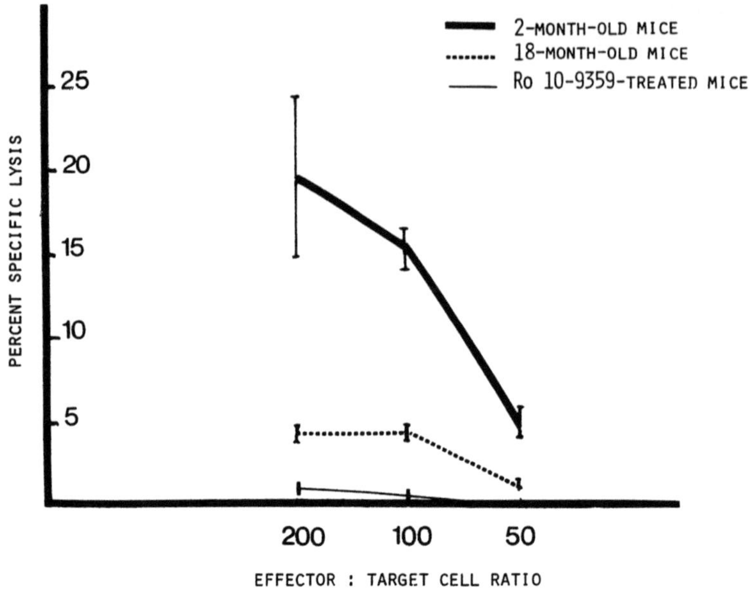

Fig. 6. Natural killer activity of spleen cells from untreated young mice, untreated aged mice, or aged mice treated with Ro 10-9359

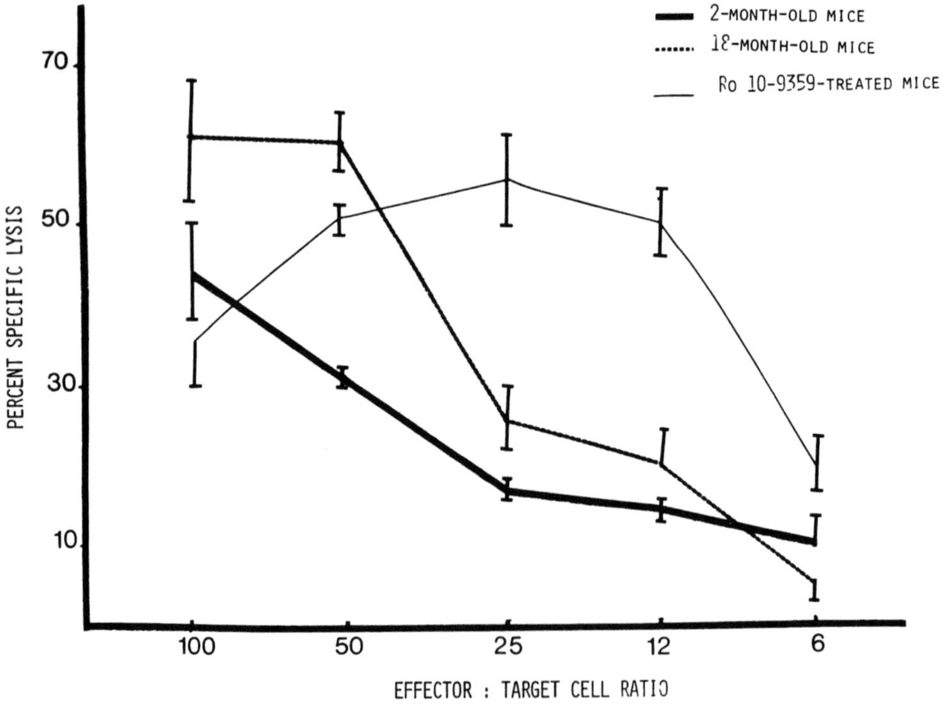

Fig. 7. Antibody-dependent cell-mediated cytotoxicity of spleen cells from untreated young mice, untreated aged mice, or aged mice treated with Ro 10-9359

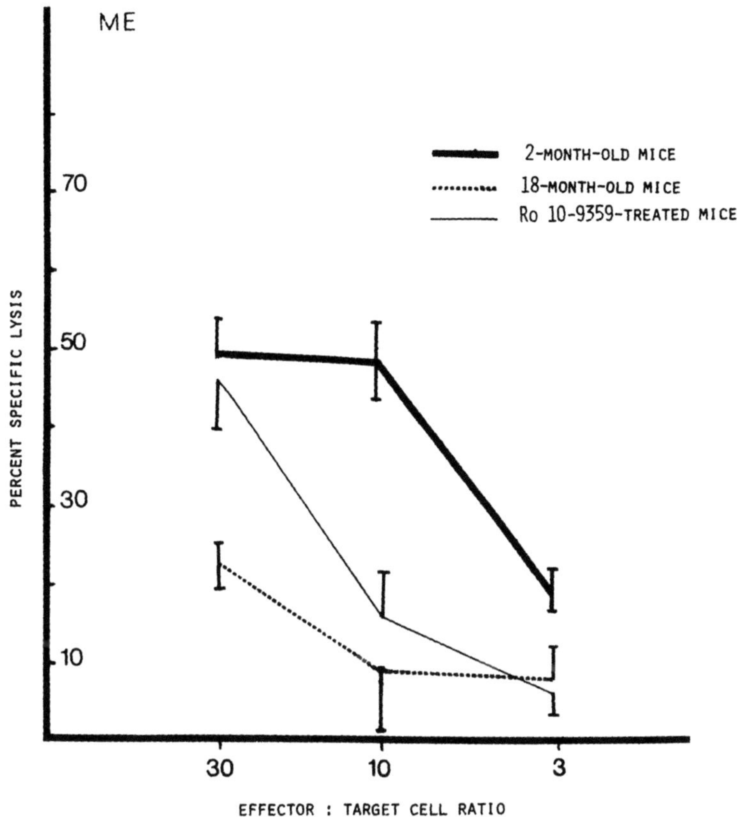

Fig. 8. Cytolytic T cell activity for P815 tumor cells of spleen cells from untreated young mice, untreated aged mice, or aged mice treated with Ro 10-9359, after in vitro allogeneic stimulation by P815 tumor cells during 4 days

rabbit anti-CRBC is elevated by aging and Ro 10-9359 permits the maintenance of this high level at lower effector to target cell ratio (Fig. 7). This result suggests either a higher number of reactive cells or a higher specific activity of the cells derived from retinoic acid-treated mice.

d) *Cytolytic T cell activity:* The capacity of spleen cells to generate cytolytic T cells after an *in vitro* allogeneic stimulation is strongly decreased when the cells originate from aged mice. Ro 10-9359 significantly enhances this activity (Fig. 8).

2. *Effect of Ro 10-9359 treatment on survival and tumor incidence:*

a) *Mortality of the animals during the treatment:* Ro 10-9359 seems to protect the mice during the first four months of treatment (6% mortality versus 22% for the controls at 16 months of age), but a cumulative toxicity (skin and liver) appears during the two last months and in this group we observed 61% mortality at 19 months of age (Fig. 9).

b) *Histological examination for spontaneous tumors:* Histological examination was performed as far as this was possible each time an animal was found moribund, or was killed for experimental testing. The numbers and the histopathological types of tumors are recorded in Table 3. Six out of 27 (22%) untreated old mice were found to bear a malignant tumor. Ro 10-9359 treatment decreases or delay significantly the tumor appearance: only one tumor, an immunoblastic lymphoma was found in this group (1/30 = 3.2%).

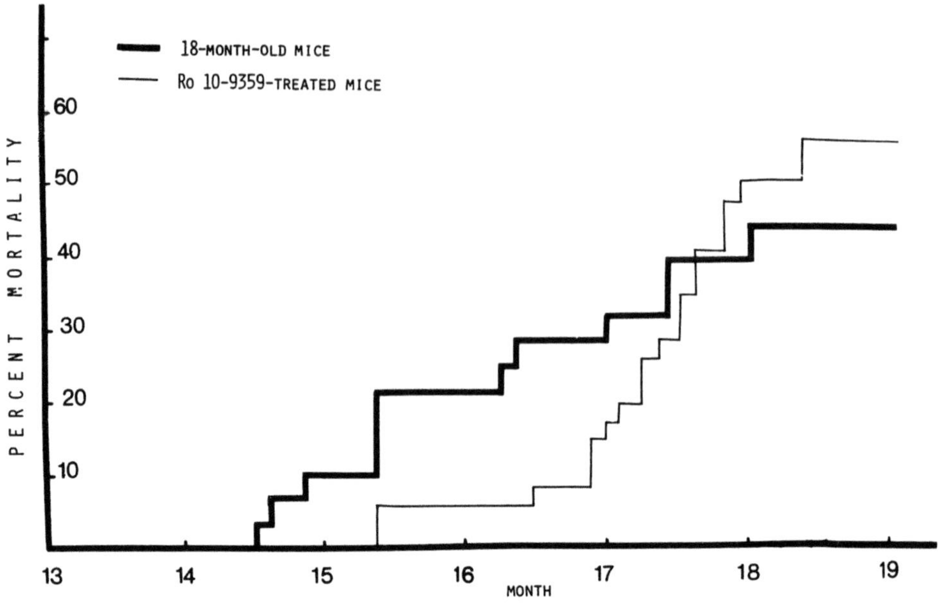

Fig. 9. Percentage of mortality related to ageing (in months) in mice either untreated or treated with Ro 10-9359

Discussion

Results presented here support the fact that retinoids are immunostimulants. We found that both derivatives induce a strong macrophage activation and stimulate the ADCC activity in young mice. However the second derivative Ro 13-6398, even administered at a much lower dose (50 times less), is more toxic for the animal (skin) and induce a suppressor cell activity

Table 3. Incidence and histological types of spontaneous tumors of aged mice. Effect of Ro 10-9359

Group of mice	Histological form of the tumor developed in aged mice	% of tumors[1]
Untreated aged mice (27 mice)	1 adenocarcinoma (genital tract) 1 undifferentiated malignant lymphoma (spleen) 1 undifferentiated malignant lymphoma (lymph node) 1 immunoblastic lymphoma (lymph node) 1 adenocarcinoma (lung) 1 malignant lymphoma unclassified (spleen)	6/27 = 22%
Ro 10-9359-treated aged mice (31 mice)	1 immunoblastic lymphoma (spleen)	1/30 = 3.2% $p < 0.05$

[1] $\% \text{ of tumors} = \dfrac{\text{number of tumor-bearing mice}}{\text{total number of mice in the group}}$

in the spleen without giving better results in the other tests. If they produce the same type of effects, the kinetic of appearance of macrophage and ADCC activation is different for the two derivatives.

No stimulation of the T cell compartment was found in young adult mice whatever the function tested: 1) T helper cell function in the production of antibodies in response to T dependent (SRBC); 2) T killer cell activity after an *in vitro* allogeneic stimulation. Results in the literature are contradictory in regard to the effect of retinoids on humoral responses but, in these studies, different antigens (BGG, DNP-Ficoll), different retinoids (retinyl palmitate or acetate) or different routes of administration were used (3, 4, 6, 8). However, Dennert and Lotan (4) demonstrated that antibody formation and delayed type hypersensitivity were not modified by retinoic acid but, in their study, the induction of specific cytotoxic T cells in response to EL_4 *in vitro* was very strongly stimulated (5). This contradiction with our work is only apparent. In their system retinoic acid was administered several times to obtain the stimulation of T killer cells (5). We did obtain similar results in aged mice which received multiple injections of Ro 10-9359 and not in young mice where only one injection was performed. In those immunorestorative experiments, stimulation of macrophage cytostatic capacity and ADCC was observed confirming the effect of Ro 10-9359 obtained in young mice.

The partial restoration of cell-mediated responses in aged mice after chronic treatment with Ro 10-9359 is followed by a decreased or delayed incidence of spontaneous tumors. These three immune effector mechanisms: macrophage cytostatism, ADCC and cytotoxic T cell could be implicated in the killing of tumor cells and may protect the host against tumor growth. However, a direct toxicity of the retinoid on the tumor cannot be excluded since some tumors have been demonstrated to be susceptible to retinoid inhibition *in vitro* (7, 11).

These results suggested a mode of action of retinoids on the immune system. They activate mainly macrophages which have an increased capacity to inhibit nonspecifically proliferation of tumor cells and to lyse cells coated with specific antibodies. In fact, it has been demonstrated that cells of macrophages series may be the major effector in ADCC of normal mice (16). However, further studies are required to determine whether retinoids directly act on macrophages which, in turn, may regulate other immune functions or conversely, whether they primarily stimulate some T cell sub-populations, and particularly, precursors of T killer cells. Macrophage activation may consequently result from lymphokine release by stimulated T cells.

Immunostimulation of host immune defenses may be one mechanism responsible for the antitumor activity of retinoids.

Summary

Two retinoids, Ro 10-9359, which is the trimethylmethoxyphenyl analog of β-retinoic acid, and Ro 13-6298, which is a more recent compound of the so-called subclass of arotinoids, were used. In a first part, two-month-old (C57BL/6xDBA/2)F1 mice were injected i.v. with a single dose of 75 mg/kg of Ro 10-9359, and 1.5 mg/kg of Ro 13-6298 and submitted to various immunological tests from day 1 to day 14 post treatment.

With both compounds we observed no significant modification of spleen cell ability: a) to produce antibodies after in vivo immunization with either thymus-dependent to thymus-independent antigens; b) to differentiate into cytolytic T-lymphocytes in response to in vitro stimulation by allogeneic tumor cells; c) to display natural cytotoxicity against YAC-1 tumor cell line. In contrast, positive results were: a) an increased capacity of treated spleen cells to lyse antibody-coated chick erythrocytes; b) a strong activation of peritoneal macrophages rendering them highly cytostatic for P815 mastocytoma cells in vitro. It should be noted that with Ro 13-6298 we observed an induction of nonspecific suppressor cells as shown by the ability of treated spleen cells to inhibit the in vitro response of normal spleen cells to PHA; this effect was not seen with Ro 10-9359.

In a second part, we have investigated the effects produced by a long-term application of Ro 10-9359 on the depressed immune functions of 18-month-old C57BL/6 mice. The results show an increase of age-impaired tumoricidal activity of peritoneal macrophages and a reduction of the already depressed NK activity of spleen cells. Ro 10-9359 increases splenic ADCC already elevated in aged mice. Cytotoxic T cell activity, diminished by age, is stimulated by Ro 10-9359. Histopathological studies revealed a significant decrease in the percentage of tumor bearing mice in the group treated by the retinoid compared to untreated mice of the same age. We confirm from these data that retinoids can stimulate antitumor immune mechanisms.

Acknowledgments. We thank Dr. Bollag from Hoffmann-La Roche for its generous gift of the different synthetic analogs of vitamin A. This work was supported by grant N° 79.67.0673 from Délégation Générale à la Recherche Scientifique et Technique (D.G.R.S.T.).

References

1. Bollag W (1972) Prophylaxis of chemically-induced benign and malignant epithelial tumors by vitamin A acid (retinoic acid). Eur J Cancer 8:689–693
2. Bollag W (1979) Retinoids and cancer. Cancer Chemother Pharmacol 3:207–215
3. Cohen BE, Cohen IK (1973) Vitamin A: adjuvant and steroid antagonist in the immune response. J Immunol 111:1376–1380
4. Dennert G, Lotan R (1978) Effects of retinoic acid on the immune system: Stimulation of T killer cell induction. Eur J Immunol 8:23–29
5. Dennert G, Crowley C, Kouba J, Lotan R (1979) Retinoic acid stimulation of induction of mouse killer T-cells in allogeneic and syngeneic systems. J Natl Cancer Inst 62:89–94
6. Dresser DN (1968) Adjuvanticity of Vitamin A. Nature 217:527–529
7. Felix EL, Loyd B, Cohn MH (1975) Inhibition of the growth and development of a transplantable murine melanoma by vitamin A. Science 189:886–887
8. Jurin M, Tannock IF (1972) Influence of vitamin A on immunological responses. Immunology 23:283–287
9. Lasnitzki I, Goodman DeWs (1974) Inhibition of the effects of methylcholanthrene on mouse prostate in organ culture by vitamin A and its analogs. Cancer Res 34:1564–1571
10. Lasnitzki I (1976) Reversal of methylcholanthrene-induced changes in mouse prostates in vitro by retinoic acid and its analogs. Br J Cancer 34:239–248
11. Lotan R, Nicolson GL (1977) Inhibitory effects of retinoic acid or retinylacetate on the growth of untransformed, transformed and tumor cells in vitro. J Natl Cancer Inst 59:1717–1722
12. Lotan R (1980) Effects on vitamin A and its analogs (retinoids) on normal and neoplastic cells. Biochem Biophys Acta 605:33–91
13. Moore T Effects of vitamin A deficiency in animals: Pharmacology and toxicology of Vitamin A. In: The vitamins, 2nd ed., Vol. 1, Sebrell WH, Harris RS (eds). Academic Press, New York, 1967, p 245–266; 280–294
14. Patek PQ, Collins JL, Yogeeswaran G, Dennert G (1979) Antitumor potential of retinoic acid; stimulation of immune mediated effectors. Int J Cancer 24:624–628
15. Sporn MB, Dunlop NM, Newton DL et al (1976) Prevention of chemical carcinogenesis by Vitamin A and its synthetic analogs (retinoids). Fed Proc 35:1332–1336
16. Tada M, Hinuma S, Abo T, Kumagai K (1980) Murine antibody-dependent cell mediated cytotoxicity; failure to detect effector cells equivalent to human K cells. J Immunol 124:1929–1936

C.E. Orfanos et al. (eds.)
Retinoids

Vitamin A Transport and Delivery and the Mechanism of Vitamin A Toxicity

DeWitt S. Goodman

Vitamin A is a generic term used for all compounds that exhibit qualitatively the biological activity of retinol. The term retinoids has been adopted recently as a general term that includes both the natural forms of vitamin A and synthetic analogs, with or without biological activity, of retinol. Vitamin A is necessary for the support of growth, health, and life of higher animals. In the absence of vitamin A, animals will cease to grow and, in time, die. Vitamin A is essential for vision, reproduction, growth, the maintenance of differentiated epithelia, and mucus secretion. The exact nature of the role of vitamin A in these functions has not been defined at the molecular level, except for its well documented role in vision (52). A general review of a number of aspects of vitamin A metabolism has recently been published (14).

Biosynthesis and Intestinal Absorption of Vitamin A

The major natural sources of vitamin A in the diet are certain plant carotenoid pigments, such as β-carotene, and the long-chain retinyl esters that are found in animal tissues. β-Carotene is converted to vitamin A primarily in the intestinal mucosa. The biosynthetic process involves two soluble enzymes; first, β-carotene-15,15′-dioxygenase, and second, retinaldehyde reductase. The first enzyme catalyzes the cleavage of β-carotene at the central double bond by a dioxygenase mechanism, to yield two molecules of retinaldehyde (19). The retinaldehyde is then reduced to retinol.

Dietary retinyl esters are hydrolyzed in the intestine, and the resulting retinol is then absorbed into the mucosal cell. Retinol in the mucosal cell (newly-absorbed or newly-synthesized from carotene) is reesterified with long-chain, mainly saturated fatty acids, and the retinyl esters are absorbed into the body, mainly in association with lymph chylomicrons. During chylomicron metabolism, virtually all of the retinyl esters remain with the chylomicron "remnant", and are removed from the circulation almost entirely by the liver (17). After uptake of the chylomicron retinyl esters, hydrolysis and reesterification occur in the liver, and the resulting retinyl esters (mainly retinyl palmitate) are stored in association with lipid droplets. From these liver stores, vitamin A is mobilized as the free alcohol, retinol, bound to a specific plasma transport protein, retinol-binding protein (RBP).

Plasma Transport: Retinol-binding Protein

Vitamin A is transported in plasma as retinol bound to RBP. Since the initial isolation of human RBP in 1968 (26), extensive studies in many laboratories have provided a considerable amount of information about the structure, metabolism, and biologic roles of this protein. RBP is a single polypeptide chain with a molecular weight close to 20,000, α_1-mobility on electrophoresis, and a single binding site for one molecule of retinol. In plasma, most of RBP normally circulates as the retinol-RBP complex (holo-RBP).

RBP interacts strongly with another protein, plasma prealbumin, and normally circulates as a 1:1 molar RBP-prealbumin complex. The usual level of RBP in plasma is about 40–50 µg/ml and that of prealbumin is about 200–300 µg/ml (46). In addition to its role in vitamin A transport, prealbumin plays a role in the binding and plasma transport of thyroid hormones. The formation of the RBP-prealbumin complex serves to reduce the glomerular filtration and renal catabolism of RBP.

During the past decade RBP has been isolated from serum of many species other than man, including the rat, monkey, pig, dog, rabbit, cattle, and chicken (see references 44, 16, 13 for earlier reviews and for references). In all of these species, RBP has been found to be a small protein of approximately 20,000 daltons weight which binds one molecule of retinol per molecule of RBP. In spite of occasional reports to the contrary, the RBP of all of these species appears to circulate in plasma as a protein-protein complex together with a larger protein. In the cases where the larger protein has been isolated, it has been found to generally resemble human prealbumin.

On the other hand, RBP isolated from fish (yellowtails) was somewhat smaller (16,000 daltons) and lacked binding affinity for prealbumin (43). The vitamin A transport system of the tadpole resembled that found in fish, but, interestingly, the adult frog was found to transport vitamin A as the RBP-prealbumin complex (43).

The vitamin A transport system provides an interesting model for the study of protein-protein and protein-ligand interactions, and of the characteristics of a specific lipid-binding and transport system.

Prealbumin Structure

Prealbumin is one of the most completely characterized human proteins. The prealbumin molecule is a stable and symmetrical tetramer, composed of four identical subunits, with a molecular weight of 54,980 (28). The complete amino acid sequence of human prealbumin is known (28), and the full three-dimensional structure of the molecule has been determined by high resolution x-ray crystallography (4, 5). These studies have shown that the subunits have extensive β-sheet structure and are linked into stable dimers, each comprising two of the four subunits. A channel runs through the center of the prealbumin molecule, in which are located two symmetry-related binding sites for iodothyronine molecules. Only one molecule of thyroxine binds to prealbumin with high affinity, however, because of negative cooperativity (4, 12).

Recent x-ray crystallographic studies have shown that the prealbumin molecule contains two surface sites with structural complementarity to double-helical DNA (3). Although the binding of prealbumin to DNA has not been reported, it has been suggested that the prealbumin molecule may serve as a model for the kind of structure that may be involved in hormone receptors with nuclear effects on DNA transcription (3).

RBP Structure

Less detailed structural information is available about RBP. Studies employing circular dichroism and optical rotary dispersion have shown that human RBP appears to have a relatively high content of unordered conformation, a significant but small complement of β-conformation, and little or no α-helix (40, 22). The RBP molecule contains no bound lipid (other than retinol) and no carbohydrate.

The complete primary structure of human RBP has been reported recently (39). RBP is cleaved by cyanogen bromide into 5 fragments; of these, the carboxy-terminal fragment represents slightly more than half the molecule. In another recent study (27), the 5 cyanogen bromide fragments were isolated and aligned, the amino acid sequences of 4 of the fragments were determined, and the sequence of the amino-terminal two-thirds of the RBP molecule was reported. Information was sought concerning the possible existence of sequence homologies between the RBP partial sequence and the amino acid sequences of other proteins whose primary structures are known. A computer search with appropriate programs failed to reveal homologies in sequence between RBP and any other known sequenced protein (27). The reported complete sequence (39) consists of 182 amino acids, with the carboxy-terminal sequence: -Gly-Arg-Ser-Glu-Arg-Asn-Leu-COOH.

RBP-Prealbumin Interaction

More information is needed about the structures and the characteristics of the binding sites on prealbumin and on RBP that are involved in the interaction between these two proteins. It is known that the interaction of RBP with prealbumin is very sensitive to ionic strength, with dissociation of the protein-protein complex occurring at low ionic strength (35, 51). The interaction of RBP with prealbumin is also strongly pH-dependent; maximum binding occurs near physiological pH and falls gradually at lower and at higher pH values (51). It has also been found that the binding of retinol to RBP appears to be stabilized by the formation of the RBP-prealbumin complex (20, 18). In contrast, there is no interdependence of the binding of thyroxine and of RBP to prealbumin.

The results of several studies strongly suggest that prealbumin contains four binding sites for human RBP (51, 34, 29). It has been suggested (29) that prealbumin possesses four identical binding sites for RBP, but that the binding (for the human proteins) is of a negative cooperative nature, largely resulting from steric hindrance by already bound RBP molecules. With the information on hand, its seems reasonable to assume that each prealbumin subunit might contain one binding site of RBP. More data are, however, needed to confirm this hypothesis.

The structures that characterize the protein-protein binding sites on RBP and prealbumin appear to be very similar across a range of species. Thus, RBPs and prealbumins of human and chicken cross-interact, and show inter-species affinities similar to those displayed by the proteins of the same species (29). Rat RBP has been isolated by affinity chromatography on human prealbumin coupled to agarose (37), and conversely rat prealbumin has been isolated by affinity chromatography on human RBP coupled to agarose (33). It appears that the structural features responsible for the protein-protein interaction were maintained during much of vertebrate evolution.

RBP-Retinol Interaction

A large number of studies have explored the binding of a variety of retinoids and related compounds to apo-RBP (see 15 for review and references). The structural features required for the binding of all-*trans*-retinol to RBP appear to be fairly, but far from absolutely, specific. A number of retinoids can bind to apo-RBP with varying degrees of effectiveness. Some of these (including all-*trans* retinoic acid) bind to RBP with an affinity similar to that of retinol. Compounds unrelated to vitamin A in structure bind minimally to RBP or not at all.

Clinical Studies

Many clinical studies have examined the effects of a variety of diseases on the plasma levels of RBP and prealbumin in humans. This topic is discussed in more detail in other reviews (44, 16, 13, 15). No disease has yet been found where RBP was totally absent or had abnormal immunological properties. Plasma RBP levels are low in patients with liver disease and are high in patients with chronic renal disease (46). These findings reflect the facts that RBP is produced in the liver and mainly catabolized in the kidneys. Several studies have examined the retinol transport system in patients with protein calorie malnutrition. Such patients have decreased concentrations of plasma RBP, prealbumin, and vitamin A. Low intake of dietary protein and calories is frequently accompanied by an inadequate intake of vitamin A. However, even in cases where there is adequate vitamin A intake, the plasma RBP and vitamin A levels are low, reflecting a functional impairment in the hepatic release of vitamin A because of defective production of RBP.

Retinol Delivery: RBP Receptors

RBP is responsible for the delivery of retinol from the liver to the extrahepatic sites of action of the vitamin. Evidence is available that this delivery process may involve cell surface receptors for RBP. Thus, studies have been reported that suggest that there are specific cell surface receptors for RBP on monkey small intestine mucosal cells (38), on bovine pigment epithelial cells (24, 6), and on chicken testicular cell membranes (2). In these studies, retinol appeared to be taken up (from holo-RBP) by the cells without a concomitant uptake of RBP. Retinol was not taken up by the pigment epithelial cells when it was presented nonspecifically bound to bovine serum albumin (6). Hence, RBP appears to deliver retinol to specific cell surface sites that "recognize" RBP, and to release retinol at these locations. The retinol then enters the cell for subsequent metabolism and action. The apo-RBP does not appear to enter the cell, but returns to the circulation, where it shows a reduced affinity for prealbumin and is selectively filtered by the renal glomeruli.

Many questions exist about the nature of the retinol delivery process and about its regulation. Information is needed about the putative "RBP receptor", including questions about its structure, metabolism, and regulation, and about its role in the release of retinol from RBP and in the uptake of retinol into the cell.

Intracellular Retinoid-binding Proteins

After delivery of retinol and its uptake into the target cell, the retinol may become associated with the intracellular binding protein for retinol (CRBP). It is now well established that a number of tissues of rats, humans, and other species contain soluble proteins with binding specificity for retinol (CRBP) or for retinoic acid (CRABP). These proteins have been purified from several tissues and partly characterized (see references 7 and 42 for recent reviews). Both CRBP and CRABP have molecular weights close to 14,600 and single binding sites for one molecule or retinoid ligand. The intracellular binding proteins differ in a number of ways from plasma RBP, and differ from each other in regard to binding specificity and immunoreactivity.

Interest in these intracellular retinoid binding proteins has been stimulated by reports suggesting a relationship between the binding affinity of the proteins for various vitamin A-related compounds and the biological activity of the compounds (7). Furthermore, a number of retinoids with anticarcinogenic activity can associate with the tissue binding proteins, and it has been reported that the binding ability tends to correlate with the biological activity for given compounds (25). Accordingly, it has been suggested that the binding proteins might be involved in some way in the biological expression of vitamin A activity within the cell.

Regulation of RBP Production and Secretion by the Liver

Vitamin A mobilization from the liver, and its delivery to peripheral tissues, is highly regulated by factors that control the rates of RBP production and secretion by the liver. A major goal of our laboratory has been to try to elucidate the cellular and molecular mechanisms involved in the regulation of RBP production and secretion. These studies have employed the rat as an animal model, and a sensitive and specific radioimmunoassay for rat RBP (31).

One factor which specifically regulates RBP secretion from the liver is the nutritional vitamin A status of the animal (31, 50, 36). Thus, retinol deficiency specifically blocks the secretion of RBP from the liver, so that plasma RBP levels fall and liver RBP levels rise. Conversely, repletion of vitamin A-deficient rats intravenously with retinol stimulates the rapid secretion of RBP from the expanded liver pool (in the deficient rat) into the plasma. This release of RBP is not blocked by inhibitors of protein synthesis, indicating that it comes from the expanded liver pool of RBP, rather than from *de novo* protein synthesis.

The block in RBP secretion seen after vitamin A depletion is highly specific for RBP. Thus, neither vitamin A depletion and deficiency, nor retinol repletion of deficient rats, significantly altered plasma levels of prealbumin (32). The secretion of RBP and prealbumin appear to be independently regulated processes, with formation of the RBP-prealbumin complex occurring in plasma, after secretion of the two proteins from the liver cell.

Studies have been conducted to explore the roles of various subcellular organelles and structures in the secretion of RBP. RBP in the liver is mainly found associated with the liver microsomes, and is particularly enriched in the rough microsomal fraction (44). The Golgi apparatus was found to contain a maximum of 23% of RBP in the liver in normal rats, and a maximum of less than 10% of the expanded pool of liver RBP in vitamin A-deficient rats (23). Presumptive evidence that the microtubules are involved in the secretion of RBP has been obtained in studies with the drug colchicine (48). These recent studies (23, 48) suggest that the Golgi apparatus and secretory vesicles are involved in the pathway of RBP secretion from the liver, but also demonstrate that the Golgi is not the major subcellular locus for RBP in either normal or vitamin A-deficient rats.

We have found two lines of differentiated rat hepatoma cells that synthesize RBP during culture *in vitro* (47). When the cells were incubated in a vitamin A serumless medium, a relatively large proportion of the RBP synthesized was retained within the cells. Addition of retinol to the medium (at levels of 0.1 or 1 μg/ml) stimulated the release of RBP from the cells into the medium and also increased the net synthesis of RBP. In contrast, retinol had no effect on either the synthesis or secretion of rat serum albumin by these cells. Thus, these cell lines appear to respond to vitamin A depletion and repletion in a similar manner as does the intact rat liver cell *in vivo*.

More recent studies, with glucocorticoid hormones, demonstrated that these hormones markedly stimulate the net synthesis of RBP by the rat hepatoma cells. When retinol and dexamethasone were added together to the incubation medium, the stimulatory effects were roughly additive. An optimal effect was obtained with approximately $5\text{–}10 \times 10^{-9}$ M dexamethasone. In addition, studies with progesterone suggest that steroid hormone receptors are involved in the dexamethasone effect. The presence of dexamethasone did not alter the stimulatory effect of retinol on the secretion of RBP from the cells into the medium.

Thus, dexamethasone and retinol appear to have distinctly separate effects on RBP metabolism by the liver cell. We believe that these isolated liver cells represent good models with which to explore the mechanisms involved in the regulation of RBP synthesis and secretion.

Vitamin A Toxicity

Excessive, chronic vitamin A intake by animals and humans produces distinct toxic manifestations, including (in humans) pseudotumor cerebri, skeletal pain, desquamative dermatitis, and other clinical signs and symptoms. Considerable information is available about the mechanism of the toxic effects of vitamin A upon tissues. Studies both in vivo and in vitro have shown that excess vitamin A results in increased lability of biological membranes (41, 10). This effect of the vitamin is believed to be due to its surface active, "membranolytic" properties (1). In particular, excess vitamin A has been shown to lead to increased synthesis and release in lysosomal enzymes, and these hydrolases have been shown to be critically involved in the effects of vitamin A on cartilage and limb-bone rudiments (10, 11, 8).

Retinol bound to RBP does not appear to manifest its surface-active effects on biological membranes. Thus, retinol bound to RBP was found to produce no discernible effects on chick limb-bone rudiments grown in organ culture (9). These observations suggested that the mode of transport of vitamin A may be an important determinant in the development of the manifestations of hypervitaminosis A.

An extensive study was carried out in rats given excessive vitamin A in doses sufficient to cause both growth disturbances and fatty livers (30). The hypervitaminotic rats showed large increases in serum vitamin A levels, which were mainly due to elevations in the circulating levels of retinyl esters, and decreased levels of serum RBP. In these toxic rats, most of the serum vitamin A and virtually all of the retinyl esters were found in association with the serum lipoproteins of hydrated density less than 1.21. It was concluded that the serum lipoproteins play an important role in the transport of vitamin A that accumulates in the serum in hypervitaminosis A. It was also suggested that serum lipoproteins may nonspecifically deliver vitamin A to biological membranes and, hence, lead to vitamin A toxicity.

Data consistent with this interpretation have been obtained in studies on vitamin A transport in human vitamin A toxicity (45). In three patients with chronic hypervitaminosis A, the toxic state in each was associated with increased plasma concentrations of total vitamin A, and particularly of retinyl esters. In contrast, plasma RBP levels were normal, and there was a molar excess of total vitamin A in relation to RBP. The data suggest that vitamin A toxicity occurs when the capacity of RBP to transport vitamin A is exceeded. Vitamin A is thus presented to cell membranes in a form other than bound to RBP, and may manifest nonspecific toxicity when so presented to them. Hence, RBP may function not only to regulate the supply of retinol to tissues, but also to protect tissues from the surface-active properties of the vitamin.

These studies have, therefore, provided considerable insight into the metabolic phenomena that may be involved in the development of vitamin A toxicity due to the "natural" form of the vitamin, retinol. It may be asked, however, whether similar considerations apply to the development of vitamin A toxicity as a result of the administration of retinoic acid, or of other retinoids.

Retinoic acid and other acidic retinoids are highly active in promoting the lysis of the extracellular matrix of cartilage grown in organ culture in vitro (21). This phenomenon is presumably caused by release of lysosomal enzymes as a result of the membrane-labilizing effects of the compounds. Thus, retinoic acid and its analogs resemble retinol in being able to cause similar toxic manifestations; in fact, retinoic acid was quantitatively more active than was retinol in producing lysis of the cartilage matrix (21).

In contrast to retinol, retinoic acid is absorbed through the portal system and is transported in plasma bound to serum albumin (49). It does not accumulate in the liver or other tissues in any appreciable amounts. Retinoic acid appears to be quite rapidly metabolized, mainly to more polar compounds, which are then largely excreted in the urine and bile.

Since retinoic acid (and other acidic retinoids) circulates bound to albumin rather than to RBP, it is likely that retinoic acid is not delivered to tissues via a specific, receptor-regulated process. Accordingly, one would anticipate that there might be a fairly close and consistent relationship between the dose of retinoic acid administered on the one hand, and the rate of tissue delivery and risk of toxicity on the other. If this is true, then the plasma level of retinoic acid (and its analogs) should correlate well with the risk and development of toxicity, and should provide a means of assessing and monitoring toxicity with these compounds in a clinical setting. Thus, detailed pharmacokinetic studies of acidic retinoids might be of particular value in providing information relevant to the question of toxicity.

Summary

Dietary vitamin A is absorbed mainly via lymph chylomicrons and stored in the liver as retinyl esters. From the liver, vitamin A is mobilized and transported in plasma as the lipid alcohol retinol, bound to a specific transport protein, retinol-binding protein (RBP). In contrast, retinoic acid (and probably other acidic retinoids as well) is absorbed through the portal system and transported in plasma as the carboxylate anion bound to serum albumin. A great deal is now known about the chemical structure, metabolism, and biological roles of RBP. Vitamin A mobilization from the liver is highly regulated by factors that control the rates of RBP production and secretion. Retinol deficiency specifically blocks the secretion of RBP, which can then be rapidly stimulated by retinol repletion. The cellular and molecular mechanisms that mediate these phenomena are under investigation. Delivery of retinol to peripheral target tissues appears to involve specific cell surface receptors for RBP. The retinol so delivered enters the target cell, where it may become associated with the intracellular binding protein for retinol (CRBP). Evidence exists that vitamin A toxicity occurs in vivo when "excess" retinol begins to circulate in plasma, and to be presented to membranes, in a form other than bound to RBP. Nonspecific and unregulated delivery of vitamin A to biological membranes may, hence, lead to vitamin A toxicity. Since retinoic acid and other acidic retinoids are probably not delivered via a specific, receptor-regulated process, it is likely that the plasma level of such retinoids would correlate well with the development of toxicity.

References

1. Bangham AD, Dingle JT, Lucy JA (1964) Studies on the mode of action of excess of vitamin A. 9. Penetration of lipid monolayers by compounds in the vitamin A series. Biochem J 90:133–140
2. Bhat MK, Cama HR (1979) Gonadal cell surface receptor for plasma retinol-binding protein. A method for its radioassay and studies on its level during spermatogenesis. Biochim Biophys Acta 587:273–281
3. Blake CCF, Oatley SJ (1977) Protein-DNA and protein-hormone interactions in prealbumin: a model of the thyroid hormone nuclear receptor? Nature 268:115–120
4. Blake CCF, Geisow MJ, Oatley SJ, Rérat B, Rérat C (1978) Structure of prealbumin: secondary, tertiary, and quarternary interactions determind by Fourier refinement at 1.8 Å. J Mol Biol 121:339–356
5. Blake CCF, Geisow MJ, Swan IDA, Rérat C, Rérat B (1974) Structure of human plasma preal-

bumin at 2.5 Å resolution. A preliminary report on the polypeptide chain conformation, quaternary structure and thyroxine binding. J Mol Biol 88:1–12
6. Chen CC, Heller J (1977) Uptake of retinol and retinoic acid from serum retinol-binding protein by retinal pigment epithelial cells. J Biol Chem 252:5216–5221
7. Chytil F, Ong DE (1979) Cellular retinol- and retinoic acid-binding proteins in vitamin A action. Fed Proc 38:2510–2514
8. Dingle JT, Barret AJ, Weston PD (1971) Cathepsin D characteristics of immunoinhibition and the confirmation of a role in cartilage breakdown. Biochem J 123:1–13
9. Dingle JT, Fell HB, Goodman DeWS (1972) The effect of retinol and of retinol-binding protein on embryonic skeletal tissue in organ culture. J Cell Sci 11:393–402
10. Fell HB (1970) The direct action of vitamin A on skeletal tissue in vitro. In: The fat soluble vitamins, DeLuca HF, Suttie JW (eds). Univ. Wisconsin Press, Madison, 187–202
11. Fell HB, Dingle JT (1971) Studies on the mode of action of excess vitamin A. 6. Lysosomal protease and the degradation of cartilage matrix. Biochem J 87:403–408
12. Ferguson RN, Edelhoch H, Saroff HA, Robbins J (1975) Negative cooperativity in the binding of thyroxine to human serum prealbumin. Biochemistry 14:282–289
13. Glover J (1973) Retinol-binding proteins. Vitam Horm 31:1–42
14. Goodman DeWS (1980) Vitamin A metabolism. Fed Proc 39:2716–2722
15. Goodman DeWS (1980) Plasma retinol-binding protein. Ann NY Acad Sci 348:378–390
16. Goodman DeWS (1974) Vitamin A transport and retinol-binding protein metabolism. Vitam Horm 32:167–180
17. Goodman DeWS, Huang HS, Shiratori T (1965) Tissue distribution and metabolism of newly absorbed vitamin A in the rat. J Lipid Res 6:390–396
18. Goodman DeWS, Leslie RB (1972) Fluorescence studies of human plasma retinol-binding protein and of the retinol-binding protein-prealbumin complex. Biochim Biophys Acta 260:670–678
19. Goodman DeWS, Olson JA (1969) The conversion of all-*trans* β-carotene into retinal. In: Methods in Enzymology. Vol. XV. Steroids and Terpenoids. Clayton RB (ed). Academic Press, New York, 462–475
20. Goodman DeWS, Raz A (1972) Extraction and recombination studies of the interaction of retinol with human plasma retinol-binding protein. J Lipid Res 13:338–347
21. Goodman DeWS, Smith JE, Hembry RM, Dingle JT (1974) Comparison of the effects of vitamin A and its analogs upon rabbit ear cartilage in organ culture and upon growth of the vitamin A-deficient rat. J Lipid Res 15:406–414
22. Gotto AM, Lux SE, Goodman DeWS (1972) Circular dichroic studies of human plasma retinol-binding protein and prealbumin. Biochim Biophys Acta 271:429–435
23. Harrison EH, Smith JE, Goodman DeWS (1980) Effects of vitamin A deficiency on the levels and distribution of retinol-binding protein and marker enzymes in homogenates and Golgi-rich fractions of rat liver. Biochim Biophys Acta 628:489–497
24. Heller J (1975) Interactions of plasma retinol-binding protein with its receptor. Specific binding of bovine and human retinol-binding protein to pigment epithelium cells from bovine eyes. J Biol Chem 250:3613–3619
25. Jetten AN, Jetten MER (1979) Possible role of retinoic acid binding protein in retinoid stimulation of embryonal carcinoma cell differentiation. Nature 278:180–182
26. Kanai M, Raz A, Goodman DeWS (1968) Retinol-binding protein: the transport protein for vitamin A in human plasma. J Clin Invest 47:2025–2044
27. Kanda Y, Goodman DeWS (1979) Partial amino acid sequence of human retinol-binding protein. Isolation and alignment of the five cyanogen bromide fragments and the amino acid sequences of four of the fragments. J Lipid Res 20:865–878
28. Kanda Y, Goodman DeWS, Canfield RE, Morgan FJ (1974) The amino acid sequence of human plasma prealbumin. J Biol Chem 249:6796–6805
29. Kopelman M, Cogan U, Mokady S, Shinitzky M (1976) The interaction between retinol-binding proteins and prealbumins studies by fluorescence polarization. Biochim Biophys Acta 439: 449–460
30. Mallia AK, Smith JE, Goodman DeWS (1975) Metabolism of retinol-binding protein and vitamin A during hypervitaminosis A in the rat. J Lipid Res 16:180–188
31. Muto Y, Smith JE, Milch PO, Goodman DeWS (1972) Regulation of retinol-binding protein metabolism by vitamin A status in the rat. J Biol Chem 247:2542–2550
32. Navab M, Smith JE, Goodman DeWS (1977) Rat plasma prealbumin. Metabolic studies on effects of vitamin A status and on tissue distribution. J Biol Chem 252:5107–5114

33. Navab M, Mallia AK, Kanda Y, Goodman DeWS (1977) Rat plasma prealbumin. Isolation and partial characterization. J Biol Chem 252:5100–5106
34. Nilsson S, Rask L, Peterson PA (1975) Studies on thyroid hormone binding proteins. II. Binding of thyroid hormones, retinol-binding protein, and fluorescent probes to prealbumin and effects of thyroxine on prealbumin subunit self-association. J Biol Chem 250:8554–8563
35. Peterson PA (1971) Studies on the interaction between prealbumin, retinol-binding protein, and vitamin A. J Biol Chem 246:44–49
36. Peterson PA, Rask L, Östberg L, Andersson L, Kamwendo F, Pertoft H (1973) Studies on the transport and cellular distribution of vitamin A in normal and vitamin A-deficient rats with special reference to the vitamin A-binding plasma protein. J Biol Chem 248:4009–4022
37. Poole AR, Dingle JT, Mallia AK, Goodman DeWS (1975) The localization of retinol-binding protein in rat liver by immunofluorescence microscopy. J Cell Sci 19:379–394
38. Rask L, Peterson PA (1976) *In vitro* uptake of vitamin A from the retinol-binding plasma protein to mucosal epithelial cells from the monkey's small intestine. J Biol Chem 251:6360–6366
39. Rask L, Anundi H, Peterson PA (1979) The primary structure of the human retinol-binding protein. FEBS Lett 104:55–58
40. Rask L, Peterson PA, Björk I (1972) Conformational studies of the human vitamin A-transporting protein complex. Biochemistry 11:264–268
41. Roels OA, Anderson OR, Lui NST, Shah DO, Trout ME (1969) Vitamin A and membranes. Am J Clin Nutr 22:1020–1032
42. Ross AC, Goodman DeWS (1979) Intracellular binding proteins for retinol and retinoic acid: comparison with each other and with serum retinol-binding protein. Fed Proc 38:2515–2518
43. Shidoji Y, Muto Y (1977) Vitamin A transport in plasma of the nonmammalian vertebrates: isolation and partial characterization of piscine retinol-binding protein. J Lipid Res 18:679–691
44. Smith JE, Goodman DeWS (1979) Retinol-binding protein and the regulation of vitamin A transport. Fed Proc 38:2504–2509
45. Smith FR, Goodman DeWS (1976) Vitamin A transport in human vitamin A toxicity. N Engl J Med 294:805–808
46. Smith FR, Goodman DeWS (1971) The effects of disease of the liver, thyroid, and kidneys on the transport of vitamin A in human plasma. J Clin Invest 50:2426–2436
47. Smith JE, Borek C, Goodman DeWS (1978) Regulation of retinol-binding protein metabolism in cultured rat liver cell lines. Cell 15:865–873
48. Smith JE, Deen Jr DD, Sklan D, Goodman DeWS (1980) Colchicine inhibition of retinol-binding protein secretion by rat liver. J Lipid Res 21:229–237
49. Smith JE, Milch PO, Muto Y, Goodman DeWS (1973) The plasma transport and metabolism of retinoic acid in the rat. Biochem J 132:821–827
50. Smith JE, Muto Y, Milch PO, Goodman DeWS (1973) The effects of chylomicron vitamin A on the metabolism of retinol-binding protein in the rat. J Biol Chem 248:1544–1549
51. van Jaarsveld PP, Edelhoch H, Goodman DeWS, Robbins J (1973) The interaction of human plasma retinol-binding protein with prealbumin. J Biol Chem 248:4698–4705
52. Wald G (1968) Molecular basis of visual excitation. Science 162:230–239

C.E. Orfanos et al. (eds.)
Retinoids

Experimental Toxicology of the Aromatic Retinoid Ro 10-9359 (Etretinate)

K. Teelmann

The therapeutic usefulness of retinoids in dermatology (9, 10) and certain cancer diseases (2, 13, 14) has been established recently. One of these compounds attracting major attention is the aromatic retinoid Ro 10-9359 (etretinate). This report reviews the results of the routine preclinical studies performed with this compound.

Material and Methods

The spray-dried form (SD) of Ro 10-9359 used in most of the tests performed is a green-yellow, odourless, homogeneous powder. It is insoluble in water. The acute systemic toxicity of Ro 10-9359 was studied by different routes of administration in mice, rats and dogs. The number of animals examined were 10 rodents/sex/group as well as one male and one female dog. For oral administrations the compound was suspended in peanut-oil, for s.c. and i.p. injections in rodents a solution in polyethylene glycol 400 (PEG 400) was used. After an observation period of 10 days the LD_{50} in rodents was calculated by the probit method (8).

The animals used for the various repeated dose tests, duration of tests and doses administered are

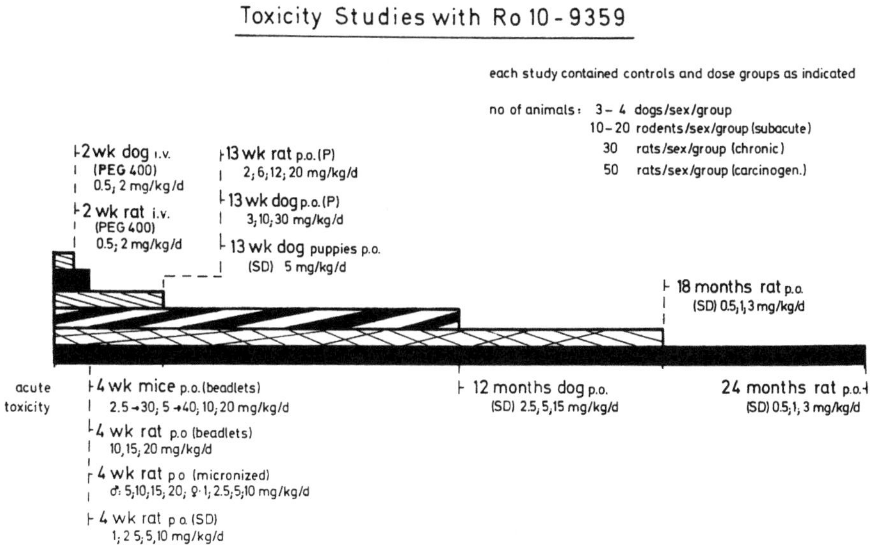

Fig. 1. Duration, route and doses of various toxicity studies performed on mice, rats and dogs with Ro 10-9359

summarized in Fig. 1. Oral administration to rodents with different pharmaceutical formulations [powdered (P), micronized, beadlet or spray-dried (SD)] was performed by means of diet admixture, while dogs received the test compound in gelatine capsules once a day. For the 2-week i.v. studies in rats and dogs, a solution containing 90% PEG 400 was used.

The parameters examined at appropriate intervals (except carcinogenicity study) were: general tolerance, food consumption, drug intake (rodents), body weight development, mortalities; haematological examinations such as: red blood counts, haemoglobin, haematocrit, mean cell volume, mean cell haemoglobin, white blood counts and differential white blood counts, platelet counts, erythrocyte sedimentation rate, reticulocyte counts and determination of thromboplastin time (dogs); blood chemistry examinations such as: GOT, GPT, AP, blood urea, glucose, cholesterol, bilirubin, sodium, potassium, calcium, total serum protein and serum electrophoresis; urinary examinations such as: colour, pH, volume, specific gravity, protein, glucose, bilirubin, haemoglobin, ketones and urinary sediment. Additional ophthalmoscopic and electrocardiographic (dogs) examinations were performed at particular times in all studies mentioned.

After termination of dosing all surviving animals were sacrificed and the macroscopically visible organ and tissue alterations noted. Organ weights were recorded for: heart, liver, lungs, spleen, kidneys, adrenals, pituitary gland, gonads and accessory sex glands, thyroids and brain. Finally all major tissues from all dogs and from 6–10 rats/sex/group (carcinogenicity study: 20 rats/sex/group) plus all tissue alterations seen at autopsy were processed and stained for histopathologic organ examinations.

Almost all group means of the test results obtained in the treated animals were compared with those of the control groups by means of statistical analysis. The tests applied were: Dunn test, Kruskal-Wallis test, analysis of variance and Student's t-test.

Results

Acute Studies in Rats, Mice and Dogs

Ro 10-9359 showed a low degree of toxicity in mice and rats after a single administration by various routes:

Species	Route	LD_{50} (mg/kg)
mice	p.o.	>4000
	i.p.	>4000
	s.c.	>4000
rats	p.o.	>4000
	i.p.	>1000
	s.c.	>1000

This tolerance changed rather dramatically with repeated doses of Ro 10-9359. The DL_{50} items after repeated oral administrations in rats and mice were:

Species	Time	DL_{50} (mg/kg)
rats	24 h after 1 admin.	>4000
	24 h after 5 admin.	310
	24 h after 10 admin.	80
	10 d after 10 admin.	50
mice	24 h after 1 admin.	>4000
	24 h after 5 admin.	220
	24 h after 10 admin.	55
	10 d after 10 admin.	45

Dogs tolerated the intravenous administration of a solution containing 0.667 mg/ml Ro 10-9359 (mixed-micelle solubilisate) in daily ascending doses of 0.5 to 4 ml/kg without side effects.

Subacute and Chronic Toxicity Studies in Rats and Dogs

The side effects noted affected mainly the weight gain of the animals, the skin and cutaneous mucous membranes, the red blood cells, the alkaline phosphatase and the skeletal system of the rats on the higher test doses.

The rat was found to be the most sensitive species. The first indication of poor tolerance usually became obvious as a reduced body weight gain. This decreased weight gain was dose-dependent; relatively high oral doses such as 10 to 15 mg/kg/day of the spray-dried form caused almost immediate body weight loss in rats with subsequent marked deterioration of the general condition. Free of side effects were doses up to 1 mg/kg/day administered for 18 or 24 months as diet admixture. Dogs were less sensitive and tolerated doses of 15 mg/kg/day relatively well during a treatment period of 12 months.

Side effects on the skin started with circumscribed reddening and erythema. The discolourations were at first noted in the face around eyes and nose as well as on the distal parts of the limbs, particularly in the dog. They appeared some 8–10 days after commencement of compound administration. The skin in these areas appeared to be slightly inflamed and thickened, but the symptoms vanished gradually after 2–3 weeks. Histologically a slight hyperplasia of the basal cell layers remained. Other areas of inflammatory skin reaction were the external ear canal with pronounced otitis externa in some dogs and the ventral inguinal and abdominal area.

Those areas with erythematous reactions showed also some hair loss and, with prolonged treatment, a hyperpigmentation of the dark pigmented skin zones (dog). The mucous production of the mucous membranes, particularly in the dog's mouth, appeared to be

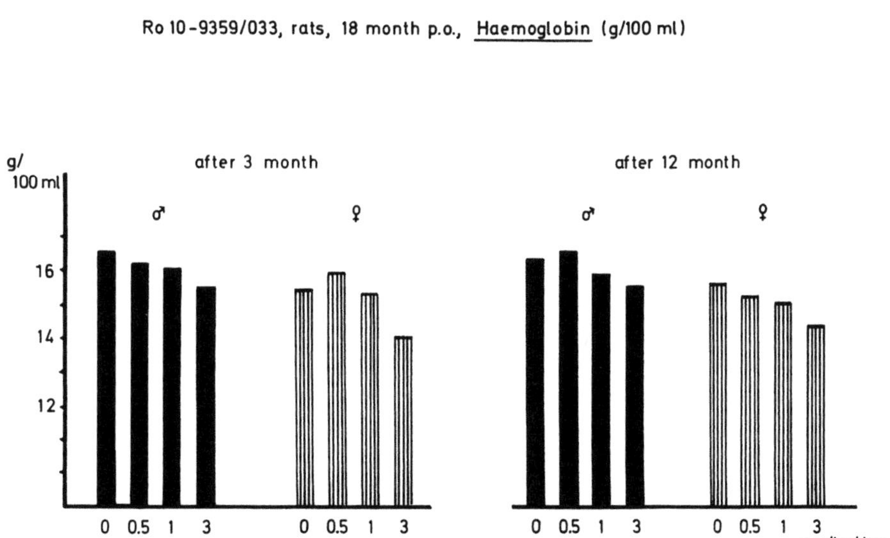

Fig. 2. Haemoglobin levels (g/100 ml) in male and female rats after 3 and 12 months of oral treatment with Ro 10-9359

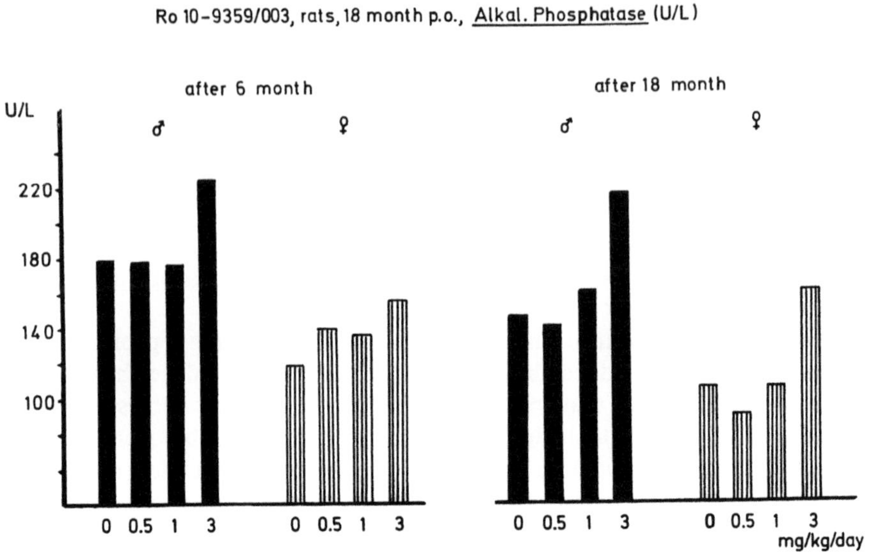

Fig. 3. Plasma alkaline phosphatase levels (U/L) in male and female rats after 6 and 18 months of oral treatment with Ro 10-9359

reduced and might have contributed to the reduced food consumption of the animals on the higher doses.

Haematologically reductions of the red blood counts and haemoglobin contents were noted in rats and dogs. These reductions were generally slight to moderate in degree, were dose-dependent and constantly noticeable throughout the studies, even in trials with long-term administration of the test compound (for example see Fig. 2). Compensation mechanisms were indicated by slightly to moderately increased reticulocyte counts as well as by some extramedullary haematopoiesis in spleen and liver of the rats.

Out of the blood chemistry parameters examined the alkaline phosphatase showed a dose-dependent elevation (for example see Fig. 3). This elevation was slight in case of dogs, somewhat more pronounced in rats and, as were the haematological changes, noticeable to the same extent throughout the studies. Other enzymes such as GPT or GOT showed only occasional elevations of transient character.

Serum electrolytes, particularly Ca^{++}, remained normal in all examinations performed.

One of the most striking side effects of overdosed vitamin A or vitamin A derivatives, bone fractures in rats, was also noted with Ro 10-9359 (Fig. 4). The duration of onset and frequency of these fractures was clearly dose-related. 10–15 mg/kg/day of the spray-dried formulation caused fractures within 10–14 days; in contrast with 3 mg/kg/day, where fractures were not observed earlier than 5–6 months after commencement of compound administration. These fractures were only an expression of a general alteration of the skeletal system. They were preceded by a markedly intensified remodelling of the bones with deformations, haemorrhages, increased periostal osteoclastic activity and thickening of the periosteum. Furthermore an augmented endostal osteoblastic activity resulting in a marked reduction of the bone diameter and increasing porosity, particularly of the long bones, was noted. Comparable bone alterations have never been observed in growing or adult dogs. The only indication of any influence of Ro 10-9359 on dog bones were occasional slight periostal haemorrhages and some slight pain sensitivity in the legs and joints. A slight sper-

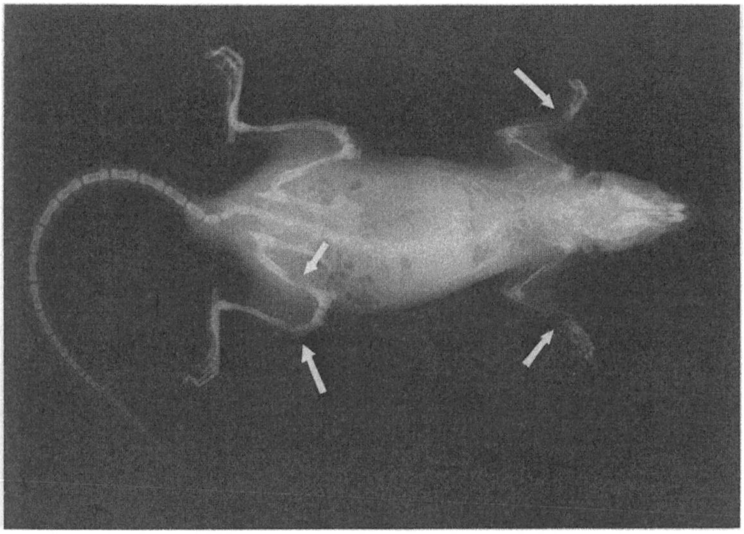

Fig. 4. X-ray film of whole rat demonstrating skeletal deformations (spine), foci of radiolucency of bones, thinning of bones and multiple fractures (arrows)

matogenic depression was noted in the testes of individual dogs on chronic treatment with the high dose (15 mg/kg/day) of Ro 10-9359.

Carcinogenic Potential

A two-year carcinogenicity study on rats revealed no carcinogenic potential of Ro 10-9359 in this species. The number of rats bearing multiple tumours was less in the intermediate- and high-dose groups than in the controls. In addition the number and variation of mammary tumours in the high-dose females (3 mg/kg/day) was significantly less than in the female controls.

Reversibility of Side Effects

All side effects mentioned above, such as reduced weight gain or weight loss, skin alterations, reduced number of red blood cells and haemoglobin, elevated alkaline phosphatase, bone alterations and spermatogenic depression, were reversible on cessation of treatment.

Discussion of Results

The acute oral toxicity of a single administration of Ro 10-9359 was very low. This changed rather dramatically when repeated doses were administered, particularly in rats. This phenomenon applies to vitamin A as well (7) and appears to be due to an overloaded or exceeded transport capacity of the retinol/retinoid-binding protein (12) and to transient incorporation of etretinate into as yet unknown storage sites of the body (perhaps liver or fat).

The pattern of side effects of overdosed etretinate resembles those of vitamin A and has therefore been called "hypervitaminosis A syndrome" (1). Changes of the skin were limited to transient erythema, circumscribed hair-loss and some hyperkeratosis primarily in the face and distal part of the limbs. This corresponds well to the findings of Rüst and Rufli (11) with Ro 10-9359 in humans, although lesions such as follicular papulae or vesicles were not seen in dogs or rats.

The haematological and biochemical alterations noted in our animal models (reduced red blood counts and haemoglobin; elevation of alkaline phosphatase) have also been reported for all-trans- and 13-cis-retinoic acid (5, 6) and to some extent for vitamin A as well (16). Another side effect found with all-trans- and 13-cis-retinoic acid: dose-dependent increased plasma triglyceride levels in rats (4) was also noted after etretinate treatment in this species (Dr. H. Lengsfeld, personal communication).

The most prominent symptoms of Ro 10-9359 treatment in rats are reduction of body weight gain and skeletal alterations. These side effects on the rat bones are fairly specific for vitamin A and its derivatives and are characterized as an enhanced bone remodelling and an increased enchondral ossification (3, 7, 15, 16). The results of this remodelling are markedly reduced diameters of the long bones, particularly the medullary cavity, reduced longitudinal growth, thinning of the epiphyseal line with premature ossification, increased bone porosity and often multiple fractures. Serum calcium is usually not elevated.

The increased serum alkaline phosphatase concentrations are partly due to the bone alterations. Intensive calcification of kidneys, heart, lungs and liver with different forms of vitamin A was found by Leelaprute et al. (7) in rats. Treatment of rats with Ro 10-9359 even for long times have never resulted in any notable tissue calcifications.

The side effects in rats on growth and bone produced by hypervitaminosis A can be almost completely prevented by pre-treatment of the animals by either spironolactone, anabolic steroids or inducers of microsomal liver enzymes particularly pregnenolone-16α-carbonitrile (17, 18). Whether this is also true for aromatic retinoids remains to be determined.

Severe skeletal side effects have never been noted in dogs or humans. The only indicators of some action of the retinoids on the bones are some increased pain sensitivity on legs and joints. Even in puppy-dogs treated for 3 months with 5 mg/kg/day of Ro 10-9359 no changes of the bones similar to those in rats could be demonstrated.

The finding that Ro 10-9359 bore no carcinogenic potential in rats and appeared to have a preventive effect on mammary tumour formation is underlined by the fact that other retinoids, e.g. retinyl methyl ether, were capable of inhibiting the progression of premalignant states of experimentally induced mammary cancer (13).

Summary

Various acute, subacute and chronic toxicity studies on mice, rats and dogs have been performed with the aromatic retinoid Ro 10-9359 (etretinate). The acute toxicity proved to be very low in rodents (> 4000 mg/kg). Repeated doses (e.g. 3–5 mg/kg/day in rats; 15–30 mg/kg/day in dogs) caused side effects such as: reduced body weight gain; transient skin erythema and slight hyperkeratosis; circumscribed hair loss; dryness of oral mucous membranes; slight to moderate reductions of red blood counts and haemoglobin; slight to moderate elevation of alkaline phosphatase and triglyceride levels; slight spermatogenic depression in some dogs; slightly increased pain sensitivity of legs and joints of dogs; enhanced remodelling of the skeletal system in rats resulting in a reduced diameter particularly of the long bones, accelerated ossification of the epiphyseal line and increased porosity of the bones with tendency to fracture. These side effects were dose-dependent and reversible after cessation of treatment.

References

1. Bollag W (1975) Prophylaxis of chemically induced epithelial tumors with an aromatic retinoid acid analog (Ro 10-9359). Eur J Cancer 11:721–724
2. Bollag W (1979) Retinoids and cancer. Cancer Chemother Pharmacol 3:207–215
3. Dämmrich K (1970) Zur formalen Pathogenese der Systemerkrankungen des Skeletts bei Tieren. Berl Münch Tierärztl Wschr 83:106–112
4. Gerber LE, Erdman Jr JW (1979) Hypertriglyceridemia in rats administered all-trans- or 13-cis-retinoic acid. Fed Proc 38:761
5. Hixon EJ, Denine EP (1978) Comparative subacute toxicity of all-trans- and 13-cis-retinoic acid in Swiss mice. Toxicol Appl Pharmacol 44:29–40
6. Hixon EJ, Burdeshaw JA, Denine EP, Harrison Jr SD (1979) Comparative subchronic toxicity of all-trans- and 13-cis-retinoic acid in Sprague-Dawley rats. Toxicol Appl Pharmacol 47:359–365
7. Leelaprute V, Boonpucknavig V, Bhamarapravati N, Weerapradist W (1973) Hypervitaminosis A in rats. Arch Pathol 96:5–9
8. Miller LC, Tainter MC (1944) Estimation of ED 50 and its error by means of logarithmic-probit graph paper. Proc Soc Exp Biol Med 57:261–264
9. Orfanos CE (1979) Retinoide – eine Breitspektrum-Dermatotherapie? Schweiz med Wochenschr 109:1909–1911
10. Peck GL (1980) Retinoids in dermatology. Arch Dermatol 116:283–284
11. Rüst O, Rufli Th (1979) Nebenwirkungen des oralen Retinoids Ro 10-9359 in der nicht erkrankten Haut des Psoriatikers: die „Retinoid-Dermatitis“. Schw med Wschr 109:1921–1925
12. Smith FR, Goodman DeWS (1976) Vitamin A transport in human vitamin A toxicity. N Engl J Med 294:805–808
13. Sporn MB (1977) Retinoids and Carcinogenesis. Nutr Rev 35:65–69
14. Sporn MB, Newton DL (1979) Chemoprevention of cancer with retinoids. Fed Proc: 38:2528–2534
15. Studer A (1950) Zur Wirkung großer Dosen von Vitamin A im Tierexperiment. Schweiz Z allg Path 13:799–802
16. Studer A, Zbinden G, Uehlinger E (1962) Hypervitaminosis A. In: Büchner F, Letterer E, Roulet F (Eds). Handbuch der allgemeinen Pathologie, Springer-Verlag, Berlin Göttingen Heidelberg, Vol. 11, Part 1, 963–976
17. Tuchweber B, Garg BD, Hatakeyama S (1970) Prevention of hypervitaminosis A by spironolactone and anabolic steroids. Int J Vitam Res 40:575–584
18. Tuchweber B, Garg BD, Salas M (1976) Microsomal enzyme inducers and hypervitaminosis A in rats. Arch Pathol Lab Med 100:100–105

C.E. Orfanos et al. (eds.)
Retinoids

Studies in Reproductive Toxicology and Mutagenicity with Ro 10-9359

H. Hummler and M.E. Schüpbach

Because of the potential risk involved during human pregnancy, Ro 10-9359 (etretinate) was tested in a series of experiments involving mice, rats and rabbits to investigate the influence on the embryo and fetus and on the general reproductive performance on these animals. Furthermore, the in vivo and in vitro experiments were performed to test for chromosome breaking or point mutation inducing activity of this compound.

Materials and Methods

Teratology

All animals used in these experiments were housed in stainless steel cages in temperature controlled rooms with a normal day/night cycle and breeding was in accordance to established protocols for each species.

Experiment I: The first series of experiments involved pregnant animals treated orally during the period of organogenesis. Mice (24, 27, 29/dose group) and rats (33–43/dose group) received daily doses of 2, 4 and 8 mg/kg b.w. between days 7–16 of pregnancy and rabbits (20/dose group) received daily doses of 0.5, 1.0, and 2.0 mg/kg b.w. between days 7–19 of pregnancy. Control animals for all experiments received rape oil i.g. during the same period and in the same volume ratio. Fetuses were either removed by C-section one day prior to parturition and examined for external, skeletal, or visceral abnormalities or the dams were allowed to birth and rear their young which were evaluated for functional defects.

Experiment II: The second series of experiments involve a fertility study where groups of 35 male or 33–35 female rats received daily doses of 1, 2.5, and 5 mg/kg b.w. during the period of gametogenesis. Females received additional treatment during mating and gestational periods to either day 14 (autopsy) or day 23 p.c. (F1). The F1-generation was mated and the resultant F2-generation examined for morphological changes.

The pre-postnatal study involved oral treatment from day 16 p.c. to day 23 p.p. with doses of 2, 4, and 8 mg/kg b.w. In each case 23–27 dams per group were allowed to birth and rear their young which were used to examine rearing behaviour. All animals were autopsied on day 23 of lactation.

Mutagenicity Studies

Part I. Ro 10–9359 Tested Alone

Micronucleus Test

3 male and 3 female mice (Füllinsdorf albino) were used per dosage group. They were treated twice p.o.

30 and 6 hours before sacrifice with 0, 250, 500 and 1000 mg/kg Ro 10-9359 in a rape oil suspension. Smears of the bone marrow of the femora were prepared and stained as described by Schmid (2). 4000 erythrocytes per animal were scored for the presence of micronuclei. Statistical analysis was performed by means of the Student's t-test.

Bacterial Strain

The *Salmonella typhimurium* strains used in our studies have been described by Ames et al. (1). The strains were obtained from Prof. B. Ames and were kept in liquid nitrogen. Single colony isolates were made for each experiment from nutrient broth agar (DIFCO) plates and checked for spontaneous reversion frequency, UV-sensitivity and R-factor.

Salmonella/rat Liver Microsome in vitro Test (Ames Test)

Testing was carried out using the plate incorporation assay technique described by Ames et al. (1) using the strains TA 1535, TA 1537, TA 1538, TA 98 and TA 100 in the absence and presence of a 9000 x *g* supernatant of rat liver (S9), previously exposed to phenobarbital. The activity of the S9 was checked by using cyclophosphamide and 3-methylcholanthrene as positive controls.

Ro 10-9359 was dissolved in dimethylsulfoxide (DMSO) at 10 and 50 µg/plate. Concentrations above 50 µg/plate precipitated and could therefore not be tested.

Host-mediated Assay

Füllinsdorf albino mice (4♂♂ and 4♀♀ per dose group) were used as host animals, strains TA 1530, TA 1532 and TA 1964 of S. typhimurium served as indicator organisms.

Suspensions of Ro 10-9359 in rape oil were applicated per os. At the same time each animal obtained 2 ml of a 90-minute culture of the corresponding bacterial strain, injected into the peritoneal cavity. After 3 hours the mice were sacrificed, the bacteria were retrieved and plated on minimal medium where only his^- to his^+ revertants can grow.

Part II. Ro 10-9359 in Combination with UV-light

Mutagenicity Tests with a UV-irradiated Solution of Ro 10-9359 in Bacteria

A solution of 500 µg/ml Ro 10-9359 in dimethylsulfoxide was irradiated for one hour with UV (254 nm) with 10.8 $J \cdot m^{-2} \cdot sec^{-1}$. The irradiated solution was then tested on strains TA 1537, TA 98 and TA 100 of S. typhimurium with and without metabolic activation by a rat liver homogenate fraction.

The Effect of Ro 10-9359 on Inactivation and Mutation Induction by UV in Bacteria

Overnight cultures of the strains G46, TA 1530 and TA 1535 were washed in saline and a suspension of ca. 2×10^9 cells was irradiated with either a germicidal lamp, emitting almost exclusively 254 nm radiation or with a sunlamp emitting in the UV-A and UV-B spectrum.

The cell suspension was stirred during irradiation and all the experiments were carried out under dim red light in order to avoid photoreactivation. After irradiation, the bacteria were plated in appropriate dilutions on complete medium (with or without Ro 10-9359) for determination of the surviving fraction and on minimal medium (with or without the retinoid) for determination of the mutation frequency.

In another set of experiments, Ro 10-9359 was present at 500 µg/ml in the overnight culture medium and in saline during irradiation as well as in the complete and minimal agar plates.

Table 1. The effect of Ro 10-9359 on the embryo

Species	Dosage mg/kg p.o.	Days of Pregnancy	Effects Embryotoxic	Effects Teratological
			General	Morphological
Mouse	0 - 2 -④-⑧	7–16	Increased resorption	Anophthalmia
			Increased stillbirth	Exencephaly
			Increased mortality	Cleft Palate
Rat	0 -②-④-⑧	7–16	of pups	Aplastic Kidney
				Aplastic Tail
Rabbit	0 - 0.5 - 1 -②	7–19		Anal Atresia
				Skeletal Anomalies

Results

Teratology

Experiment I: After administration of 2 mg/kg of Ro 10-9359 in the mouse there were no drug-related effects observed and all parameters were within the control range. The rat was more susceptible to low doses as indicated by the increase in skeletal variation (61.3%) and postnatal mortality (29.6%). In the 9 mg/kg group skeletal variation increased in the rat (77.2%) as did postnatal mortality (33.1%). The mouse showed an increase in skeletal variations (29.5%), stillbirths (38%) and cleft palate (27.3%). Embryotoxic and teratogenic effects in the mouse after 8 mg/kg were an increase in prenatal mortality (43.5%) and examination of the remaining fetuses revealed an increased incidence of defects of the vitamin A-type such as cleft palate, exencephaly, anophthalmia etc. (Table 1). In the rat 25% of all examined fetuses possess the same defects as the mouse, however, the skeletal variation is more severe (90%). Postnatal mortality from days 1–23 p.p. was increased to 54%.

In the rabbit no adverse effects were observed at doses of up to 1.0 mg/kg. Doses of 2 mg/kg resulted in increased resorptions (35%) and postnatal mortality. Skeletal variations were also increased but confined to digits and there was a 6.6% occurrence of cleft palate.

Experiment II: In the fertility study doses of 1, 2.5 and 5 mg/kg had no effect on the dams or embryos examined on day 14 p.c. However, at 5 mg/kg the number of the viable newborn pups per litter was lower in the F1-group (7.7) than the control (8.8) and postnatal weight

Table 2. The effect of Ro 10-9359 on general reproductive performance in the rat

Experiment	Dosage mg/kg p.o.	Treatment days	Results
		♂&♀:	
Fertility Study	0 - 1 - 2.5 -⑤	throughout gametogenesis	Increase in fetal resorptions
		♀: duration of pregnancy to the end of lactation	Reduced survivability and weight development of neonates
		♀:	
Peri-postnatal Study	0 - 2 - 4 -⑧	last 1/3 of pregnancy to the end of lactation	Increased stillbirths Reduced survivability of neonates (< 10% of control)

development reduced. Postnatal mortality between days 23–65 p.p. was increased at 20% and markedly higher than control values (< 1%) (Table 2).

The mating success of the F1 females was lower (35.3%) than control values (64.1%) and the postnatal weight development of the F2 animals slightly reduced during the lactation period.

Mutagenicity

Part I. Ro 10-9359 Tested Alone

Micronucleus Test

The average percentage of erythrocytes containing one or more than one micronucleus was 0.054 ± 0.02 for the control group. After twofold application per os of 250, 500 and 1000 mg/kg, the mean values of micronuclei containing erythrocytes was 0.050 ± 0.02, 0.054 ± 0.02 and 0.050 ± 0.02, respectively.

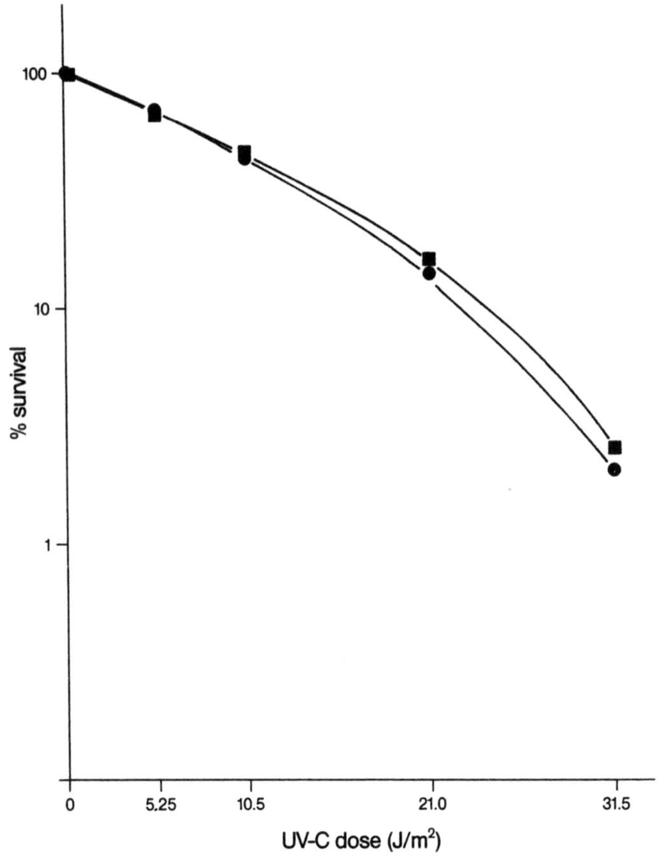

Fig. 1. Inactivation of S. typhimurium G 46 after irradiation with UV-C
● Plating medium: Nutrient Broth
■ Plating medium: Nutrient Broth + Ro 10-9359 (50 μg/plate)

Thus no indication of chromosome damaging or non-disjunction inducing effects of Ro 10-9359 was observed in this system.

Salmonella/rat Liver Microsome in vitro Test (Ames Test)

None of the 5 tester strains TA 1535, TA 1537, TA 1538, TA 98 and TA 100 of Salmonella typhimurium showed any increase in the number of revertants (mutations from histidine auxotrophy to prototrophy) at concentrations of 10 µg/plate and 50 µg/plate. No effect was observed whether or not a rat liver homogenate (S-9 fraction) was included into the top agar layer. All the values were in the range of spontaneous reversion frequencies of the corresponding strain.

Host-mediated Assay Mouse/Salmonella

Strains TA 1530, TA 1532 and TA 1964 of Salmonella typhimurium were used as indicator organisms, mice as host animal. At oral doses of 250, 500 and 1000 mg/kg of Ro 10-9359, no increase of the spontaneous reversion frequency was observed after a three-hour treatment.

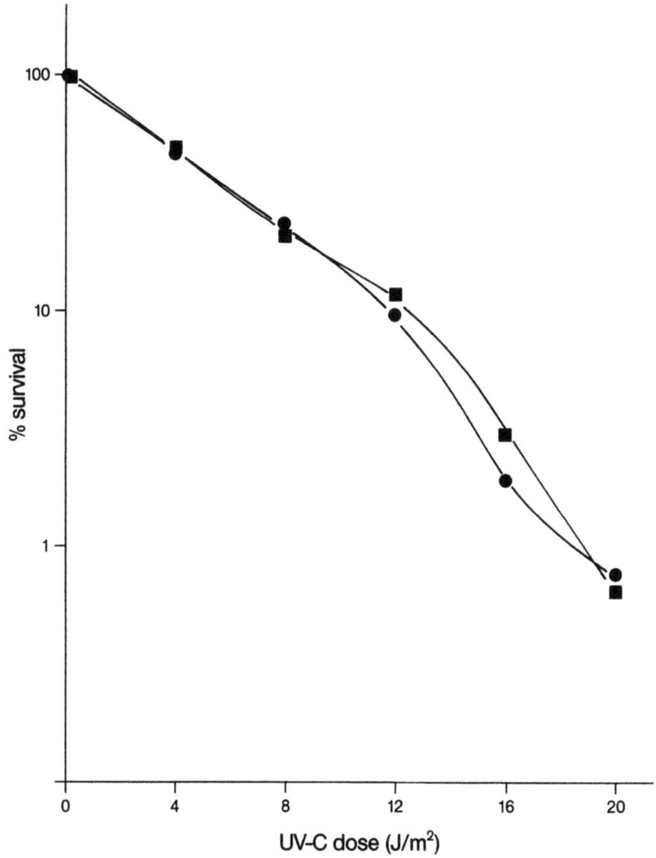

Fig. 2. Inactivation of S. typhimurium TA 100 after irradiation with UV-C
●Plating medium: Nutrient Broth
■ Plating medium: Nutrient Broth + Ro 10-9359 (50 µg/plate)

Part II. Ro 10-9359 in Combination with UV-light

Mutagenicity Tests with a UV-irradiated Solution of Ro 10-9359 in Bacteria

No effect was observed with a UV-irradiated solution of the compound in any of the 3 tester strains TA 1537, TA 98 and TA 100 of S. typhimurium at a concentration of 50 μg/plate (calculation based on the untreated compound).

The Effect of Ro 10-9359 on Inactivation and Mutation Induction by UV in Bacteria

Figs. 1, 2 and 3 show the survival curves after irradiation with UV (254 nm) of

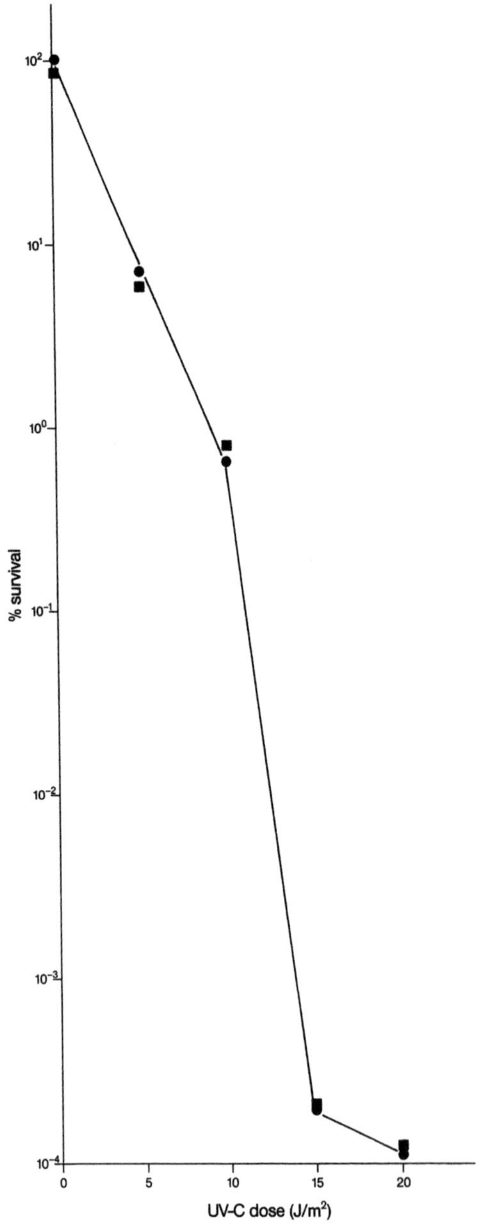

Fig. 3. Inactivation of S. typhimurium TA 1535 after irradiation with UV-C
●Plating medium: Nutrient Broth
■ Plating medium: Nutrient Broth + Ro 10-9359 (50 μg/plate)

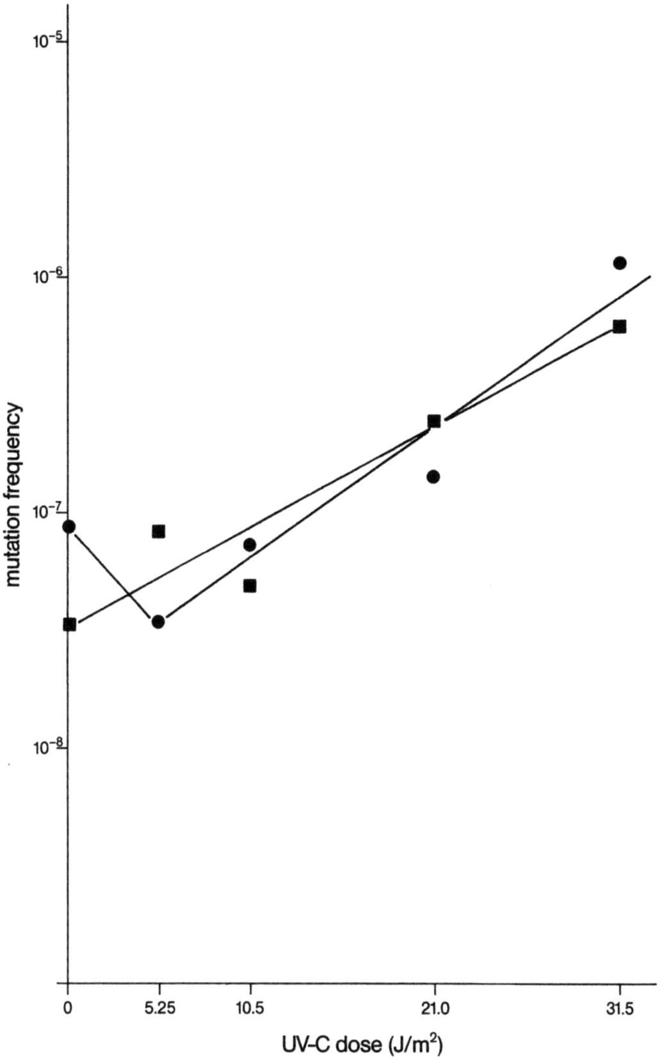

Fig. 4. Mutation-induction curve after UV-C treatment of S. typhimurium G 46
● Plating medium: Nutrient Broth
■ Plating medium: Nutrient Broth + Ro 10-9359 (50 µg/plate)

S. typhimurium strains G 46, TA 1535 and TA 100. The curves show that the inactivation kinetics remains the same whether Ro 10-9359 (50 µg/plate) is present or absent in the complete medium on which the cells were plated after irradiation.

Mutation induction curves with UV (254 nm) are shown in Figures 4, 5 and 6. In the 3 strains G 46, TA 1535 and TA 100 with different capacities in repairing DNA lesions, the frequencies of UV-induced revertants (mutations from his^- to his^+) were the same in presence or in absence of Ro 10-9359 from the minimal medium used for plating the bacteria after irradiation.

Thus Ro 10-9359 does not influence UV-induced mutagenesis in S. typhimurium.

The same conclusion was also made from experiments in which Ro 10-9359 was present

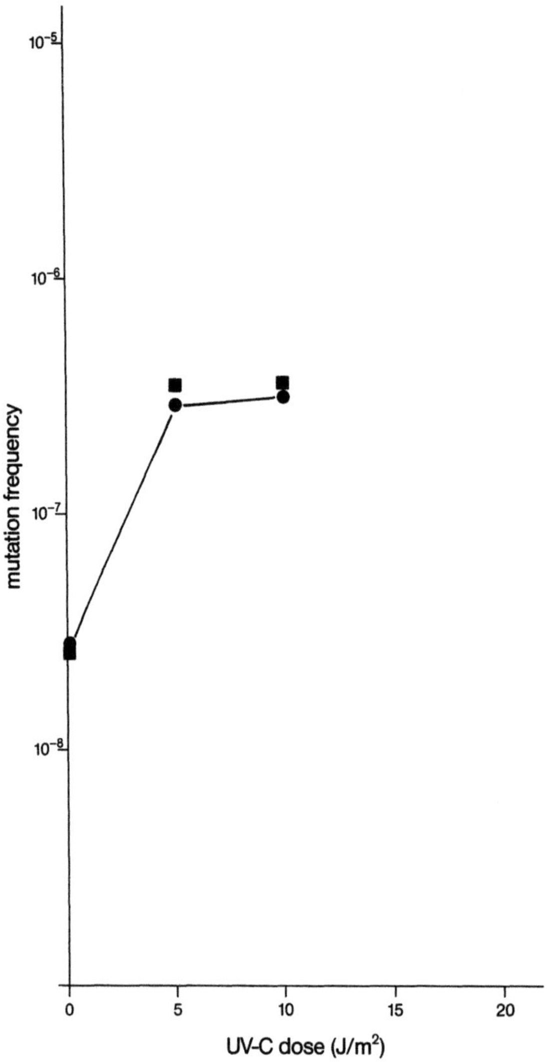

Fig. 5. Mutation-induction curve after UV-C treatment of S. typhimurium TA 1535
● Plating medium: Nutrient Broth
■ Plating medium: Nutrient Broth + Ro 10-9359 (50 µg/plate)

in the overnight culture medium as well as in the buffer solution during irradiation and in the post irradiation medium.

There was also no effect observed if a sunlamp with UV-A, UV-B spectrum was used instead of the 254 nm lamp.

Discussion

Teratology

It is obvious that this compound has severe teratogenic properties when administered on

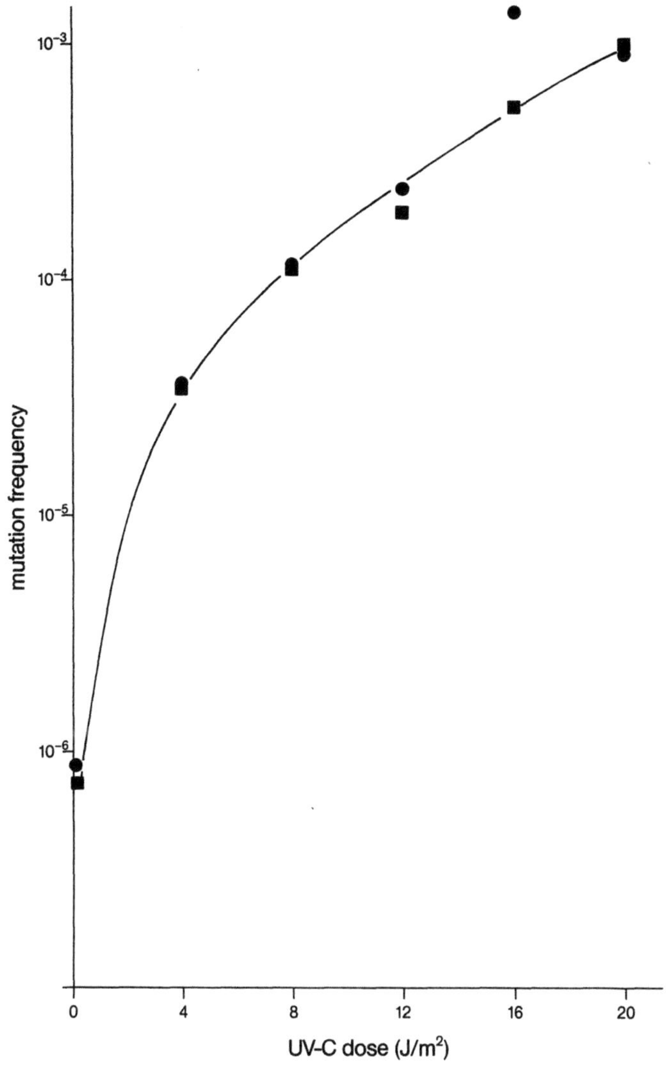

Fig. 6. Mutation-induction curve after UV-C treatment of S. typhimurium TA 100
● Plating medium: Nutrient Broth
■ Plating medium: Nutrient Broth + Ro 10-9359 (50 µg/plate)

both short- and long-term basis at levels as low as the human therapeutic dose. The morphological defects exhibited are similar to vit. A-type defects such as anophthalmia, exencephaly, cleft palate, aplastic kidney and tail, anal atresia and skeletal abnormalities.

A collective view of the fertility and peri-postnatal data suggest two important points: 1) etretinate has a potentially long half-life and can remain active in the maternal system for several months after therapy ceases to influence postnatal development (Paravicini U., p. 13) and 2) treatment on exposure late in gestation produces fetal toxicity resulting in still-birth or early postnatal death.

The extrapolation of experimental results from laboratory animals to human conditions is very difficult. However, an overview of this experimental data clearly demonstrates the teratogenic potential of etretinate in very low doses.

Mutagenicity

In contrast to the findings obtained by teratology studies, no indication for adverse side effects was obtained from in vivo and in vitro mutagenicity tests. The results of the micronucleus test show that even at doses as high as 2 × 1000 mg/kg no chromosome breaks or mitotic non-disjunction were induced. Results obtained from a host-mediated assay and in vitro tests on S. typhimurium (Ames test) suggest that Ro 10-9359 also has no point mutation-inducing activity.

Studies on a possible interaction between Ro 10-9359 and UV-light showed all negative results. Irradiation of the compound and subsequent treatment of the bacteria with the irradiated solution did not have any effect on mutation frequencies in S. typhimurium, indicating that no breakdown by UV-light into mutagenic products occurs.

Also UV (UV-A + B as well as UV-C) inactivation and mutation induction curves for 3 strains of S. typhimurium with different DNA repair capacities, were identical in presence and in absence of Ro 10-9359. An interaction of the compound with DNA repair – as far as it can be detected by bacterial systems – can therefore be excluded.

Conclusions

Teratology

Etretinate (Ro 10-9359), a retinoid compound used to clinically treat psoriasis, is obviously teratogenic at the suggested human therapeutic dose of 2 mg/kg b.w. in rats and rabbits. Mice require slightly higher levels to induce a teratogenic response. Prenatal effects are manifested by increased resorptions, stillbirths, and skeletal variations and postnatal effects by reduced survivability and weight development of the neonates during the lactation period. Because of the prolonged half-life of this compound, long-term exposure results in the accumulation of the drug in the maternal system, which can be considered a potential teratogenic risk in conceptions closely following cessation of treatment.

Mutagenicity

In contrast to the results from teratology studies, it can be assumed that Ro 10-9359 has no adverse side effects towards mutagenicity. In vivo and in vitro mutagenicity tests with the compound revealed no chromosome breaking or point mutation-inducing activity. Furthermore in vitro tests on bacteria with Ro 10-9359 in combination with UV-light gave no indication for an interaction with DNA repair or for mutagenic UV-breakdown products.

Summary

Ro 10-9359 was tested in a series of experiments involving rats, mice and rabbits to investigate the influence on the development of the embryo and fetus and on the general reproductive performance of these animals. The teratological part of these studies involved pregnant animals that were treated orally during the period of organogenesis. Mice and rats received dosages of 0, 2, 4 and 8 mg/kg between days 7–16 of pregnancy, and rabbits received dosages of 0, 0.5, 1 and 2 mg/kg between days 7–19 of pregnancy. The fetuses were removed from the dams by C-section one day before the expected delivery date. At autopsy the fetuses were examined for external and for skeletal and visceral abnormalities.

Embryotoxic and teratogenic effects were observed after 2 mg/kg in rats and rabbits, and after 4 mg/kg in mice. The malformations were of the same type as found in hypervitaminosis A-induced teratogenesis which included eye abnormalities, cleft palate, craniofacial malformations, and defects of the axial and appendicular skeleton.

Mutagenicity studies were performed in reversion assays on several histidine auxotrophic strains of Salmonella typhimurium: 1) An in vivo host-mediated assay with strains TA 1530, TA 1532 and TA 1964 as indicator-bacteria in the peritoneum of the mouse. Ro 10-9359 was given orally at 250, 500 and 1000 mg/kg. No mutation-induction was observed in any of the 3 tester strains. 2) In vitro studies were performed in Salmonella typhimurium strains G 46, TA 1535 and TA 100 to examine a possible interaction with UV-light. The results suggested that both UV survival- and mutation induction-curves were not affected by Ro 10-9359, present in the pre- and/or post-irradiation medium.

The effect on induction of cytogenetic damage was studied by means of the micronucleus test in the mouse. No increase in the number of micronuclei in the bone marrow cells was observed after twofold oral application of 250, 500 and 1000 mg/kg, indicating that neither chromosome breaks nor non-disjunction is induced by Ro 10-9359.

References

1. Ames BN, McCann J, Yamasaky E (1975) Methods for detecting carcinogens and mutagens with the Salmonella/mammalian-microsome mutagenicity test. Mutat Res 31:347–364
2. Schmid W (1975) The micronucleus test. Mutat Res 31:9–15

C.E. Orfanos et al. (eds.)
Retinoids

Cytogenetic Studies in Patients Treated with Oral Retinoid Ro 10-9359

R. Happle and A. Niedworok

It is well known that there is a close relationship between chromosomal instability and cancer (3). If a new drug is found to induce chromosome breakage, it must be regarded as potentially harmful in terms of mutagenicity and carcinogenicity. The fact that retinoic acid and its analogs have shown to prevent chemical carcinogenesis (1, 10), does not necessarily exclude a carcinogenic effect of these compounds. We therefore determined the rate of chromosomal breakage in cultured peripheral blood lymphocytes obtained from patients treated with the aromatic retinoid Ro 10-9359 (etretinate).

Chromosomal breakage can be observed, in a low frequency, in cells cultured from normal individuals (7). The frequency of chromosome breaks found in normal cells may vary considerably between different laboratories, and at different times in the same laboratory (4, 5). This may be due to different culture conditions, but also to the fact that it is difficult to standardize the analysis of chromosome breakage. Therefore, adequate controls are essential.

Patients and Method

The study comprised 9 patients treated with the retinoid Ro 10-9359 for various skin diseases (Table 1). The mean age of this group was 36.7 years. The patients were treated for at least 4 weeks with 1 mg/kg body weight of the drug. In some patients, the duration of treatment was considerably longer. For continuous therapy these patients received 0.5–1.0 mg/kg. All of the patients showed, at the time of chromosome analysis, dryness and desquamation of the lips. This was taken as a sign that the patients had taken the drug regularly.

The control group comprised 6 patients with various skin diseases and one healthy individual (Table 2). The mean age of this group was 33.0 years. Blood samples were taken at the same time from patients of the retinoid group and from controls of approximately the same age, and they were handled in the same way. There were only 7 control persons because, on two occasions, blood samples were taken simultaneously from two patients treated with retinoid and from only one control for parallel cultures.

For the analysis of chromosomes in mitosis, a modification of the well-established method of Moorhead was used (6, 8). 30 ml of venous blood were mixed with 10,000 I.U. of Vetren. Separation of the leucocyte fraction was obtained in Ficoll. The leucocytes were diluted to 2000 cells/mm^3 in McCoy 5 a medium. 8 µg/ml concanavalin A were added to individual portions of 8 ml of the suspension. After incubation for 72 hours, colcemid (0.5×10^{-6} g) was added. After hypotonic treatment and fixation of cells, spreading of chromosomes was achieved by air drying. The preparations were examined for well-spread and intact metaphases. These metaphases were scored for the following chromosome aberrations: gaps (achromatic regions without dislocation of the chromatid), chromatid or isochromatid breaks (dislocation of the broken segment), acentric fragments including double minutes, and structural rearrangements (dicentric chromosomes, ring chromosomes and interchange figures) (Fig. 1a-e).

Table 1. Structural chromosome abnormalities in lymphocyte cultures from 9 patients treated with Ro 10-9359

Case No.	Sex	Age	Diagnosis	Duration of retinoid treatment	Number of metaphases examined	Gaps	Chromatid or isochromatid breaks	Acentric fragments	Dicentric chromosomes	Ring chromosomes	Interchange figures	Percentage of aberrant metaphases
1	M	22	Acne vulgaris	8 weeks	101	-	-	-	-	1	-	1.0%
2	M	36	Psoriasis vulgaris	4 weeks	118	3	-	1	-	-	-	3.4%
3	F	41	Psoriasis vulgaris	15 weeks	104	-	-	2	1	-	-	2.9%
4	F	23	Psoriasis vulgaris	4 weeks	81	-	-	-	-	-	-	0.0%
5	F	40	Monilethrix	10 weeks	97	-	-	-	1	-	-	1.0%
6	F	20	Monilethrix	10 weeks	102	2	-	-	-	-	-	2.0%
7	M	30	Psoriasis vulgaris	21 weeks	97	-	-	-	-	1	-	1.0%
8	F	56	Lichen planus	4 weeks	23	-	1	-	-	-	-	4.3%
9	F	63	Lichen planus	4 weeks	69	1	-	-	-	-	-	1.4%

The cytogenetic analysis was performed as a blind study. The preparations were coded, using random numbers. All of the metaphases selected for examination were scored by two observers who did not know whether they were examining a preparation from the retinoid group or from controls. The aim was to examine about 100 metaphases in each individual, but in some cultures the number of intact metaphases was lower (Tables 1 and 2).

Results

The results are summarized in Tables 1 and 2. In the retinoid group, the frequency of

Table 2. Structural chromosome abnormalities in lymphocyte cultures from 7 control persons

Case No.	Sex	Age	Diagnosis	Number of metaphases examined	Gaps	Chromatid or isochromatid breaks	Acentric fragments	Dicentric chromosomes	Ring chromosomes	Interchange figures	Percentage of aberrant metaphases
1	M	28	Lichen planus	120	1	-	-	-	-	-	0.8%
2	M	37	Rosacea	104	-	-	-	1	-	1	1.9%
3	F	38	Normal	101	-	-	1	-	-	-	1.0%
4	F	24	Psoriasis vulgaris	107	-	-	2	1	-	-	2.8%
5	F	22	Atopic eczema	84	-	-	1	-	-	-	1.2%
6	M	27	Pigmented nevus	43	-	-	1	-	-	1	4.7%
7	F	55	Contact dermatitis	99	1	-	1	1	-	-	3.0%

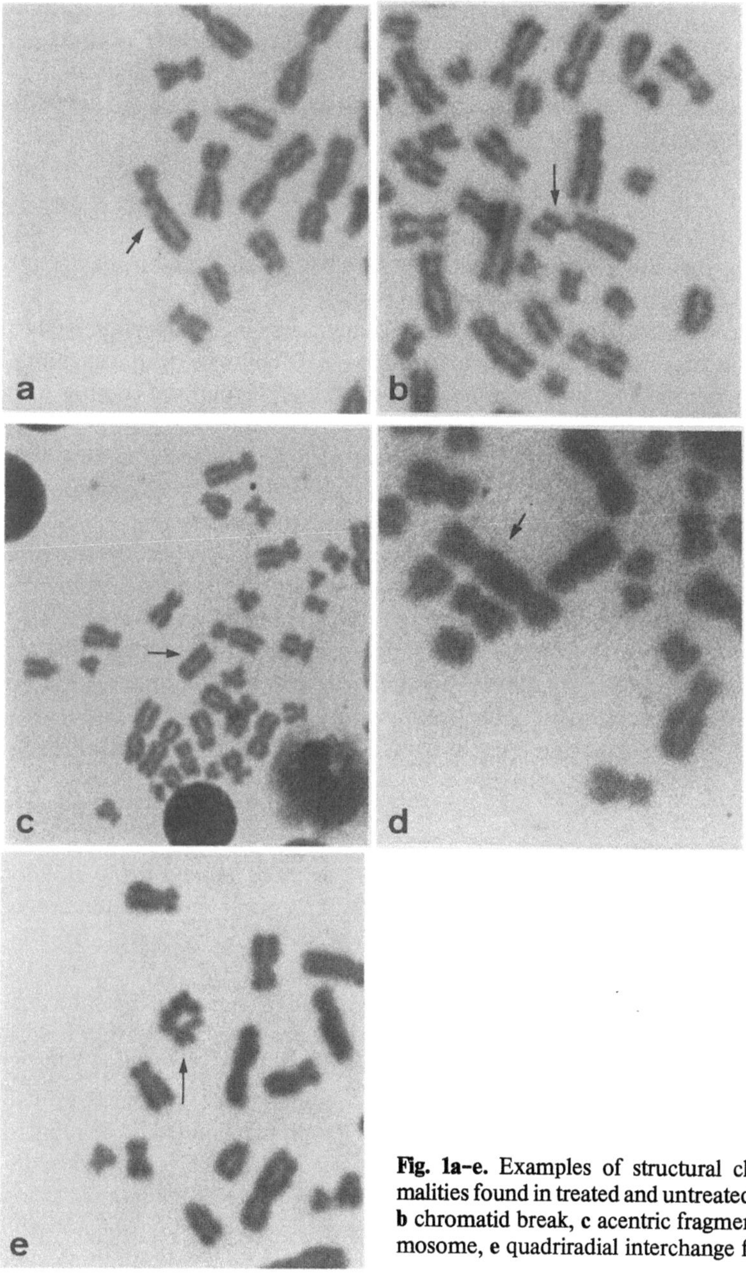

Fig. 1a–e. Examples of structural chromosome abnormalities found in treated and untreated individuals. **a** Gap, **b** chromatid break, **c** acentric fragment, **d** dicentric chromosome, **e** quadriradial interchange figure

Table 3. Comparison of cytogenetic data obtained after pooling of the metaphases examined in treated and untreated individuals

	Number of cases	Total number of metaphases examined	Number of aberrant metaphases
Retinoid group	9	792	14 (1.8%)
Control group	7	658	13 (1.9%)

aberrant metaphases varied from 0% to 4.3%. In the control group, the rate of aberrant metaphases varied from 0.8 to 4.7%. Simple chromosome breaks as well as structural rearrangements were equally distributed in both groups. When the examined metaphases were pooled, the frequency of aberrant mitoses was 1.8% in the retinoid group versus 1.9% in the control group (Table 3).

Discussion

The results indicate that the aromatic retinoid Ro 10-9359, given orally in therapeutic dosage, does not induce chromosomal breakage in man.

In this study, the frequency of two-break rearrangements was higher than observed by other investigators in larger series of normal individuals (4, 5). This may be due to culture conditions because there was no difference between the retinoid group and controls with regard to this finding.

This study, however, does not exclude with certainty potential mutagenic and carcinogenic effects of the drug, in view of the fact that scoring for chromosome breakage is a rather gross method to determine mutagenicity and carcinogenicity. Nevertheless, our results obtained in patients treated with Ro 10-9359 may be important because other investigators found that this drug induces sister chromatid exchanges in vitro when added to human fibroblasts (2). These authors assumed that there is a correlation between the dose-related induction of sister chromatid exchanges and a potential cancer-promoting effect of retinoids. This problem, however, should also be studied in vivo. For example, it is known that vitamin C induces sister chromatid exchanges in vitro, but not in vivo (9). Further cytogenetic studies may show whether the same is true for the aromatic retinoid Ro 10-9359.

Summary

A cytogenetic study was performed in 9 patients treated with the retinoid Ro 10-9359 for psoriasis or other skin diseases, and in 7 control persons of the same age. The duration of retinoid treatment ranged from 4 to 21 weeks. The drug was given in daily doses of 1.0 mg/kg body weight for at least 4 weeks, and subsequently the patients received 0.5–1.0 mg/kg. Blood samples were taken from patients of the retinoid group and controls at the same time and handled in the same way. Scoring for chromosome breakage was performed on metaphases of blood lymphocytes stimulated with concanavalin A and cultured for 72 hours. The preparations were coded, using random numbers, and examined by two observers who did not know whether they were scoring a preparation from the retinoid group or from the control group. The number of cells selected for analysis varied in different individuals from 23 to 120. A total number of 792 metaphases of the retinoid group and 658 metaphases of the control group was scored for gaps, chromatid or isochromatid breaks, acentric fragments and structural rearrangements. In the retinoid group, the frequency of cells with an aberration was 1.8%, and in the control group it was found to be 1.9%. In the retinoid group, the frequency of aberrant metaphases varied in different individuals from 0% to 4.3%, and in the control group it varied from 0.8% to 4.7%. These results indicate that the retinoid Ro 10-9359, given orally in therapeutic dosage, does not induce chromosomal breakage in man.

References

1. Bollag W (1972) Prophylaxis of chemically - induced benign and malignant epithelial tumors by vitamin A acid (retinoic acid). Eur J Cancer 8:689–693
2. Juhl HJ, Schürer CC, Bartram CR, Kohl F-V, Melderis H, Wichert P von, Rüdiger HW (1978) Retinoids induce sister-chromatid exchanges in human diploid fibroblasts. Mutat Res 58:317–320
3. German J (ed.) (1974) Chromosomes and cancer. John Wiley & Sons, New York London Sydney Toronto
4. Littlefield LG, Goh KO (1973) Cytogenetic studies in control men and women. I. Variations in aberration frequencies in 29,709 metaphases from 305 cultures obtained over a three-year period. Cytogenet Cell Genet 12:17–34
5. Lubs HA, Samuelson J (1967) Chromosome abnormalities in lymphocytes from normal human subjects. Cytogenet Cell Genet 6:402–411
6. Moorhead PS, Nowell PC, Mellman WJ, Battips DM, Hungerford DA (1960) Chromosome preparations of leukocytes cultured from human peripheral blood. Exp Cell Res 20:613–616
7. Passarge E (1974) The human karyotype. Analysis of chromosomes in mitosis and evaluation of cytogenetic data. In: Methods in human cytogenetics. Schwarzacher HG, Wolf U, Passarge E (eds). Springer, Berlin Heidelberg New York, pp 135–205
8. Pfeiffer RA (1974) Cell cultures from blood and bone marrow. In: Methods in human cytogenetics. Schwarzacher HG, Wolf U, Passarge E (eds). Springer, Berlin Heidelberg New York, pp 1–37
9. Speit G, Wolf M, Vogel W (1980) The SCE-inducing capacity of vitamin C: investigations in vitro and in vivo. Mutat Res 78:273–278
10. Sporn MB, Dunlop NM, Newton DL, Smith JM (1976) Prevention of chemical carcinogenesis by vitamin A and its synthetic analogs (retinoids). Fed Proc 35:1332–1338

C.E. Orfanos et al. (eds.)
Retinoids

Chromosomal Analysis in Patients Treated with the Aromatic Retinoid Ro 10-9359

G. Obe and D. Tsambaos

Recent clinical trials have demonstrated the efficiency of the oral aromatic retinoid Ro 10-9359 (etretinate) in the treatment of severe psoriasis, ichthyosis and other keratinization disorders. Possible long-term hazards of the retinoid therapy, which at the moment are almost entirely unknown, should be thoroughly investigated and clearly defined, before the drug is introduced on a large scale.

One of the major concerns is whether the aromatic retinoid Ro 10-9359 has the potential to induce mutations. In this paper we report on the results of chromosomal analyses performed in the peripheral lymphocytes of patients under oral treatment with Ro 10-9359. The rationale behind this investigation is that an elevation of chromosomal aberrations in humans under treatment with a certain drug may be regarded as an effect of the drug. Agents inducing chromosomal aberrations are also capable of producing point mutations, which cannot be seen at the chromosomal level. Since the same mechanisms are responsible for the induction of mutations in both somatic and germ cells, mutations occurring in somatic cells, e.g., lymphocytes, can be taken as an indication, that mutations have also been induced in germ cells, which can transfer them to the progeny. Agents which are inducing an elevation of chromosomal aberrations in the peripheral lymphocytes, are most likely also cancerogenic in man, examples for this are tobacco smoking and alcohol consumption (5, 6, 9, 10).

The peripheral blood of a healthy human contains some 10×10^9 lymphocytes, most of which have a half-life time of about three years (14, 15). The peripheral lymphocytes are in a resting phase (Gô) of the cell cycle and their chromosomes contain one DNA double helix. Upon in vitro stimulation, they pass through the G_1 phase into the phase of DNA synthesis (S). The S phase is followed by the G_2 phase, in which each chromosome contains two DNA helices. After the G_2 phase the lymphocytes enter mitosis. Up to the metaphase, their chromosomes contain two DNA helices, one in each chromatid. In the anaphase the chromatids are separated and arranged at the cell poles.

Only few agents can directly lead to chromosomal aberrations in the G_0 or G_1 phase of the cell cycle. Such aberrations are replicated in the S phase and appear as chromosome type aberrations in the following metaphase. Typical chromosome type aberrations are dicentric chromosomes (Dic), in which break in two different chromosomes healed up, and ring chromosomes (Rings), in which two breaks in one chromosome healed together. Therapeutic agents which are known to induce chromosome type aberrations are X-rays and bleomycin. Most chemical mutagens react with the DNA in the G_0 or G_1 stage of the cells, but they are not directly inducing chromosomal aberrations. However, when the affected cells are passing the S phase, lesions induced in the DNA can lead to aberrations by means of mistakes during DNA synthesis. In the following metaphase these aberrations occur in the chromatids and are called chromatid-type aberrations. Chromatid translocations (RB′), formed when two breaks in the chromatids of two different chromosomes heal together, belong to this type and can only be obtained when lymphocytes containing lesions in their DNA are stimulated in vitro. A chronic exposure of the peripheral lymphocytes to DNA damaging agents will result in a permanent induction of DNA lesions, counteracted by cellular repair. Thus, only few lesions are expected to persist in the cells and to be transformed into chromatid-type aberrations in vitro. To avoid selection against aberrant cells, it is necessary to investigate chromosomes from lymphocytes cultivated for 48 h, when most of them undergo their first in vitro mitosis (see 2, 4, 7, 8).

Another genetic end point originating from DNA lesions that persist until the S phase is reached, is the sister chromatid exchange (SCE). SCEs can be demonstrated in chromosome preparations from lymphocytes cultivated in the presence of bromodeoxyuridine (BrdU). After two cell cycles, BrdU (B) is incorporated instead of thymidine (T) into the DNA of the two chromatids of a chromosome, resulting in a TB – BB constitution of the DNA in the two chromatids. The chromatids are differentially stained, and switches between them, i.e., SCEs, can be recognized in the light microscope. Chemicals inducing chromatid type aberrations in the S phase are also raising the frequency of SCEs (see 11, 13, 16).

Material and Methods

Blood samples were obtained from 18 patients of both sexes, who suffered from psoriasis (13 patients), lichen planus (3 patients) and Darier's disease (2 patients). All patients were treated orally with the aromatic retinoid Ro 10-9359 in daily doses ranging between 25 mg and 75 mg (Table 1). Blood cultures were set up with Ham's F-10 medium supplemented with 10% fetal bovine serum, antibiotics, and the

Table 1. Age, sex, types of dermatoses, details of treatment with Ro 10–9359 and chromosomal aberrations of the chromatid type (chromatid translocations: RB′) and of the chromosome type (dicentric chromosomes: Dic; ring chromosomes: Ring) in 18 patients

Patient	Age, sex	Type of dermatosis	Daily dose of Ro 10–9359 (mg/kg)	Duration of treatment (weeks)	Number of metaphases analyzed	Aberrations
1	55, F	Psoriasis	50	4	200	1 Ring
2	27, M	Psoriasis	75	12	200	1 Dic
3	67, M	Psoriasis	50	8	200	0
4	75, M	Psoriasis	50	4	200	0
5	65, F	Psoriasis	50	12	200	1 Dic
6	46, M	Lichen planus	50	24	200	0
7	72, M	Lichen planus	25	18	400	0
8	69, F	Psoriasis	50	4	132	2 RB’
9	69, M	Lichen planus	35	8	200	0
10	51, F	Psoriasis	50	4	200	0
11	67, F	Darier's disease	50	12	200	0
12	56, M	Psoriasis	75	4	91	0
13	51, F	Psoriasis	50	8	57	0
14	49, M	Psoriasis	50	24	200	0
15	43, M	Psoriasis	50	24	200	0
16	39, M	Psoriasis	75	12	128	0
17	52, F	Psoriasis	75	8	200	3 Dic, 1 Ring
18	59, F	Darier's disease	75	16	200	1 RB′, 1 Ring

mitogen phytohemagglutinin. The cultures were incubated for 48 h at 37 °C, including a 4.5-hour treatment with colcemid to arrest the metaphases. Metaphases were prepared after a standard protocol and stained with Giemsa stain. The metaphases were analyzed with respect to chromosome type (Dic and Rings) and chromatid type (RB') aberrations. In addition, in 8 out of the 18 patients the rate of sister chromatid exchanges (SCEs) was determined from blood cultures incubated for 72 h in the presence of BrdU (10^{-5} *M* final concentration). The chromosomes were stained differentially according to the method of Perry and Wolff (12).

Results and Discussion

In 3408 metaphases of lymphocytes derived from the retinoid-treated patients, we found 3 chromatid translocations (RB':8.8×10^{-4}), 5 dicentric chromosomes (Dic: 14.7×10^{-4}) and 3 ring chromosomes (Rings: 8.8×10^{-4}) (see Table 1). In 14,652 metaphases from 83 healthy individuals used as controls, we detected 12 RB' (8.2×10^{-4}), 5 Dic (3.4×10^{-4}) but no Rings. These results clearly show that under therapy with Ro 10-9359, no elevation in the rate of RB', i.e., of S-dependent aberrations occurs in the retinoid-treated patients, as compared to the controls. The frequency of S-independent aberrations, i.e., Dic and Rings, is elevated in the lymphocytes of the retinoid-treated patients. It seems to be highly improbable that the elevation of the S-independent aberrations has been induced by Ro 10-9359. The chronic character of the dermatoses of our patients makes two to three rehospitalizations per year necessary. This leads to a higher frequency of diagnostic X-irradiations in these patients as compared to healthy people. This higher than normal irradiation load may be one explanation for the higher than normal rate of chromosome type aberrations (see 1). Probands 5, 12, and 17 are heavy smokers (≧ 40 cigarettes/day) and this is known to induce aberrations (6, 10).

The SCE analyses in 8 patients revealed values of 2.96 ± 0.24 up to 4.66 ± 0.38 SCEs per metaphase (Table 2), which are clearly within the control range found in our and in other laboratories. Nevertheless, Juhl et al. (3) reported that Ro 10-9359 in a concentration of 5 µg/ml doubles the rate of SCEs in human diploid fibroblasts in vitro. In conclusion our results indicate that treatment with the oral aromatic retinoid Ro 10-9359 does not lead to an elevation of chromosomal aberrations and sister chromatid exchanges in the peripheral lymphocytes. Our analysis does not answer the question whether Ro 10-9359 is capable of producing point mutations in man. Our findings are in agreement with the negative results of Happle and Niedworok (p. 61) and are consistent with the observations of Hummler

Table 2. Frequencies of sister chromatid exchanges (SCE) found in the peripheral lymphocytes of patients with dermatoses treated orally with Ro 10–9359 (see Table 1 for details)

Patient	Number of metaphases analyzed	SCE per metaphase (± SE)
2	50	4.48 (0.35)
5	50	3.36 (0.28)
6	50	4.50 (0.37)
10	36	4.13 (0.51)
11	50	3.20 (0.31)
13	50	4.32 (0.40)
14	55	2.96 (0.24)
15	50	4.66 (0.38)

Control values from our laboratory are around 5 SCE per metaphase and Schüpbach (p. 49), who were unable to detect chromosomal aberrations in the mouse and point mutations in Salmonella typhimurium after application of Ro 10-9359.

Summary

Recent clinical trials have demonstrated the efficacy of the oral aromatic retinoid Ro 10-9359 in the treatment of severe psoriasis and other keratinization disorders. However, relatively little is known about the possibility of long-term hazards of oral retinoid therapy.

In the present study we investigated the chromosomes of the peripheral blood lymphocytes from 18 psoriatic patients being under treatment with Ro 10-9359 for 4–24 weeks (25–75 mg/day), with respect to exchange-type aberrations. Whole blood cultures were incubated for 48 hrs in order to ascertain that most cells were in their first in vitro mitosis. The frequency of exchange-type aberrations was found to be at the control level. In 8 patients we found no elevation of the rate of sister chromatid exchanges.

References

1. Banduhn N, Obe G, Müller-Oerlinghausen B (1980) Is Lithium mutagenic in man? Pharmakopsychiatr Neuropsychopharmakol 13:218–227
2. Beek B, Obe G (1979) Sister chromatid exchanges in human leukocyte chromosomes: Spontaneous and induced frequencies in early- and late-proliferating cells in vitro. Hum Genet 49:51–61
3. Juhl HJ, Schürer CC, Bartram CR, Kohl F-V, Melderis H, Wichert P v, Rüdiger HW (1978) Retinoids induce sister-chromatid exchanges in human diploid fibroblasts. Mutat Res 58:317–320
4. Natarajan AT, Obe G (1980) Screening of human populations for mutations induced by environmental pollutants: Use of the human lymphocyte system. Ecotox Env Safety 4:468–481
5. Obe G (1980) Mutagenicity of alcohol and tobacco smoke. In: Research Advances in Alcohol and Drug Problems, Vol VI. Israel Y, Glaser FB, Kalant H, Popham RE, Schmidt W, Smart RG (eds). Plenum, New York, in press
6. Obe G, Herha J (1978) Chromosomal aberrations in heavy smokers. Hum Genet 41:259–263
7. Obe G, Madle S (1980) Prüfung der Mutagenität von Medikamenten beim Menschen. Prax Klin Pneumonol, in press
8. Obe G, Natarajan AT (1980) Umweltbedingte Mutationen beim Menschen. Klinikarzt 9:271–289
9. Obe G, Ristow H (1979) Mutagenic, cancerogenic and teratogenic effects of alcohol. Mutat Res 65:229–259
10. Obe G, Göbel D, Engeln H, Herha J, Natarajan AT (1980) Chromosomal aberrations in peripheral lymphocytes of alcoholics. Mutat Res 73:377–386
11. Perry P, Evans HJ (1975) Cytological detection of mutagen-carcinogen exposure by sister chromatid exchange. Nature 258:121–125
12. Perry P, Wolff S (1974) New Giemsa method for the differential staining of sister chromatids. Nature 251:156–158
13. Shiraishi Y, Sandberg AA (1980) Sister chromatid exchange in human chromosomes, including observations in neoplasia. Cancer Genet Cytogenet 1:363–380
14. Trepel F (1975) Kinetik lymphatischer Zellen. In: Lymphozyt und klinische Immunologie. Theml H, Begemann H (eds). Springer, Berlin Heidelberg New York, pp 16–26
15. Trepel F (1976) Das lymphatische Zellsystem: Struktur, allgemeine Physiologie und allgemeine Pathophysiologie. In: Handbuch der inneren Medizin, Bd. 2, Blut und Blutkrankheiten. Begemann H (ed). Springer, Berlin Heidelberg New York, pp 1–191
16. Wolff S (1977) Sister chromatid exchange. Annu Rev Genet 11:183–201

Biological Effects of Retinoids

C.E. Orfanos et al. (eds.)
Retinoids

Retinoids: New Developments in Their Mechanism of Action as Related to Control of Proliferative Diseases

M.B. Sporn

Although there has been recent concern that improper use of retinoids can induce a proliferative reaction in various types of cells (10), there can be little doubt that the basic, physiological role of retinoids is to control proliferative activity in the various secretory and ductular epithelial tissues of the body. This has been known since the original classic observations of Wolbach and Howe (15) on the pathogenesis and histogenesis of vitamin A deficiency in the rat, and is nowhere better stated than in their original paper. They noted that "growth activity of (retinoid-deficient) epithelium is not diminished. On the contrary, there is convincing evidence that it is greatly augmented. In (some of the retinoid-deficient) animals, the behavior of the replacing epithelium in respect to numbers of mitotic figures and response on the part of the connective tissue and blood vessels suggests the acquisition of neoplastic properties ... It is highly probable that the epithelium of gland ducts, respiratory mucosa, and genitourinary tract have secretory functions, so that we conclude that the [retinoid] deficiency results in loss of specific chemical functions of the epithelia concerned, while the power of growth becomes augmented."

In most situations in which retinoids have been shown to have a proliferative effect on secretory or ductular cells of epithelial origin, one may suspect that these cells have been exposed to an unduly high, borderline toxic, dose of retinoid. Recent studies by Levine and Ohuchi (8) suggest that toxic levels of several retinoids induce lipid deacylation and prostaglandin production in dog kidney cells; conversely, some of the toxic effects of retinoic acid can be prevented *in vivo* by administration of inhibitors of prostaglandin synthesis, such as aspirin (6) or several of the non-steroidal anti-inflammatory agents which inhibit cyclo-oxygenase (7). We will not discuss these toxic proliferative reactions any further in this article, and instead will focus on some new studies which relate to the physiological antiproliferative action of retinoids, and in particular to their mechanism of action in this regard.

The proliferation of normal cells is controlled in large part by the interactions between several polypeptide hormones and hormone-like growth factors that are present in body fluids, together with lower molecular weight substances such as steroids and retinoids. We have previously discussed three mechanisms whereby a proliferative polypeptide hormone or hormone-like substance may reach a target cell: 1) in the case of typical hormones, the polypeptide is secreted by some distant producer cell and then is transported to the target cell via the bloodstream (endocrine secretion); 2) the polypeptide may be secreted by a nearby regulatory cell and then reach the target cell by local diffusion through the extracellular space (paracrine secretion); and 3) the polypeptide may be secreted by the target cell itself, in which case the same cell that produces the proliferative polypeptide also has functional external receptors for that peptide (autocrine secretion, 11). Recent studies indicate that all three types of proliferative mechanisms (endocrine, paracrine, and autocrine)

involving polypeptide agents can be blocked by retinoids, and we shall discuss each of these in turn.

Our initial interest in the interaction between retinoids and proliferative polypeptide hormones derived from studies performed collaboratively with Moon et al. (9), in which both 4-hydroxyphenyl retinamide and retinyl acetate were found to have a potent antiproliferative effect on mammary epithelium when they were fed chronically in the diet

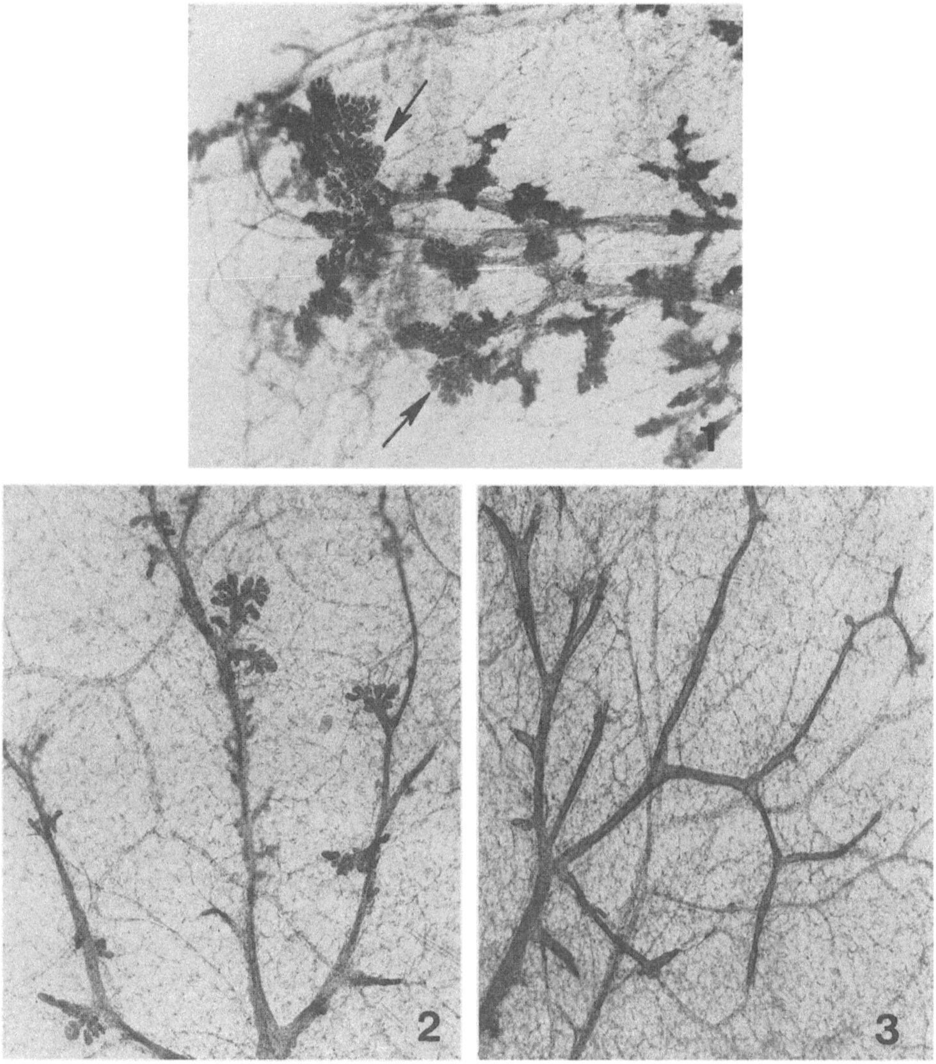

Fig. 1–3. Representative areas of mammary gland whole mounts from virgin female rats, fed special diets from age 2 months to 8 months.
1. Control diet. Note the marked end-bud proliferation (arrows). Alum carmine, × 30
2. Retinyl acetate (328 mg/kg of diet). A marked decrease in end-body proliferation is noted. Compare to Fig. 1. Alum carmine, × 30
3. 4-Hydroxyphenyl retinamide (782 mg/kg of diet). An almost total absence of end-bud proliferation is noted. Compare to Fig. 1. Alum carmine, × 30
Reprinted, with permission, from Moon et al. (9)

of Sprague-Dawley female rats, as shown in Figures 1, 2, and 3. Mammary whole mounts from rats treated with retinoids for 6 months showed decreased ductal branching and decreased end-bud proliferation. The effect of feeding the retinoids on the structure of the mammary gland was similar to that found previously in animals that had been prolactin-suppressed by means of the dopamine antagonist, bromocriptine (14); and indeed, in subsequent studies it has been reported that retinyl acetate and bromocriptine exert a marked synergistic action in prevention of mammary cancer induced in rats by injection of nitrosomethylurea (13). Although studies in whole animals cannot prove that retinoids directly antagonize prolactin, recent studies in organ culture (Mehta and Moon, personal communication) indicate that such is the case; in these latest experiments 4-hydroxyphenyl retinamide has been found to block the combined proliferative effects of insulin and prolactin upon mammary epithelium growing in vitro. In summary, then, a variety of studies on mammary epithelium, both in vivo and in vitro, indicate that retinoids can block a proliferative response caused by an endocrine polypeptide.

Paracrine mechanisms of proliferation are receiving increasing attention, particularly with the immense recent interest in the role of lymphokines and monokines in many types of proliferative diseases. Recent studies on the etiology of rheumatoid arthritis have emphasized the proliferative nature of the basic rheumatoid lesion (4) and have stressed the importance of paracrine polypeptide factors, such as lymphokines and monokines, in both the proliferative and destructive components of the disease (5). One of the enzymes induced by a lymphokine such as mononuclear cell factor is collagenase (2), which is believed to be critically involved in the destruction which occurs in the rheumatoid joint. Using human rheumatoid synovial cells in culture as their assay system, Brinckerhoff et al. (1) have shown that retinoic acid is a potent inhibitor of collagenase production induced by mononuclear cell factor. Whether other responses of a more proliferative nature induced by this paracrine polypeptide can also be inhibited by retinoic acid remains to be determined. Similarly, the possible application of this finding to prevention of rheumatoid arthritis in either an experimental animal or man also remains to be determined.

Finally, autocrine mechanisms of peptide action have become the subject of intensive study with the discovery of sarcoma growth factor (SGF) by De Larco and Todaro (3). SGF is an acid-stable, low-molecular-weight polypeptide which is a direct, reversible effector of cellular transformation. SGF is believed to be endogenously produced within the very same transformed cell which also has functional external receptors for this mitogenic, growth-promoting polypeptide; this type of autocrine self-stimulation confers a definite selective growth advantage upon a transformed cell. When applied exogenously to a phenotypically normal cell, SGF rapidly causes the appearance of properties characteristic of the transformed state, such as anchorage-independent growth in soft agar and overgrowth of neighboring cells in monolayer culture. The transforming activity of low concentrations of SGF on phenotypically normal NRK rat fibroblasts can be blocked by several different retinoids (12). When NRK fibroblasts were treated with SGF and nanogram levels of retinoids (retinoic acid, retinyl acetate, retinyl methyl ether, and retinylidene dimedone at $1.0–2.0 \times 10^{-8}$ M), the transforming activity of SGF was inhibited. This included a suppression of anchorage-independent growth in soft agar, as well as a suppression of overgrowth in monolayer culture. While normal NRK fibroblasts treated with SGF alone formed multiple layers and criss-crossed each other in a fashion resembling virally transformed cells, those treated with both retinyl acetate and SGF did not have a disordered growth pattern and did not have an increased saturation density in monolayer culture. In all of the experiments performed, the effect of the retinoids was clearly not a cytotoxic one, since, at the concentrations used, they inhibited neither normal rat fibroblastic growth in monolayer nor the ability of rat or mouse cells which had been permanently transformed by an oncogenic virus to form colonies in soft agar.

Summary

We have briefly reviewed new evidence which suggests that a variety of proliferative responses induced by polypeptide hormones or hormone-like agents can be blocked by various retinoids. Whether the endogenous, physiological anti-proliferative effects of retinoids in controlling epithelial cell differentiation also involve modulation of the action of various polypeptide hormones is unknown. However, it is clear that in several disease states, particularly in malignancy, there is enhanced activity of proliferative polypeptide hormones, and that retinoids have already been shown to be useful antagonists of this proliferative action. In turn, this antagonism of proliferative polypeptides may help to explain some of the useful experimental and clinical results that have been obtained in prevention or treatment of various disease states with the retinoids.

Acknowledgments. I am indebted to Drs. Richard C. Moon and Peter J. Becci for Figures 1, 2, and 3. Ms. Ellen Friedman provided expert assistance with the manuscript.

References

1. Brinckerhoff CE, McMillan RM, Dayer J-M, Harris ED Jr (1980) Inhibition by retinoic acid of collagenase production in rheumatoid synovial cells. N Engl J Med 303:432–436
2. Dayer J-M, Russell RG, Krane SM (1977) Collagenase production by rheumatoid synovial cells: stimulation by a human lymphocyte factor. Science 195:181–183
3. De Larco JE, Todaro GJ (1978) Growth factors from murine sarcoma virus-transformed cells. Proc Natl Acad Sci USA 75:4001–4005
4. Harris ED Jr (1976) Recent insights into the pathogenesis of the proliferative lesion in rheumatoid arthritis. Arthritis Rheum 19:68–72
5. Harris ED Jr (1980) Pathogenesis of rheumatoid arthritis. In: Textbook of rheumatology. Kelley WN, Harris ED Jr, Ruddy S, Sledge CB (eds). Saunders, Philadelphia, pp 896–922
6. Harrison SD, Hixson EJ, Burdeshaw JA, Denine EP (1977) Effect of aspirin administration on retinoic acid toxicity in mice. Nature 269:511–512
7. Hixson EJ, Denine EP (1978) Effect of nonsteroidal anti-inflammatory agents on toxicity of retinoic acid in mice. Toxicol Appl Pharmacol 45:317
8. Levine L, Ohuchi K (1978) Retinoids as well as tumor promoters enhance deacylation of cellular lipids and prostaglandin production in MDCK cells. Nature 276:274–275
9. Moon RC, Thompson HJ, Becci PJ, Grubbs CJ, Gander RJ, Newton DL, Smith JM, Phillips SL, Henderson WR, Mullen LT, Brown CC, Sporn MB (1979) N-(4-hydroxyphenyl) retinamide, a new retinoid for prevention of breast cancer in the rat. Cancer Res 39:1339–1346
10. Schroder EW, Black PH (1980) Retinoids: tumor preventers or tumor enhancers? J Natl Cancer Inst 65:671–674
11. Sporn MB, Todaro GJ (1980) Autocrine secretion and malignant transformation of cells. N Engl J Med 303:878–880
12. Todaro GJ, De Larco JE, Sporn MB (1978) Retinoids block phenotypic cell transformation produced by sarcoma growth factor. Nature 276:272–274
13. Welsch CW, Brown CK, Goodrich-Smith M, Chiusano J, Moon RC (1980) Synergistic effect of chronic prolactin suppression and retinoid treatment in the prophylaxis of *N*-methyl-*N*-nitrosourea-induced mammary tumorigenesis in female Sprague-Dawley rats. Cancer Res 40:3095–3098
14. Welsch CW, Nagasawa H (1977) Prolactin and murine mammary tumorigenesis: a review. Cancer Res 37: 951–963
15. Wolbach SB, Howe PR (1925) Tissue changes following deprivation of fat-soluble A vitamin. J Exp Med 42:753–777

C.E. Orfanos et al. (eds.)
Retinoids

The Effects of Retinoids on Stratum Corneum. Structure and Function

R. Marks, A. Finlay, S. Nicholls and S. Barton

There is no doubt now that the retinoids offer new hope for patients with a variety of persistent and disabling skin disorders. Their effectiveness in such diverse disorders as erythrokeratodermia variabilis (7, 17), lamellar ichthyosis (7, 14), epidermolytic hyperkeratosis (3, 7), Darier's disease (5, 7), pityriasis rubra pilaris (5, 7), psoriasis (11, 15) and acne (13) is gratifying but puzzling. How can such different disorders with presumably different underlying biochemical faults and structural abnormalities respond similarly to the same type of treatment? We believe that an answer to this question will considerably advance development of this important group of drugs. Our aim in this study has been to determine whether Ro 10-9359 exerts particular and specific effects on keratinization and on stratum corneum structure and function.

Patients and Methods

The details of the 25 patients treated and their responses are given in Table 1. The side effects experienced by these patients are annotated in Table 2. All patients were investigated initially and after 4 weeks treatment with 1 mg/kg/day (in two divided doses). The investigations performed before and after 4 weeks treatment are outlined in Table 3. Where possible, both uninvolved and involved skin was studied.

1. Results

The clinical results and side effects are set out in Tables 1 and 2, respectively. Overall, 6 patients were graded as "excellent", 7 patients were graded as "good", 2 were graded as intermediate between "fair and good", 5 were graded as "fair", 3 were graded as "poor", 2 were graded as "worse". As a group, patients with erythrokeratodermia variabilis (EKV) responded most satisfactorily.

Routine biochemical and haematological checks revealed no significant changes indicative of serious marrow, hepatic or renal toxicity.

2. Histological Observations

There were no signs of epidermal cell damage that could be attributable to the treatment in the biopsies taken after 4 weeks. There were no obvious morphological alterations in the uninvolved skin after treatment. Neither was there any remarkable change in the post-treatment biopsies of patients with EKV, lamellar ichthyosis, pityriasis rubra pilaris (PRP), tylosis, persistent palmo-plantar keratolysis or follicular ichthyosis. The epidermis of the post-

Table 1. Patients treated with Ro 10-9359

Patient	Disease	Age	Sex	Duration	Result
1	EKV*	20	F	Since age 6 weeks	Excellent
2	EKV	17	F	Since shortly after birth	Excellent
3	EKV	20	M	Since early infancy	Excellent
4	Darier's Disease	16	M	5 years	Excellent
5	Darier's Disease	47	M	15 years	Fair
6	Darier's Disease	52	F	5 years	Fair
7	Lamellar ichthyosis	8	F	Since age 3 weeks	Fair/Good
8	Lamellar ichthyosis	9	M	Present at birth	Fair/Good
9	Tylosis	23	F	Since age 5 years	Good
10	Follicular ichthyosis	24	F	Since early childhood	Good
11	Follicular ichthyosis	12	M	Since early childhood	Poor
12	Localized EH+	14	F	Since age 7 months	Good
13	Localized EH+	23	F	Present since birth	Fair
14	PRPø	41	M	Present 4 months	Poor
15	PRPø	24	M	Past 11 years	Good
16	PRPø	56	M	Previous 4 months	Good
17	Dominant ichthyosis	56	M	Since early infancy	Fair
18	Dominant ichthyosis	46	F	Since birth	Fair
19	Dominant ichthyosis	55	M	Since early childhood	Good
20	Dominant ichthyosis	55	M	Since birth	Poor
21	Psoriasis	51	F	Past 25 years	Good
22	Psoriasis	45	M	Past 20 years	Excellent
23	Psoriasis	43	M	Past 8 years	Worse
24	Psoriasis	56	M	Past 4 years	Worse
25	Pustulosis palms/soles	58	F	Past 20 years	Excellent

* Erythrokeratodermia variabilis ø Pityriasis rubra pilaris + Epidermolytic hyperkeratosis

treatment biopsies from the patients with autosomal dominant ichthyosis (ADI) were somewhat thicker than the pre-treatment specimens and a granular layer became evident in two out of the three examples examined. There was less clefting and dyskeratosis in the post-treatment biopsies from the patients with Darier's disease. The post-treatment biopsies of the 4 patients with psoriasis and the one with pustular psoriasis of the palms and soles showed considerable reduction in the amount of epidermal thickening and absence of permeation by polymorphs. They did not appear different from the appearance of healing psoriasis due to other treatments.

Table 2. Side effects in 25 patients treated with Ro 10-9359

Side effect	Numbers Affected	Comment
1. Cheilitis: dryness of lips, nose or mouth	24	Mostly minor but intolerable in two
2. Hair loss	7	Transient in all cases
3. Pruritus	7	Particularly in ichthyotics
4. Rash	3	Urticarial - 1; morbilliform - 2
5. Buccal leukokeratosis	1	Asymptomatic
6. Headaches	2	Minor and transient
7. Episodic drowsiness	1	Not proven
8. Nose bleeds	2	Minor and transient

Table 3. Summary of special tests performed before and after four-week Ro 10-9359 treatment

Test	Comment	Parameter	Ref.	Information obtained
1. Histological	Routine techniques	Descriptive	-	Microscopic pathology
2. Histometric	Projection techniques	Epidermal thickness in absolute terms (μm) and code number (MET)	6	Measure of epidermal structure
3. Cell kinetic	Incubation of biopsy fragment in presence of tritiated thymidine for 4-hour period	Labelling Index (per cent labelled cells)	16	Measure of epidermal proliferation
4. Histochemical	Quantitative enzyme histochemistry using microdensitometric evaluation on Quantimet 720 image analyzing computer	Optical density units	12	Epidermal metabolic activity
5. Electron microscopy	Routine techniques of fixation and embedding for transmission electron microscopy	Descriptive	-	Ultrastructural pathology
6. Corneocyte sizing	Projection techniques	Mean corneocyte area (μm²)	6	Measure of corneocyte size
7. a) Intracorneal cohesion	a) Technique of cohesography employing specially built instrument	a) g force	9	Measures of stratum corneum function
b) Transepidermal water loss	b) Technique of evaporimetry employing specially built evaporimeter	b) g/m² body surface/hour	10	
c) Forced desquamation	c) Technique employing scrub apparatus, specially built to deliver standardized stimulus to skin surface	c) Cells removed in 10 sec scrub	9	
8. Surface structure of corneocytes	a) Differential interference microscopy of isolated corneocytes	Descriptive		Detailed structural alteration of surface of corneocytes
	b) Scanning electron microscopy of isolated corneocytes	Descriptive		

3. Histometric Results

The mean epidermal thicknesses in cell number (MET) and in absolute terms (μm) are given in Table 4. It can be seen that in many of the disease groups – in both involved and uninvolved skin – there is an increase in epidermal thickness. Taking mean keratinocyte height (MKH) (which is $\frac{\mu m}{MET}$) as an index of keratinocyte size, it can be seen that there are no special changes in this parameter. No attempts were made to take measurements from the involved skin in patients with Darier's disease, epidermolytic hyperkeratosis, or psoriasis.

Table 4. Histometric data (means and standard deviation)

Condition	Numbers available for analysis	Pre-treatment MET	Pre-treatment µm	Pre-treatment MKh	Post-treatment MET	Post-treatment µm	Post-treatment MKh
Autosomal dominant ichthyosis	4	4.7 ± 0.5	51.3 ± 2.6	10.9 ± 0.6	6.0 ± 1.3	6.60 ± 17.7	10.9 ± 1.4
PRP	2	9.0	88.0	9.8	9.9	92.5	9.2
Darier's disease (uninvolved)	3	4.2 ± 0.9	51.5 ± 19.0	12.0 ± 2.4	5.5 ± 1.9	56.1 ± 14.9	10.4 ± 1.1
EKV	2	5.6	53.5	9.7	6.7	59.5	9.3
Overall	11	5.49 ± 1.97	58.41 ± 18.11	10.79 ± 1.46	6.70 ± 2.26*	66.92±21.11^ø^	10.17±1.42

N.B.
* $0.01 > p > 0.0001$
ø $0.1 > p > 0.05$

4. Cell Kinetic Findings

No changes in thymidine autoradiographic epidermal labelling indices were detected in either the involved or uninvolved skin of patients with Darier's disease or EKV after treatment with Ro 10–9359. Neither were any alterations found in labelling index in patients with lamellar ichthyosis, PRP or autosomal dominant ichthyosis (Table 5).

5. Quantitative Enzyme Histochemical Studies

No marked changes in the distribution or density of reaction product within the epidermis were found in the post-treatment specimens for the respiratory enzyme activities. There was an obvious reduction in the density of formazan reaction product due to the glucose-6-phosphate dehydrogenase reaction in the post-treatment specimens within the granular cell layer of the 14 patients with disorders of keratinization so examined (pre Ro 10-9359: 0.54 ± 0.08 O.D. units; post Ro 10-9359: 0.47±0.13 O.D. units; $0.05 < p < 0.02$). These results will be reported in full elsewhere (4).

Table 5. Labelling indices.
Percentage basal and suprabasal cells autoradiographically labelled of 1000 basal epidermal cells counted

Condition	n	Before	After
Dominant ichthyosis	4	6.03 ± 2.23	8.58 ± 1.23
Darier's disease (involved)	2	11.22	13.48
Darier's disease (uninvolved)	3	6.85 ± 0.59	6.26 ± 2.64
PRP	2	25.12	20.59
EKV (involved)	3	14.17 ± 7.26	13.82 ± 3.40
EKV (uninvolved)	2	6.88	7.65
Lamellar ichthyosis	2	17.86	16.09

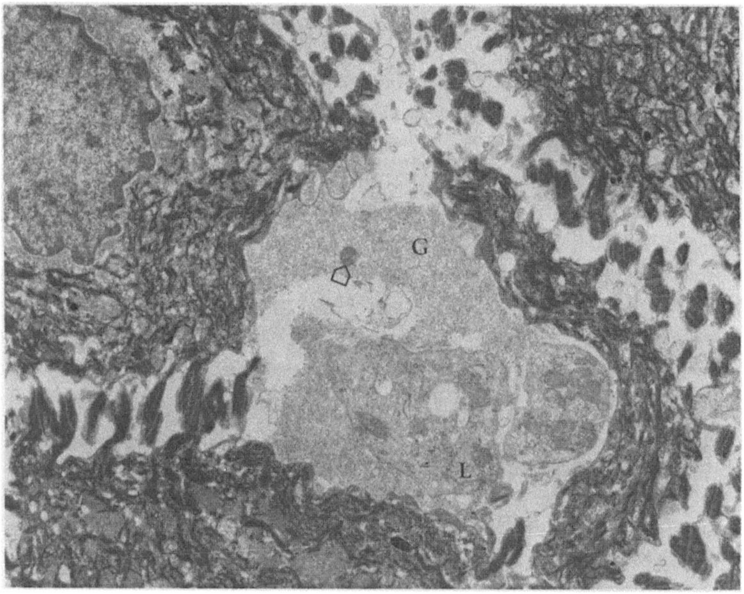

Fig. 1. Extracellular granular material (G) seen in the epidermis of a patient with autosomal dominant ichthyosis treated with Ro 10-9359. Mitochondrion (arrowed) within this material suggests that cytolysis has occurred. (L: Langerhans' cell). Magnification × 4100

6. Ultrastructural Findings

Thus far specimens from 9 of the patients have been examined before and after 4 weeks of treatment. The most striking feature in the post-treatment specimens was the accumulation of a granular material between the epidermal cells (Fig. 1). The material consisted of both fine and coarse granules. This material was not confined to the intercellular spaces of the epidermis but was also found beneath the basal lamina and in smaller amounts between the horny cells of the stratum corneum. In some of the pre-treatment specimens there was also a small amount of the same material. The ultrastructural findings will be reported in full elsewhere (1).

7. Studies on Corneocytes

No gross alterations were detected in shape or surface markings of corneocytes either by scanning electron microscopy or by differential interference phase microscopy. The area of corneocytes was increased following Ro 10-9359 treatment in the 18 subjects examined by this technique (pre Ro 10-9359: $748.0 \pm 191.8\ \mu m^2$; post Ro 10-9359: $893.4 \pm 252.6\ \mu m^2$; $0.01 > p > 0.0001$).

8. Studies on Stratum Corneum Function

No consistent changes were found after Ro 10-9359 treatment in transepidermal water loss (TEWL), intracorneal cohesion measurements or the number of cells that could be removed by a standardized "scrub stimulus". In some cases even marked clinical improvement was not matched by changes in the measurements of function.

Comment

Despité the quite dramatic change in clinical state of many of the patients in this study our investigations revealed that the alterations in the epidermis following treatment were quite subtle. However, it should be remembered that our post-treatment investigations were conducted four weeks after starting Ro 10-9359 and there may have been more marked changes earlier on that we could not observe. The lack of morphological change or alteration in rate of epidermal cell production in the four-week specimens plus the decreased glucose-6-phosphate dehydrogenase and increase in corneocyte area indicate that the bulk of the change after retinoid administration is in the process of keratinization.

It is perhaps not surprising that no consistent change was revealed by the tests of stratum corneum function. Even the most minor epidermal disturbance results in changes in these tests and these patients while, dramatically improved still showed the pre-treatment intrinsic epidermal abnormalities.

It is less easy to characterize the type of change in keratinization that has occurred. It seems most unlikely that granular cell glucose-6-phosphate dehydrogenase is concerned with the supply of pentose sugars for DNA synthesis as it is in other tissues, and clearly it is impossible to comment on the change in activity of this enzyme following treatment without firm knowledge of its role in epidermal differentiation. The change in corneocyte area (no observations on corneocyte volume were made) could indicate a change in conformation of the membrane proteins so that they were less rigid and allowed the corneocyte to become flatter. It is interesting in this respect that the retinoids have been found to have a marked effect on membrane glycoprotein synthesis (2).

The accumulation of granular material within the epidermis following retinoid treatment is of considerable interest. It may represent plasma membrane alterations or may be the result of cytolysis (8) occurring early on after retinoid administration, but may not be evident subsequently.

The retinoids offer great hope for patients for whom previously there was no effective treatment. However, much work is required before there is full understanding of their effects and of their mode of action.

Summary

A total of 25 patients (20 with disorders of keratinization, 5 with psoriasis) have been treated with Ro 10-9359 and studied with particular reference to the effects on keratinization before and four weeks after treatment. Significant increases were found in epidermal thickness and corneocyte area in skin from patients with disorders of keratinization after treatment. A significant decrease in glucose-6-phosphate dehydrogenase activity in the granular cell layer was also demonstrated. There was a striking increase of granular material between epidermal cells which appeared heterogenous in character. This material was found throughout the epidermis but only occasionally within the stratum corneum. No change was found in corneocyte structure ultrastructurally or by light microscopy.

References

1. Barton S, Marks R (1980) Ultrastructural changes in the epidermis of patients with disorders of keratinization after treatment with an oral retinoid (Ro 10-9359). In preparation
2. De Luca LM, Bhat PV, Sasak W, Adamo S (1979) Biosynthesis of phosphoryl and glycosyl phosphoryl derivatives of vitamin A in biological membranes. Fed Proc 38:2535–2539

3. Fritsch P, Hönigsmann H, Jaschke E (1978) Epidermolytic hereditary palmoplantar keratoderma. Br J Dermatol 99:561–568
4. Gaskell S, Marks R (1980) Effects of an oral retinoid (Ro 10-9359) on epidermal metabolism in patients with disorders of keratinization. A quantitative enzyme histochemical study. In preparation
5. Gilgor RS, Chiarmonti A, Goldsmith LA, Lazarus GS (1980) Evaluation of 13-cis retinoic acid in lamellar ichthyosis, pityriasis rubra pilaris and Darier's Disease. Cutis 25:380–385
6. Holt PJA, Marks R (1976) Epidermal architecture, growth and metabolism in acromegaly. Br Med J 1:496–497
7. Marks R, Finlay AY, Holt PJA (1980) Skin changes in patients with congenital disorders of keratinization treated with Ro 10-9359, Abstract. Br J Dermatol 103 (suppl 18):11–12
8. Matter A, Bollag W (1977) A fine structural study of the therapeutic effect of aromatic retinoids on chemically induced skin papillomas of the mouth. Eur J Cancer 13:831–838
9. Nicholls S, Marks R (1977) Novel techniques for the estimation of intracorneal cohesion in vivo. Br J Dermatol 96:595–602
10. Nilssen GE (1977) Measurement of water exchange through skin. Med Biol Eng Comput 15: 209
11. Orfanos CE, Mahrle G, Goerz R, Happle R, Hofbauer M, Landes E, Schimpf A (1979) Laboratory investigations in patients with generalized psoriasis under oral retinoid treatment. Dermatologica 159:62–70
12. Pearse AD, Marks R (1977) Actinic keratoses and the epidermis on which they arise. Br J Dermatol 95:513–518
13. Peck GL, Olsen TG, Yoder FW, Strauss JS, Downing DT, Pandya M, Butkus D, Arnaud-Battandier J (1979) Prolonged remissions of cystic and conglobate acne with 13-cis retinoic acid. N Engl J Med 300:329–333
14. Pehamberger H, Neumann H, Holubar K (1978) Oral treatment of ichthyosis with an aromatic retinoid. Br J Dermatol 99:319–324
15. Pettit JHS (1979) Oral retinoid for psoriasis. A report of a double blind study. Acta Derm Venerol (Stockh) 59 (suppl 85):133–136
16. Shahrad P, Marks R (1976) Hair follicle kinetics in psoriasis. Br J Dermatol 94:7–12
17. Wateren van der AR, Cormane RH (1977) Oral retinoic acid as therapy for erythrokeratodermia variabilis. Br J Dermatol 97:83–85

C.E. Orfanos et al. (eds.)
Retinoids

Light and Electron Microscopic Changes of Human Epidermis Under Oral Retinoid Treatment

U. Schultz-Ehrenburg and C.E. Orfanos

Oral administration of retinoids shows clinically a basic beneficial influence in various skin diseases with disorders of keratinization, regardless to their pathogenesis and their particular histological substrate. It seems that retinoids act as a general regulator of epidermal phenomena related to dysfunction of (a) epidermal cell differentiation, (b) keratin synthesis and (c) desquamation of corneocytes. This is the result of our clinical and experimental experience with this group of drugs over one decade.

Up to now only a few investigations were performed showing the light and electron microscopic changes taking place in the diseased epidermis under oral retinoid therapy (2, 3, 4). In the present paper we are summarizing our observations in human skin over the last 5 years.

Materials and Methods

Light and electron microscopic investigations were performed on the epidermis of 12 patients with oral retinoid treatment (4 x psoriasis, including the pustular type Zumbusch, 2 x Darier's disease, 2 x lichen planus, 1 x ichtyosis vulgaris, 1 x circumscribed scleroderma, 1 x arsenic keratosis and 1 x multiple basal cell cacinoma, BCC). Additionally, non-involved skin in psoriasis, psoriasiform dermatitis in Darier's disease, and healthy skin of a volunteer were also examined and evaluated for this study.

Biopsies were taken, as a rule, before and 1–6 weeks after oral administration of aromatic retinoid Ro 10-9359 (75 mg/d for 3 weeks, then reduction of the daily dose to 50 mg); in most patients more than one control biopsies were taken after treatment at different time intervals.

For light microscopy, sections embedded in paraffin were stained with hematoxylin-eosin, with van Gieson and PAS stains. Specimens for electron microscopy were fixed in 0.1 M glutaraldehyde/paraformaldehyde solution (2.5 : 4.5 %, buffered with sodium cacodylate pH 7.2), were postfixed in 1 % osmium tetroxide solution, were dehydrated in rising series of acetone and were then embedded in Araldite. The ultrathin sections were stained with uranyl acetate and with lead citrate.

Results

The findings showed that oral retinoid therapy has a distinct influence on (a) epidermal keratinocytes, (b) the Langerhans' cells and (c) the inflammatory cell infiltrate invading the epidermis in skin diseases; whereas, no significant changes were observed on the number and the ultrastructure of the melanocytes.

In biopsies performed after one week of treatment, striking changes were seen showing detachment of the lower corneal layers and significant loss of corneocytes. The living keratinocytes showed *cytotoxic alterations* in all skin disorders examined by us, including non-involved or normal skin. They were, however, temporary since they decreased rapidly in the 2nd and 3rd week of treatment. Only in cases of neoplastic disorders cytotoxic effects seem-

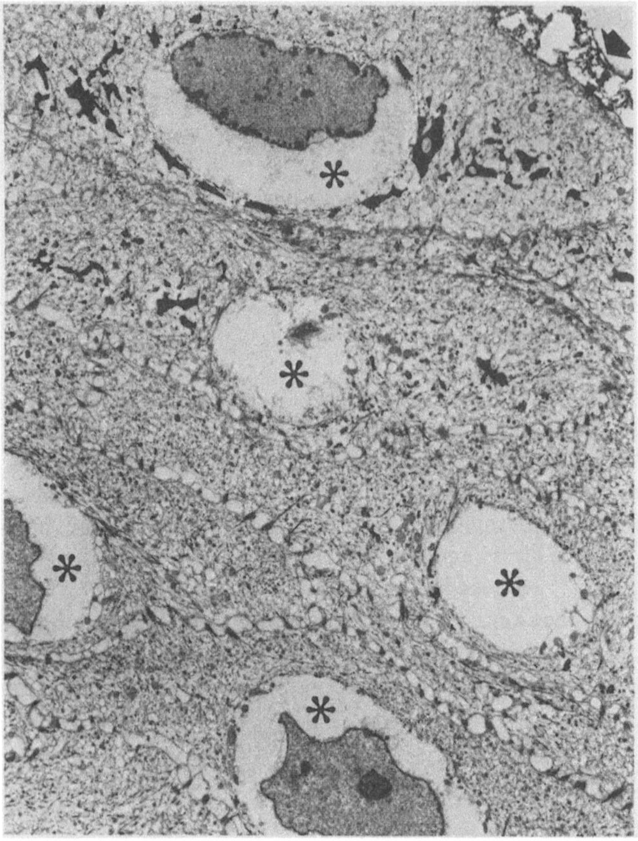

Fig. 1. *Psoriasis; non-involved skin,* one week after onset of treatment, showing the typical pattern of retinoid-induced cytotoxic effect: Marked perinuclear edema with glykogen-like particles (asterisks) in all epidermal layers. Arrow = loosened corneocyte. × 5,300

ed to persist even longer. Retinoid-induced cytotoxicity is characterized by a typical pattern of ultrastructural changes consisting of perinuclear edema, cytoplasmic accumulation of fluid and glycogen, or glycogen-like particles, and swelling of mitochondria (Fig. 1). Occasionally, moderate numbers of lysosomes can be seen. In some instances, a number of cells with small vacuolar cytoplasmic degeneration and scattered individual cell necroses were found in the malpighian layers, obviously representing the final stages of retinoid-induced cytotoxicity.

The other structural changes induced by retinoid in human epidermis varied not only from disease to disease, but sometimes also from case to case and from area to area. A prominent finding was in most cases the appearance of a *mucus-like material (MLM)* in the diseased epidermis, previously described under various conditions in animals and in human (3, 4). In patients with psoriasis examined here, MLM was found in the 1st or 2nd week after treatment, occasionally later (Fig. 2). It seemed that in early stages MLM occurred intracellularly in the cisterns of the endoplasmic reticulum, and is accumulated later in larger vacuoles which were often seen in perinuclear position. At places, the cytoplasm appeared nearly completely filled with MLM and nearly all other cytoplasmic organelles disappeared. In later stages, finally, MLM accumulations were seen in the extracellular spaces and the epider-

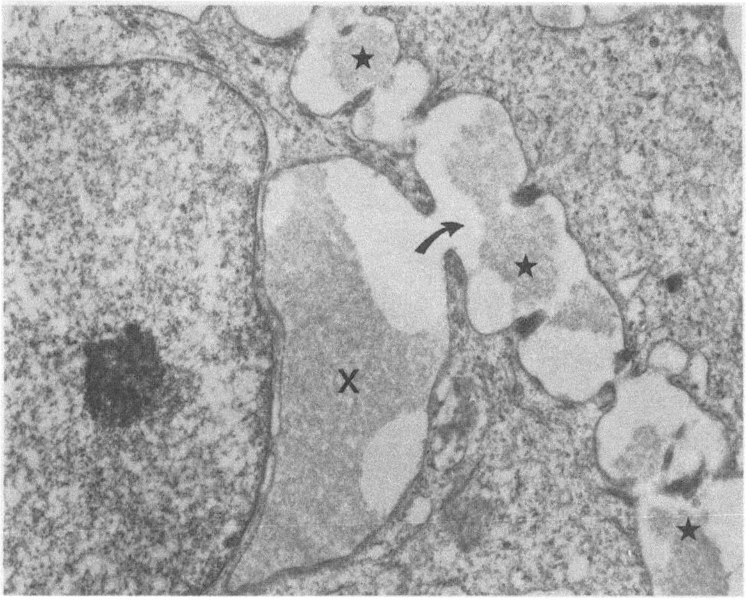

Fig. 2. *Psoriasis (involved skin)*; 2 weeks after onset of treatment: Appearance of mucus-like material in a large paranuclear vacuole (cross) and in the intercellular spaces (asterisks). Some desmosomes are separated or disrupted. × 20,000

mis revealed a spongiotic appearance, containing abundant amounts of MLM. The material preserved its amorphous ultrastructural appearance and seemed sometimes to adhere at the cell surfaces. Occasionally, melanocytes were surrounded by MLM floating in it like in a lake. The regions mostly affected were the lower epidermal layers, occasionally the stratum granulosum and only rarely the lower part of stratum corneum.

The quantities of MLM appearing after retinoid varied greatly from epidermal area to epidermal area. It was detected in psoriatic lesions of 3 patients and also in non-involved skin. In contrast to this, we did not find MLM in a patient with psoriasis treated with retinoid who did not improve clinically. Epidermal keratinocytes are obviously able to produce MLM without retinoid under certain circumstances, since we also found it to some degree in basal cell carcinoma before treatment, during the course of which it then increased (Figs. 3 and 4). No or rather little MLM, compared to psoriasis, was detected by us in patients with Darier's disease and in one patient with ichthyosis.

The other activities of mature epidermal keratinocytes such as *biosynthesis of keratin precursors*, revealed different alterations, varying from disease to disease: Tonofilaments and keratohyalin granules were found increased in disorders in which they have been diminished before treatment. Newly synthesized keratohyalin granules showed an unusual star-like or reticular configuration, particularly in psoriasis. This irregular shape was pronounced after 2 weeks of treatment and it then returned to normal. Surprisingly enough, the amount of keratohyalin granules and the thickness of the granular layer varied greatly under oral retinoid: In psoriatic parakeratosis without keratohyalin the granular layer reappeared under oral treatment, in a patient with BCC retinoid-induced hypergranulosis was seen and in lichen planus with preexistent hypergranulosis the changes were normalized after 3 weeks, i.e. the number of keratohyalin granules was reduced. The

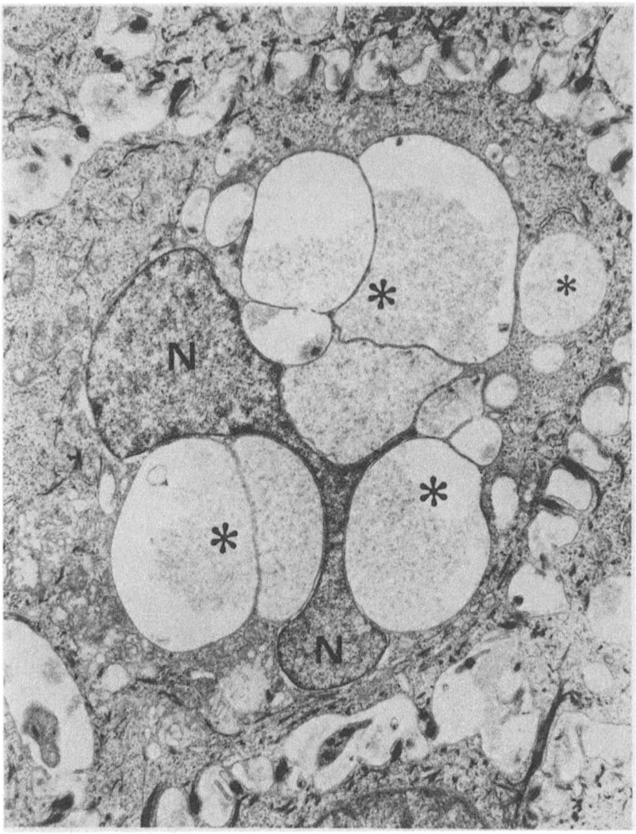

Fig. 3. *Basal cell carcinoma*, 6 weeks after onset of treatment: Keratinocyte in stratum malpighii showing large multiple cytoplasmic vacuoles containing MLM (asterisks), leading to compression and deformation of the cell nucleus (N). Some MLM is also seen in the intercellular spaces. × 13,000

keratinosomes seemed to increase in the first 3 weeks in all examined cases including a case of ichthyosis in which they were almost completely lacking before treatment.

After *initial keratolysis* induced by retinoid, e.g. in psoriasis, the corneal layer showed a tendency to return to orthokeratosis. It may, however, happen that parakeratotic changes remain or even newly appear. In ichthyosis treated with retinoid we have observed parakeratotic transformation of the previously orthokeratotic horny layer, with persisting nuclear remnants and loosening of the keratin pattern. In one patient with Darier's disease some clinical worsening occurred during oral retinoid treatment and the lesions became erythematous with some oozing; histological examination revealed a *psoriasiform dermatitis*, showing loss of dyskeratosis and appearance of psoriasiform acanthosis with parakeratosis and only a few keratohyalin granules. Some suprabasal clefts here and there still evidenced the former changes indicative for Darier's disease.

The epidermal *mitotic activity* seemed to increase during oral retinoid treatment: A considerable amount of normal mitoses was seen in retinoid-treated epidermis, however, no pathologic changes of any type were seen ultrastructurally in these cells. Acanthosis occurred in all treated patients examined by light microscopy. It regressed only gradually and, in most cases, it persisted longer than 6 weeks after onset of treatment.

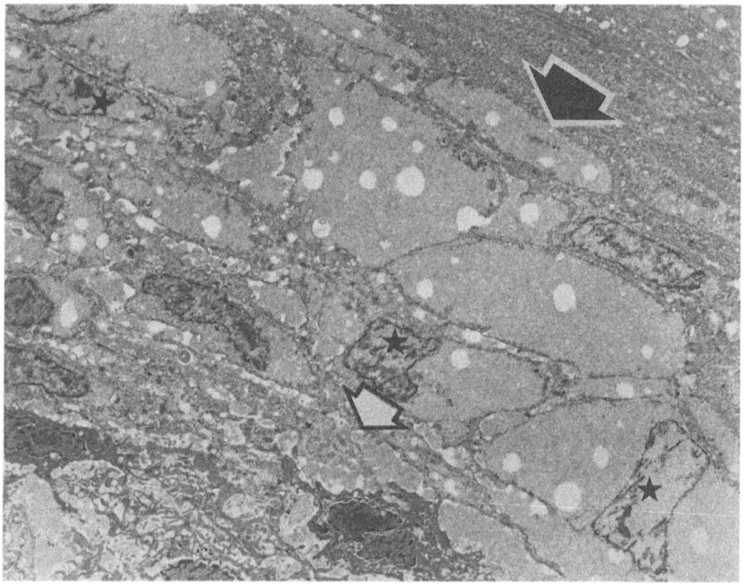

Fig. 4. *Basal cell carcinoma*, 5 weeks after onset of treatment: Excessive amounts of MLM in intra- and extracellular position in the upper epidermis and the lower part of stratum corneum (arrows). It seems that larger epidermal areas undergo mucinous degeneration. The cells in these areas show edematous degeneration of the nuclei (asterisks) and loss of cytoplasmic organelles. × 5,300

During the course of therapy, *epidermal Langerhans' cells* showed frequently signs of stimulation. We found increased number of organelles and membrane profiles in their cytoplasm, several Golgi zones and, occasionally, remnants of phagocytosed material.

As far as the intraepidermal *inflammatory cells* are concerned, the most remarkable finding was a rapid regression of granulocytic invasion, which already became visible after one week. Furthermore, we sometimes observed Sézary-like lymphocytes and activated macrophages in psoriatic epidermis after 3 weeks of oral retinoid treatment, a finding which may be related to the stimulation of dermal Langerhans' cells, to be reported later in another paper from our laboratory.

Discussion

The epidermal alterations seen by light and electron microscopy under retinoid treatment suggest that the retinoid-induced changes regularly follow a certain temporal course. The main changes are:

1st week: Keratolysis; decrease of granulocytic invasion; cytotoxic effects.

1st/2nd week: Intracellular synthesis of mucus-like material (MLM), accumulation in the intracellular spaces; numerous normal mitoses, development of acanthosis.

2nd/3rd week: Normalization of tonofilaments and keratohyalin granules, normalization of various keratinization disorders; appearance of stimulated Langerhans' cells, activated macrophages and Sézary-like lymphocytes.

6th week and later: Regression of the inflammatory cell infiltrate; gradual disappearance of acanthosis.

These changes frequently appear focally in some areas and may evidence distinct quantitative differences. It seemed to us that the site of the lesions and also the site chosen for biopsy may be of considerable significance. Additionally, the morphological changes may be more or less pronounced because of different clinical responsiveness to the drug.

Of particular interest is undoubtedly the question of how one and the same medicament can induce such different and sometimes controversial effects as the following: Reappearance of keratohyalin granules in psoriasis and reduction of hypergranulosis in lichen planus, or, normalization of hyperkeratosis in ichthyosis, dyskeratosis in Darier's disease and parakeratosis in psoriasis, but induction of parakeratotic changes in other disorders or individual cases (psoriasiform dermatitis in Darier's disease, parakeratotic signs in ichthyosis). The answering of this question seems to have a key position in the problem of what is the mode of action of the drug at all.

The *initial cytotoxic changes* described above may only represent an undesirable side effect of the drug; however, they may also signify a selection of cells resistant to the cytotoxic action of retinoid, being able to launch hyperproliferation of normal keratinocytes after 3 weeks (1). At any case it is obvious that cytotoxic changes are visible during the first week of treatment only and that the new population of keratinocytes appearing under treatment is somehow better protected or adapted to the influence of the drug. The signs of cytotoxicity disappear (4). Increased keratolysis and desquamation help to remove the old population of diseased cells.

The most prominent effect of retinoid, however, seems to be its remarkable influence on the phenomena of cell differentiation; we called this effect *modulation of differentiation*, since it cannot be described either as a stimulatory or an inhibitory effect (Fig. 5). During its course, a change in epithelial differentiation occurs leading to the synthesis of MLM. It is not clear whether this new material may have a special function itself, p.e. protection from toxic drug-induced changes, or similar. It appears, however, that the keratinocytes are conditioned into a state of embryonal immaturity; thus inherent ontogenetic properties of epidermal cells may reappear. Some similarities may be found indeed between MLM-synthesis and the secretory function of periderm in embryonal life. In other words, the synthetic capacities of the new population of keratinocytes appearing under retinoid treatment are shifted to another metabolic pathway, namely, from synthesis of keratin into synthesis of mucin or mucopolysaccharides.

The adaptation of epidermal keratinocytes to retinoid and the modulation of their differentiation by the drug lead to *restoration of normal structure and function*, regardless to the cause of the previous individual dermatosis in particular. One may suggest that the in-

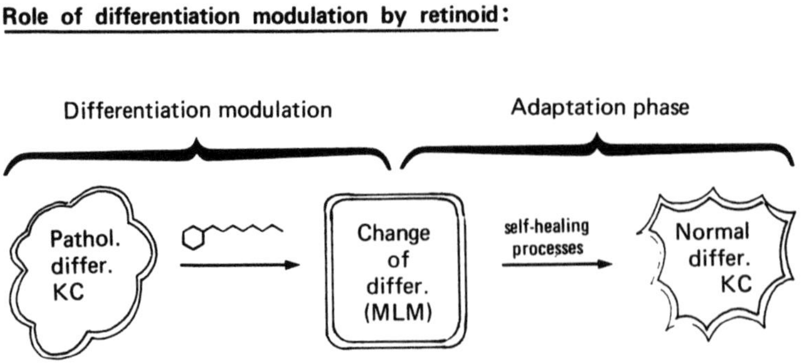

Fig. 5

fluence of retinoid on epidermal cell differentiation interrupts some general feedback mechanisms which maintain and control formal pathogenesis. Thus, selfhealing processes enable the cell to overcome various disorders of keratinization, irrespective to their basic cause, during or after their adaptation phase and to reestablish normal function. Since modulatory influences most likely take place at the molecular level, the appearance of MLM is merely one visible marker but not necessarily a precondition for the selfhealing phase. As a fact, under the influence of retinoid a new population of epidermal keratinocytes reacts again to the stimuli of normal growth and differentiation and results into clinical improvement.

The stimulatory effect of retinoid on epidermal Langerhans' cells and its influence on dermal cells invading the epidermis may also play a role in skin diseases with keratinization disorders, however, this is still subject for further investigation. Interestingly enough, melanocytes did not reveal any particular ultrastructural changes under retinoid treatment. Nevertheless, the action of retinoid is not restricted to cells of epithelial origin as a target tissue.

Conclusions

Oral retinoid treatment induces marked morphological changes in human epidermis which can be seen under the light and the electron microscope. The therapeutic result apparently consists of a mixture of

(a) actual retinoid effects which appear in nearly all cases representing the pharmacological action of the drug, and
(b) consecutive cell reactions which are only indirectly related to the drug and which can vary from disease to disease.

A few days after onset of treatment increased keratolysis, desquamation and temporary cytotoxic changes are seen, followed by stimulation of proliferation and modulation of differentiation of a new population of keratinocytes. In addition, the aromatic retinoid obviously exerts stimulating influences on Langerhans' cells and on the inflammatory cell infiltrate; furthermore, an early finding is the rapid regression of the epidermal granulocytic invasion, particularly in psoriasis pustulosa.

A most prominent effect of retinoid seems to be *the modulation of cellular differentiation* in human and animal epidermis, which finds its clearest morphological expression in the synthesis of a new, mucus-like material (MLM). The synthetic activities of the cells are apparently directed into another metabolic pathway, obviously resulting in an interruption of the feedback control mechanisms which maintain formal pathogenesis. In other words, the keratinocytes are put into an early state of development, being able to react again to the stimuli of *normal* differentiation. Depending on whether this is successful, selfhealing mechanisms develop leading to restoration of normal architecture and, therefore, to clinical improvement.

Summary

Light- and electron microscopic investigations were performed on the epidermis of 12 (9) patients before and 1–6 weeks after treatment with oral retinoid (4 × psoriasis including pustular Zumbusch type; 2 × Darier's disease; 2 × lichen ruber; 1 × vulgar ichthyosis; 1 × circumscribet scleroderma; 1 × arsenic keratosis; 1 × multiple basal cell carcinoma (BCC). Additionally, non-involved skin in psoriasis, psoriasiform dermatitis in Darier's disease, and healthy skin in patient with eczema were also examined. In most patients several biopsies at different time intervals were evaluated. The findinds revealed definite morphological changes of keratinocytes, Langerhans cells and the intraepidermal cell infiltrate. No significant changes of the melanocytes were seen.

(1) A striking finding was the detachment of stratum corneum in its lower part. The living keratinocytes showed initial intracellular perinuclear edema, mitochondrial swelling, occasional vacuolar degeneration and individual cell degradation. In psoriasis and in BCC significant amounts of mucus-like material (MLM) were seen intra- and extracellularly after 1–3 weeks, being most likely synthesized in the lower malphighian layers. MLM occasionally occurred in the granular, and rarely, in the horny layer. No or little MLM was detected in Darier's disease and in ichthyosis.

(2) Langerhans cells showed increased numbers of cytoplasmic organelles and membrane profiles indicating higher levels of cytoplasmic stimulation.

(3) The number of dermal cells invading the epidermis was definitely reduced after treatment. In particular, decreased granulocytic migration was clearly evident in pustular psoriasis as early was 1 week after onset of treatment. After 3 weeks some Sézary-like lymphocytic cells and macrophages were found in the epidermis.

As clinical response progressed, controversial effects were seen: Reappearing of variably shaped keratohyalin granules in psoriasis, reduction of hypergranulosis in lichen planus, normalization of hyperkeratosis, dyskeratosis and parakeratosis in various conditions, but induction of some parakeratosis in others. Acanthosis remained last to be influenced under oral retinoid or persisted longer than 6 weeks. These oberservations indicate that oral retinoid (a) has a particular effect on human epidermal keratinocytes modulating their differentiation and leading to desquamation. It normalizes disorders of keratinization of different types by inducing growth of a new population of normal appearing keratinocytes, (b) exerts a stimulatory influence on Langerhans cells and (c) inhibits intraepidermal granulocytic migration.

References

1. Dierlich E, Orfanos CE, Pullmann H, Steigleder GK (1979) Epidermale Zellproliferation unter oraler Retinoid-Therapie bei Psoriasis. Arch Dermatol Res 264:169–177
2. Matter A, Bollag W (1977) A fine structural study on the therapeutic effect of an aromatic retinoid on chemically induced skin papillomas of the mouse. Eur J Cancer 13:831–838
3. Orfanos CE, Runne U (1978) Tissue changes in psoriatic plaques after oral administration of retinoid. Dermatologica 157 (Suppl. 1):19–25
4. Tsambaos D, Mahrle G, Orfanos CE (1980) Epidermal changes induced by oral excess of aromatic retinoid in guinea pigs. Arch Dermatol Res 267:141–152

C.E. Orfanos et al. (eds.)
Retinoids

Retinoid-Stimulated Material in Psoriatic Epidermis During Ro 10-9359 Therapy

Ch.N. Ellis, R.C. Gold, R.C. Grekin, N.A. Swanson, Th.F. Anderson and J.J. Voorhees

Cell surface molecules modulate the cell-to-cell interactions which may control cell proliferation. Psoriasis is a disease in which abnormal epidermal cell interactions may play a pertinent role (13). Retinoids, which are known to be effective in psoriasis therapy, exert profound effects on squamous epithelia in cell culture and in vivo as manifested by mucous metaplasia and alterations in cell proliferation (10). Whether these biological effects are the result of differences in cell interactions induced by retinoids is unknown.

Ro 10-9359, an aromatic retinoid used orally in the treatment of psoriasis, has been associated with a finely-granular intercellular material in psoriatic epidermis as first reported by Orfanos and Runne (12). A similar substance has been seen ultrastructurally in the intercellular space of various tissues exposed to retinoids (2, 9, 14, 17). The nature and biologic activity of this retinoid-stimulated material (RSM) are unknown. This study was undertaken to further examine the ultrastructural changes in the involved and uninvolved skin of psoriatic patients taking Ro 10-9359.

Materials and Methods

Patients: Ten patients were selected for either extensive psoriasis (at least 20% of total body surface area involved) or significant disability. All patients were part of a multi-center research trial of Ro 10-9359 for treatment of psoriasis. Various disease types were represented: 3 patients had large-plaque type psoriasis, 3 had pustular psoriasis, 1 had generalized erythrodermic psoriasis, 1 had "guttate" (chronic small-plaque type) psoriasis, and 2 had "inverse-seborrheic" (mainly intertriginous) psoriasis.

Prior to entry into the study, patients discontinued all systemic therapies (PUVA, methotrexate, etc.) for at least 1 month and all topical treatments, except bland emollients, for at least 2 weeks. Ro 10-9359 was initiated at a dose of 1.0 mg/kg/day for 1 week, and then decreased to 0.5 mg/kg/day for two weeks. Subsequently, doses were adjusted from 0.5 mg/kg/day to 1.5 mg/kg/day to achieve maximum clinical response. Patients avoided sunlight and used only bland emollients as adjunctive therapy.

Active psoriatic lesions and uninvolved regions (when possible) were biopsied pre-treatment and at weeks 2, 12, and 16 during the administration of Ro 10-9359. Skin from five normal volunteers taking no medications was also biopsied.

Electron Microscopy: Biopsies were prepared for transmission electron micrographic study as follows. Tissue was fixed at 4 °C for 24 hours in freshly-prepared 4.5% formaldehyde - 2.5% glutaraldehyde solution in 0.025 M sodium cacodylate buffer, pH 7.2. Specimens were postfixed for 1.5 hours in 1% osmium tetroxide in s-Collidine buffer, pH 7.4, dehydrated in rising concentrations of acetone, embedded in Epon-Araldite epoxy resins, and cured 72 hours at 60 °C. Samples were thin-sectioned with a LKB ultratome III ultramicrotome and DuPont diamond knife, mounted on 3-mm nickel grids, stained with 2% uranyl acetate and Reynolds lead citrate, and examined under a Philips 300 electron microscope.

Results

Clinical response: Nine of ten patients taking Ro 10-9359 had very good to excellent clearing of psoriasis during the 16-week trial. One patient, with large-plaque type psoriasis, failed to respond satisfactorily. Typical side effects of cheilitis, peeling of the skin of palms and soles, and hair loss were seen, but no patient discontinued Ro 10-9359 as a result. The multi-center data will be reported elsewhere.

Ultrastructural findings: In electron micrographs (EMs) of involved and uninvolved psoriatic skin, we detected a finely-granular substance (retinoid-stimulated material, RSM). Biopsies were considered positive if the material could be demonstrated unequivocally in the intercellular space.

In general, the substance was found in the epidermal intercellular space adjacent to the cell membrane; a typical example is shown in Figure 1. The material is readily visualized, and it fills the intercellular space, except where it apparently has been lost during processing. The intercellular spaces were widened in positive biopsies compared to negative samples. The material was detected in all levels of involved psoriatic epidermis, but was concentrated in the thickened stratum spinosum.

At high magnification (Figure 1, inset), RSM is an amorphous substance containing randomly distributed, darkly staining granules of unknown composition. The granules do not have the ultrastructural appearance of ribosomes, organelles, or membrane fragments, however.

Occasionally, the material was seen in what appeared to be an intracellular location (Figure 2). We did not detect any vacuoles containing the substance in continuity with the cell membrane.

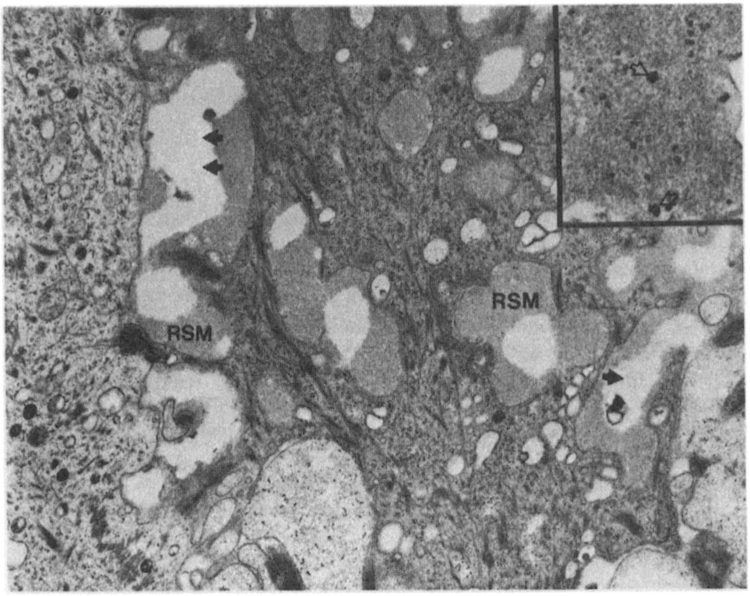

Fig. 1. Ultrastructural features of human epidermis treated with Ro 10-9359. Retinoid-stimulated material (RSM) is seen in the widened intercellular space. Empty areas within the intercellular space may be due to loss of RSM during processing (solid arrows). Insert depicts RSM at a high magnification. There are randomly distributed darker-staining granules of unknown composition (open arrows). Figure: 8,600 × Insert: 54,800

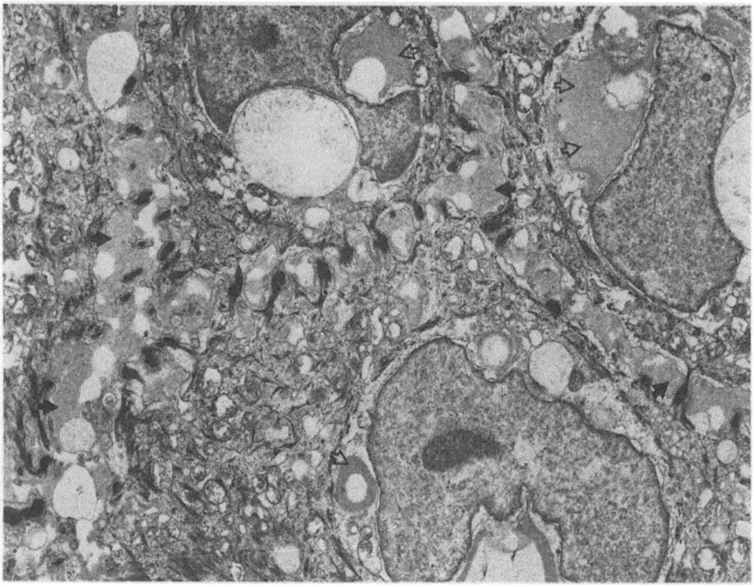

Fig. 2. Low magnification photo depicting intracellular (open arrows) and intercellular (solid arrows) retinoid-stimulated material (RSM). The intracellular material appears to be contained in a membrane-bound structure. 4,650 ×

All ten patients showed intercellular material in at least one skin biopsy. Among the patients who were positive, the substance could not be detected in all sampled areas from a single biopsy, nor was it apparent in every biopsy subsequent to a positive one. The staining density of the RSM varied from patient to patient, and from biopsy to biopsy within a single patient. This variability, coupled with the lack of quantitative electron microscopic technology, made it impossible to evaluate individual patient increases or decreases of RSM.

Table 1. Intercellular amorphous material in electron micrographs of skin from patients taking Ro 10-9359

Case	Age	Sex	Type of Psoriasis[a]	Week on Therapy 0[b]	2	12	16
1	32	F	Plaque	–	–	NA	+
2	70	M	Guttate	–	–	NA	+[c]
3	58	M	Plaque	–	–	+	–
4	46	M	Inverse	–	+	+	–
5	55	M	Inverse	–	+	–	–
6	52	F	Pustular	+	–	+	+
7	57	M	Erythrodermic	–	–	+	–
8	21	M	Pustular	–	–	NA	+
9	49	M	Pustular	NA	+	+	–
10	54	M	Plaque	–	NA	NA	–[c]

Key: amorphous intercellular material in psoriatic lesional skin:
+, seen; –, not seen; NA, biopsy not available.
[a]: see text
[b]: week 0 is pre-therapy
[c]: patients with material seen in uninvolved skin after 12th week.

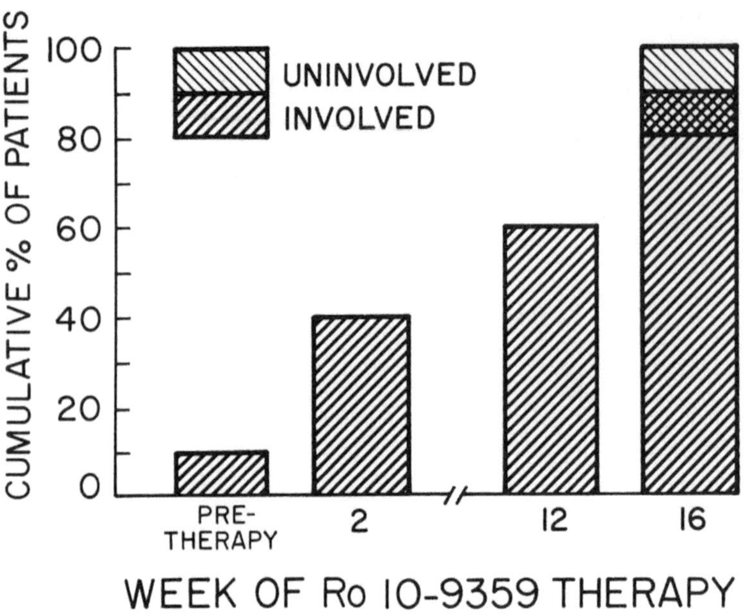

Fig. 3. Cumulative percent of patients who have demonstrated intercellular amorphous material in skin biopsies during Ro 10-9359 therapy

In one patient, the material was found in involved skin prior to as well as during retinoid therapy. The intercellular material was seen in only two biopsies from normal-appearing uninvolved skin; in both cases, this occurred after the 12th week of retinoid therapy. However, as patients improved during therapy, it frequently became difficult to distinguish involved and uninvolved skin. As a result, we suspect that the RSM seen in uninvolved skin in two patients actually represented positive findings in skin with sub-clinical psoriatic involvement. The data are summarized in the Table 1 and presented graphically in Figure 3. No abnormal intercellular material was seen in biopsies from 5 untreated controls.

Clinical correlation: Onset of RSM was not temporally associated with overall clearing in our patients. Clinical improvement was noted in all patients within the first two weeks of therapy, at which point only 4 of our patients demonstrated RSM. Interestingly, the single patient with pre-therapy deposition of RSM had the most rapid response to Ro 10-9359, with nearly complete resolution of pustular psoriasis of the palms and soles within two weeks. Nevertheless, the only patient who failed to respond satisfactorily to Ro 10-9359 showed RSM in lesional skin. In general, therefore, detection of RSM is not a predictor of clinical response. Side effects and laboratory abnormalities, while mild or minimal, did not relate to onset of RSM.

Comment

This study shows that the aromatic retinoid, Ro 10-9359, is associated with the deposition of a finely granular, amorphous appearing material in the skin of psoriatic patients which is readily visible in EMs. Skin biopsies of nine patients did not show the substance prior to retinoid administration, yet eight of these patients demonstrated deposition of the material in lesional psoriatic skin, and the ninth had deposits in normal-appearing skin, during Ro 10-

9359 therapy. In our tenth patient, the substance was observed in pre- and post-therapy biopsies.

Vitamin A and retinoid derivatives are known to induce mucous metaplasia in many epithelial tissues (1, 15, 17, 18, 19). RSM may well be a glycoconjugate elaborated by the keratinocyte as proposed by other authors (12, 14, 17, 20), although proof that this is indeed the case is not conclusive. Such theories about the composition of RSM are based on non-specific histochemical techniques for staining such glycoconjugates. Further studies will be required to determine whether RSM represents an alteration of the normal protein synthesis by epidermal cells.

Alternatively, RSM may be non-epidermal in origin; for example, plasma proteins exuded from the dermis. Since plasma proteins have frequently been demonstrated in psoriatic lesions (5, 6, 7, 8), it is possible that RSM is a serum component. If Ro 10-9359 causes increased fenestrations in the basal lamina as shown for vitamin A and retinoic acid (4, 14, 16), dermal substances could enter the epidermal intercellular spaces, appearing as RSM. This study showed RSM in intracellular membrane-bound collections, which may indicate active pinocytosis by cells.

Finally, RSM may be a cell surface product of epidermal cells. The epidermal intercellular substances are thought to be formed by interacting cell surface molecules, which may be glycoconjugates integral or peripheral to epidermal cell membranes (3). RSM may accumulate in the intercellular space by increased production within epidermal cells for transport to the cell surface, or by increased synthesis at the cell membrane.

RSM, or substances with a similar appearance in EMs, has been demonstrated pre-therapy by us and others (5, 11, 12); thus, the material may represent a component of psoriatic epidermis which is secondarily increased or produced in greater quantities during Ro 10-9359 therapy. However, it would be of significant concern if RSM occurs in serum, in other epithelial tissues, or in other organs. Further investigation is required to elucidate the chemical nature and biologic activity of RSM.

Conclusions

1. Ro 10-9359, an effective therapy for psoriasis, caused increased amounts of a finely-granular amorphous material to be deposited in epidermal intercellular spaces.

2. The substance, which we term retinoid-stimulated material (RSM), can rarely be seen pre-therapy.

3. It has not been possible to correlate RSM directly with clinical response.

4. Although the nature of RSM has not been elucidated, it may represent a) altered cell products; b) secondary infiltration of material into dilated intercellular spaces; or c) cell-surface glycoconjugates.

Summary

The aromatic retinoid, Ro 10-9359, was given orally to ten patients for the treatment of varying types of psoriasis. Skin biopsies from all patients undergoing Ro 10-9359 therapy demonstrated a finely-granular amorphous material in epidermal intercellular spaces by electron microscopic technique. This retinoid-stimulated material (RSM) was seen pre-therapy in only one patient. Nine of ten patients had very good or excellent clearing of psoriasis with Ro 10-9359, but clinical response did not correlate with the appearance of RSM. Studies are underway to establish the nature of RSM.

Acknowledgment. Ro 10-9359 was supplied by Hoffmann-La Roche, Inc., Nutley, N.J. (Drs. Dorothy B. Windhorst and Carl W. Ehmann).

References

1. Bellows CG, Hardy MH (1977) Histochemical evidence of mucosubstances in the metaplastic epidermis and hair follicles produced *in vitro* in the presence of excess vitamin A. Anat Rec 18: 257-272
2. Bundino S, Zina AM (1980) Disseminated porokeratosis Mibelli treated with Ro 10-9359. Dermatologica 160:328-336
3. Diaz LA (1979) Molecular structure of the epidermal extracellular spaces. Int J Dermatol 18: 434-442
4. Hardy MH, Sweeny PR, Bellows CG (1978) The effects of vitamin A on the epidermis of the fetal mouse in organ culture - an ultrastructural study. J Ultrastruct Res 64:246-260
5. Kimura S (1977) Composition and mechanism of deposition of the intercellular substance in parakeratotic psoriatic epidermis. J Dermatol (Tokyo) 4:179-185
6. Kimura S, Nishikawa T (1978) An immunohistochemical analysis of the deposited immunoglobulins of fibrinogen in parakeratotic psoriatic horny layer and pemphigus skin lesions. Arch Dermatol Res 261:55-62
7. Kimura S, Nishikawa T (1980) A further study on the mechanism of deposition of plasma protein in psoriasis scale. Arch Dermatol Res 268:79-84
8. Krogh HK, Tønder O (1973) Antibodies in psoriatic scales. Scand J Immunol 2:45-51
9. Matter A, Bollag W (1977) A fine structural study on the therapeutic effect of an aromatic retinoid on chemically-induced skin papilloma of the mouse. Eur J Cancer 13:831-838
10. Mayer H, Bollag W, Hänni R, Ruegg R (1978) Retinoids, a new class of compounds with prophylactic and therapeutic activities in oncology and dermatology. Experientia 34:1105-1119
11. Nagy-Vezekényi C, Zs-Nagy I (1971) Studies on the ultrastructure of psoriasis and of the "normal" skin of psoriatics. Acta Derm Vener (Stockh) 51:435-443
12. Orfanos CE, Runne U (1978) Tissue changes in psoriatic plaques after oral administration of retinoid. Dermatologica 157 (Suppl. 1):19-25
13. Orfanos CE, Schaumburg-Lever G, Mahrle G, Lever WF (1973) Alterations of cell surfaces as a pathogenetic factor in psoriasis. Arch Dermatol 107:38-46
14. Peck GL, Elias PM, Wetzel B (1977) Effects of retinoic acid on embryonic chick skin. J Invest Dermatol 69:463-476
15. Prutkin L (1975) Mucus metaplasia and gap junctions in the vitamin A acid-treated skin tumor, keratoacanthoma. Cancer Res 35:364-369
16. Sagami S, Kitano Y (1970) Electron microscopic study of the effect of vitamin A on the differentiation of reconstructed embryonic chick skin. Br J Dermatol 83:565-571
17. Tsambaos D, Mahrle G, Orfanos CE (1980) Epidermal changes induced by oral excess of aromatic retinoid in guinea pigs. Arch Dermatol Res 267:141-152
18. Wilkoff LJ, Peckham JC, Dulmadge EA, Mowry RW, Chopra DP (1976) Evaluation of vitamin A analogs in modulating epithelial differentiation of 13-day chick embryo metatarsal skin explants. Cancer Res 36:964-972
19. Wong YC (1975) Mucous metaplasia of the hamster check pouch epithelium under hypervitaminosis A. Exp Mol Pathol 23:132-143
20. Williams ML, Elias PM (1980) The pathogenesis of skin fragility from systemic retinoids is epidermal in origin. Clin Res 28:585A (Abstract)

C.E. Orfanos et al. (eds.)
Retinoids

Effects of Oral Retinoid on Dermal Components in Human and Animal Skin

D. Tsambaos and C.E. Orfanos

In the past few years, a vast amount of evidence has demonstrated the profound influence of oral aromatic retinoid Ro 10-9359 on the growth and differentiation of epithelial cells (2, 15, 19, 22). Though some experimental observations have led to the suggestion that also the dermis may be a target tissue for retinoids, little attention has been paid to dermal changes under oral retinoid therapy. Thus, the effects of Ro 10-9359 on the dermis remained almost entirely unknown.

The object of this paper is to present data derived from the morphological approach to the interesting aspect of oral aromatic retinoid action on dermal tissue. We have ourselves been concerned with the study of structural alterations occurring in normal guinea pig dermis under excessive doses of oral Ro 10-9359 and in psoriatic dermis under therapeutic doses of this compound.

Material and Methods

Animal experiments with excessive doses: Aromatic retinoid Ro 10-9359* (15 mg/kg/day in arachis oil) was orally administered to 10 male albino guinea pigs (300 g) for a period of two weeks. 10 control animals received corresponding quantities of arachis oil. Skin biopsies taken from the snout, ears, back and from the flank area of retinoid-treated and control guinea pigs were embedded in paraffin, stained with hematoxylin-eosin and PAS stains and were finally examined by light microscopy.
Application of therapeutic doses in psoriasis: Skin biopsies were obtained from typical lesions of 4 patients with chronic stationary psoriasis and of 1 patient with pustular psoriasis before and 1, 2 and 3 weeks after the beginning of oral treatment with the aromatic retinoid (1 mg/kg/day). The specimens were fixed in 4% formaldehyde and 2.5% glutaraldehyde, buffered with sodium cacodylate (pH 7.2) and were postfixed in 1% osmium tetroxide solution. After dehydration in rising concentrations of acetone, the samples were embedded in Araldite.

Ultrathin sections stained with uranyl acetate and lead citrate were examined with Zeiss EM 9A and EM 10 C electron microscopes.

Results

Guinea pig skin: After two weeks of oral retinoid administration the treated animals developed erythema, edema and scaling of the skin, whereas the controls showed no obvious clinical alteration. There were clear quantitative differences in the expression of retinoid-induced changes in various skin regions of the same animal; they were more

---

* The aromatic retinoid Ro 10-9359 was kindly supplied by Dr. R. Hennes (Hoffmann-La Roche AG, Grenzach-Wyhlen).

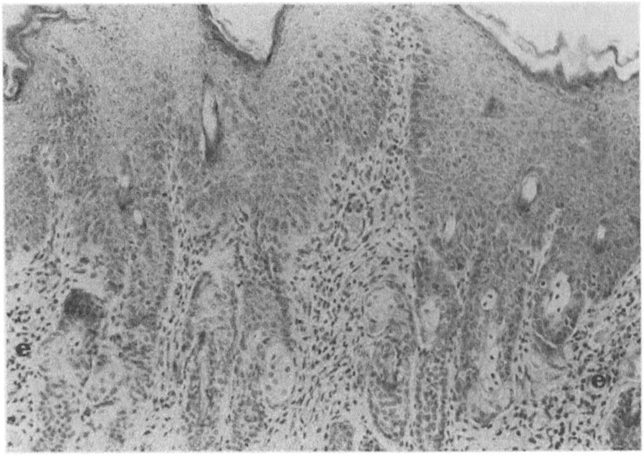

Fig. 1. A relatively dense cellular infiltrate with numerous eosinophils (e) can be seen under an acanthotic epidermis with focal parakeratosis. Guinea-pig skin: snout region; after 2 weeks of retinoid administration

pronounced at the ear and snout than at the back and flank area, as assessed by clinical and histological criteria. On light microscopy, the epidermis revealed increased desquamation, hypergranulosis and acanthosis with psoriasiform elongation of the rete ridges. Particularly in specimens obtained from the snout a parakeratotic horny layer could be clearly seen. Dermal vessels were often dilated and mildly engorged with erythrocytes. The density of the cellular infiltrate in the upper and mid-dermis varied greatly from site to site. It was minimal in the back skin and prominent in the snout region (Fig. 1); the infiltrate consisted of polymorphonuclear neutrophils, histiocytes, some lymphocytic cells and numerous eosinophils (Fig. 2). In several specimens the dermis was clearly thickened showing a marked fibroplasia with numerous fibrocytes arranged in a parallel array and densely packed collagen fibers.

Psoriatic (involved) skin: After one week of retinoid administration psoriatic dermis was

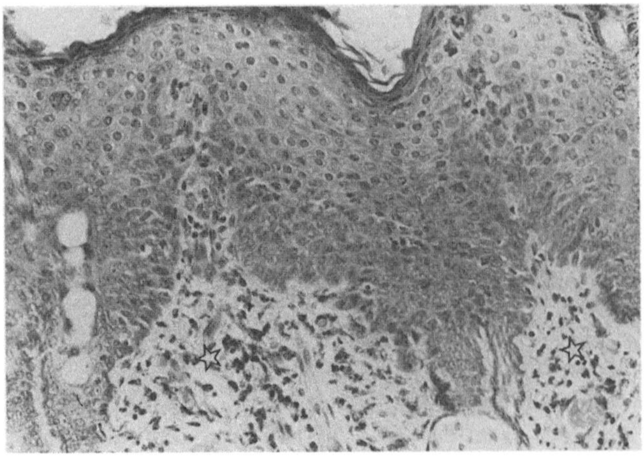

Fig. 2. Large numbers of eosinophils (stars) and spindle-shaped connective tissue cells can be observed in the papillary and upper dermis. Guinea-pig skin; snout region; after 2 weeks of retinoid administration

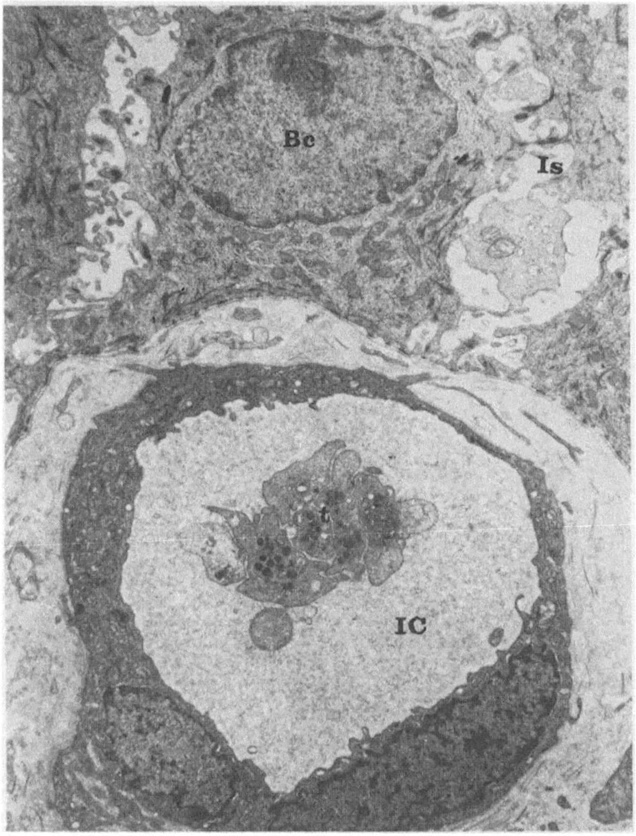

Fig. 3. Psoriasis vulgaris (after 3 weeks of treatment): Intrapapillary capillary (IC) revealing a moderate dilatation and an almost normal microarchitecture (Bc = basal epidermal cell; Is = intercellular space; t = thrombocytes: × 6,400

still edematous. In the dermoepidermal junction a focal rarefaction of the anchoring fibrils and an amorphous granular material, possibly exudate, could be observed.

The vessels in the papillary and upper dermis were still thin-walled, abnormally dilated and revealed endothelial gaps and fenestrations, as in the pretreatment phase. After two and three weeks of therapy, however, dermal edema was less pronounced and tendency to vascular normalization was clearly seen (Fig. 3). Dilatation was reduced; gaps and fenestrations were less frequent than before treatment.

In an attempt to estimate the Ro 10-9359 effects on vascular dilatation in psoriasis, we determined the outside endothelial diameter of the crest in 15 intrapapillary capillary loops before and in 23 after 3 weeks of treatment. It was found that the diameter of the crest measured 12.3 ± 4.8 nm in the untreated psoriatic dermis and had been reduced to 9.1 ± 3.7 nm after 3 weeks of oral retinoid administration.

In the untreated dermis of pustular psoriatic lesions migration of neutrophils was evident (Fig. 4). Large numbers of neutrophils passed through the endothelial walls into the dermis. After one week of retinoid therapy numerous neutrophils were still seen in the lumen of the vessels but their migration into the dermis was clearly reduced, although dermal vessels were not normalized (Fig. 5). Migration of neutrophils was further progressively reduced within the second and third week of therapy.

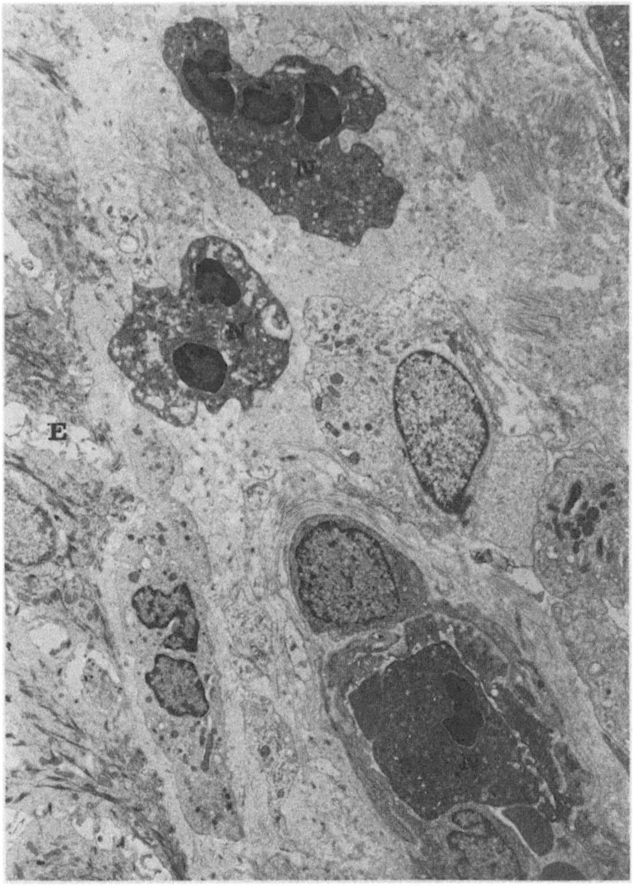

Fig. 4. Pustular psoriasis (before treatment): Migration of neutrophils (N) through the endothelial walls into the dermis is evident (E = epidermis; × 3,470)

In chronic psoriatic plaques, the density of the cellular infiltrate remained unchanged during the first 3 weeks of retinoid therapy. However, some alterations were found in its composition. In the retinoid-treated psoriatic dermis, lymphocytic cells with deeply indented nuclei, resembling Sézary cells (Fig. 6), could be seen in increased number, as compared to the pretreatment phase. Also large monocytic cells with differentiation into activated macrophages were found to be increased under retinoid treatment. In their cytoplasm, phagolysosomes, myelin figures, lipid droplets, vesicles, crystalloid inclusions and worm-like structures were present. Dermal Langerhans' cells, which were rare before therapy, were quite frequent under retinoid (Fig. 7), revealed prominent cytoplasmic activity and, in some instances, more than one nuclear profiles (Fig. 8). The considerable cytoplasmic activity of fibroblasts in the untreated psoriatic skin seemed to be markedly enhanced under retinoid treatment. The numbers of mast cells remained unchanged, as compared to the pretreatment phase. After therapy, however, membrane fusion of their granules, degranulation figures and lipid droplets were more often seen.

Discussion

The molecular mechanisms by which aromatic retinoid Ro 10-9359 exerts its modulating

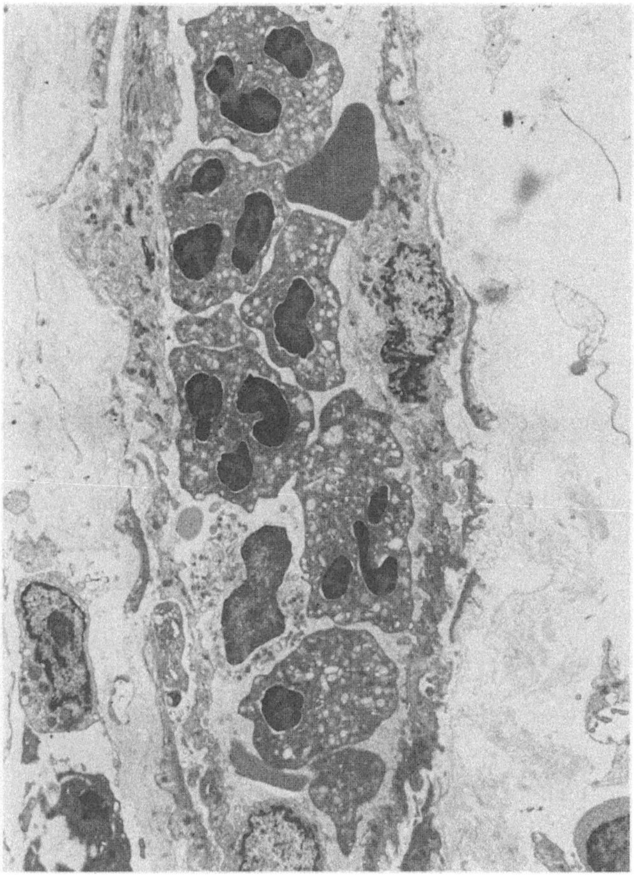

Fig. 5. Pustular psoriasis (after 1 week of treatment): The lumen of a post-capillary venule is filled with neutrophils; however, migration of neutrophils is not seen (× 3,490)

effect on epithelial differentiation are far from being clearly understood. The results of the present study point out that, apart from the epidermis, also the dermis undergoes distinct alterations under oral administration of this compound. Considering the possible interactions between epithelial cells and cellular or fibrous components of the mesenchyme, it may be suggested, that the effects of Ro 10-9359 on dermal tissue may have far-reaching implications in the mechanisms of retinoid action on normal and pathological skin.

In guinea pigs, a two-week administration of excessive oral doses of Ro 10-9359 induced a psoriasiform dermatitis, which was clinically characterized by erythema, edema and scaling of the skin. There were marked quantitative differences in the expression of these changes in various skin regions of the treated animals; they were more pronounced at the snout and ears, suggesting a higher susceptibility of these areas to the drug. However, with regard to the prominent changes at the snout, it cannot be ruled out that during oral application small amounts of Ro 10-9359 may have also exerted some local effect on this region. On light microscopy, under a hyperplastic and focally parakeratotic epidermis, dermis revealed prominent vessels, a cellular infiltrate of varying density and in some places intense fibroplasia. The large number of eosinophils present in the retinoid-treated dermis was remarkable. Since in our experiments eosinophils were rare in the dermis of control

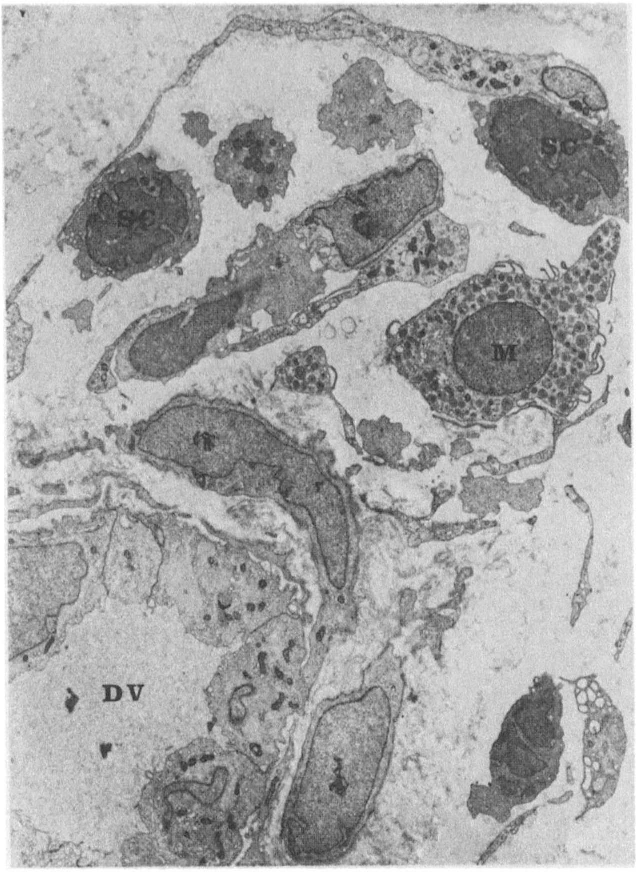

Fig. 6. Psoriasis vulgaris (after 3 weeks of treatment): In the close vicinity of a dermal vessel (DV), Sézary-like lymphocytic cells (SC) with deeply indented nuclei and mast cell (M) with fusion of granule membranes and reduced electron density of granule content (× 3,390)

animals, an implication of the vehicle (arachis oil) in the enhancement of eosinophil migration observed under retinoid seems unlikely. It may be postulated, therefore, that excessive doses of oral retinoid may result to a release of eosinophilic chemotactic factors in normal guinea-pig dermis (14) or to an enhancement of receptor sites for chemotactic factors at the eosinophils (1).

The intense fibroplasia observed in some instances after Ro 10-9359 administration cannot be definitely regarded as a retinoid effect, because the phases of the hair cycle in these regions have not been considered. A possible retinoid-induced stimulation of fibroblasts in guinea-pig dermis under the present experimental conditions should be, however, kept in mind, if one takes into account that the main metabolite of Ro 10-9359 stimulates in vitro fibroblastic cell lines by increasing the number of the available receptor sites for epidermal growth factor (10).

We do not consider the above described changes to be specific for Ro 10-9359. At least some of the other retinoids may induce similar, even identical alterations, if they are administered in sufficient quantities. However, we cannot exclude the possibility that the changes produced by excessive retinoid doses in the dermis, traditionally regarded as

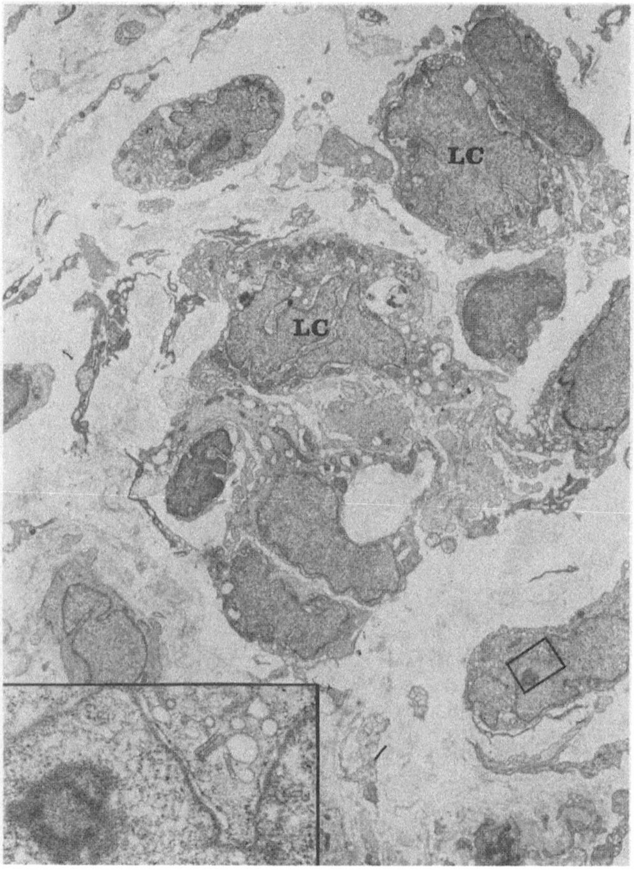

Fig. 7. Psoriasis vulgaris (after 2 weeks of treatment): Langerhans' cells (LC) in the dermal infiltrate of psoriatic lesions, showing prominent cytoplasmic activity (× 3,340) and typical Langerhans' granules (inset; × 18,250)

simple "toxic irritant" effects, may be implicated in the mechanisms of retinoid action on the epidermis.

The most important ultrastructural changes in psoriatic dermis under oral treatment with the aromatic retinoid Ro 10-9359 were a) the partial restoration of psoriatic vascular abnormalities, b) the inhibition of neutrophil migration (in pustular psoriasis) and c) the increase of Sézary-like lymphocytic cells, activated macrophages and dermal Langerhans' cells in the cellular infiltrate. The effects of retinoid therapy on dermal vessels in psoriasis may be not specific for the drug, since they have been also observed under topical treatment with dithranol and other antipsoriatic agents (Unpublished data). On the other hand, the impressive inhibition of neutrophil migration, already after one week of retinoid administration before a tendency towards vascular normalization became evident, seems to represent evidence for neutrophils being targets of retinoid action. One can speculate that aromatic retinoid may interact with neutrophil surface receptors or may suppress mechanisms, which lead to the production of neutrophil chemotactic factors; alternatively, it may induce the release of diverse factors with inhibitory effect on the chemotactic responsiveness and migration of neutrophils. The mechanisms leading to the accumulation of neu-

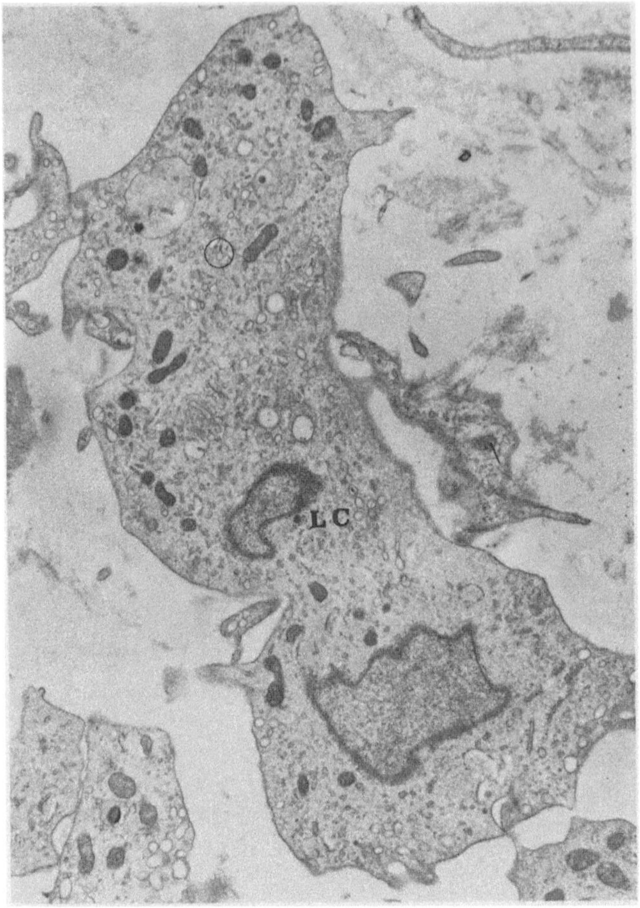

Fig. 8. Psoriasis vulgaris (after 3 weeks of treatment): Large dermal Langerhans' cell (LC) with two nuclear profiles, numerous vesicles and Langerhans' granules (circle) (× 8,420)

trophils in psoriatic lesions (4), particularly in the pustular ones, are not yet fully understood. However, it seems to be beyond doubt that neutrophils are of importance in the pathogenesis of this disease (8). Thus, it is possible that the dramatic efficacy of oral aromatic retinoid in pustular psoriasis may be due, at least in part, to the reduction in the numbers of neutrophils migrating into the dermis and epidermis. – Sézary-like cells may occur in normal epithelial tissues and are considered to originate from lymphocytes; they are probably of T-cell nature since they reveal membrane receptors for uncoated sheep erythrocytes (7). Increased numbers of Sézary-like cells have been observed in oral mucosa in mice subsequent to antigenic challenge (3). In human dermis accumulation of these cells occurs under pathological conditions, particularly in those with concomitant antigenic persistence, such as mycosis fungoides. They can be occasionally seen in psoriatic dermis before treatment (5) and were also described in psoriasis after local treatment with retinoic acid (16). The increase of these cells in psoriatic dermis under oral administration of aromatic retinoid, as shown in the present study, may represent an enhanced differentiation of lymphocytes into this cell line due to a) a direct effect of the drug or b) to the influence of changes induced by the retinoid in the microenvironment of lymphocytes.

For a long time the origin and the function of skin Langerhans' cells have remained an unresolved enigma. Recently it has been shown that Langerhans' cells are most likely immunocompetent cells derived from a mobile cell pool, which originates in the bone marrow (11). Monocytes seem to be their precursors, since Langerhans' cells possess surface markers of the monocyte-histiocyte-macrophage series expressing Fc-IgG and C_3 receptors (21). Furthermore, Langerhans' cells circulating between epidermis, dermis and vessels can obviously function both as stimulators in a mixed lymphocyte reaction and as antigen-presenting cells (20). An increased number of Langerhans' cells has been reported in the human and animal dermis in contact allergic hypersensitivity reactions (18). The increased number of dermal Langerhans' cells and activated macrophages in psoriasis under treatment with Ro 10-9359 suggests that this drug may be capable of stimulating the monocytes to further differentiation in tissue. This speculative hypothesis is consistent with the accelerating effect of retinoid on allogeneic graft rejection (13), in which Langerhans' cells are considered to have an important role (11). Interestingly enough, topical excess of vitamin A on the mouse tail scale skin results: 1. to the conversion of the parakeratotic epidermis into an orthokeratotic one and 2. to the stimulation of dermal cells (9) with features of Langerhans' cells, which invade the epidermis (17).

The data presented here, though purely morphological, suggest that Ro 10-9359 may affect immunocompetent cells in psoriasis modulating the immune response. In recent years, there has been growing evidence that some defect of the immune-inflammatory cell function including T-lymphocytes may occur in psoriasis (6, 12). However, the relationship between these abnormalities and the pathogenesis of epidermal hyperproliferation in this disease is far from being clearly understood. It remains to be elucidated, therefore, whether a possible immunomodulatory activity of aromatic retinoid may be of importance for its therapeutic effect in psoriasis.

Conclusions and Summary

Retinoids are known to elicit various biological and biochemical responses from epithelial tissues in vivo and in vitro. In human skin, distinct structural alterations of normal and pathological keratinocytes have been reported under therapeutic doses of the aromatic derivative Ro 10-9359. We have also described marked epidermal changes in guinea-pig epidermis after high dosage of this compound (Tsambaos et al. 1980). Further investigations under similar conditions (15 mg/kg/day p.o. in arachis oil) in guinea pigs and careful evaluation of several biopsies embedded for light- and electron microscopy under oral retinoid treatment (75 mg/d) in humans showed that well defined alterations of dermal components also regularly occur. In guinea pigs, skin biopsies taken from the snout, flank, back and ear after 2 weeks of retinoid administration revealed dilated and hyperemic dermal vessels, some cellular infiltrate of mononuclear cells and eosinophils, and increasing amount of connective tissue cells with focal swelling of collagen. These changes were more pronounced in certain skin regions, e.g. ears and snout. Dermal components of diseased human skin, particularly in psoriasis, underwent distinct alterations under treatment with the oral retinoid: The dermoepidermal junction showed edematous changes with rarefication of the anchoring fibrils; the vessels were still abnormally dilated and showed some endothelial swelling, but the overall changes including gaps and fenestrations seemed to be less pronounced after 3 weeks of therapy; the cellular infiltrate showed activated macrophages and fibroblasts, the numbers of granulocytes were decreased, and increasing numbers of Sézary-like lymphocytic cells and dermal Langerhans' cells were detected. Finally, some edematous disintegration of collagen fibres and accumulation of amorphous ground substances were clearly present after 3 weeks in the upper dermis. These observations indicate that the oral retinoid Ro 10-9359, additionally to its action on the epidermis, exerts two distinct influences on dermal components in guinea-pig and in human skin at different dose levels: (a) It leads to dermal edema increasing the amorphous ground substances and (b) it modulates the cellular tissue response due to stimulation of macrophages, lymphocytic cells and dermal Langerhans' cells.

Acknowledgment. We thank Mrs. E. Bodeux, Köln, and Miss M. Hoffmann, Berlin, for their skilful technical assistance. - Part of these results were published in the Brit J Dermatol (1981).

References

1. Anwar ARG, Kay AB (1978) Enhancement of human eosinophil complement receptors by pharmacologic mediators. J Immunol 121:1245–1250
2. Bollag W, Hanck A (1977) From Vitamin A to retinoids. Modern trends in the field of oncology and dermatology. Acta Vitaminol Enzymol (Milano) 31:113–123
3. Burkhardt A, Bos IR, Löning T, Gebbers JO, Otto HF, Seifert G (1979) Interepithelial cells of the oral mucosa in mice. An ultrastructural classification with reflections on the origin of the Langerhans cells. Virchows Arch [Pathol Anat] 384:223–244
4. Cormane RH, Hunyadi J, Hamerlinck F (1976) The role of lymphoid cells and polymorphonuclear leukocytes in the pathogenesis of psoriasis: Proceedings of the Second International Symposium. Farber EM, Cox AJ (eds). Yorke Medical Books. New York, pp 47–54
5. Flaxman BA, Zelazny G, Van Scott EJ (1971) Nonspecificity of characteristic cells in mycosis fungoides. Arch Dermatol 104:141–147
6. Glinski W, Obalek S, Langner A, Jablonska S, Hafted M (1978) Defective function of T lymphocytes in psoriasis. J Invest Dermatol 70:105–110
7. Gupta S, Safai B, Good RA (1978) Subpopulations of human T lymphocytes. IV. Quantitation and distribution in patients with mycosis fungoides and Sézary syndrome. Cell Immunol 39:18–26
8. Jabłońska S, Beutner EH, Binder WL, Jarząbek-Chorzelska M, Rzesa G, Chowaniec O (1979) Immunopathology of psoriasis. Arch Dermatol Res 264:65–71
9. Jarrett A, Wrench R, Mahmoud B (1979) Granular layer induction following the topical application of proliferating agents. Arch Dermatol Res 264:143–151
10. Jetten AM (1980) Retinoids specifically enhance the number of epidermal growth factor receptors. Nature 284:626–629
11. Katz SI, Tamaki K, Sachs DH (1979) Epidermal Langerhans cells are derived from cells originating in bone marrow. Nature 282:324–326
12. Krueger GG, Hill HR, Jederberg WW (1978) Inflammatory and immune cell function in psoriasis - a subtile disorder. I. In vivo and in vitro survey. J Invest Dermatol 71:189–194
13. Mayer H, Bollag W, Hänni R, Rüegg R (1978) Retinoids, a new class of compounds with prophylactic and therapeutic activities in oncology and dermatology. Experientia 34:1105–1119
14. Olsson I, Venge P (1979) The role of the eosinophil granulocyte in the inflammatory reaction. Allergy 34:353–367
15. Orfanos CE (1979) Retinoide - eine Breitspektrum- Dermatotherapie? Schweiz med Wochenschr 109:1909–1911
16. Orfanos CE, Schmidt HW, Mahrle G, Gartmann H, Lever WF (1973) Retinoic acid in psoriasis: its value for topical therapy with and without corticosteroids. Brit J Dermatol 88:167–182
17. Schweizer J, Marks F (1977) A developmental study of the distribution and frequency of Langerhans cells in relation to formation of patterning in mouse tail epidermis. J Invest Dermatol 69: 198–204
18. Silberberg I, Baer RL, Rosenthal SA (1976) The role of Langerhans cells in allergic contact hypersensitivity. A review of findings in man and guinea pigs. J Invest Dermatol 66:210–217
19. Sporn MB, Dunlop NM, Newton DL, Henderson WR (1976) Relationship between structure and activity of retinoids. Nature 263:110–113
20. Stingl G, Katz CI, Clement L, Green I, Shevach EM (1978) Immunologic functions of Ia-bearing epidermal Langerhans cells. J Immunol 121:2005–2013
21. Stingl G, Wolff-Schreiner EC, Pichler W, Gschnait F, Knapp W, Wolff K (1977) Epidermal Langerhans cells bear Fe and C_3 receptors. Nature 268:245–246
22. Tsambaos D, Mahrle G, Orfanos CE (1980) Epidermal changes induced by oral excess of aromatic retinoid in guinea pigs. Arch Dermatol Res 267:141–152

C.E. Orfanos et al. (eds.)
Retinoids

Retinoid-binding Proteins and the Plasma Transport of Etretinate (Ro 10-9359) in Man

A. Vahlquist, G. Michaëlsson, A. Kober, I. Sjöholm, G. Palmskog and U. Pettersson

Retinoids (vitamin A and its analogs) are too hydrophobic to be dissolved in water. In biological fluids they form complexes with proteins and lipids. In plasma, the naturally occurring retinyl esters are associated with the lipoproteins until they reach the liver (9). Retinol is released from the liver bound equimolarily to the retinol-binding protein (RBP) (6) and cell-surface receptors for RBP are involved in the delivery of the vitamin to epithelia (14).

Retinoic acid, an active metabolite of retinol, has been detected in plasma in small amounts (2). In rats given this retinoid, albumin has been found to be a main plasma carrier (18). This is surprising in view of the high affinity between RBP and retinoic acid observed in vitro (1), but is explained by the fact that retinoic acid is not taken up by the liver and therefore not incorporated into RBP in situ (11).

A prolonged supplementation of rats with retinoic acid is claimed to cause a lowering of the plasma retinol level and a concurrent increase in the liver vitamin A concentration (7). The opposite effect, a rise of plasma vitamin A, was observed, however, in patients treated systemically with retinoic acid (5). The interactions between natural and artificial retinoids have thus been a matter of controversy.

Retinoids other than retinol probably enter the cells from a pool of free molecules. Their affinity to extracellular proteins will accordingly affect the availability of the compounds. Protein interactions will also influence the pharmacodynamics of systemic retinoid treatment. The binding and plasma transport of etretinate (Ro 10-9359), the ethyl ester of an aromatic analog of retinoic acid, has not been reported in man. It is also unknown whether this compound alone or its main metabolite, the free acid (Ro 10-1670), is responsible for the biological effect of the drug.

This paper deals with the pharmacokinetics of etretinate in healthy controls and in patients with psoriasis with special regards to the affinity of the aromatic retinoids to plasma proteins. The effects of etretinate therapy on the serum levels of retinol and RBP are also reported.

Material and Methods

Patients: In six male patients with psoriasis (aged 22–46 years; body weight 65–90 kg) the pharmacokinetics of a single oral dose of etretinate was studied. Five of the patients, all of whom had a widespread psoriasis, participated also in a multiple-dose study two months later. In two of the patients the elimination of the drug was additionally studied after 6 and 12 months, respectively, of etretinate treatment with a daily dosage of 50 mg. Apart from their psoriasis the patients were healthy and had only indifferent topical treatment.

Controls: Five healthy men (aged 24–34 years, body weight 65–85 kg) took part in the single-dose pharmacokinetic study. They used no drugs.

Pharmacokinetic Protocol

Single-dose study. At 8.00 am 75 mg of etretinate in three capsules were taken with 200 ml water before breakfast. No food had been allowed after midnight. A light breakfast was taken within half an hour after ingestion of the drug. Controls and patients stayed in the hospital during the study and had the same types of meal. Blood was drawn under dim-red light before the capsules were taken and at various times thereafter up to 24 hours.

Multiple-dose study. One 25-mg capsule of etretinate was taken three times daily for 10 days. On day 11 the drug was taken only in the morning. Blood samples were drawn before the first capsule and then twice daily before and 3 hours after the morning capsule. On day 11 and on the following 1–3 days blood was drawn repeatedly.

Materials

Tritium-labeled Ro 10-9359 and 10-1670 (200 mCi/mmole) and the corresponding unlabeled drugs were obtained from Hoffmann-La Roche, Basle. The radiochemical purity always exceeded 98%. Human serum albumin was purchased from KABI AB, Sweden, and was used without further purification. RBP was prepared from human urine (19). The purity was 80% and about 50% of the protein contained retinol. Other chemicals were of analytical grade.

Serum Analysis

Retinol was determined by a fluorometric procedure as outlined earlier (20). RBP was measured using radial immunodiffusion (10). The aromatic retinoids were analyzed by high-pressure liquid chromatography (HPLC) as described separately (12). There was no interference between retinol and the aromatic retinoids in the assays.

Gel chromatographic separations of plasma proteins were accomplished on a column of Sephadex G-100 (50 × 1.5 cm) equilibrated with 0.02 M Tris-HCl (pH 7.4) + 0.2 M NaCl. The collected fractions (3 ml) were assayed for proteins by the absorption at 280 nm and for retinoids by HPLC and fluorometry (see above).

Protein-binding

Microparticles containing albumin, RBP or a mixture of human serum proteins were prepared (3). The binding of ^{3}H-retinoids to the immobilized proteins was studied using different amounts of retinoids added in a physiologically buffered water-ethanol (5%) solution under protection from light. The radioactivity remaining in the supernatant after equilibration was measured (8). Appropriate controls with microparticles devoid of protein were included. The data were analyzed according to Scatchard (17) or Rosenthal (15).

Results

Pharmacokinetics

In Fig. 1 the plasma levels of Ro 10-9359 and Ro 10-1670 at various times after a single oral dose of etretinate are shown for one of the controls. Six subjects (one patient and five controls) were studied long enough to permit a calculation of the β-slope. The mean half-lives ($t_{1/2}$) of Ro 10-9359 and Ro 10-1670 were 8.3 and 8.9 hours, and the median volumes of dis-

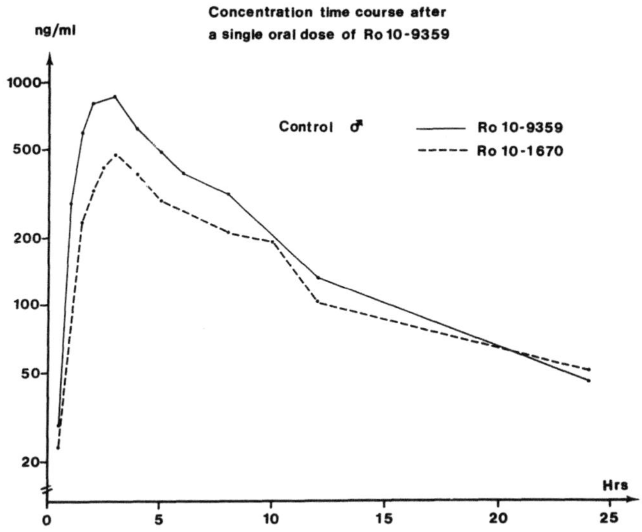

Fig. 1. A semi-logarithmic plot of the plasma concentrations of the aromatic retinoids at various times (hours) after the ingestion of etretinate (75 mg)

tribution 150 and 210 l, respectively. In Table 1 the maximal serum concentrations of the two retinoids after 3–6 hours are given. It can be seen that the concentrations of Ro 10-9359 in the psoriatic patients were always lower than those of the controls. The difference between the mean values is highly significant ($p < 0.001$). In the patients the concentration of Ro 10-1670 sometimes exceeded that of Ro 10-9359, but again the psoriatics had a lower mean level than the controls although the difference was not statistically significant.

In the multiple-dose study, the serum retinoid values (measured before the morning dose) reached a maximum by the third day (4–600 ng/ml for Ro 10-9359 and 2–300 ng/ml for Ro 10-1670). When the treatment was stopped after 11 days, the $t\frac{1}{2}$ was 17 hours for Ro 10-9359 in the patient studied long enough to permit a prediction of the final slope.

The elimination rate of the two retinoids at the end of a one year maintenance treatment

Table 1. Maximal serum concentrations of aromatic retinoids after a single dose of etretinate (75 mg) in male volunteers

Order by magnitude of Ro 10-9359 values	Diagnosis	Maximal concentration (ng/ml) Ro 10-9359		Ro 10-1670	
1	Psoriasis	294	$\bar{x} = 545$	271	$\bar{x} = 470$
2	Psoriasis	454		510	
3	Psoriasis	487		515	
4	Psoriasis	520		573	
5	Psoriasis	726		423	
6	Psoriasis	788		533	
7	Healthy control	855	$\bar{x} = 930$	397	$\bar{x} = 583$
8	Healthy control	865		764	
9	Healthy control	927		697	
10	Healthy control	969		517	
11	Healthy control	1030		542	

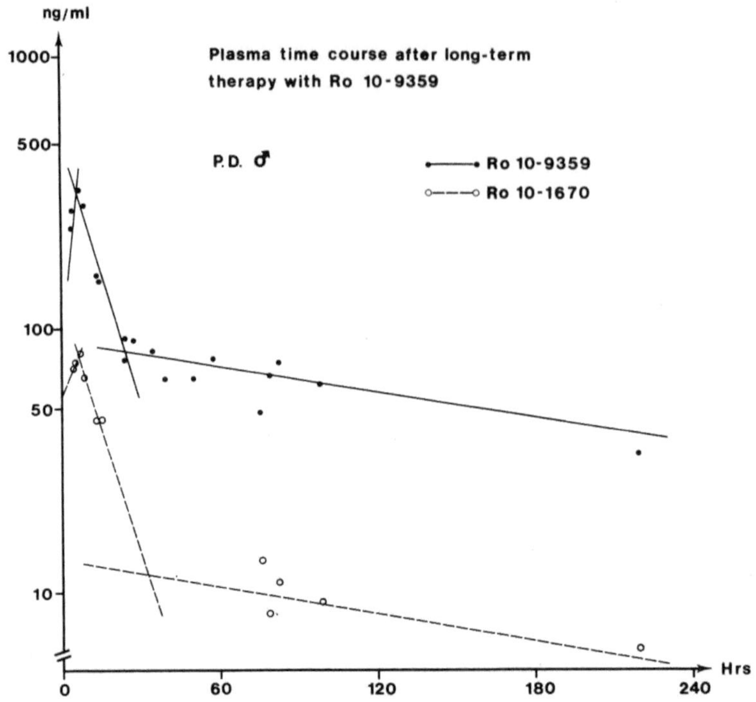

Fig. 2. The plasma disappearance of aromatic retinoids during 10 days after cessation of etretinate therapy. The last dose (25 mg) of a one-year schedule was taken at time zero. The exponentials drawn in the figure are the regression lines

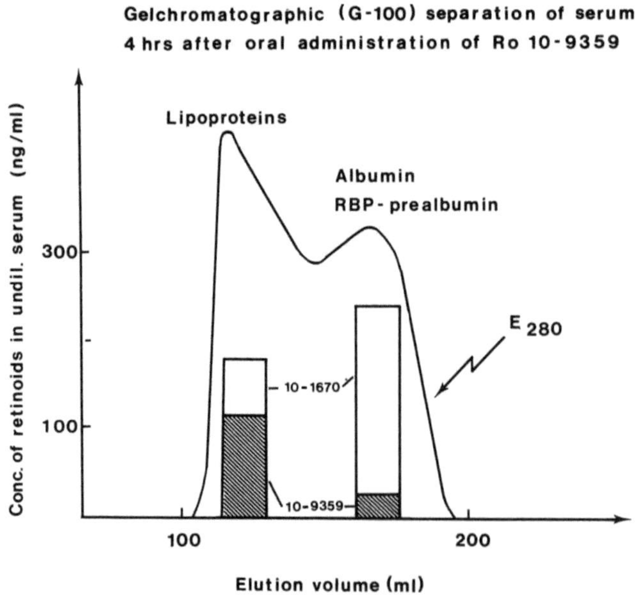

Fig. 3. Gel chromatography of plasma from a patient treated with etretinate (50 mg daily). The full-drawn curve indicates the protein profile (extinction units omitted). The bars indicate the concentration of aromatic retinoids in pooled fractions recalculated to undiluted plasma

Table 2. Percentual distribution of aromatic retinoids and retinol in two main protein fractions obtained by gel chromatography of fasting plasma[a]

Fraction	Ro 10-9359 %	Ro 10-1670 %	Retinol %
"Lipoproteins"	85	33	5
"Albumin/ RBP"	15	67	95

[a]Mean values of 4 samples from different persons and at various times after the administration of etretinate

with etretinate is shown in Fig. 2. This patient received a total of 16 g of etretinate and the $t^1/_2$ of the last slope observed within 10 days was 136 hours for Ro 10-9359. For the other patient the $t\frac{1}{2}$ was 76 hours after receiving a total of 8 g of the drug during 6 months.

Binding of Aromatic Retinoids to Plasma Proteins

Fig. 3 shows a chromatography of plasma proteins obtained from a psoriatic patient 4 hours after the oral administration of 50 mg of etretinate (maintenance treatment). The two retinoids were found in fractions containing lipoproteins and albumin, respectively. The distribution of the retinoids between these two plasma fractions differed for Ro 10-9359 and Ro 10-1670. In Table 2 the results from repeated experiments are summarized. The distribution of natural vitamin A (retinol) is shown for reference. RBP did not separate from albumin by the chromatography. This necessitated a further characterization in vitro of the affinity of the aromatic retinoids to various purified proteins (Table 3). Serum albumin seemed to have a strong primary binding site for 10-9359. Several secondary sites were also active (not shown) having about the same affinity for Ro 10-9359 as the binding sites for Ro 10-1670. The binding of Ro 10-9359 to RBP exhibited an association constant (K_a) similar to that of its interaction with albumin. However, a calculation of the total binding capacity at physiological concentrations of the two proteins, reveals that albumin is by far the main carrier since its concentration is a 1000-fold higher than that of RBP. The coinciding results

Table 3. Some characteristics of the binding of aromatic retinoids to human plasma proteins[a]

Retinoid	Protein	$n \cdot K_a$[b] $(M^{-1}) \times 10^6$	n	K_a $(M^{-1}) \times 10^6$
Ro 10-9359	Albumin	3.6	1.0	3.6
Ro 10-1670	Albumin	0.9	2.0	0.45
Ro 10-9359	RBP	3.0	--[d]	--
Ro 10-9359	Serum proteins[c]	3.2	1.2	2.7
Ro 10-1670	Serum proteins[c]	0.9	1.2	0.75

[a]The binding was measured in vitro with the proteins immobilized in microparticles at pH 7.4 and 22 °C. K_a denotes the association constant and n the number of sites
[b]The accumulated association constant
[c]Not containing lipoproteins. The data were calculated on the basis of a protein concentration equal to albumin
[d]Analysis according to Rosenthal (15); therefore only data for the accumulated binding available

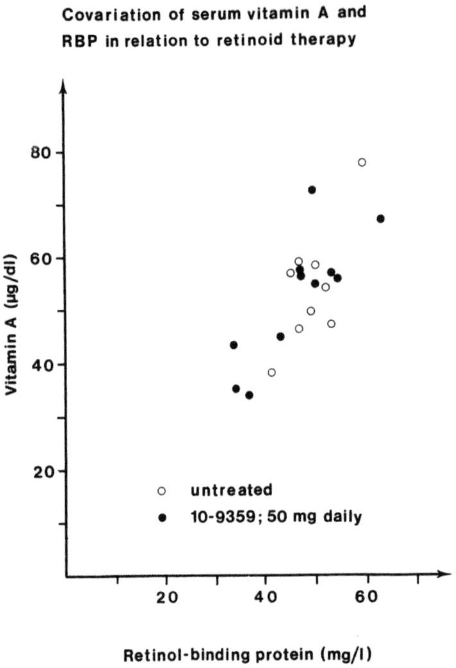

Fig. 4. Correlation between plasma levels of RBP and vitamin A (retinol) in patients before and during etretinate treatment (fasting blood samples)

obtained with albumin and the mixture of serum proteins unequivocally show that albumin is the predominant retinoid-binding protein apart from the lipoproteins.

Effects of Retinoid Treatment on the Levels of RBP and Vitamin A

Serum samples from 11 patients were examined before and after the initiation of etretinate treatment. The correlation between the serum concentrations of vitamin A and RBP was unaffected by the treatment (Fig. 4). Also, the mean RBP level did not change significantly during the treatment (Table 4).

Discussion

Several studies have emphasized the rapid turnover in plasma of retinoic acid (11). In the present study of an aromatic analog of retinoic acid (Ro 10-9359) the $t\frac{1}{2}$ of the ß-slope after a

Table 4. Effects of etretinate treatment on the serum RBP level

Schedule & No. of patients[a]		RBP (mg/l) (mean ± SD)		
Short-term (25 mg x 3 n = 4)	Pre-treatment 44.8 ± 8.2	4 days 41.0 ± 7.1	7 days 42.3 ± 6.1	11 days 44.3 ± 7.3
Long-term (25 mg x 2 n = 7)	Pre-treatment 44.3 ± 4.6	1 month 46.5 ± 8.2	2-3 months 49.3 ± 7.2	4-6 months 44.7 ± 7.1

[a] Male patients suffering from psoriasis and Darier's disease

single dose was found to be about 8 hours. The main metabolite, Ro 10-1670, appeared in plasma shortly after Ro 10-9359 and its concentration subsequently paralleled that of the latter compound. Some subjects had higher levels of Ro 10-1670 than of Ro 10-9359. This was only seen in the psoriatic patients who at the same time had peak values of Ro 10-9359 consistently lower than the controls. We do not know if this reflects a poorer absorption of the drug in the psoriatics of perhaps a different mode of transport and metabolism of retinoids.

The pharmacokinetics changed when the treatment with etretinate was extended for several weeks. In one patient treated for 1 year, the $t^1/_2$ for the elimination of the loast dose was twenty times higher than after a single dose. This indicates that the drug accumulates in some "deep" compartment as has been suggested by Paravicini (personal communication). The distribution volume of etretinate after a single dose was about 150 l. This points to a pronounced tissue binding of the drug which is remarkable considering its high binding degree in plasma (less than 2% of the drug occurs in its free form).

The microparticle technique used to study the protein binding in vitro offers several advantages over conventional techniques (3, 8). Unspecific interactions of retinoids with surfaces can be corrected for. A drawback is that lipoproteins are likely to be denaturated during the preparation of the microparticles from a mixture of serum proteins. Therefore, to obtain information about the binding of the retinoids to lipoproteins, gel chromatography experiments were undertaken. Our results show that Ro 10-9359, in spite of a high affinity for albumin also found by others (16), is predominantly bound to the lipoproteins. Ro 10-1670, like retinoic acid (18), is bound mainly to albumin. None of the aromatic retinoids is to an appreciable amount transported by RBP. One reason for this is that retinol, the natural ligand of RBP is already firmly attached to the protein when it is secreted from the liver and the amounts of apo-RBP in plasma available for the interaction with other retinoids is exceedingly small (13).

In the therapeutic situation the molar concentration of the aromatic retinoids will be less than 1% that of serum albumin. Also, several sites are involved in the binding of the retinoids to albumin. Therefore, it is highly unlikely that significant amounts of the retinoids can be displaced by other compounds.

In the patients treated with etretinate no significant changes of the plasma levels of vitamin A and RBP occurred. This might indicate that etretinate, in contrast to retinoic acid in rats (4, 7) does not interfere with the transport of vitamin A (at least not in the therapeutic range of concentration). Data are missing, however, regarding the turn over and metabolism of vitamin A during etretinate treatment. It is therefore premature to determine whether or not the aromatic retinoids function independently of vitamin A.

Summary

The pharmacokinetics and the protein-binding of etretinate (Ro 10-9359) were studied in psoriatic patients and healthy controls. The maximal plasma concentration of the retinoid was attained 3–6 hours after a single oral dose and was markedly lower in the psoriatics than in the controls ($p<0.001$). The rate of disappearance ($t^1/_2$) was 8 hours after the single dose, 17 hours after treatment for 10 days and 136 hours after one year of treatment. The main metabolite, Ro 10-1670, had similar kinetics but its plasma concentration was usually lower than for the parent retinoid. Both compounds were to $>98\%$ bound to the plasma proteins. The lipoproteins were the main carriers for Ro 10-9359 (the retinoid ester) whereas albumin carried most of the free retinoid. The K_a for the interaction with albumin was in the order of 10^6 M^{-1}. During treatment with etretinate there seemed to be no interference with the plasma transport of vitamin A and retinol-binding protein.

Acknowledgments. We wish to thank Ass. Prof. L. Rask for providing RBP and Mrs. E. Hagforsen, I. Phil-Lundin, I.L. Backlund and Mrs. S. Gebre-Medhin for skilful technical assistance. This study was supported by the Swedish Medical Research Council (grant no. B 81-03x-05174-04 A), the Swedish Psoriasis Foundation and the Welander Foundation.

References

1. Cogan U, Kopelman M, Mokady S, Shinitzky M (1976) Binding affinities of retinol and related compounds to retinol-binding proteins. Eur J Biochem 65:71–78
2. De Ruyter MG, Lambert WE, De Leeuheer AP (1979) Retinoic acid: An endogenous compound of human blood. Anal Biochem 98:402–409
3. Ekman B, Sjöholm I (1978) Improved stability of proteins immobilized in microparticles prepared by a modified emulsion polymerization technique. J Pharm Sci 67:107–109
4. Gerber LE, Erdman JE (1980) Comparative effects of all-trans and 13-cis retinoic acid administration on serum and liver lipids in rats. J Nutr 110:343–351
5. Günther S, Alston W (1973) Follicular keratoses. Dermatologica 147:274–283
6. Kanai M, Raz A, Goodman De WS (1968) Retinol-binding protein: the transport protein for vitamin A in human plasma. J Clin Invest 47:2025–2044
7. Keilson B, Underwood BA, Loerch JD (1979) Effects of retinoic acid on the mobilization of vitamin A from the liver in rats. J Nutr 109:785–797
8. Kober A, Ekman B, Sjöholm I (1978) Direct and indirect determination of binding constants of drug-protein complexes with microparticles. J Pharm Sci 67:693–696
9. Krinsky NI, Cornwell DG, Oncley JL (1958) The transport of vitamin A and carotenoids in human plasma. Arch Biochem Biophys 73:223–246
10. Michaëlsson G, Vahlquist A, Juhlin L, Mellbin T, Bratt L (1976) Zinc and vitamin A. Serum concentrations of zinc and RBP in healthy adolescents. Scand J Clin Lab Invest 36:827–832
11. Ott DB, Lachance PA, Lachance MS (1979) Retinoic acid – a review. Am J Clin Nutr 32:2522–2531
12. Palmskog G (1980) Determination of plasma levels of two aromatic retinoic acid analogues with antipsoriatic activity by high-performance liquid chromatography. J Chromatogr 221:345–351
13. Peterson PA, Nilsson JF, Östberg L, Rask L, Vahlquist A (1974) Aspects on the metabolism of retinol-binding protein and retinol. Vitam Horm 32:181–214
14. Rask L, Peterson PA (1976) In vitro uptake of vitamin A from the retinol-binding plasma protein to mucosal epithelial cells from monkey's small intestine. J Biol Chem 251:6360–6366
15. Rosenthal HE (1967) A graphic method for the determination and presentation of binding parameters in a complex system. Anal Biochem 20:525–532
16. Sani BP, Titus BC, Banerjee CK (1978) Determination of binding affinities of retinoids to retinoic acid-binding protein and serum albumin. Biochem J 171:711–717
17. Scatchard G (1949) The attraction of proteins for small molecules and ions. Ann NY Acad Sci 51:660–692
18. Smith JE, Milch PO, Muto Y, Goodman De WS (1973) The plasma transport and metabolism of retinoic acid in the rat. Biochem J 132:821–827
19. Vahlquist A, Nilsson SF, Peterson PA (1971) Isolation of the human retinol-binding protein by affinity chromatography. Eur J Biochem 20:160–168
20. Vahlquist A, Michaëlsson G, Juhlin L (1978) Acne treatment with oral zinc and vitamin A: Effects on the serum levels of zinc and RBP. Acta Derm Venerol (Stockh) 58:437–442

C.E. Orfanos et al. (eds.)
Retinoids

Biochemical Mechanism of Modulation of Skin Carcinogenesis by Retinoids

Ajit K. Verma

Vitamin A acid (retinoic acid), a major metabolite of retinol or retinyl esters (8, 11, 16), is required to maintain normal growth and differentiation of epithelial tissues (54, 58), but it cannot replace retinal to support the visual function and reproduction (15, 19). Epidemiological study and evidence from experimental animals indicate a close association between retinoic acid deficiency and enhanced susceptibility to chemical carcinogenesis of the respiratory system, bladder, and colon (30, 42). Retinoic acid has been used in experimental animals to prevent and treat cancers of a variety of epithelial tissues (bronchi and trachea, stomach, intestine, uterus, kidney and bladder, testis, prostate, pancreatic ducts, and skin), the target sites of the origin of cancer (3, 26, 32, 42, 51). The pharmacological use of natural retinoids in chemoprevention of cancer is handicapped by their toxic effects (hypervitaminosis syndromes) (3). Recently, a number of retinoids have been synthesized in an attempt to obtain compounds with less host toxicity and with greater antitumorigenicity, which have been found to be superior in the prevention of cancer of skin, lung, bladder, and breast in animals (3, 33, 41). In addition, retinoids have therapeutic effects in skin diseases such as acne, psoriasis, and ichthyosis (1, 35). Retinoids reverse carcinogen-induced lesions in tissue culture (13, 28) and influence the growth of tumor cell lines (24).

The molecular mechanism of prevention of chemical carcinogenesis by retinoids is not clear. It is known that there is a relationship between the role of vitamin A in controlling epithelial cell differentiation and the development of malignancy in epithelial tissues. Intracellular cytosolic retinoic acid-binding protein, which is distinct from well-known serum retinol-binding protein, is probably involved in the transport of retinoic acid to specific sites within the cell for biochemical effects (36, 38). Retinol and retinoic acid play a role in the incorporation of mannose into glycoproteins of mammalian membranes, which fulfill a variety of biological functions, including cell adhesion, growth, and the reception of specific hormones (6, 10, 56). A direct relationship between glycosaminoglycan synthesis by chondrosarcoma chondrocytes and inhibition of tumor growth has been shown (40). Retinoic acid suppresses the production of interferon produced by virus by blocking the transcriptional step, suggesting that the site of action of retinoic acid is at the gene level (2). Furthermore, evidence indicates that the antineoplastic activity of retinoids may be mediated via stimulation of the host-immune response to tumor antigens (25). Our results (46–49, 51) of the effect of retinoic acid on skin tumor promotion by TPA indicate that one of the possible mechanisms of its inhibition of skin tumor promotion is via its inhibitory effect on ornithine decarboxylase (ODC, EC 4.1.1.17) induction by TPA, which will be the focus of this chapter. Data showing the effect of retinoids on TPA-induced polyamine biosynthesis, DNA synthesis, and hyperplasia will be presented, and the results that imply that the effect of retinoic acid on skin carcinogenesis is not universal will be summarized (53).

Experiments and Results

The experiments and results section will be divided into six subsections. The first will deal with the two-stage model of skin carcinogenesis. The second will review biochemical processes linked to tumor promotion by TPA. The third will summarize the effect of retinoids on TPA-induced polyamine biosynthesis and tumor promotion by TPA. The fourth will review the mechanism of inhibition by retinoic acid of ODC induction. The fifth will summarize the effect of retinoic acid on DNA synthesis, and hyperplasia caused by TPA. Finally, the evidence indicating that the effect of retinoic acid on skin carcinogenesis is not universal will be presented.

I. The Two-stage Model of Mouse Skin Carcinogenesis

The two-stage model of mouse skin carcinogenesis is a useful model system in which biochemical events unique to either initiation (first stage) or promotion (second stage) can be studied and related to cancer formation (4). Initiation can be accomplished by a single topical application of a carcinogen (e.g., 7, 12-dimethylbenz[a]anthracene (DMBA)) at a sufficiently small dose so that it will not lead to the development of visible tumors during the life span of the animal. However, many tumors result following repeated and prolonged applications to the initiated skin of another chemical known as a tumor promoter. Tumor promoters are not carcinogenic themselves; it is only their application following initiation that elicits tumors. 12-0-Tetradecanoylphorbol-13-acetate (TPA), a component of croton oil, is a very potent and useful tumor promoter (Fig. 1) (4, 52). The two-step model is an excellent quantitative model for the investigation of the biochemical mechanism of the action of agents, auch as retinoids, which modify tumor formation.

II. Biochemical and Biological Processes Linked to Tumor Promotion by TPA

The biochemical mechanism of tumor promotion by TPA has been extensively reviewed

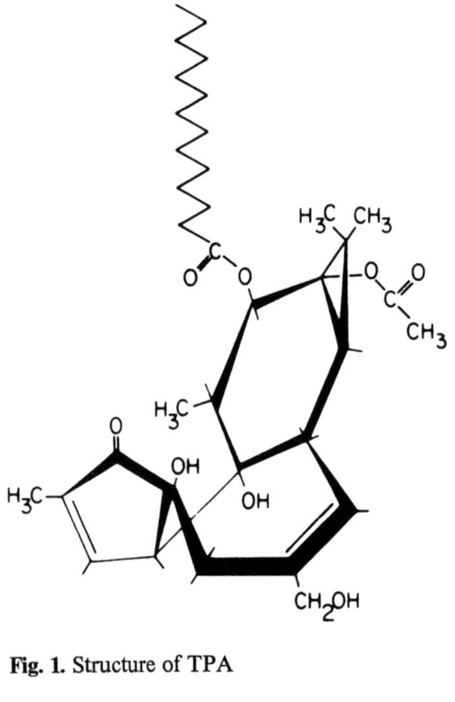

Fig. 1. Structure of TPA

(4, 12). Briefly, a single topical application of TPA to mouse skin leads to enhanced incorporation of ^{32}P into phospholipids, increased accumulation of prostaglandins, and to sequential activation of RNA, protein, and DNA synthesis. Other biochemical changes observed following TPA treatment include enhanced phosphorylation of nuclear histones, decreased histidase activity, altered cyclic nucleotide metabolism, induction of ODC and S-adenosylmethionine decarboxylase (SAMD, EC 4.1.1.50) activities, and accumulation of putrescine and spermidine in mouse epidermis (4, 12). Among the numerous biological effects of TPA in mouse epidermis are hyperplasia, altered terminal differentiation, and the induction of dark keratinocytes (12, 22).

Among the biochemical changes observed following TPA treatment to mouse skin, the induction of ODC activity is prominent (5, 34). Evidence from dose-response and structure-response studies showed a good correlation between the ability of an agent to induce ODC activity and to promote tumor formation (5, 34). The most convincing evidence to strengthen the concept that ODC induction is an important component of the mechanism of tumor promotion by TPA stemmed from the findings that retinoic acid applied in conjunction with TPA inhibits both the induction of ODC activity and tumor formation (46–49, 51).

III. Effects of Retinoids on TPA-stimulated Polyamine Biosynthesis and Tumor Promotion by TPA

ODC, which decarboxylates ornithine to putrescine, is the first and probably the rate-limiting step in the pathway of polyamine biosynthesis. S-Adenosyl-L-methionine decarboxylase, a second enzyme in the polyamine biosynthetic pathway, decarboxylates S-adenosyl-L-methionine; the propylamine moiety derived from S-adenosyl-L-methionine condenses with putrescine to form spermidine and with spermidine to form spermine (21).

The activities of the polyamine biosynthetic enzymes, especially ODC, and the levels of their biosynthetic products putrescine, spermidine, and spermine are elevated in various tissues stimulated to growth (21, 37). Several lines of evidence suggest that increased ODC activity and polyamine accumulation are important for the regulation of the synthesis of nucleic acid and protein (30). Furthermore, the polyamines and the enzymes that synthesize polyamines are implicated in neoplastic growth (21, 37, 51).

Accumulating evidence indicates that the induction of epidermal ODC activity is an important component of the mechanism of skin tumor promotion by TPA; this has been a

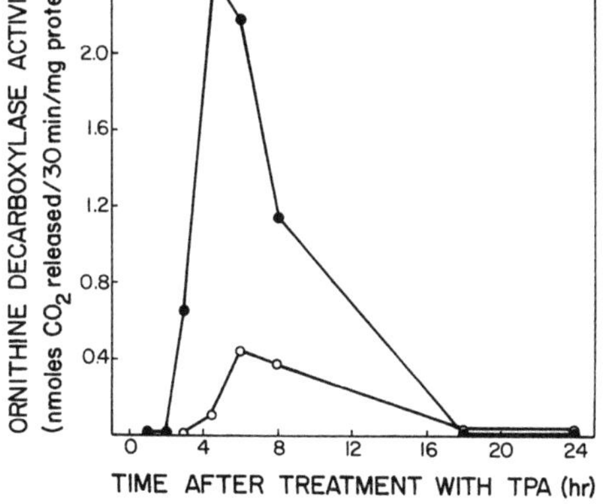

Fig. 2. The effect of pretreatment with retinoic acid on the induction of epidermal ODC activity by TPA. Groups of mice were treated with 1.7 nmoles of retinoic acid (○) or acetone (●) 1 h before treatment with 17 nmoles of TPA. Mice were killed for enzyme assay at the indicated times after application of TPA. Each point on the graph represents the average of triplicate determinations of enzyme activity from soluble epidermal extracts prepared from 4 mice

Table 1. The effect of various retinoids on the induction of epidermal ODC and S-adenosyl-L-methionine decarboxylase activities, and tumor promotion by TPA

All mice were initiated by topical application to skin of 0.2 µmol of DMBA in 0.2 ml of acetone; 2 weeks after initiation, mice were treated twice a week with either 0.2 ml of acetone or a retinoid in 0.2 ml of acetone 1 h before each treatment with 8 nmol of TPA. The analyses were made after the seventh TPA treatment and the tumor data were recorded at the twentieth week of promotion. For determination of ODC and S-adenosyl-L-methionine decarboxylase activities, mice were killed 4.5 and 24 h after TPA treatment, respectively. Each value represents the mean ± S.E. of determinations of enzyme activity from 3 groups of mice, and each group contained the combined supernatant prepared from 3 or 4 mice

Treatment	Dose (nmol)	ODC activity	S-adenosyl-L-methionine decarboxylase activity	A 20 weeks of promotion	
		($nmol\ CO_2$/30 min/mg protein)		Pa[a]/mouse	% with Pa[a]
None		0.02	0.04 ± 0.01	None	None
Acetone		3.5 ± 0.4	0.14 ± 0.01	9.9	90
β-Retinoic acid	34	0.04	0.12 ± 0.00	1.7	54
13-cis-Retinoic acid	34	0.5 ± 0.1	0.14 ± 0.01	3.7	48
TMMP[b] analog of ethyl retinoate	140	0.5 ± 0.1	0.14 ± 0.01	1.5	42
TMHP[c] analog of ethyl retinoate	140	3.3 ± 0.7	0.14 ± 0.01	12.9	92
13-Trifluoromethyl-TMMP analog of ethyl retinoate	140	3.8 ± 0.7	0.13 ± 0.01	9.6	100

[a]papillomas [b]trimethylmethoxyphenyl [c]trimethylhydroxyphenyl

topic of recent reviews (5, 51) and all will not be presented here. In this section, will review the findings that the mechanism of inhibition by retinoic acid of tumor promotion by TPA involves its ability to inhibit the induction of ODC activity and the resultant accumulation of putrescine (46–49, 51).

1. Application of retinoic acid 1 h before application of 17 nmol of TPA inhibited the induction of ODC activity in a dose-dependent manner (46). Retinoic acid pretreatment did not alter the time course of ODC induction by TPA (Fig. 2, reference 46).

Retinoic acid also inhibited skin tumor promotion by TPA in a dose-dependent manner. Thus, application of 1.7 and 17 nmol of retinoic acid 1 h prior to each promotion treatment with TPA to DMBA-initiated skin resulted in 57% and 75% reduction in the number of papillomas per mouse respectively. A similar dose-dependent inhibitory effect was observed on carcinoma incidence (46, 48, 49).

2. Application of certain retinoids in conjunction with TPA inhibited the induction of ODC activity as well as skin tumor formation, but none of them was more active than retinoic acid (Table 1). Retinoids, which inhibited skin tumor promotion, inhibited the accumulation of putrescine, but inhibited neither the induction of SAMD activity nor spermidine by TPA (Tables 1 and 2).

3. Recently (9, 27), it has been shown that 5,6-epoxyretinoic acid may be an active metabolite of retinoic acid. We compared the effect of 5,6-epoxyretinoic acid with retinoic acid and 5,6-dihydroretinoic acid on both the induction of ODC activity and tumor promotion by TPA (49). Application of 5,6-epoxy-retinoic acid 1 h after each application of TPA to the initiated mouse skin inhibited the formation of skin tumors as effectively as did

Table 2. Effects of treatment with retinoids on TPA-caused accumulation of polyamines

Acetone or a retinoid in acetone was applied 1 h before application of 17 nmoles TPA to the shaved backs of CD-1 mice. Control mice were not treated at all. The levels of polyamines were determined 8 h after TPA treatment as described (47)

Treatment	Dose of retinoids (nmoles)	Polyamines (nmoles/mg DNA)		
		Putrescine	Spermidine	Spermine
Control		26 ± 2[a]	70 ± 2	45 ± 5
Acetone		83 ± 8	105 ± 11	60 ± 5
β-Retinoic acid	17	31 ± 7	124 ± 23	48 ± 4
13-cis-Retinoic acid	17	34 ± 3	124 ± 5	52 ± 2
TMMP analog of ethyl retinoate	68	36 ± 4	129 ± 1	63 ± 4
TMHP analog of ethyl retinoate	68	63 ± 3	143 ± 10	68 ± 10

[a] Each value represents the mean ± S.E. of determinations carried out on 3 groups of mice with 3 mice/group

retinoic acid. Furthermore, 5,6-dihydroretinoic acid, which is a poor substrate for epoxidation, also inhibited skin tumor promotion. A similar effect was seen on the induction of ODC activity by TPA (Table 3). These results indicate that epoxidation of retinoic acid at the 5,6-position is not a rare-limiting modification for the antipromoting activity of retinoic acid.

4. Additional evidence to support the concept that ODC induction is relevant to tumor promotion by TPA and the mechanism of inhibition by retinoic acid of skin tumor promotion involves its ability to inhibit ODC induction, emerged from the experimental results described herein. Groups of mice were treated with 34 nmol of retinoic acid 24 h after each treatment with 8 nmol of TPA, the time point when maximum ODC induction had passed and ODC levels had completely returned to original control values (Fig. 3). This retinoic

Table 3. Inhibition by retinoids of the induction of ODC activity and skin tumor promotion by TPA

CD-1 mice were intitiaed with 0.2 µmol of DMBA in 0.2 ml of acetone. Beginning 2 weeks after initiation, mice were treated twice weekly with 5 nmol of TPA for the duration of the experiment (22 weeks). Mice were treated with retinoids in 0.2 ml of acetone 1 h after each treatment with TPA. Control mice were treated with acetone only. To test for ODC induction, separate groups of mice were used which were treated only once with the retinoid 1 h after treatment with 5 nmol of TPA and were killed for ODC assay 4.5 h after TPA treatment

Treatment	Dose (nmol)	ODC activity (nmol CO_2/30 min/mg protein	Papillomas/ mouse	% with papillomas
Acetone		2.92 ± 0.11[a]	3.5	65
Retinoic acid	17	0.50 ± 0.20	0.22	15
5,6-Epoxyretinoic acid	17	0.48 ± 0.06	0.19	12
5,6-Dihydroretinoic acid	17	0.72 ± 0.25	0.68	36

[a] Mean ± S.E. of determination carried out from 3 groups of mice with 3 mice/group

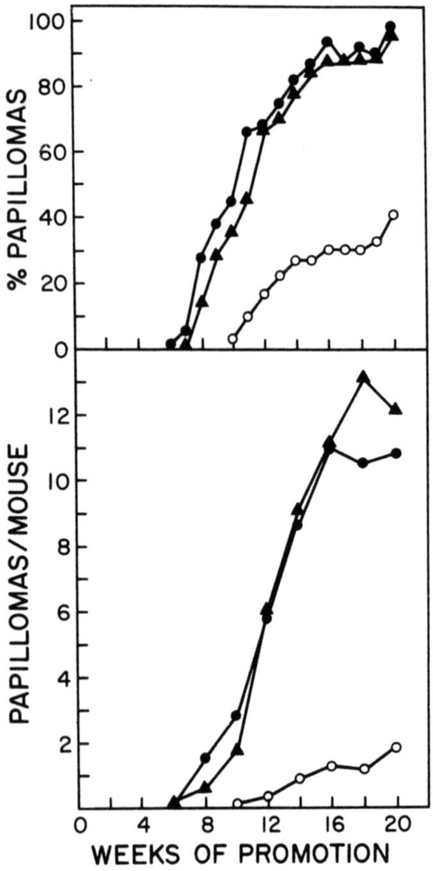

Fig. 3. The effect of retinoic acid treatment on the formation of skin tumors. All mice were initiated with a single topical application of 0.2 μmol of DMBA to mouse skin. After 2 weeks, retinoic acid, 17 nmol (○) or acetone (●) was applied 1 h before each promotion with 8 nmol of TPA twice weekly; retinoic acid, 17 nmol was applied 24 h after each TPA treatment (▲)

acid treatment did not affect the tumor incidence, whereas in the same experiment, the same solution of retinoic acid applied 1 h before each TPA promotion treatment produced an 84% reduction in the number of papillomas per mouse and there were only 42% papilloma-bearing mice (Fig. 3).

5. Topical application of retinoic acid in conjunction with an initiating dose of DMBA fails to inhibit tumor formation elicited by repeated applications of TPA (48, 51).

IV. How Does Retinoic Acid Inhibit the Induction of ODC Activity by TPA?

The exact biochemical mechanism by which retinoic acid inhibits the induction of ODC activity by TPA is not clearly understood. However, some clues about the retinoic acid mechanism will be summarized in this section.

1. The inhibitory effect of retinoic acid on ODC induction was not the result of nonspecific cytotoxicity, because retinoic acid treatment inhibited the induction of ODC activity and failed to affect S-adenosylmethionine decarboxylase induction measured in the epidermal extracts prepared from the same groups of mice (Table 1, reference 46).

2. Retinoic acid treatment may not lead to the production of a soluble inhibitor of the ODC enzyme.

a) Soluble supernatants from mouse epidermis treated with either acetone or as much as 68 nmol of retinoic acid before application of either acetone or TPA were prepared, and

Table 4. ODC activity in mixed soluble epidermal extracts prepared from acetone- or TPA-treated mouse epidermis pretreated with either acetone or retinoic acid

Mice were treated with acetone or 68 nmoles of retinoic acid in acetone 1 h before application of acetone or 10 nmoles of TPA in acetone. Mice were killed 4.5 h after the latter treatment; soluble epidermal extracts were prepared, and ODC activity in extracts was determined. Each value is the mean of triplicate determinations of enzyme activity from 4 groups of mice; each group contained the combined extracts from 3 mice

Treatment	ODC activity (nmoles CO_2 released/30 min)
A. Retinoic acid - Acetone	0.010
B. Acetone - TPA	0.318
C. Retinoic acid - TPA	0.012
A + B	
Calculated	0.328
Experimental	0.337
B + C	
Calculated	0.330
Experimental	0.362

ODC activity in individual and mixed supernatants was determined. A mixture of extracts prepared from retinoic acid and acetone-treated mouse epidermis gave simple additive ODC activity (Table 4). This argues against the production of a soluble inhibitor of the ODC enzyme. However, further experimentation is required to refute that retinoic acid treatment does not lead to the production of an antizyme as reported by Heller et al. (20) in H-35 rat hepatoma cells in culture after treatment with putrescine.

b) Retinoic acid-caused inhibition of TPA-induced ODC activity could not be reversed

Table 5. Effect of retinoic acid on incorporation of tritiated histidine and leucine into mouse epidermal protein

Mice were treated with acetone or 17 nmol of retinoic acid (RA) in acetone 1 h before application of acetone or 10 nmol of TPA in acetone to the shaved backs of mice. Mice were killed at the indicated times after the latter treatment. Tritiated precursor was injected intraperitoneally 1 h before sacrifice. Incorporation of tritiated precursors into epidermal proteins was determined as described before (50).

Time	Fold-increase over acetone control			
	^{3}H-histidine incorporation		^{3}H-leucine incorporation	
h	Acetone[a]	RA[b]	Acetone[a]	RA[b]
3	1.60	1.51	1.46	1.20
6	1.92	2.00	1.89	2.09
12	2.68	2.58	-	-
24	2.99	2.74	1.83	1.69
48	2.82	-	1.56	-
60	2.92	-	1.54	-
72	1.85	1.80	1.41	1.34

[a] $\frac{\text{Acetone - 1 h - TPA}}{\text{Acetone - 1 h - Acetone}}$ [b] $\frac{\text{RA - 1 h - TPA}}{\text{RA - 1 h - Acetone}}$

by extensive dialysis of epidermal extracts. In this experiment, groups of mice were treated with acetone or 17 nmol of retinoic acid 1 h before application of 5 nmol of TPA, and epidermal supernatants were prepared. Epidermal supernatants were dialyzed against three changes (200 ml) of 50 mM sodium phosphate buffer (pH 7.2) containing 0.1 mM EDTA and 0.1 mM pyridoxal phosphate. ODC activity in acetone and retinoic acid treatment groups were 2.5 and 0.2 nmol CO_2/30 min/mg protein respectively.

3. Inhibition of ODC induction was not the result of an inhibitory effect of retinoic acid on general protein synthesis. The results are shown in Table 5. In this experiment, mice were treated with acetone or 17 nmol of retinoic acid in acetone 1 h before application of 17 nmol of TPA. Incorporation of tritiated leucine or histidine into epidermal proteins was determined at the indicated times after TPA treatment. TPA treatment resulted in about a 2- to 3-fold increase in amino acid incorporation as early as 6 h following treatment. Retinoic acid pretreatment did not inhibit increased protein synthesis at any of the time points studied. These results indicate that retinoic acid may be selectively inhibiting the synthesis of the ODC protein.

4. Although it remains to be determined whether in mouse skin retinoic acid interferes with the early effects of TPA such as membrane interaction (binding of TPA with membrane protein, glycoprotein, and phospholipid synthesis), the findings (Fig. 4) that retinoic acid inhibits the induction of ODC activity by 80% even when applied 2 h after TPA strongly argues against such en effect. We have shown that TPA-caused accumulation of PGE_2 plays a role in the induction of ODC activity because indomethacin, an inhibitor of prostaglandin synthesis, inhibits the induction of ODC activity by TPA, and this inhibition can be overcome by concurrent application of PGE_2 with TPA (50). The results shown in Table 6 indicate that the inhibition of the induction of ODC activity by retinoic acid may not involve synthesis of PGE_2.

5. TPA-caused increase in ODC activity is inhibited by inhibitors of protein (cycloheximide) and RNA (5-azacytidine) synthesis (34). This suggests that ODC induction involves new protein and RNA synthesis. It is not known whether retinoic acid inhibits ODC induction at the transcriptional and/or posttranscriptional levels. To prove that retinoic acid inhibits the synthesis of the ODC enzyme caused by TPA, one has to demonstrate a decrease in immunoprecipitable protein after treatment with antibodies monospecific to ODC. The results (Fig. 5) of the effect of retinoic acid treatment on the kinetic parameters (apparent K_m and V_{max}) for the enzyme induced by TPA suggest that retinoic acid may inhibit the synthesis of the ODC enzyme. In this experiment, mice

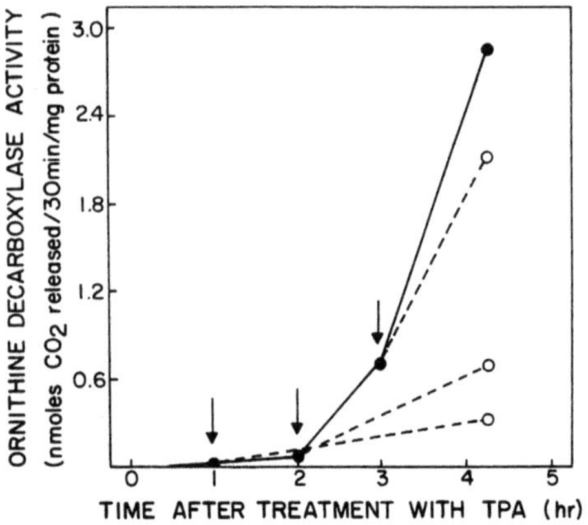

Fig. 4. The effect of posttreatment with retinoic acid on TPA-induced epidermal ODC activity. Mice were killed at the indicated times after application of 17 nmoles of TPA (●). In other groups, 1.7 nmoles of retinoic acid was applied at 1, 2, or 3 h after treatment with 17 nmoles of TPA as indicated by arrows. Mice were killed at 4.25 h after application of TPA (O) for enzyme assay. Each point represents the mean of triplicate determinations of enzyme activity from combined epidermal extracts prepared from 4 mice

Table 6. Effect of PGE_2 on indomethacin- or retinoic acid-caused inhibition of the induction of ODC activity

Groups of mice were treated with acetone, 280 nmol of indomethacin, or 0.17 nmol of retinoic acid 2 h prior to treatment with 5 nmol of TPA or 5 nmol of TPA containing 70 or 140 nmol of PGE_2. Mice were killed 4.5 h after the last treatment, and soluble epidermal ODC activity was determined. Each value represents the mean ± S.E. of determinations carried out on 3 groups of mice with 3 mice/group

Treatment	ODC activity ($nmol/CO_2/30$ min/ mg protein)	% of control
Acetone + acetone	0.02	
Acetone + TPA	5.81 ± 0.15	100
Indomethacin + TPA	1.38 ± 0.41	24
Indomethacin + TPA + PGE_2[a]	6.37 ± 0.78	110
Retinoic acid + TPA	0.85 ± 0.08	15
Retinoic acid + TPA + PGE_2[a]	1.18 ± 0.14	20
Retinoic acid + TPA + PGE_2[b]	0.85 ± 0.14	15
Indomethacin + retinoic acid + TPA	0.14 ± 0.08	2

[a] 70 nmol PGE_2
[b] 140 nmol PGE_2

were treated with acetone or 17 nmol of retinoic acid 1 h before application of 17 nmol of TPA. ODC activity in the epidermal extracts was determined with various concentrations of ornithine in the assay mixture. The Lineweaver and Burk plot analysis indicates that retinoic acid treatment did not alter the apparent K_m, but V_{max} was decreased by 73%. This suggests that retinoic acid did not affect the affinity of the enzyme to substrate ornithine, but probably affects the net amount of the ODC enzyme.

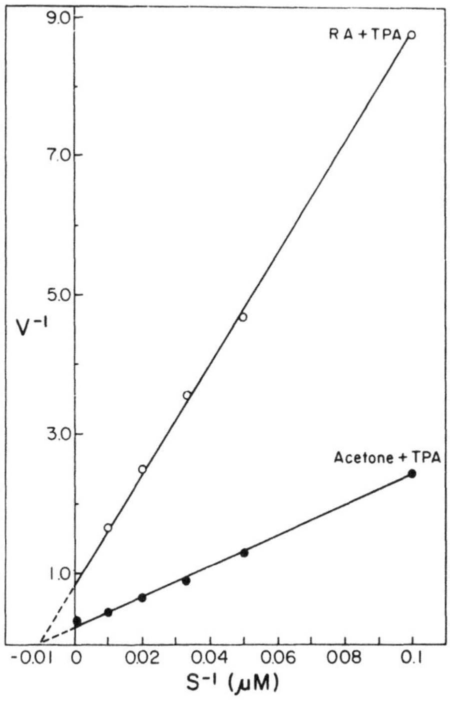

Fig. 5. Effect of retinoic acid pretreatment on the apparent K_m and V_{max} of soluble mouse epidermal ODC. Mice were treated with acetone or 1.7 nmol of retinoic acid 1 h before application of 17 nmol of TPA to mouse skin. Soluble epidermal extracts were prepared 4.5 h after TPA treatment; ODC activity was determined at various ornithine concentrations (S) in the assay mixture. Apparent K_m and V_{max} were determined from intercepts from a plot of 1/V versus 1/S. Apparent K_m; 100 μmol; V_{max} from acetone and retinoic acid pretreated skin was 4.54 and 1.25 nmol CO_2/30 min/mg protein, respectively

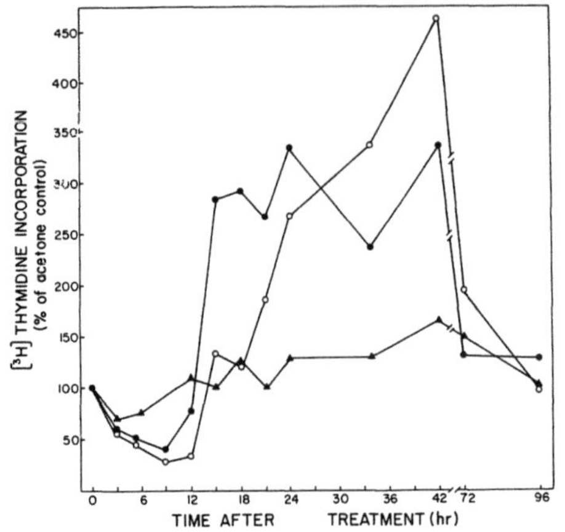

Fig. 6. Effect of retinoic acid on the time course of incorporation of thymidine after application of acetone or TPA to mouse skin. Mice were treated with acetone or 17 nmol of retinoic acid 1 h before treatment with acetone or 17 nmol of TPA. Mice were given i.p. tritiated thymidine (1 µCi/g body weight) 30 min before sacrifice at the indicated times after the latter treatment. Each point is the mean of determinations carried out on four groups of mice with two mice per group. (●), acetone was applied 1 h before TPA; (○), retinoic acid was applied 1 h before TPA; T▲), retinoic acid was applied 1 h before acetone

V. Effect of Retinoic Acid on DNA Synthesis and Hyperplasia Caused by TPA

Application of 17 nmol of TPA to mouse skin resulted in an initial depression followed by three peaks of DNA synthesis at about 18, 24, and 42 h after treatment (Fig. 6). Application of 17 nmol of retinoic acid 1 h before treatment with 17 nmol of TPA completely inhibited the 18 h peak but failed to inhibit the late peaks (after 21 h) of DNA synthesis. Application of 17 nmol retinoic acid alone 1 h before acetone treatment caused about a 70% increase in thymidine incorporation at 42 h following acetone treatment (Fig. 6).

Application of 17 nmol of retinoic acid 1 h before treatment with 17 nmol TPA failed to affect increased cell proliferation normally observed at days 1 and 3 following TPA treatment. The number of interfollicular epidermal cell layers with or without retinoic acid pretreatment was 4 or 5.

The relationship among TPA-induced ODC activity, resultant accumulation of putrescine, and enhanced DNA synthesis is not clear. The dose of retinoic acid that inhibited the induction of ODC activity and the accumulation of putrescine inhibited the early peak of DNA synthesis but augmented the late peaks of DNA synthesis. Furthermore, retinoic acid treatment did not inhibit TPA-induced hyperplasia of mouse epidermis. Application of 17 nmol of retinoic acid alone did not induce ODC activity but resulted in enhanced thymidine incorporation at 32 and 42 h following treatment (Fig. 6).

A similar observation indicative of dissociation between ODC induction and cell proliferation is the finding that TPA did not induce ODC activity in mice kept on a vitamin B_6-deficient diet, but caused increased epidermal cell proliferation (31). Furthermore, cell proliferation, but not ODC activity, was increased by simple massage of mouse skin (7). In contrast, application of indomethacin 2 h before TPA treatment inhibited the induction of ODC activity, accumulation of putrescine, enhanced incorporation of thymidine, and cell proliferation by TPA (18, 50). Furthermore, intraperitoneal administration of DL-α-hydrazino-α-aminovaleric acid (DL-HAVA) has been shown to inhibit both ethylphenylpropiolate-stimulated polyamine biosynthesis and DNA synthesis (43).

VI. Is the Effect of Retinoic Acid on Skin Carcinogenesis Universal?

As shown in the preceding section, retinoic acid is a potent inhibitor of the induction of ODC activity as well as skin tumor promotion by TPA. It was of interest to know whether

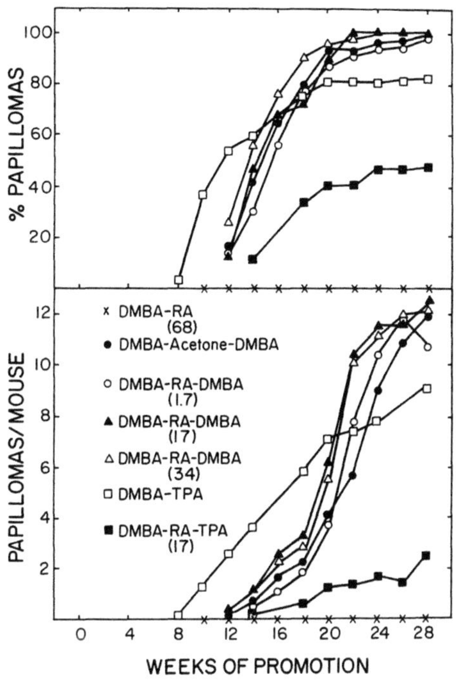

Fig. 7. Effect of retinoic acid (RA) on skin tumor formation by either DMBA or TPA. 0.2 µmol of DMBA in 0.2 ml acetone was applied to the shaved backs of CD-1 mice. Beginning 2 weeks after initiation, mice were treated twice weekly with 68 nmol of RA only, acetone or the indicated dose of RA 1 h before once weekly application of 0.2 µmol of DMBA or twice weekly applications of 5 nmol of TPA

the inhibitory effect of retinoic acid on both the induction of ODC activity and on the formation of skin tumors is common to other agents, such as DMBA, which elicit skin tumors.

The experiments summarized below provide evidence that indicates the failure of retinoic acid to inhibit ODC induction as well as tumor formation by DMBA (53).

1. Induction of skin tumors elicited by a single large dose (3.6 µmol) of DMBA could not be inhibited by application of a dose as large as 68 nmol of retinoic acid. However, application of 367 nmol of 7,8-benzoflavone inhibited quite effectively both DMBA-induced ODC activity and tumor formation (53).

2. Topical application of various doses of retinoic acid did not inhibit tumor formation by weekly repeated doses of 0.2 µmol of DMBA (Fig. 7). In the same experiment, the same solution of retinoic acid inhibited tumor promotion by TPA applied to DMBA-initiated skin.

a) In an experiment where retinoic acid was applied both 1 h before and 24 h after each DMBA treatment, a paradoxical augmentation of DMBA carcinogenesis was observed (53).

b) Application of 34 nmol of retinoic acid 30 min before each twice weekly application of 1, 10 or 50 nmol of DMBA did not inhibit tumor formation.

c) Intraperitoneal administration of retinoic acid in corn oil 30 min before each weekly application of 0.2 µmol of DMBA failed to inhibit, but rather potentiated DMBA carcinogenesis (53).

3. Retinoic acid not only failed to inhibit tumor formation by the carcinogen DMBA, but it also failed to inhibit tumor formation by twice weekly applications of 0.1 µmol of either 3-methylcholanthrene or benzo(a)pyrene.

Conclusions

1. The mechanism of inhibition of tumor promotion by TPA is due to its ability to inhibit the induction of ODC activity and the resultant accumulation of putrescine. If retinoic acid prevents skin carcinogenesis by the alteration of epidermal differentiation, it seems reasonable to assume that putrescine is a critical determinant of control of cellular differentiation (44, 51).

2. Although an effect of retinoic acid on the plasma membrane cannot be excluded, it seems to affect the late events induced by TPA (i.e., nuclear events, gene transcription, or translation). In this context, the work of Tryfiates and Krause (45) and Schwartz (39) is noteworthy. Vitamin A deficiency influences both qualitatively and quantitatively the synthesis of mRNA in liver (45). Topically applied all-trans-retinoic acid changes the relative amount of iso-accepting arginyl-tRNA in the epidermis of guinea pigs (39).

3. In mouse epidermis, the relationship between polyamine biosynthesis and enhanced cell proliferation is not clear.

4. a) The protective effect of retinoic acid on skin carcinogenesis is not universal.

b) The mechanism of induction of ODC activity and tumor formation by the complete carcinogen appears to be different from that of the tumor promoter TPA.

c) DMBA-induced ODC activity may be an important component of the mechanism of DMBA carcinogenesis.

Perspectives

Although there is a wealth of data that indicates the efficacy of retinoids in the prevention of cancers in experimental animals (3, 26, 29, 32, 42, 51), accumulating evidence indicates that retinoids may enhance the effects of carcinogens (14, 17, 23, 55, 57). Similarly, our results show the inability of retinoic acid to inhibit tumor formation by DMBA. Under some experimental conditions retinoic acid treatment augmented DMBA carcinogenesis. It appears obvious that the promoting component in DMBA carcinogenesis (if any) is different from that of TPA promotion. Thus it appears that – depending on the carcinogenic agent and target tissue – retinoids can either inhibit, have no effect, or enhance tumor formation. The cause of manifold biological effects of retinoid on carcinogenesis is unclear. It may be related to the dose, schedule, or mode of administration, or the transport and availability of retinoid to the target tissue as well as the mode of action of the carcinogen. Obviously, more research is essential to understand the basic mechanism of action of retinoids in the modification of carcinogenesis before they can be used for prophylaxis against certain human cancers.

Summary

1. Topical application of retinoic acid 1 h before application of TPA to mouse skin *inhibits:*

a) the induction of ODC activity and the resultant accumulation of putrescine; and

b) enhanced accumulation DNA synthesis at 18 h, but not at 24 and 42 h;

does not inhibit:

a) the induction of S-adenosylmethionine decarboxylase activity and the accumulation of spermidine or spermine,

b) the incorporation of tritiated leucine or histidine into mouse epidermal proteins;

c) the induction of cyclic AMP phosphodiesterase activity (data not shown);

d) the accumulation of prostaglandins E and F (data not shown);

e) hyperplasia observed at 1 and 3 days after TPA treatment.

2. Application of 17 nmol of retinoic acid alone did not result in a detectable increase in polyamine biosynthesis, but did result in an increased thymidine incorporation at 42 h following treatment.

3. Application of retinoic acid in conjunction with an initiating dose of DMBA did not affect tumors elicited by repeated applications of TPA. In contrast, retinoic acid treatment in conjunction with each TPA treatment to initiated skin inhibited the formation of skin papillomas as well as carcinomas. Application of as much as 68 nmol of retinoic acid alone to DMBA-initiated skin did not elicit skin tumors.

4. Application of retinoic acid in conjunction with a single 3.6 μmol dose or weekly repeated 0.2 μmol doses of DMBA inhibited neither the induction of epidermal ODC activity nor tumor formation.

Acknowledgments. The authors thank E.A. Conrad and G. Rymer for technical assistance. This investigation was supported by US Public Health Service Grants CA-22484 and CA-07175 from the National Cancer Institute, NIH. The encouragement of Dr. R.K. Boutwell throughout the course of this work is gratefully acknowleged.

References

1. Ashton H, Stephenson CJ, Frenk E (1971) Retinoic acid. Br J Dermatol 85:500–503
2. Blalock J, Gifford GE (1977) Retinoic acid (vitamin A acid) induced transcriptional control of interferon production. Proc Natl Acad Sci USA 74:5382–5386
3. Bollag W (1975) Therapy of epithelial tumors with an aromatic retinoic acid analog. Chemotherapy 21:236–247
4. Boutwell RK (1974) The function and mechanisms of promoters of carcinogenesis. CRC Crit Rev Toxicol 2:419–443
5. Boutwell RK (1977) The role of the induction of ornithine decarboxylase activity in tumor promotion. In: Origins of Human Cancer, Book B. Hiatt HH, Watson JD, Winsten JA (eds). Cold Spring Harbor, NY: Cold Spring Harbor Laboratory 1977, pp 773–783
6. Clark JN, Marchok AC (1979) The effect of vitamin A on cellular differentiation and mucous glycoprotein synthesis in long-term rat tracheal organ cultures. Differentiation 14:175–183
7. Clark-Lewis I, Murray AW (1978) Tumor promotion and induction of epidermal ornithine decarboxylase activity in mechanically stimulated mouse skin. Cancer Res 38:494–497
8. Crain FD, Lotspeich FJ, Krause RF (1967) Biosynthesis of retinoic acid by intestinal enzymes of rats. J Lipid Res 8:249–254
9. DeLuca HF (1979) Retinoic acid metabolism. Fed Proc 38:2519–2523
10. DeLuca LM, Bhat PV, Sasak W, Adama S (1979) Synthesis of phosphoryl and glycosyl phosphoryl derivatives of vitamin A in biological membranes. Fed Proc 38:2535–2539
11. Deshmukh DS, Malathi P, Ganguly J (1965) Rapid conversion of retinal (vitamin A aldehyde) to retinoic acid (vitamin A acid) in the living rat. Biochim Biophys Acta 107:120–122
12. Diamond L, O'Brien TG, Baird WM (1980) Tumor promoters and the mechanism of tumor promotion. Adv Cancer Res 32:1–74
13. Dickens MS, Custer RP, Sorof S (1979) Retinoids prevent mammary gland transformation by carcinogenic hydrocarbon in whole-organ culture. Proc Natl Acad Sci USA 76:5891–5895
14. Dicker P, Rozengurt E (1979) Retinoids enhance mitogenesis by tumor promoter and polypeptide growth factors. Biochem Biophys Res Commun 91:1203–1210
15. Dowling JE, Wald G (1960) The biological function of vitamin A acid. Proc Natl Acad Sci USA 46:587–608
16. Emerick RJ, Zile M, DeLuca HF (1967) Formation of retinoic acid from retinol in the rat. Biochem J 102:606–611
17. Forbes PD, Urbach F, Davies RE (1979) Enhancement of experimental photocarcinogenesis by topical retinoic acid. Cancer Lett 7:85–90
18. Fürstenberger G, Marks F (1978) Indomethacin inhibition of cell proliferation induced by the phorbol ester TPA is reversed by prostaglandin E_2 in mouse epidermis in vivo. Biochem Biophys Res Commun 84:1103–1111
19. Goodman DS (1979) Vitamin A and retinoids: recent advances, introduction, background, and general overview. Fed Proc 38:2501–2503

20. Heller JS, Fong WF, Canellakis ES (1976) Induction of a protein inhibitor to ornithine decarboxylase by the end products of its reaction. Proc Natl Acad Sci USA 73:1858–1862
21. Jänne J, Pösö H, Raina A (1978) Polyamines in rapid growth and cancer. Biochim Biophys Acta 473:241–293
22. Klein-Szántó AJP, Major SK, Slaga TJ (1980) Induction of dark keratinocytes by 12-0-tetradecanoylphorbol-13-acetate and mezerein as an indicator of promoting efficiency. Carcinogenesis 1:399–406
23. Levine L, Ohuchi K (1978) Retinoids as well as tumor promoters enhance deacylation of cellular lipids and prostaglandin production in MDCK cells. Nature 276:274–275
24. Lotan R (1979) Different susceptibilities of human melanoma and breast carcinoma cell lines to retinoic acid-induced growth inhibition. Cancer Res 39:1014–1019
25. Lotan R, Dennert G (1979) Stimulatory effects of vitamin A analogs on induction of cell-mediated cytotoxicity in vivo. Cancer Res 39:55–58
26. Mayer H, Bollag W, Hänni R, Rüegg R (1978) Retinoids, a new class of compounds with prophylactic and therapeutic activities in oncology and dermatology. Experientia 34:1105–1119
27. McCormick AM, Napoli JL, Yoshizawa S, DeLuca HF (1980) 5,6-Epoxyretinoic acid is a physiological metabolite of retinoic acid in the rat. Biochem J 186:475–481
28. Merriman RL, Bertram JS (1979) Reversible inhibition by retinoids of 3-methylcholanthrene-induced neoplastic transformation in C3H/10T $\frac{1}{2}$ clone 8 cells. Cancer Res 39:1661–1666
29. Moon RC, Grubbs CJ, Sporn MB (1976) Inhibition of 7,12-dimethylbenz(a)anthracene-induced mammary carcinogenesis by retinyl acetate. Cancer Res 36:2626–2630
30. Moore T (1967) Effects of vitamin A deficiency in animals: pharmacology and toxicology of vitamin A. In: The Vitamins, second edition, Vol. 1. Sebrell WH, Harris RS (eds). Academic Press, New York, pp 245–266 and 280–294
31. Murray AW (1978) Induction of epidermal cell proliferation by a tumor promoter in vitamin B_6-deficient mice. Experientia (Basel) 34:691
32. Nettesheim P (1980) Inhibition of carcinogenesis by retinoids. Can Med Assoc J 122:757–765
33. Newton DL, Henderson WR, Sporn MB (1980) Structure-activity relationships of retinoids in hamster tracheal organ culture. Cancer Res 40:3413–3425
34. O'Brien TG (1976) The induction of ornithine decarboxylase as an early, possibly obligatory, event in mouse skin carcinogenesis. Cancer Res 36:2644–2653
35. Orfanos CE, Runne U (1976) Systemic use of a new retinoid with and without local dithranol treatment in generalized psoriasis. Br J Dermatol 95:101–103
36. Ross AC, Goodman DS (1979) Intracellular binding proteins for retinol and retinoic acid: comparison with each other and with serum retinol-binding protein. Fed Proc 38:2515–2518
37. Russell DH, Durie BGM (1978) Polyamines as markers of normal and malignant growth. Russell DH (ed). Raven Press, New York
38. Sani BP, Corbett TH (1977) A retinoic acid-binding protein in normal and experimental tumors. Cancer Res 37:209–213
39. Schwartz E (1978) Changes in the relative amounts of iso-accepting arginyl-tRNA in the epidermis of guinea pigs under treatment with retinoic acid. Dermatologica 157 (Suppl 1):54–56
40. Shapiro SS, Bishop M, Poon JP, Brown PW (1976) Effect of aromatic retinoids on rat chondrosarcoma glycosaminoglycan biosynthesis. Cancer Res 36:3702–3706
41. Sporn MB, Newton DL (1979) Chemoprevention of cancer with retinoids. Fed Proc 38:2528–2534
42. Sporn MB, Dunlop NM, Newton DL, Smith JM (1976) Prevention of chemical carcinogenesis by vitamin A and its synthetic analogs (retinoids). Fed Proc 35:1332–1338
43. Takigawa M, Inoue H, Gohda E, Asada A, Takeda Y, Mori Y (1977) The role of putrescine in cell proliferation of the skin of mice induced by ethylphenylpropiolate. Exp Mol Path 27:183–196
44. Takigawa M, Ishida H, Takano T, Suzuki F (1980) Polyamine and differentiation: induction of ornithine decarboxylase by parathyroid hormone is a good marker of differentiated chondrocytes. Proc Natl Acad Sci USA 77:1481–1485
45. Tryfiates GP, Krause RF (1971) Altered messenger RNA synthesis in vitamin A deficient rat liver. Life Sci 10:1097–1103
46. Verma AK, Boutwell RK (1977) Vitamin A acid (retinoic acid), a potent inhibitor of 12-0-tetradecanoylphorbol-13-acetate-induced ornithine decarboxylase activity in mouse epidermis. Cancer Res 37:2196–2201
47. Verma AK, Rice HM, Shapas BG, Boutwell RK (1978) Inhibition of 12-0-tetradecanoylphorbol-13-acetate-induced ornithine decarboxylase activity in mouse epidermis by vitamin A analogs (retinoids). Cancer Res 38:793–801

48. Verma AK, Shapas BG, Rice HM, Boutwell RK (1979) Correlation of the inhibition of retinoids of tumor promoter-induced mouse epidermal ornithine decarboxylase activity and of skin tumor promotion. Cancer Res 39:419–425
49. Verma AK, Slaga TJ, Wertz PW, Mueller GC, Boutwell RK (1980) Inhibition of skin tumor promotion by retinoic acid and its metabolite 5,6-epoxyretinoic acid. Cancer Res 40:2367–2371
50. Verma AK, Ashendel CL, Boutwell RK (1980) Inhibition by prostaglandin synthesis inhibitors of the induction of epidermal ornithine decarboxylase activity, the accumulation of prostaglandins, and tumor promotion caused by 12-0-tetradecanoylphorbol-13-acetate. Cancer Res 40:308–315
51. Verma AK, Boutwell RK (1980) Inhibition of tumor promoter-induced mouse epidermal ornithine decarboxylase activity and prevention of skin carcinogenesis by vitamin A acid and its analogues (retinoids). In: Polyamines in Biomedical Research. Gaugas JM (ed). John Wiley & Sons, New York, Chapter 12, pp 185–202
52. Verma AK, Boutwell RK (1980) Effect of dose and duration of treatment with the tumor promoting agent, 12-0-tetradecanoylphorbol-13-acetone on mouse skin. Carcinogenesis 1:271–276
53. Verma AK, Conrad EA, Boutwell RK (1980) Induction of mouse epidermal ornithine decarboxylase activity and skin tumors by 7, 12-dimethylbenz[a]anthracene: modulation by retinoic acid and 7,8-benzoflavone. Carcinogenesis 1:607–611
54. Walback SB, Howe PR (1925) Tissue changes following deprivation of fat-soluble vitamin A. J Exp Med 42:753–778
55. Wilson EL, Reich E (1978) Plasminogen activator in chick fibroblasts: induction of synthesis by retinoic acid; synergism with viral transformation and phorbol ester. Cell 15:385–392
56. Wolf G, Kiorpes TC, Masushige S, Schreiber JB, Smith MJ, Anderson RS (1979) Recent evidence for the participation of vitamin A in glycoprotein synthesis. Fed Proc 38:2540–2542
57. Yarita T, Nettesheim P, Mitchell TJ (1980) Failure of two retinoids to inhibit tracheal carcinogenesis in hamsters. Carcinogenesis 1:255–265
58. Zile M, DeLuca H (1968) Retinoic acid: some aspects of growth promoting activity in the albino rat. J Nutr 94:302–308

C.E. Orfanos et al. (eds.)
Retinoids

Mitogenic Properties of Aromatic Retinoids: in vivo and in vitro Effects on Epidermal Cells

J. Pohl and E. Christophers

Retinoic acid (RA) is a potent stimulator of epidermal DNA synthesis and mitosis in vivo and in vitro (2–4, 8). In vivo repeated application of RA leads to epidermal hyperplasia, which shows psoriasiform changes in the guinea pig ear (2, 8). In vitro the presence of RA in the culture medium increases the attachment of epidermal cells and causes rapid expansion and growth of the cell cultures (3).

The enhancement effects of RA on epidermal cell proliferation as well as the concomitant changes in keratinization may be the basis for the known clinical effects of the drugs. This may also include the tumor-promoting capacity of RA as shown in hairless albino mice (1, 6). Recent studies revealed that small changes of the RA molecule clinically caused modified responses in skin. We therefore thought it worthwhile to investigate the new aromatic retinoids (Ro 10-9359, Ro 10-1670 and ro 11-1430) in comparison to RA in several model systems in which the stimulation of epidermal cell proliferation can be measured quantitatively.

Material and Methods

The following systems have been chosen:

1. Guinea Pig Epidermal Cell Cultures

The method has been published previously (7). The following substances were added to the growth medium:

Table 1. Counts per min (cpm) ± standard deviation of incorporated thymidine after incubation of guinea pig epidermal cell cultures with different concentrations of Ro 10-9359 and Ro 10-1670 after 24 h and 48 h of incubation. Four animals were used for every determination

Concentration of 8-MOP	cpm after 24 h incubation Ro 10-9359	Ro 10-1670	cpm after 48 h incubation Ro 10-9339	Ro 10-1670
Control	2439 ± 189	4483 ± 1316	4545 ± 123	5864 ± 1533
0.01 µg/ml	3024 ± 489	6157 ± 2013	4489 ± 342	8021 ± 1374
0.1 µg/ml	2561 ± 469	7156 ± 1097	5441 ± 1474	7357 ± 178
1.0 µg/ml	2910 ± 516	6933 ± 1016	7389 ± 1054	8486 ± 1183
10.0 µg/ml	2559 ± 311	1388 ± 155	6259 ± 1731	4425 ± 881
50.0 µg/ml	734 ± 176	71 ± 50	2152 ± 463	52 ± 5

1.1. Dimethylsulfoxide (DMSO), 0.2% (control).
1.2. Retinoic acid (RA) in concentrations of 0.01, 0.1, 1.0, 10.0 and 50.0 µg/ml in the growth medium. RA was first dissolved in DMSO. The final concentration of DMSO in the growth medium was always 0.2%.
1.3. Ro 10-9359, Ro 10-1670 and Ro 11-1430 in concentrations of 0.01, 0.1, 1.0, 10.0, 50.0 µg/ml, applied in the same way as described in 1.2.
After incubation times of 24 h and 48 h (s. Figs. 1–2 and Table 1) ^{3}H-thymidine (2 µCi/ml, Amersham, specific activity 5 Ci/mmole) was added to 1 ml cell cultures. Two hours later, i.e. 24 h and 48 h after the beginning of the experiment, the incorporation of the labelled thymidine was measured by a liquid scintillation counter (Packard Spectrometer) and calculated as counts per minute (cpm) per culture. The stimulatory effect was expressed in % of the corresponding solvent control (= 100%). Every determination was based on 4 cell cultures.

2. Guinea Pig Ear Skin, in vivo

The following solutions were painted daily in quantities of 0.1 ml on an area of 3 cm^2 of the ear skin for 14 days:
2.1. Ethanol 94%/propylene glycol $\overline{aa}$ (= solvent).
2.2. Retinoic acid 0.05% in the solvent.
2.3. Ro 11-1430 0.05% in the solvent.
The thickness of the epidermis was measured by planimetry in histological sections and determination of the number of labelled epidermal cells 40 min after intracutaneous injection of 0.1 ml (10 µCi) of ^{3}H-thymidine was performed in the autoradiographed sections. In the autoradiographs (Kodak AR 10, stripping film) the number of ^{3}H-labelled cells was counted per basement membrane length (mm) in at least 10 sections. Determinations were done on days 2, 4, 6, 8, 10, 12 and 14, using 3 animals for every time period and every preparation 2.1, 2.2, and 2.3. The stimulatory effect was expressed in % of the solvent controls.

3. Human Skin, in vivo

Three volunteers were treated topically on an area of 3 cm^2 of the back skin for 10 days with 0.1 ml of the following solutions:
3.1. Ethanol 94%/propylene glycol $\overline{aa}$ (= solvent).
3.2. Retinoic acid 0.05% in the solvent.
3.3. Ro 11-1430 0.05% in the solvent.
The proliferation was measured by planimetry of the thickness of the epidermis in histological sections and by autoradiographic determination of the number of ^{3}H-thymidine-labelled cells. For this purpose, the biopsies taken at the end of the treatment were incubated in a solution of ^{3}H-thymidine for 1 h (37 °C) and then rinsed, fixed and processed for autoradiography (Kodak AR 10). The ^{3}H-thymidine concentration was 4 µCi/ml in Earle's solution. The number of labelled cells per mm of basement membrane length was determined by autoradiography.

Results

1. Guinea Pig Epidermal Cell Cultures

In Figures 1 and 2 the effects of RA and Ro 11-1430 on growing epidermal cells after 24 h and 48 h of incubation are shown. From these figures it can be seen that after 24 h 10 µg/ml RA caused an increased uptake of ^{3}H-TdR (260% of the control radioactivity), whereas with Ro 11-1430 no change was produced at the tested concentrations. After 48 h a concentration of 0.01 µg RA per ml induced the ^{3}H-TdR incorporation to increase (160% of the controls), whereas with Ro 11-1430 only an approximately 100-fold higher dose showed equivalent values (1 µg/ml, Fig. 2). As presented in Table 1 there was a small stimulation of epidermal

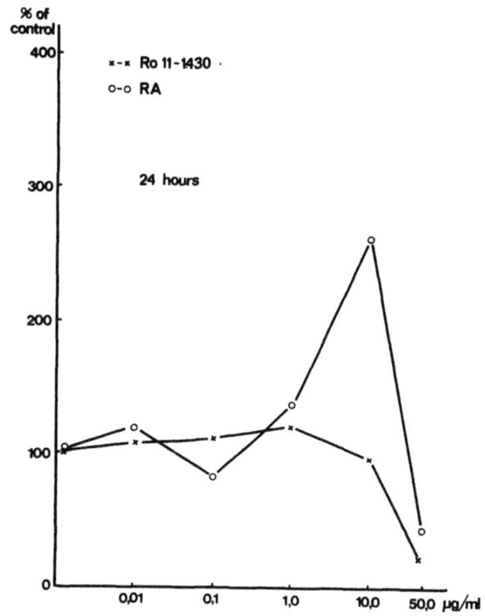

Fig. 1. Stimulatory effect (% of control) of RA and Ro 11-1430 after 24 h of incubation on epidermal ^{3}H-TdR uptake in guinea pig epidermal cell cultures

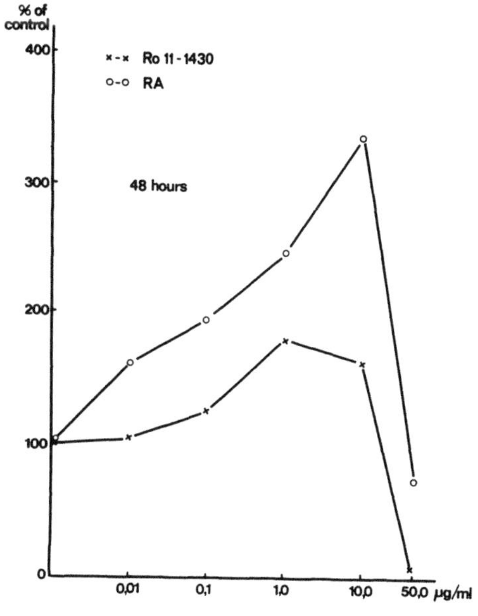

Fig. 2. Stimulatory effect (% of control) of RA and Ro 11-1430 after 48 h of incubation on ^{3}H-TdR uptake in guinea pig epidermal cell cultures

cell proliferation with Ro 10-9359 and Ro 10-1670 similar to Ro 11-1430. At a concentration of 1 µg/ml these drugs led to an increased thymidine uptake by epidermal cells by 150%.

2. Guinea Pig Ear Skin, in vivo

Figures 3 and 4 show the thickness of the epidermis and the number of labelled cells/mm after different periods of daily administration of the solvent as well as RA and Ro 11-1430.

It is evident that in vivo RA leads to an increased thickness of the epidermis and to an increased number of labelled cells dependent upon the length of treatment. On the other hand, Ro 11-1430, like the solvent, did not cause any such effect.

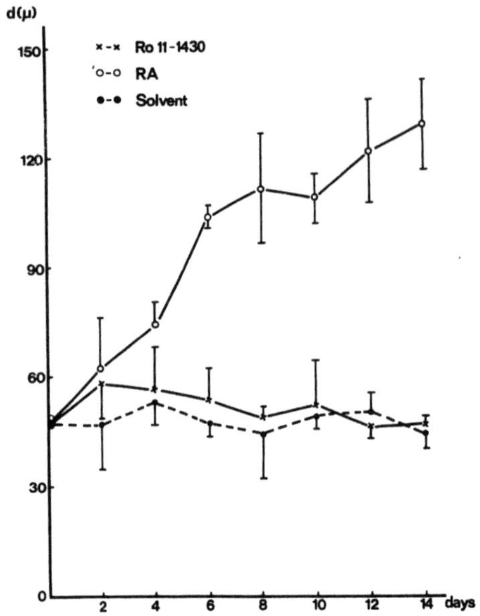

Fig. 3. Thickness of guinea pig epidermis after different durations of daily administration of the solvent as well as RA and Ro 11-1430. Bars represent standard deviations

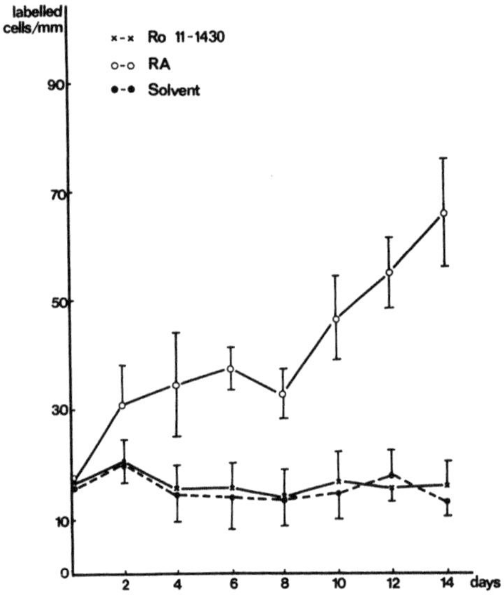

Fig. 4. Number of labelled cells in guinea pig epidermis after different durations of daily administration of the solvent as well as RA and Ro 11-1430. Bars represent standard deviations

3. Human Skin, in vivo

Figures 5 and 6 show the thickness of human epidermis and the number of labelled cells after 10 days. These results confirm the data obtained in guinea pigs, i.e. the considerable increase of epidermal thickness and the marked increase of the number of labelled cells produced by RA. On the other hand, Ro 11-1430 was ineffective with respect to both parameters. The values obtained with this drug were identical to those of the solvent.

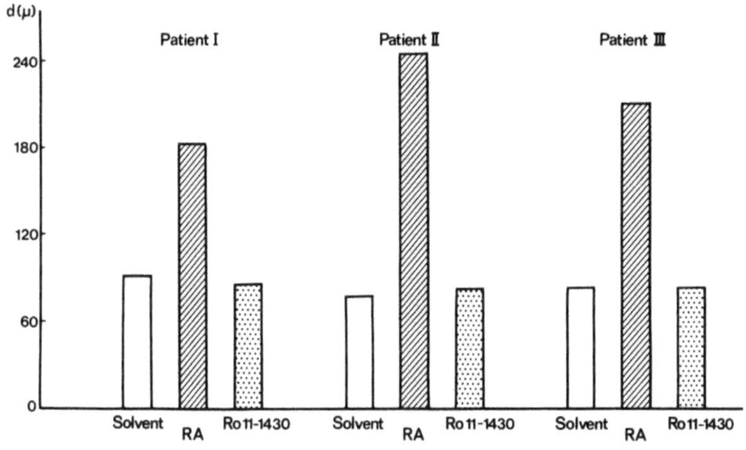

Fig. 5. Thickness of human epidermis after 10 daily applications of the solvent as well as RA and Ro 11-1430

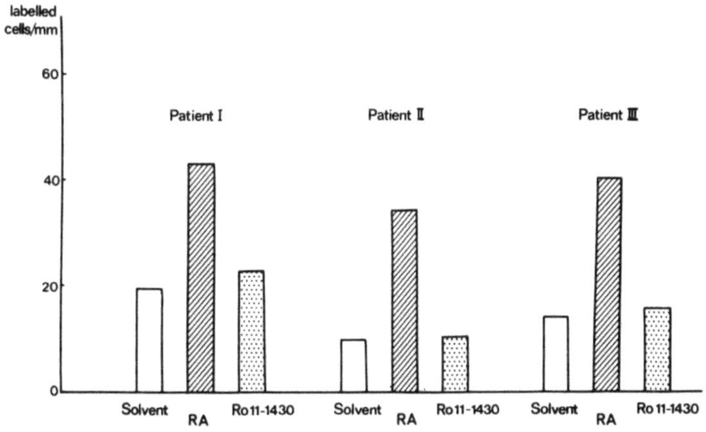

Fig. 6. Labelled cells/mm in human skin after 10 daily applications of the solvent as well as RA and Ro 11-1430

Conclusions

The three systems used in the present experiments led to consistent results. The well-known stimulation of cell proliferation by topical retinoic acid (RA) was confirmed on the basis of the increased incorporation of labelled thymidine - as a parameter of DNA synthesis - in vitro and in vivo. Further support is given by the increased thickness of the epidermis in guinea pigs and in men. In contrast to RA, Ro 11-1430 was indistinguishable from the solvent in both in vivo-studies. In the case of guinea pig epidermal cell cultures it was less effective than RA by a factor of about 100.

Generally the mechanism whereby some of the retinoids stimulate epidermal DNA synthesis and cell proliferation is poorly understood. The information available at present indicates that the mitogenic property of RA is species-nonspecific however tissue-specific for keratinizing epithelia. Possibly the tumor-promoting capacity of RA may be linked to its mitogenic activity thus resembling promoting activity similar to phorbol esters (5). It is of interest, that small molecular changes grossly result in a loss of mitogenic property of the resulting compound. This may have interesting bearings considering the clinical effects of these drugs.

Summary

In vitro and in vivo studies in man and guinea pigs were performed in order to study the influence of retinoic acid (RA) as well as new synthetic retinoids (Ro 10-9359, Ro 10-1670 and Ro 11-1430) on epidermal cell proliferation. In vivo, RA (0.05%) and Ro 11-1430 (0.05%) were painted daily (0.1 ml) on 3 cm^2 ear skin of guinea pig or back skin of man for 14 days. Cell proliferation was measured every second day by planimetry of the thickness of the epidermis in histological sections and by autoradiographic determination of the number of labelled cells after injection of ^{3}H-TdR (guinea pig) or after ^{3}H-TdR incubation of biopsies taken at various intervals (man). RA led to increased thickness of the epidermis and to an increased number of labelled cells. This was dependent upon the length of treatment and was observed in guinea pig skin as well as in man. Ro 11-1430 did not cause such effects.

In epidermal cell cultures 10 µg/ml RA 24 h and 48 h lead to an increase of 260–330% of thymidine incorporation. Ro 11-1430 (1 µg/ml, 48 h) produced an increase of 160% compared to controls. Ro 10-9359 and Ro 10-1670 showed no significant stimulatory effect upon ^{3}H-TdR incorporation.

The three systems used in the present experiments led to consistent results. The well-known stimulation of cell proliferation by topical RA was confirmed in guinea pig and man. In contrast, Ro 11-1430 was less effective, Ro 10-9359 and Ro 10-1670 were ineffective in altering the proliferative activity of epidermal cells.

References

1. Bollag W (1971) Therapy of chemically-induced skin tumors of mice with vitamin A palmitate and vitamin A acid. Experientia 27:90–92
2. Braun-Falco O, Christophers E (1969) Psoriasiforme Epidermisreaktion der Meerschweinchenhaut durch örtliche Vitamin A-Säure-Applikation. Arch klin exp Derm 234:70–86
3. Christophers E (1974) Growth stimulation of cultured postembryonic epidermal cells by vitamin A acid. J Invest Dermatol 63:450–455
4. Christophers E, Braun-Falco O (1968) Stimulation der epidermalen DNS-Synthese durch Vitamin A-Säure. Arch klin exp Derm 232:427–433
5. Dicker Ph, Rozengurt E (1979) Retinoids enhance mitogenesis by tumor promotor and polypeptide growth factors. Biochem Biophys Res Comm 91:1203–1210
6. Feigg M, Torhorst J (1977) Autoradiographic and histopathologic studies on the mode of action of an aromatic retinoid (Ro 10-9359) on chemically induced epithelial tumors in Swiss mice. J Natl Cancer Inst 58:1365
7. Laurence EB, Christophers E (1976) Selective action of hydrocortisone on postmitotic epidermal cells in vivo. J Invest Dermatol 66:222–229
8. Wolff HH, Christophers E, Braun-Falco O (1970) Beeinflussung durch Vitamin A-Säure. Eine elektronenmikroskopische Untersuchung. Arch klin exp Derm 237:774–795

C.E. Orfanos et al. (eds.)
Retinoids

On The Effects Induced by Aromatic Retinoid Ro 10-9359 on Explants of Skin from Psoriatic Patients

L. Rusciani, P. Massaro, P. Orlando, F.P. Spinnato, A. Venier and F. Serri

The recent introduction in therapeutical practice of retinoids derived from vitamin A has promoted a whole series of studies which have shown how retinoic acid and its analogs, besides regulating both the growth and differentiation of the epithelial cells (8), also have an anti-tumoral effect and are able to influence the immunological phenomena by stimulating the humoral as well as the cellular immunological responses.

Recently aromatic retinoids have been used in the treatment of many dermatoses characterized by an alteration of normal keratinization. One of the diseases in which very encouraging results have been obtained is psoriasis.

The aim of this research was to evaluate, through incorporation of tritiated thymidine, the effects induced by the retinoid on the mitotic activity of skin cells in cultures from psoriatic patients.

Materials and Methods

The study was made on patients suffering from diffuse psoriasis in evolution; the patients had not undergone any type of general or topical therapy for about two months.

Two samples, one of apparently healthy skin and one of psoriatic skin, were taken from areas which were not photo-exposed.

The explants, removed under sterile conditions with a Castrovejo keratotome after disinfection with ether, were always taken at the same time and from the same parts (right gluteus and thigh).

Each explant was divided into 3 parts which were then put into TC 199 (Difco) culture medium containing 0, 300 and 600 ng/ml, respectively, of Ro 10-9359, to which 6-^{3}H thymidine (S.A. 2 Ci/mmole) 10 Ci/ml was added. The cultures were incubated for 6 h at 37 °C in air atmosphere of 5% CO_2.

After incubation the samples were washed in physiological solution to remove the non-incorporated marked thymidine, dried on bibulous paper and weighed, and homogenized with a Polytron homogenizer.

After homogenization, scintillating liquid (Instagel) was added and the samples were counted in Tricarb (Packard) Mod. 3385 liquid phase scintillation counters.

Incorporated radioactivity of each sample was determined in disintegration per minute (d.p.m.) per mg of tissue. The data obtained were elaborated with Student's t-test.

Results

The results obtained (Table 1) show how thymidine incorporation, expressed in d.p.m. per mg, in the cultures of apparently healthy skin, rose from a mean value of 7254 ± 1000 in the culture with no drug added, to 7770 ± 800 in those with 300 ng/ml, and to 8080 ± 1180 in those with 600 ng/ml of Ro 10-9359, showing a slight increase in the mitotic activity of the cells under observation.

Table 1. Influence of thymidine on apparently healthy and psoriatic skin in culture with A) no drugs added and B) and C) with Ro 10–9359

	Ro 10–9359 ng/ml	d.p.m./mg mean values		Δ	t	2P
		normal	7254 ± 1000			
A	0			2400 (33%)	3.23	< 1%
		psoriatic	9655 ± 1700			
		normal	7770 ± 800			
B	300			1760 (23%)	2.8	< 2%
		psoriatic	9430 ± 750			
		normal	8080 ± 1180			
C	600			630 (8%)	1.2	N.S.
		psoriatic	8720 ± 765			

The increase in the mean values of thymidine incorporation by the cultures with 300 and 600 ng/ml of the drug, tested with Student's t-test, was not significant compared to the control cultures.

The cultures of psoriatic skin showed a different behaviour: the mean values recorded were: 9655 ± 1700 in the cultures with no drug added; 9430 ± 750 in the cultures with 300 ng/ml concentration and 8720 ± 765 in the ones with 600 ng/ml of Ro 10-9359.

In other words, psoriatic skin showed a decrease in thymidine incorporation, indication of a reduction in the mitotic activity of the cells under examination. Also in this case the decrease in average values of thymidine incorporation by the cells is not significant if tested with Student's t-test compared to the control cultures.

On the contrary, comparison of the mitotic activity of normal and psoriatic skin in cultures without Ro 10-9359 and with the drug at the two different concentrations, shows that in the former the psoriatic skin has a mitotic activity which is 33% higher than that of the apparently healthy skin. The difference between the two means is highly significant ($2\,p < 1\%$).

In the cultures containing Ro 10-9359 the difference between psoriatic and apparently healthy skin tends to decrease progressively: from surplus 23% in psoriatic skin in cultures with 300 ng/ml to surplus 8% in cultures with 600 ng/ml of Ro 10-9359. This difference between the two means, evaluated with Student's t-test, is no longer significant.

In short, it is evident that Ro 10-9359 at the higher concentrations balanced the mitotic activity of the apparently healthy and of the psoriatic cells by a slight but plain stimulation of the former and a depression of the latter.

In the graph (Fig. 1) this action of the retinoid is clearly visualized.

The effect is more apparent in the curves of the ratio between the average values of thymidine incorporation in psoriatic skin and in apparently healthy skin in cultures with the drug at different concentrations. The ratio, which is about 1.4 in the control cultures, decreases to 1.2 in those with 300 ng/ml and to 1.0 in those with 600 ng/ml of Ro 10-9359 (Table 2).

Graphical representation of these ratios (Fig. 2) shows clearly that the drug tends to level out the mitotic activity of the cells of psoriatic and of apparently healthy skin.

Discussion

The results obtained seem to show that Ro 10-9359 induced a different action according to

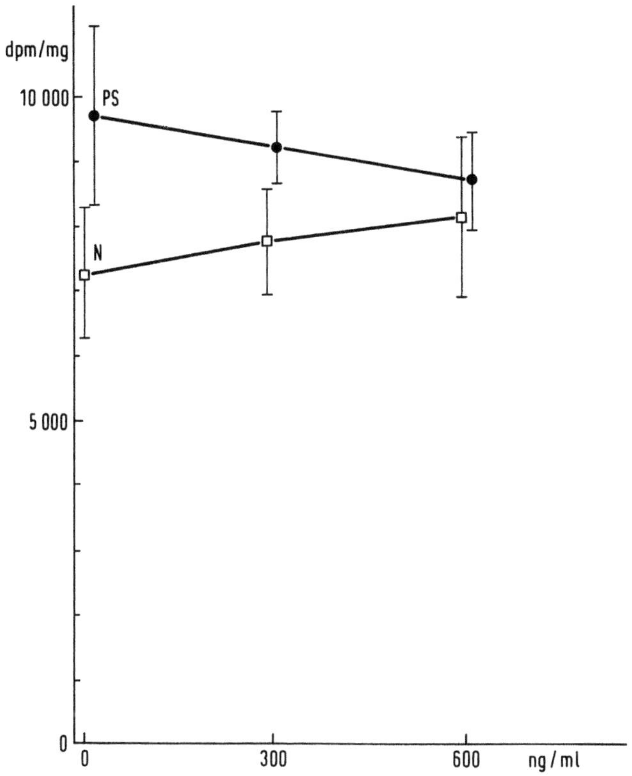

Fig. 1. Balance by Ro 10-9359 of the mitotic activity of apparently healthy and of psoriatic cells

whether it was added to cultures of apparently healthy or of psoriatic skin taken from one and the same patient. In fact, it stimulated the healthy skin and depressed the mitotic activity of the psoriatic skin. Both these effects seem to be related to the concentration of the drug: the stimulation of the healthy skin and the depression of the psoriatic skin are both more evident in the cultures with a higher concentration of Ro 10-9359.

Our current knowledge of the drug does not permit an easy interpretation of these results. In fact, although the drug's mechanism of action is not known, many phenomena which can be attributed to it have been observed, such as the break-up of lysosomal membranes (4), the breakup of gap junction formations (13), a damaging action on cell membranes,

Table 2. Values of thc comparison between control culture (A) and cultures with the concentrations of Ro 10–9359 as indicated (B–C)

	Ro 10–9359 ng/ml	RATIO $\frac{\text{DPM/mg psoriatic skin}}{\text{DPM/mg normal skin}}$ mean values	t	2P
A	0	1.4 ± 0.1		
B	300	1.2 ± 0.1	2.13	< 5%
C	600	1.0 ± 0.1	2.15	< 5%

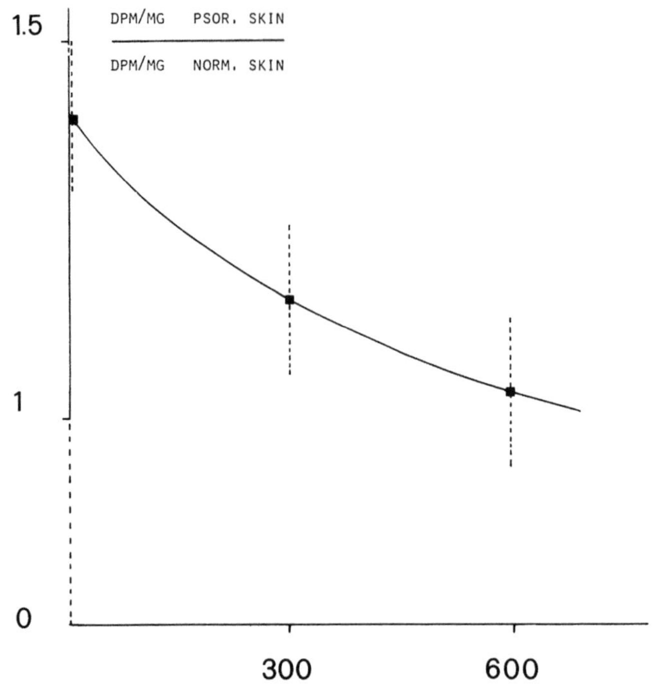

Fig. 2. Efficacy of Ro 10-9359 in levelling out the mitotic activity of cells of psoriatic and apparently healthy (normal) skin

inhibition of the production of interferon (2). Also some apparently contrasting actions of the drug have been described. It has been shown, in fact, that vitamin A is able to increase in vitro the synthesis of mucopolysaccarids in explants of skin of chicken embryos, guinea pigs and humans (1–7).

On the contrary, vitamin A added to cultures of cartilage determines a destruction of the protein matrix as a consequence of the breakup of the lysosomes (5-6). Also the action on cultures of tumoral cells is not always univocal: as we know, vitamin A and its analogs are able to inhibit the proliferation of cell lines and of S91 and B16 melanomas in mice, whereas it stimulates cultures of cells of human melanoma (9–11).

In our study we found that the drug had a different effect on cultures of skin from the same subject but in different clinical situations, i.e. pathological and apparently normal. In short, the action of stimulation exerted on epithelial tissues has been confirmed, while on psoriatic skin the same inhibiting action exerted on cultures of tumoral tissues has been observed.

As far as the latter are concerned, the function of mediating the antitumoral effect (3–12) has been attributed to a cell protein which is able to bind with the drug. Most probably a similar mechanism of action takes place in psoriasis.

Summary

Ro 10-9359 exerts an evident therapeutical effect on dermatoses characterized by altered keratinization, and on psoriasis in particular.

The authors studied the effects induced by the drug on the kinetics of healthy and psoriatic cells in culture, by means of incorporation of tritiated thymidine.

The results obtained seem to show that Ro 10-9359 depresses the mitotic activity of psoriatic cells, whereas it exerts a stimulating effect on the apparently healthy skin cells.

References

1. Barker SA, Cruickshank CH, Webb T (1964) The effect of vitamin A, hydrocortisone and citral upon sulphate metabolism in skin. Exp Cell Res 35:255–261
2. Blalock JE, Gifford GE (1977) Retinoic acid (vitamin A acid) induced transcriptional control of interferon production. Proc Natl Acad Sci USA 74:5382–5386
3. Chytil F, Ong DE (1978) Cellular vitamin A binding proteins. Vitam Horm 36:1–32
4. Dingle JT, Lucy JA (1965) Vitamin A, carotenoids and cell function. Biol Rev 40:422–461
5. Fell HB, Dingle JT (1963) Studies on the mode of action of excess of vitamin A. 6. Lysosomal protease and the degradation of cartilage matrix. Biochem J 87:403–408
6. Fell HB, Mellanby E (1952) Effect of hypervitaminosis A on embryonic limb-bones cultivated in vitro. J Physiol (Lond) 116:320–349
7. Fell HB, Mellanby E (1953) Metaplasia produced in cultures of chick ectoderm by high vitamin A. J Physiol (Lond) 119:470–488
8. Harris CC, Sporn MB, Kaufman DG, Smith JM, Frank BA, Jackson FE, Saffiotti U (1972) Histogenesis of squamous metaplasia in the hamster tracheal epithelium caused by vitamin A deficiency or benzo-[a-]pyrene-ferric oxide. J Natl Cancer Inst 48:743-761
9. Lotan R (1979) Different susceptibilities of human melanoma and breast carcinoma cell lines to retinoic acid-induced growth inhibition. Cancer Res 39:1014–1019
10. Lotan R, Giotta G, Nork E, Nicolson GL (1978) Characterization of the inhibitory effects of retinoids on the in vitro growth of two malignant murine melanomas. J Natl Cancer Inst 60:1035-1041
11. Lotan R, Nicolson GL (1977) Inhibitory effects of retinoic acid or retinyl acetate on the growth of untransformed, transformed, and tumor cells in vitro. J Natl Cancer Inst 59:1717–1722
12. Ong DE, Chytil F (1976) Presence of cellular retinol and retinoic acid binding proteins in experimental tumors. Cancer Lett 2:25–30
13. Prutkin L (1975) Mucous metaplasia and gap junctions in the vitamin A acid-treated skin tumor, keratoacanthoma. Cancer Res 35:364–369

C.E. Orfanos et al. (eds.)
Retinoids

Effects of Retinoids on Keratinocytes in vitro

G.O. Mahrle, D.I. Wilkinson and E.M. Farber

Retinoids control proliferation and differentiation of keratinizing and non-keratinizing epithelia. But there are some confusing, seemingly contradictory results on their effects and their mode of action.

Retinoids are used to inhibit cell growth of epidermal tumors and of hyperproliferative disorders of the skin (10, 11, 16). On the other hand, they have been shown to stimulate the proliferation of normal epidermis and they may even act as tumor promoters (6, 13). They have been reported to increase as well as to decrease DNA synthesis of cultured keratinocytes (2, 16). They influence markers of differentiation in a divergent way since they reduce the formation of keratin, whereas they induce the production of keratohyalin (17).

In order to get more information on the effects of retinoids we treated cultured guinea pig epidermal cells grown on collagen-coated dishes, on which these cells grow well (18). We compared the effects of two retinoids, vitamin A acid and aromatic retinoid, in various concentrations in long-term cell cultures after a single initial dose and during continuous treatment.

Material and Methods

Tissue Treatment and Cell Culture Procedures. Ears of adult albino guinea pigs were prepared as described previously (18). They were sliced to a depth of 0.2 mm with a keratotome and epidermal cells were isolated in GKN solution containing 0.3% trypsin. Cells were suspended in McCoy's 5A Medium (Flow Laboratories) supplemented with 9% newborn calf serum, containing 15 mM Hepes, 50 µg/ml gentamycin, 5 U/ml Mycostatin (Gibco) and 100 µg/ml carbenicillin. They were plated at a density of 15.6×10^4 cells/cm^2 onto plastic petri dishes (35 x 10 mm), which were coated with a thin layer of collagen (8).

Vitamin A acid (VAA) was obtained from Sigma and the aromatic retinoid Ro 10-9359 (AR) was kindly supplied by Hoffmann-LaRoche. VAA and AR were dissolved in acetone. Stock solutions (0.25; 1; 5 mg/ml VAA and 0.25; 1; 6 mg/ml AR) were freshly prepared for each experiment and stored at -80° C. The final concentrations used were: 1.7×10^{-6} M, 6.7×10^{-6} M, 3.3×10^{-5} M VAA and 0.2% acetone each, 1.4×10^{-6} M, 5.6×10^{-6} M, 3.4×10^{-5} M AR and 0.2% acetone each and as control 0.2% acetone only. VAA and AR were added to the medium at plating, once as a single initial dose or subsequently at every change of the medium.

Cells were maintained at 37° C in humidified atmosphere of 6% CO_2 and 94% air. They were fed the day after plating and then on alternate days with McCoy's Medium completed as described above but without carbenicillin.

Harvesting of Cells and Cell Counting. All investigations were performed in duplicates or triplicates. The number of detached cells was calculated in the aspirated medium using a hemocytometer. The attached cells were then exposed to ^{3}H-thymidine and ^{14}C-leucine containing medium, as described below, washed twice with PBS, and harvested from the dish with a trypsin-EDTA solution. The number of attached cells was determined and an equal volume of cold 10% TCA added to the dispersed cell suspension.

Labelling and DNA Determination. The attached cells were incubated with medium containing ^{3}H-thymidine (2 μ Ci/ml, specific activity 6 Ci/mM, Schwartz/Mann) and ^{14}C-leucine (0.5 μ Ci/ml, specific activity 250 m Ci/mM, ICN Pharmaceuticals) for 2 h at 37° C. After harvesting of the cells, determination of the cell number and treatment with 10% TCA, the precipitates were stored at -80° C for less than three weeks until enough material was collected to proceed.

The material was then homogenized and the precipitate collected by centrifugation for 20 min at 8,000 rpm in a refrigerated centrifuge. The supernatant was discarded and the final pellet was dissolved in 0.8 ml formic acid.

Duplicates of 0.25 ml were removed for scintillation counting. Each duplicate was precipitated with cold 5% TCA, filtered through Whatman GF/A glass fiber filters, and extensively washed with cold 5% TCA. The glass fiber papers were placed in scintillation vials and air-dried. Protosol 0.5 ml (New England Nuclear) was added and the vials were heated in a water bath at 60° C for 30 min. They were then allowed to cool. 20 μl of glacial acetic acid and 10 ml of ACS (Amersham) were added to each vial. The activity was measured in a Beckman liquid scintillation counter.

The rest (0.3 ml) was reprecipitated with TCA, centrifuged, and dissolved in 1 M perchloric acid for DNA determination by the method of Leyva and Kelley (7).

Demonstration of Lectin-reactive Sugars. Fluorescein-labelled lectins were obtained from Vector Lab. (Burlingame, Ca.). The following lectins were applied in molar fluorescein/lectin ratios as indicated, concanavalin A (ConA, F/P 6.3), wheat germ agglutinin (WGA, F/P 2.1), soy bean agglutinin (SBA, F/P 3.2), Dolichos biflorus agglutinin (DBA, F/P 4.0), Ulex europaeus agglutinin I (UEA I, F/P 4.8), peanut agglutinin (PNA, F/P 5.5), and Ricinus communis agglutinin (RCA_{120}, F/P 4.6). The lectins were reconstituted as prescribed (4 mg/ml).

Cell cultures were treated with an initial dose of 3.3×10^{-5} M VAA only or in addition 24 h and 72 h after plating and compared with controls fed with 0.2% acetone. Staining was performed 24, 72 and 110 h after plating. The medium was decanted, the cells were rinsed twice with PBS, dried for 30 min at 37° C, incubated with lectin-FITC (200 μg/ml) for 30 min at room temperature, washed shortly with PBS, once more dried for 30 min at 37 °C and rinsed with PBS for 30 min and finally covered with FA Mounting Fluid (Difco). The preparations were examined with a Zeiss fluorescence microscope using excitation filters LP 455 plus SP 490 and a barrier filter of LP 520.

Results

Growth Pattern. The growth curve of normal epidermal cells showed a lag phase of 5 days during which the number of attached cells decreased, followed by a proliferative phase of approximately 17 days, and a plateau phase (Fig. 1a). VAA given continuously reduced the number of attached cells during the lag phase and, in concentrations of 10^{-6} M, it accelerated and stimulated the proliferation resulting in higher cell density. During the plateau phased VAA depressed the number of attached cells below the control level. With increasing concentrations of VAA this depression started earlier and was more pronounced.

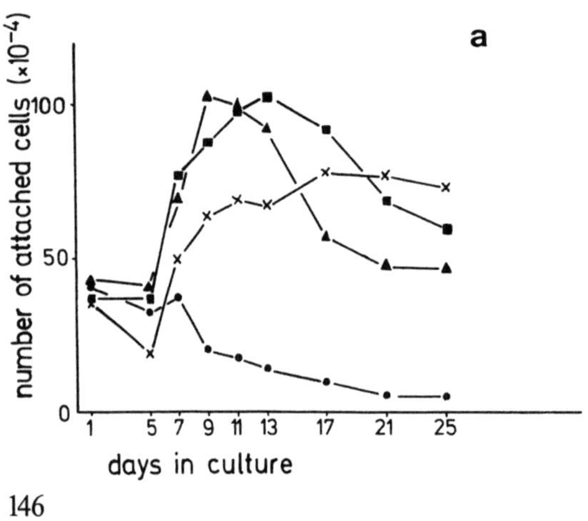

Fig. 1a

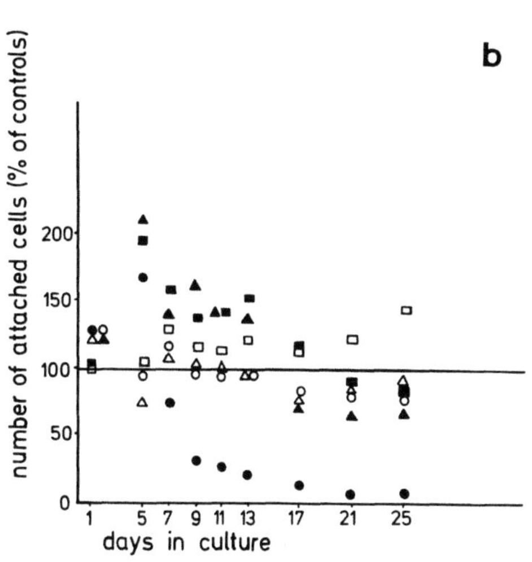

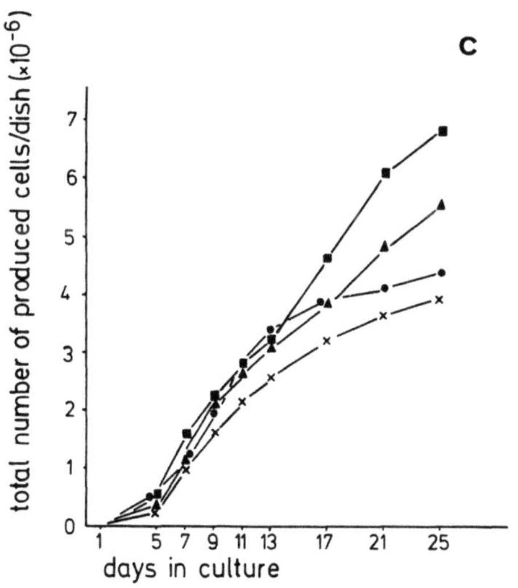

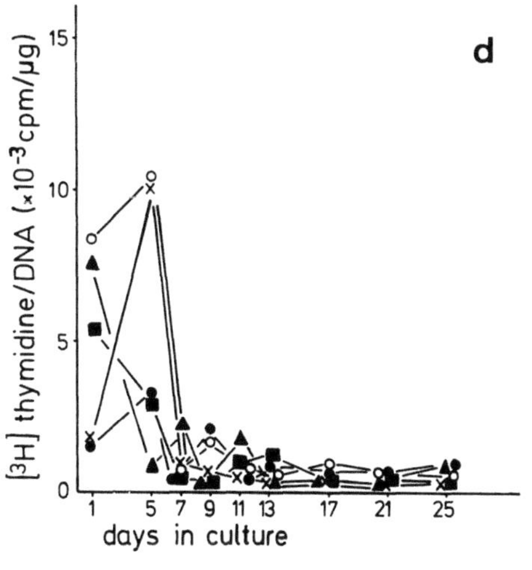

Fig. 1a. Growth of guinea pig epidermal cells determined by direct count of the cell number of attached cells. **b** Growth pattern of cell cultures treated with various concentrations of vitamin A acid (VAA) and aromatic retinoid (AR). **c** Total cell production including the number of attached cells and the sum of all cells until this time released into the medium and determined at each change of the medium. **d** ^{3}H-TdR incorporation into DNA of the attached epidermal cells. (x) control; (■) 1.7 x 10^{-6} M VAA; (▲) 6.7 x 10^{-6} M VAA; (●) 3.3 x 10^{-5} M VAA; (□) 1.4 x 10^{-6} M AR; (△) 5.6 x 10^{-6} M AR; (○) 3.4 x 10^{-5} M AR

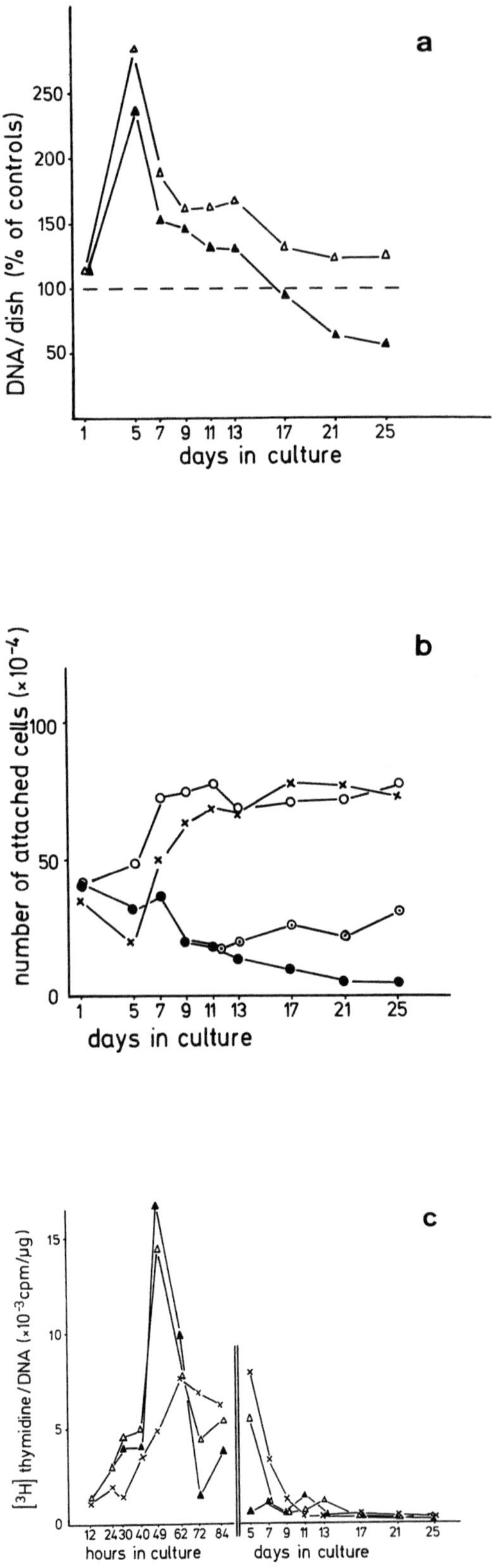
a
DNA/dish (% of controls)
250
200
150
100
50
1 5 7 9 11 13 17 21 25
days in culture
b
number of attached cells (×10⁻⁴)
100
50
0
1 5 7 9 11 13 17 21 25
days in culture
c
[³H] thymidine/DNA (×10⁻³cpm/µg)
15
10
5
0
12 24 30 40 49 62 72 84
hours in culture
5 7 9 11 13 17 21 25
days in culture

Figs. 2a-c

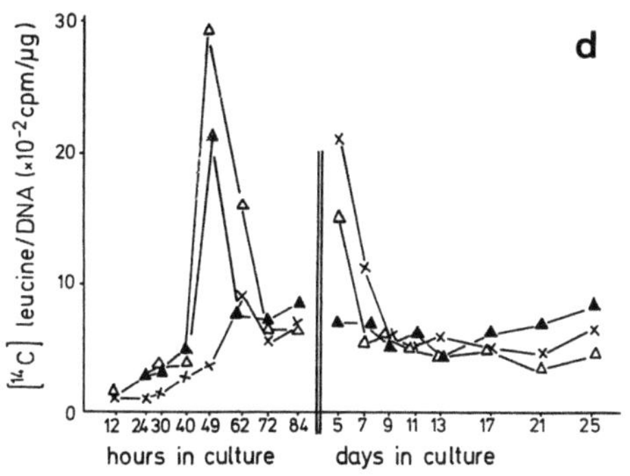

Fig. 2a. Growth of guinea pig epidermal cells determined by change in DNA content and **b** by count of the number of attached cells. Comparison of cell growth under continuous treatment with 6.7 x 10^{-6} M VAA (▲) and 3.3 x 10^{-5} M VAA (●) with cell cultures treated with a single equimolar dose at plating (△, ○). Growth curve after cessation of continuous high dosage treatment with VAA at day 9 (⊙). **c** Uptake of ^{3}H-TdR into DNA of attached cells and **d** incorporation of ^{14}C-leucine related to DNA in comparison to control (x)

We compared these findings with the results which we obtained from cell cultures treated with nearly equimolar concentrations of AR. VAA was more effective in raising and depressing the number of attached cells than AR, as is indicated in Fig. 1b by larger amplitudes from the control level.

The influence of VAA given continuously (VAA cont.) on the total cell production is shown in Fig. 1c. The values include the number of attached cells at a certain day and of all detached cells produced up to that day. In particular low concentrations of VAA cont. increased the proliferation of the cells. At these concentrations (1.7 and 6.7 x 10^{-6} M VAA) the ratio of attached to detached cells (A/D ratio, not indicated) was higher than the controls 5 to 17 days after plating and it was lower than the controls from day 17 to 25 after plating. Even though 3.3 x 10^{-5} M VAA cont. depressed the number of attached cells, the total cell production was evidently not reduced, because of a high rate of detachment of cells. At this relatively high concentration of VAA, the A/D ratio was above the control only at the beginning of the culture period at day 5. It was then lower than the control up to the end of the culture period.

A single initial dose of VAA (VAA I) overcame the retardation of cell growth during the lag phase more effectively and stimulated cell proliferation more extensively than VAA cont. (Fig. 2a and b). There was no depression of the number of attached cells below the control level within the time of observation. Low concentrations of VAA I (6.7 x 10^{-6} M) were even able to maintain the high number of attached cells above the control until the end of the experiment. Cessation of high dosage treatment with 3.3 x 10^{-5} M VAA cont. resulted in decreased desquamation (Fig. 2b).

Labelling Indices. Retinoids increased the incorporation of ^{3}H-TdR into DNA when measured one day after plating and decreased ^{3}H-TdR incorporation when measured five days after plating (Fig. 1d). There were two exceptions; 3.3 x 10^{-5} M VAA cont. showed no increase of ^{3}H-TdR incorporation at day 1, and 3.4 x 10^{-5} M AR cont. did not differ from the control at day 5.

The maximum stimulation of the incorporation of ^{3}H-TdR by 6.7 x 10^{-6} M VAA I and VAA cont. occurred 49 h after plating (Fig. 2c). The incorporation of ^{3}H-TdR in the controls started later, was less intense, and lasted longer. The incorporation of ^{14}C-leucine was similarly stimulated by VAA (Fig. 2a). ^{14}C-leucine was incorporated during the whole length of the experiment, whereas the incorporation of ^{3}H-TdR was negligible later than 9 days after plating.

Lectin-reactive Sugars. A specific fluorescence could be detected at the cell membrane with most of the applied lectins (Table 1). The cell culture treated with VAA showed a reduced membrane fluorescence with soy bean agglutinin, Dolichos biflorus agglutinin,

Table 1. Lectin-reactive groups at the cell surface of attached epidermal cells 24 to 110 h after plating with 3.3 x 10^{-5} M vitamin A acid (VA) in comparison to control (C). Explanation of the abbreviations of lectins used see under material and methods

Lectin	Saccharide specifity	Fluorescence of attached polygonal cells		Fluorescence of attached round cells	
		C	VA	C	VA
Con A	α-D-mannosyl α-D-glucosyl	∅	∅	++	++
WGA	NAc-glu-NH_3	(+)	(+)	+	+
SBA	NAc-gal-NH_3	++	+	++	+
DBA	NAc-gal-NH_3	+	+	+	−
UEA I	L-fucose	∅	∅	(+)	(+)
PNA	α-D-gal-NAc-gal	+	+	++	(+)
RCA_{120}	β-D-galactosyl	(+)	(+)	++	++

and peanut agglutinin indicating a depletion of the galactosamine and galactosyl containing cell surface sugars. This effect was observed 24, 72 as well as 110 h after plating using VAA I or VAA cont.. The effect of AR on the lectin binding has not been studied.

Discussion

In equimolar concentrations AR was less effective in stimulating proliferation and less toxic than VAA under the conditions of this study. Concerning inhibition of keratinization and stimulation of RNA synthesis in tracheal epithelium VAA was about one hundred to one thousand times more effective than AR (15).

Two principal effects could be observed in this study when epidermal cells were incubated with VAA. VAA-stimulated cell growth at a concentration of 10^{-6} M as is demonstrated by the accelerated and increased incorporation of ^{3}H-TdR into DNA, by the shortening of the lag phase and higher cell density (attached cells) and by the increased total cell production (attached cells plus detached cells). The narrow peak of ^{3}H-TdR incorporation two days after plating with 6.7 x 10^{-6} M VAA indicated a synchronizing effect of VAA on cell growth (VAA cont. > VAA I). When cells were incubated with high concentrations of VAA (10^{-5} M), they showed less activity of DNA synthesis measured by the incorporation of ^{3}H-TdR one day and five days after plating.

The other important effect was the influence of VAA on the attachment of cells on collagen and/or the detachment of cells into the medium. It has been reported that VAA facilitates cell attachment and increases cell density in the first hours after seeding on plastic dishes (2). However, we did not observe an increase of plating efficiency due to VAA or AR during the first 24 h in cell cultures (unpublished data). The collagen film in the dishes used seemed to facilitate the attachment of untreated epidermal cells and to equal the retinoid effect. Therefore, it is not likely that the increased attachment of cells in the prereplicative phase of the cell cycle is a condition sine qua non for the stimulation of the cell growth in VAA-treated cultures. Nevertheless, we observed an increased attachment rate and a higher A/D ratio during the replicative and proliferative phase indicating a direct relation between attachment and proliferation.

Since a constant equilibrium establishes between cell division and cell loss (3) a higher rate of cells sloughing off into the medium could be expected in the presence of VAA early in the culture period. Concentrations of 10^{-5} M VAA seemed to be cytotoxic, reducing the attached cell fraction in favor of the detached cell fraction already starting seven days after plating. Prolonged presence of VAA in lower concentrations (10^{-6} M) evidently facilitated the detachment of advanced keratinized cells, if we accept that cell cultures become multilayered with age and that the upper layers consist of more mature cells than the deep layer (5). From the observation that detached cells are more differentiated than attached cells (9) it might be suggested that the detachment of cells in vitro represents an equivalent to the shedding in vivo. In this respect the action of VAA on epidermal cell cultures is consistent with the loss of stratum corneum under systemic treatment with retinoids (17).

To examine protein synthesis we exposed the cells to ^{14}C-leucine. Compared to ^{3}H-TdR incorporation ^{14}C-leucine was incorporated during the whole length of the experiment. Concentrations of 10^{-6} M VAA stimulated the incorporation of ^{14}C-leucine about two days after plating. Since it has been claimed that the uptake of ^{14}C-leucine in epidermal cells correlates with the biogenesis of tonofilaments (1), it seems that VAA stimulated the synthesis of keratin precursors. Nevertheless, on the other hand, vitamin A compounds inhibit the formation of tonofilaments in attached cells of isolated epidermal cell cultures (19). This suggests an inhibitory effect of VAA on the maturation process of tonofilaments and/or an accelerated detachment of premature cells.

The mechanism by which retinoids act on cell growth, cell attachment in vitro, and shedding is not yet understood. They stimulate glycoprotein synthesis (4), but do not alter biosynthesis of sulfated glycosaminoglycans in epidermal cells (14). The present studies with lectins showed a depletion of galactosamine and galactosyl containing sugars at the cell surface in VAA-treated cells. These findings are consistent with the findings on the intact epidermis after systemic treatment with retinoids (12). Therefore it is likely that the effect of VAA is mediated by an alteration of the polysaccharide rich surface coat of keratinocytes.

Summary

The effects of vitamin A acid (VAA) and aromatic retinoid Ro 10-9359 (AR) on the growth pattern of epidermal cells from guinea pigs were investigated in long-term cell culture.

VAA in concentrations of 1.7 and 6.7 x 10^{-6} M given continuously every second day stimulated cell growth as demonstrated by accelerated, increased, and synchronized incorporation of ^{3}H-TdR into DNA, by shortening of the lag phase of cell growth after plating, and by increase of total cell production. VAA also stimulated incorporation of ^{14}C-leucine indicating a higher activity of protein synthesis. VAA raised the number of attached cells absolutely and in relation to the number of detached cells (A/D ratio) resulting in higher cell density during the replicative and proliferative growth phase. It facilitated the detachment of cells and reduced the A/D ratio during the plateau phase of cell growth.

VAA given as a single initial dose at plating increased cell proliferation but did not cause a higher rate of detachment during the plateau phase. VAA applied continuously in concentrations of 3.3 x 10^{-5} M seemed to be cytotoxic. AR given in about equimolar concentrations was less or not effective.

Studies with FITC-labelled lectins gave evidence that VAA causes depletion of galactosamine and galactosyl containing sugars at the cell surface of epidermal cells.

Acknowledgments. The studies were performed during the tenure of a Max Kade Postdoctoral Research Grant by Dr. Mahrle at Stanford University School of Medicine, Department of Dermatology. This work was supported by Deutsche Forschungsgemeinschaft (Ma 674/1) and by the International Psoriasis Research Foundation, P.O. Box V, Stanford, Ca. 94305.

We thank Hoffmann-La Roche, Grenzach, W.-Germany, and Nutley, New Jersey, USA, for their kind support.

The technical assistance of Mrs. B. Gray and Mrs. T. Tomashevsky is gratefully acknowledged.

References

1. Brysk MM, Gray RH, Bernstein IA (1977) Tonofilament protein from newborn rat epidermis. Isolation, localization, and biosynthesis of marker of epidermal differentiation. J Biol Chem 252:2127–2133
2. Christophers E (1974) Growth stimulation of cultured post-embryonic epidermal cells by vitamin A acid. J Invest Dermatol 63:450–455
3. Davison P, Liu S, Karasek M (1979) Limitations in the use of ^{3}H-thymidine incorporation into DNA as an indicator of epidermal keratinocyte proliferation in vitro. Cell Tissue Kinet 12:605–614
4. DeLuca L, Yuspa SH (1974) Altered glycoprotein synthesis in mouse epidermal cells treated with retinyl acetate in vitro. Exp Cell Res 86:106–110
5. Green H (1977) Terminal differentiation of cultured human epidermal cells. Cell 11:405–416
6. Kripke ML, Glassman HN (1980) Retinoic acid and photocarcinogenesis workshop. J Am Acad Dermatol 2:439–442
7. Leyva A, Kelley WN (1974) Measurement of DNA in cultured human cells. Anal Biochem 62:173–179
8. Liu S, Karasek MA (1978) Isolation and serial cultivation of rabbit skin epithelial cells. J Invest Dermatol 70:288–293
9. Liu S, Eaton MJ, Karasek MA (1979) Growth characteristics of human epidermal keratinocytes from newborn foreskin in primary and serial cultures. In Vitro 15:813–822
10. Mahrle G, Berger H (1978) Protective effect of aromatic retinoic acid analog on skin tumor. J Invest Derm 70:235
11. Mahrle G, Meyer-Hamme S, Ippen H (1981) Systemic treatment of keratinizing disorders of the skin and the mucous membrane with aromatic retinoid (Ro 10-9359). Comparative study on 113 patients. Arch Dermatol, in press
12. Nemanic MK, Elias PM Influence of retinoids on membrane glycosylation in epidermis. J Invest Dermatol, in press
13. Pullmann H, Lennartz KJ, Steigleder GK (1975) Die Proliferationskinetik normaler Epidermis vor und nach äußerlicher Anwendung einer 1%igen Vitamin A-Säure-Lösung. Arch Dermatol Res 253:71–76
14. Shapiro SS, Poon JP (1978) Effect of retinyl acetate on sulfated glycosaminoglycan biosynthesis in dermal and epidermal cells in vitro. Connect Tissue Res 6:101–108
15. Sporn MB, Dunlop MN, Newton DL, Henderson WR (1976) Relationships between structure and activity of retinoids. Nature 263:110–113
16. Stüttgen G, Ippen H, Mahrle G (1977) Oral vitamin A acid in treatment of dermatoses with pathologic keratinization. Int J Dermatol 16:500–502
17. Tsambaos D, Mahrle G, Orfanos CE (1980) Epidermal changes induced by oral excess of aromatic retinoid in guinea pigs. Arch Dermatol Res 267:141–152
18. Wilkinson DI (1978) Effect of vitamin A acid on the growth of keratinocytes in culture. Arch Dermatol Res 263:75–81
19. Yuspa SH, Harris CC (1974) Altered differentiation of mouse epidermal cells treated with retinyl acetate in vitro. Exp Cell Res 86:95–105
20. Yuspa SH, Elgjo K, Morse MA, Friedrich JW (1977) Retinyl acetate modulation of cell growth kinetics and carcinogen-cellular interaction in mouse epidermal cell cultures. Chem Biol Interact 16:251–264

C.E. Orfanos et al. (eds.)
Retinoids

Influence of Retinoid on Human Blood Cells in vitro. TMMP-Retinoid Inhibits the Mitogenic Properties of Lectins and Modulates the Lymphocytic Response

R. Bauer and C.E. Orfanos

Natural and synthetic retinoids apparently have marked effects on epithelial tissues. However, we have only little information on the effect of retinoids on mesenchymal cells. In this paper, an attempt will be made to elucidate some effects of retinoids on this particular tissue. To start with, several findings have been obtained in vitro on fibroblasts (Table 1) (1, 6, 8, 13). In addition to these investigations, a few publications have appeared during the last few years and months indicating some influence of various retinoids on blood cells, lymphocytes and monocytes (Table 2) (2, 3, 7, 15). Summarizing these findings, it appears reasonable to believe that retinoids may exert particular influences on mesenchymal cells, altering their functional properties in vitro.

In our laboratory, we investigated some possible interactions between the aromatic retinoid derivative Ro 10-9359, which has been introduced into dermatotherapy to large extent (9–11), and human peripheral blood lymphocytes.

Only a few hours after oral intake of the aromatic retinoid Ro 10-9359, its free acid trimethylmethoxyphenyl-retinoic acid (TMMP-RA, Ro 10-1670) appears in the blood (5).

Table 1

↑	Cell adhesion Contact inhibition of growth
↓	Proliferation Malignant transformation Microviscosity of the plasma cell membrane Effect of sarcoma growth factor

Table 2

↓	Humoral response to SRBC in vitro Comitogenic influence of TPA Interferon activity
↑	Cell-mediated cytotoxicity T-killer cells Blood monocytes

Table 3

Solvent	Solubility of TMMP-retinoic acid in g/100 ml
Ethanol 94%	0.07
Propylene glycol	0.02
Polyethylene glycol 400	0.25
Ethanol/propylene glycol	0.1
Acetone	0.013
Glycofurol	0.25
Dimethyl sulfoxide	1.5
H_2O	0

TMMP-RA obviously represents the main effective metabolite of the oral compound. Therefore, we preferred this substance for our experiments.

Addition of Retinoid Ro 10-1670 in Culture

For testing a drug in cell culture in vitro, it is necessary to solve the substance. Reproducible results and quantitative information on the real effective dosage of the drug will only be obtained if the system is stable. In Table 3 the solubility of TMMP-RA in various solvents shows that TMMP-RA is practically insoluble in aqueous environments.

Substance quantities solved in DMSO precipitated immediately on having been added to the culture medium RPMI 1641, apparently because the aqueous phase was present in excess. Even with various solutes, we did not succeed in maintaining the TMMP-RA solved in culture medium. We finally realized that TMMP-RA remained partly in solution only if bound to protein. For this reason, we incubated the TMMP-RA in complete culture medium RPMI 1640 for 1 h at 37 °C.

The samples were then centrifuged for 10 min at 3000 rpm, so that non-bound TMMP-RA was separated by sedimentation. The supernatant still contained considerable amounts of TMMP-RA bound to protein, as shown by difference spectra between loaded and non-loaded culture media, written in the range of 240 to 400 nm. The presence of TMMP-RA was indicated by an absorption maximum at 340 nm.

Experiments with ^{3}H-labelled TMMP-RA revealed that, after addition of 25 µg/ml RPMI 1640, approximately 20 µg TMMP-RA is bound to protein, being actually effective in the in vitro experiments. The culture medium thus enriched with TMMP-RA was used for our further experiments.

Lymphocytes Cultures

Influence of TMMP-RA on Cultured Lymphocytes Without Addition of Lectins

A possible direct influence of non-stimulated lymphocytes was carefully checked. No dose-dependent effect of the TMMP-RA on blast transformation was measurable in concentrations ranging from 3 ng/ml to 20 µg/ml culture medium when compared with non-stimulated controls; whereas phytohemagglutinin (PHA-P) alone showed a good stimulation index.

Evaluation of Cytotoxicity

Cell vitality was evaluated by trypan dye exclusion and by measurements of the intracellular ATP-content in tests at 72 h. No alteration was found in concentrations ranging from 3 ng to 20 µg TMMP-RA per ml culture medium when compared with cultures without lectin.

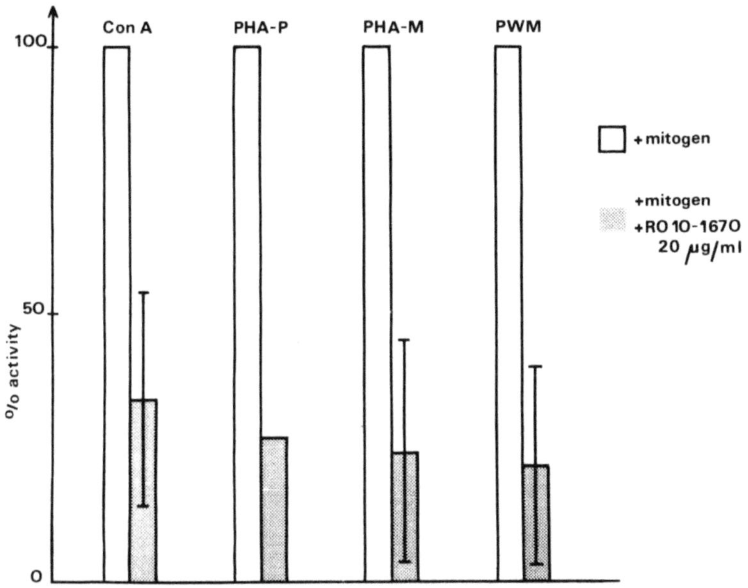

Fig. 1. Mitosis-inhibiting effect of TMMP-RA on four tested mitogens. The simultaneous administration of mitogen and 20 µg TMMP-RA per ml culture medium reduced the DNA-synthesis of cultivated lymphocytes in comparison with control cultures without TMMP-PA to values between 21 and 34%. The columns represent the mean values of several cultures; for ConA n = 6, for PHA-P n = 1, for PHA-M n = 7, for PWM n = 7. Each culture was measured in 3-fold assays. Lymphocyte cultures: 5×10^5/ml lymphocytes were cultivated in RPMI 1640 with 20 mM Hepes, 200 mM L-glutamine, 10% calf serum, 10 µg/ml neomycin and 0.5 U/ml bacitracin in a total volume of 0.5 ml. Mitogens were set at maximal stimulation values. After a 48-h incubation period, 3 µC of ^{3}H-thymidine (specific activity 6.7 C/mmol) were added per test assay for the next 18 h for radioactive labelling of the DNA-synthesis

Influence of TMMP-RA on Cultured Lymphocytes with Addition of Lectins

Numerous lymphocyte cultures were carried out in retinoid-enriched medium under simultaneous addition of mitogens. Figure 1 shows that TMMP-RA exerts a clearly inhibiting effect onto the proliferation of lymphocytes in the presence of four different mitogens. Addition of 20 µg TMMP-RA per ml culture medium inhibited, in its protein-bound form, the lectin-induced stimulation of DNA-synthesis in vitro. This retinoid effect was found to be clearly dose-dependent (Fig. 2).

The illustration in Fig. 3 presents one possibility of how TMMP-RA suppresses the proliferation of lymphocytes induced by lectins: Namely, the activity of lectins may be inhibited due to the binding of TMMP-RA to the plasma cell membrane, by blocking its lectin receptors. The following experiment supports this suggestion: Human lymphocytes were pretreated 24 h with 20 µg TMMP-RA per ml mitogen-free culture medium. They were washed thoroughly in buffer solution, and were then exposed to various lectins in fresh medium devoid of retinoid. No stimulation of DNA-synthesis was measured in this experiments. This finding shows clearly that TMMP-RA may interact with lymphocytes and block their response to lectins in vitro.

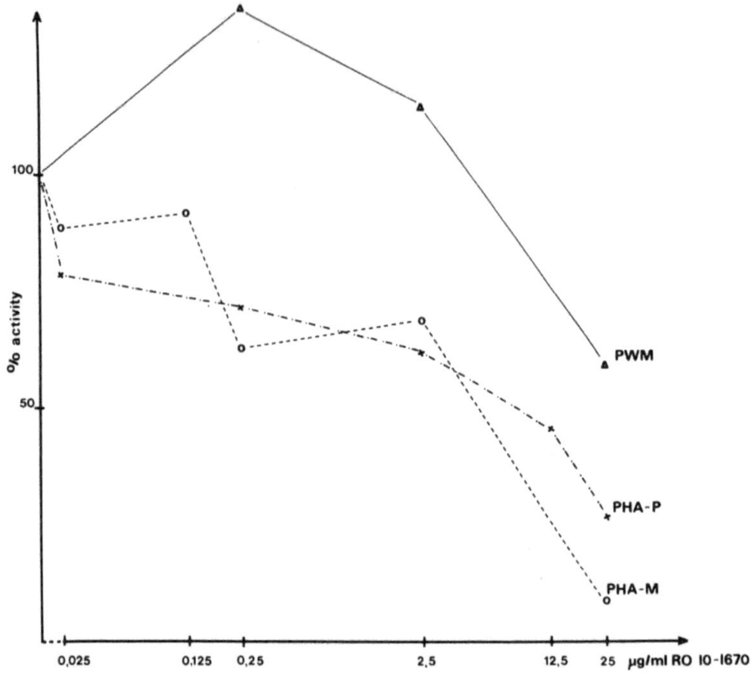

Fig. 2. Dose dependence of mitosis inhibition by TMMP-RA for the concentration range of 0.025–25 µg/ml. Between 1–2 µg/ml there is already a visible inhibition of the DNA-synthesis. This concentration corresponds to the plasma level at 3 h after oral administration of 2.5 mg/kg Ro 10-9359

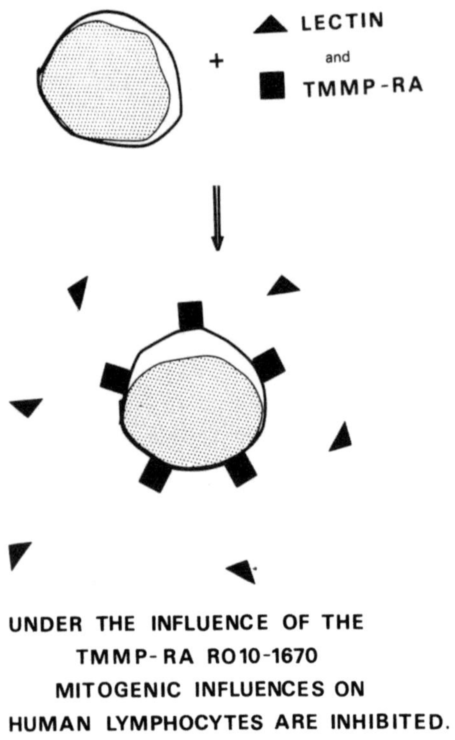

Fig. 3. A possible mechanism of how TMMP-RA suppresses the proliferation of lymphocytes as induced by lectins

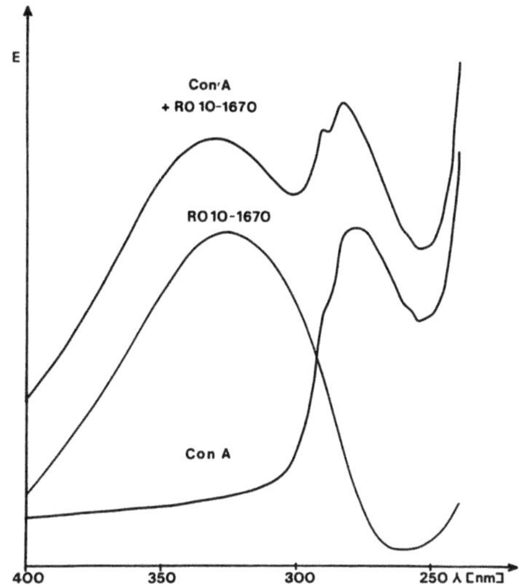

Fig. 4. Lectin-TMMP-RA interaction. After binding of TMMP-RA to concanavalin A the UV-spectrum of the lectin changes, showing an absorption maximum in the range of 340 nm. A difference spectrum between loaded and non-loaded concanavalin A shows only the UV-spectrum of TMMP-RA

Autoradiography

Autoradiography experiments with ^{3}H-labelled TMMP-RA revealed that lymphocytes obviously accumulate the drug and suggest that TMMP-RA may be localized on their plasma cell membrane.

Lectin-retinoid Interaction

Another interaction of TMMP-RA in mitogen-stimulated culture of lymphocytes relates to the fact that lectins obviously possess retinoic acid-binding capacities.

This binding of TMMP-RA to lectins is easily measurable: lectins have no absorption maximum in the UV-range of 340 nm. After incubation of lectins with TMMP-RA and separation of non-bound TMMP-RA by centrifugation, the UV-spectrum changes, showing a strong absorption maximum in the range of 340 nm (Fig. 4). This obviously indicated that TMMP-RA is being bound. The binding most likely occurs to a hydrophobic part of the lectin molecule. Moreover, a difference spectrum between loaded and non-loaded lectin shows only the typical UV-spectrum of TMMP-RA.

In additional experiments we found that all four tested lectins are able to bind TMMP-RA, their affinity being approximately 20- to 30-fold higher than that of calf serum.

Conclusions

It can be stated that retinoids may lead to different results acting on keratinocytes and on peripheral blood lymphocytes: Keratinocytes seem to proliferate in vivo and also in vitro under various retinoids, whereas lectin-induced proliferation of lymphocytes is clearly inhibited in this range of concentration. This adverse effect can possibly be explained by a different mode of action of the drug: In the first case the retinoid may be transferred to the nucleus of keratinocytes, as has been reported in liver cells (14) stimulating DNA-synthesis and cell proliferation. In the other case TMMP-RA may obviously not penetrate into the cell, reacting with the plasma membrane of lymphocytes and with the lectin molecule (Fig. 5a, b). The retinoid-plasma cell membrane interaction does not exert any visible or measurable

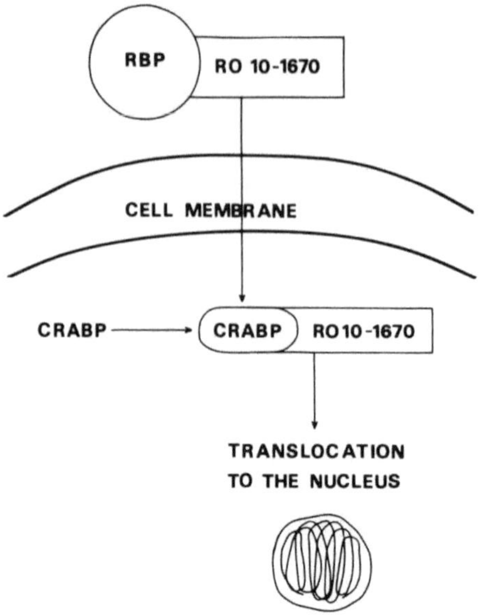

Fig. 5a. Transfer of retinoid to the nucleus stimulating DNA-synthesis and cell proliferation in liver cells

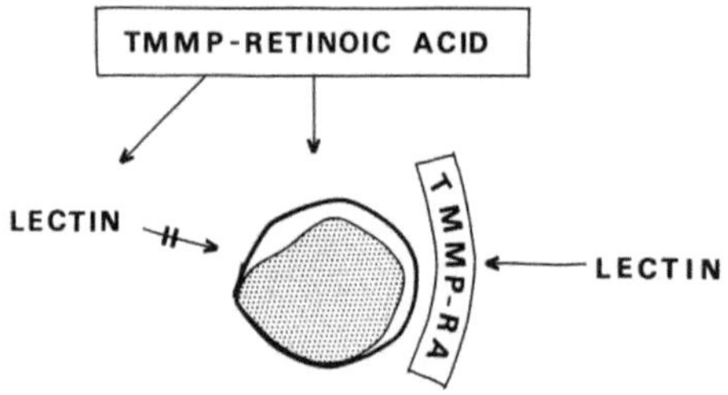

Fig. 5b. Interaction of TMMP-RA with the plasma membrane of lymphocytes and with the lectin molecule

reaction of the lymphocytes and is not cytotoxic at this concentration. However, a stimulation of the cells by lectins is not longer possible because the lymphocytes do not receive the lectin signal. Moreover, the lectin seems to be blocked by the retinoid-lectin interaction, most likely at the molecular level. Near the carbohydrate-binding site of the ConA molecule there is a non-polar region forming by hydrophobic amino acid residues (4). This region binds aromatic aglycones, for instance phenyl-β-D-glycopyranoside, leading to a functional change of the lectin (12). This part of the lectin molecule may also be the actual binding site for TMMP-RA.

We suggest, therefore, that the mechanism for the effects of retinoids on tissue cells can be attributed *to their influence on regulating proteins, by interaction with polypeptide chains.* This suggestion would explain the inhibition of interferon activity, the blocking of sarcoma growth factor, the blocking of proliferative effects of prolactin on mammary epithelium, etc.

Summarizing these findings, our studies revealed that TMMP-RA may be bound to lectins and plasma cell membrane of lymphocytes, leading to interruption of the lectin-cell interaction in vitro. The response of human peripheral blood lymphocytes to mitogenic stimuli is thus inhibited. Therefore, the main metabolite of Ro 10-9359 exerts in vitro modulating properties on immunocompetent cells, additionally to its influence on keratinizing tissues.

This effect may have some significance for its therapeutic efficacy in vivo.

Summary

The aromatic retinoid Ro 10-9359 obviously exerts a definite effect on peripheral blood lymphocytes in vitro. Since only a few hours after oral intake of this drug its free acid trimethylmethoxyphenyl-retinoid (TMMP, Ro 10-1670) appears in the blood of treated patients, we selected this metabolite for our in vitro studies. The following findings were obtained: (1) TMMP-retinoid is in an aqueous environment practically insoluble; in RPMI 1640 culture medium it remains in solution only if bound to protein. The binding curve is biphasic.

(2) Experiments with ^{3}H-labelled retinoid revealed that after addition of 25 µg/ml RPMI 1640 approximately 20 µg TMMP-retinoid is bound to protein, being actually effective in the in vitro cell culture.

(3) TMMP-retinoid has no influence on DNA-synthesis on human peripheral blood lymphocytes in concentrations between 3 ng-20 µg/ml culture medium, if added in vitro without lectin. Cell vitality evaluated by trypan blue dye exclusion and by measurements of the intracellular ATP-content showed no alterations.

(4) Human peripheral blood lymphocytes cultivated in vitro with lectins (Con A, PHA-M, PWM) in presence of TMMP-retinoid showed marked inhibition or no stimulation of DNA-synthesis.

(5) Human lymphocytes pretreated 24 h with TMMP-retinoid, washed in buffer solution and then exposed to lectins showed no stimulation of DNA-synthesis. Experiments with ^{3}H-labelled TMMP-retinoid revealed that the lymphocytes obviously accumulate the drug and suggest that TMMP-retinoid may be localized on the plasma cell membrane.

(6) Similarly, no stimulation occurs if lectins are pretreated with TMMP-retinoid and then added to the cell culture. The retinoid seems then to be bound to an hydrophobic part of the lectin molecule. The affinity of different lectins to retinoids varies, however, their binding capacity for TMMP-retinoid being approximately 20- to 30-fold higher than that of serum.

In conclusion, our studies revealed that TMMP-retinoid may be bound to lectins and plasma cell membranes, leading to interruption of the lectin-cell interaction in vitro. The response of human peripheral blood lymphocytes to mitogenic stimuli is thus inhibited. Therefore, the main metabolite of Ro 10-9359 exerts in vitro modulating properties on immunocompetent cells, additionally to its influence on keratinizing tissues. This effect may have some significance for its therapeutic efficacy in vivo.

References

1. Adamo S, Akalowsky I, De Luca LM (1978) Retinoic acid induced changes in saturation density and adhesion of transformed mouse fibroblasts. Proc Am Ass Cancer Res 19:27
2. Blalock JE, Gifford GE (1976) Inhibitor of interferon action by vitamin A. J Gen Virol 29:315–324
3. Dennert G, Lotan R (1978) Effects of retinoic acid on the immune system: stimulation of T-killer-cell induction. Eur J Immunol 8:23–29
4. Edelman GM, Cunningham BA, Reeke GN, Becker JW, Waxdal MJ, Wang JL (1972) The covalent and three-dimensional structure of concanavalin. Proc Natl Acad Sci USA 69:2580–2584
5. Hänni R (1978) Pharmacokinetic and metabolic pathways of systemically applied retinoids. Dermatologica 157 (Suppl 1):5–10
6. Jetten AM, Jetten MER, Shapiro SS, Poors JP (1979) Characterization of the action of retinoids on mouse fibroblast cell lines. Exp Cell Res 119:283–289
7. Kensler ThW, Mueller GC (1978) Retinoic acid inhibition of comitogenic action of mezerein and phorbol esters in bovine lymphocytes. Cancer Res 38:771–775
8. Meeks RG, Chen RF (1979) The effect of membrane detergents and retinoic acid on membrane microviscosity. Fed Proc 38:540

9. Orfanos CE (1979) Retinoide - Eine Breitspektrum-Dermatotherapie. Schweiz Med Wochenschr 109:1909–1911
10. Orfanos CE (1980) Retinoids - present status. Br J Dermatol 103:473–481
11. Orfanos CE, Pullmann H, Runne U, Kurka M, Strunk V, Künzig M, Dierlich E (1979) Behandlung der Psoriasis mit Vitamin A, Vitamin A-Säure und oralen Retinoiden. Hautarzt 30: 124–133
12. Poretz RD, Goldstein IJ (1971) Protein-carbohydrate interaction. On the mode of binding of aromatic moieties to concanavalin A, the phytohemagglutinin of the jack bean. Biochem Pharmacol 20:2727–2739
13. Sporn MB, Newton DL (1978) Chemoprevention of cancer with retinoids. Fed Proc 38:2528–2534
14. Takase S, Ong DE, Chytil F (1979) Cellular retinol-binding protein allows specific interaction of retinol with the nucleus in vitro. Proc Natl Acad Sci USA 76:2204–2208
15. Wertz PhW, Kensler ThW, Müller GC, Verma AK, Boutwell RK (1979) 5,6-Epoxyretinoic acid opposites the effects of 12-0-tretradecanoyl-phorbol-13-acetate in bovine lymphocytes. Nature 277: 227–229

C.E. Orfanos et al. (eds.)
Retinoids

Ro 10-9359 Retinoid Inhibits Both in vitro Epidermal Cell Proliferation and Differentiation

K. Madison, Ph.S. Tong, C.L. Marcelo and J.J. Voorhees

Summary

The TMMP analog of retinoic acid (Ro 10-9359) is successfully used in the treatment of psoriasis, a hyperproliferative scaling disorder. Primary neonatal mouse keratinocyte cultures that grow at 32 °C were used to study the effect of the retinoid on epidermal cell proliferation and fibrous protein (keratins) synthesis. ^{3}H-TdR uptake into isolated DNA fractions (cpm/µg DNA) was used to quantitate proliferation. ^{3}H-histidine (^{3}H-his) pulse-labelling of the cells followed by serial extraction with 4 buffers. Lowry protein analyses and SDS polyacrylamide gel electrophoresis (PAGE) were used to quantitate the synthesis of 5 categories of epidermal proteins. 8M urea + reducing agent soluble and insoluble fibrous proteins are two of these categories. The cultures were treated with Ro 10-9359 in 0.2% DMSO on day 3 after plating and with every medium change. The doses were: 12 µg/ml (34 µM), 6, 3, 0.05, 0.01 and 0.005 µg/ml (14 nM) (N = 15). There was no change in cpm/µg DNA one or 5 days after treatment. After 9 days of growth in the analog, there occurred an approximately 50% decrease in ^{3}H-TdR cpm/µg DNA with 12, 6 and 3 µg/ml of the retinoid. Thirty percent, 12% and 5% decreases in cpm/µg DNA were seen with 0.05, 0.01 and 0.005 µg/ml of the drug. No changes in total culture DNA were noted and the DMSO vehicle did not affect culture proliferation. Cultures treated with 12 µg/ml of the drug (day 3) were pulse-labelled for 4 h with 2 µCi/ml ^{3}H-his after 1, 5 and 9 days of drug treatment. Analyses of the different protein fractions showed an effect on day 1 by the Ro 10-9359: the synthesis of the 8M urea + reducing agent soluble fibrous protein fraction was inhibited approximately 50%. The inhibitory effect was also observed on the 5th and 9th day after treatment. PAGE showed no changes in the band patterns of the fractions and documented a decrease in normally synthesized fibrous proteins. The DMSO vehicle also affected the synthesis of these fibrous proteins but only at the later time points. We conclude that Ro 10-9359 can inhibit both the proliferation and fibrous protein synthesis (differentiation) of isolated epidermal cells in culture. Although the differentiation effect apparently occurred at an earlier time point than the proliferation effect, we do not know at present whether the two effects of this retinoid are independent or related in a cause-effect manner. It is possible that Ro 10-9359 is beneficial in psoriasis through similar proliferation and differentiation control mechanisms.

Application of Oral Retinoids in Psoriasis

C.E. Orfanos et al. (eds.)
Retinoids

Aromatic Retinoids in Psoriasis: Clinical, Histological, Histochemical, Electron Microscopical and Immunological Investigations

S. Jablonska, H. Wolska, J. Dąbrowski, M. Haftek, M. Groniowska and M. Jarząbek-Chorzelska

The aim of the studies was to evaluate the clinical efficacy of Ro 10-9359, and to correlate the histological and ultrastructural changes at various times of treatment. The further aim was to find out whether retinoids modify the antigenicity of the stratum corneum (SC), which is the substrate for reaction with SC antibodies both in psoriatic plaques (immune deposits detected by direct immunofluorescence), and in in vitro IF reaction using normal human serum with a high titer of SC antibodies (1, 2). Indirect IF method makes it possible to assess whether the antigenicity of SC is preserved.

Material and Methods

Clinical Trial

Ro 10-9359 (Tigason) was used in 40 psoriatic patients in a double blind study (20 treated with Ro 10-9359, 20 with placebo) and in an additional 22 patients in open trial. Most of them suffered from very severe, widespread disease. Patients with a smaller extent of skin lesions were treated with Tigason, if the disease was very resistant to other treatment or if concomitant arthralgia or arthropathy was very pronounced. The psoriatic area and severity index (PASI), as reported by Fredriksson and Pettersson (6), extended to patients with pustules, was assessed every week.

The dose of 1 mg/kg body weight was given until a satisfactory response (marked improvement: clearing of $\geqq 50\%$ of skin lesions or almost complete remission: clearing of $\geqq 90\%$ of lesions) was obtained. After that, in patients with marked improvement the dose was usually decreased to 0.6 mg/kg.

In patients with complete clearing, the maintenance dose was 0.2–0.8 mg/kg, depending on response. In some patients with severe or troublesome side effects it was necessary to reduce dosage before satisfactory results were achieved.

Histological and Histochemical Studies

Histological and histochemical investigations (PAS, alcian blue and peroxidase staining) were performed in 14 patients before and after 3 weeks of treatment; in 5 of them examinations were also made after 10 days and in 8 after 6 weeks of treatment.

Additionally, in 12 of these patients healthy skin at the same periods of treatment was examined.

Ultrastructural Studies

Electron microscopical examinations were performed in 6 patients before and after 3 and 6 weeks of treatment; in two cases the seemingly uninvolved skin was examined also.

Immunofluorescent (IF) Studies

IF studies of psoriatic plaques were performed in 12 patients before and at various times between 10 and 56 days of treatment. In some cases studies were performed also in the uninvolved skin, using the indirect and direct IF methods, as described by Beutner et al. (1).

Results and Comments

Clinical Results

The results of treatment in 42 patients are shown in Table 1. Thirteen of these patients, 8 of them with erythroderma, were under treatment for less than 4 months.

There was a prevalence of satisfactory responses in cases with widespread and/or erythrodermic psoriasis, and even more striking effects in pustular psoriasis of von Zumbusch type, as noted also by other investigators (7, 8, 14, 16, 18). All 4 cases of generalized pustular psoriasis were never before free of skin lesions until after this therapy. This is more evident in the double-blind study (Table 2), which, however, did not show a statistically significant difference in the PASI score (index of severity and extent of lesions) before and after treatment in erythrodermic patients. But the data covered a smaller number of only 6 patients in comparison with 17 now under or after treatment (Table 1), and included cases of congenital psoriasis and erythroderma lasting for more than 10 years, which did not respond to any methods of treatment.

A comparison of PASI scores in patients with psoriasis vulgaris after 4 months of the treatment with Tigason and placebo showed a statistically significant difference in favour of Tigason, as reported also by Lassus (11). However, the response to Tigason in psoriasis vulgaris was slower than in erythroderma and much slower than in pustular psoriasis.

In the latter, clearing of lesions was observed even within 1–2 weeks of treatment.

In 5 of 42 patients treated with Tigason, it was necessary to continue therapy with other methods (tar, anthralin, PUVA) because of unsatisfactory results after 4 months of treatment.

In 16 patients, when satisfactory results were obtained, the treatment was discontinued. Seven of these patients are still without skin lesions (the time of observation ranging from

Table 1. Results of treatment with Ro 10-9359

Type of psoriasis	Number of patients	No change	Minimal improvement	Marked or moderate improvement	Fast complete remission	Complete remission
Widespread disseminated p. vulgaris	19	1	5	6	5	2
Erythroderma	17	2	2	6	7	
P. pustulosa von Zumbusch	4				2	2
Pustular palmoplantar psoriasis	2			1*	1	
Total	42	3	7	13	15	4

* Two weeks of treatment

Table 2. PASI score in patients treated with Ro 10-9359 (double-blind study)

Treatment	Type of psoriasis (number of patients)	PASI score (mean ± SD) Before treatment	After treatment	p-value (t-test)
Ro 10-9359	P. vulgaris (10)	18.63 ± 8.5[a]	7.02 ± 5.06[a]	0.02
	P. erythrodermica (6)	28.6 ± 7.35	12.77 ± 12.31	NS
	P. pustulosa (4)	23.1 ± 6.92	1.43 ± 1.66	0.02
	Total (20)	22.51 ± 8.7[b]	7.62 ± 8.31[b]	0.001
Placebo	P. vulgaris (18)	18.10 ± 7.15[a]	17.40 ± 9.39[a]	NS
	P. erythrodermica (1)	26.6	52.5	-
	P. pustulosa (1)	15.6	19.6	-
	Total (20)	18.48 ± 7.05[b]	19.26 ± 8.31[b]	NS

[a] $p < 0.01$
[b] $p < 0.02$

2.5 to 6 months). In 9 patients, relapses occurred after different periods of remission (Table 3).

It is worth stressing that a patient with generalized pustular psoriasis, who was completely free of skin lesions for 7 months for the first time in 10 years, was cleared after a new course of therapy. Another patient with severe erythroderma was also treated successfully with Tigason and PUVA after a relapse had occurred 4 months after the treatment has been discontinued.

In 8 patients the maintenance therapy was continued for 3–8 months, including 3 patients with generalized pustular psoriasis, in whom mild relapses were observed whenever alternate day treatment was attempted. Maintenance therapy was well tolerated, as reported also by others (8, 11, 17). The response to Tigason in one patient with pustular palmo-plantar psoriasis was the best observed during the last 8 years. Favourable results in pustular palmo-plantar psoriasis have been reported also by others (5, 6).

Psoriatic Arthropathy

Of the 7 cases of psoriatic arthropathy and the 2 cases of arthralgia marked improvement was noted in 5 and 2, respectively. The placebo had no effect in two cases (Table 4). Good response of psoriatic arthropathy has been reported earlier (20).

Table 3. Relapse after discontinuation of treatment with Ro 10-9359 (9 patients)

Time of relapse	Psoriasis vulgaris	Psoriasis erythrodermica	Psoriasis pustulosa	Total	Further treatment
≦ 1 month	2			2	Tar or anthralin
≦ 3 months	1	2		3	PUVA or tar or anthralin
≦ 6 months	1	2		3	Ro 10-9359 + PUVA or tar
≦ 9 months			1	1	Ro 10-9359 (complete clearing)

Table 4. Effect of the treatment with Ro 10-9359 and placebo on arthralgia and psoriatic arthropathy

	Ro 10-9359		
	Marked improvement	Slight improvement	No change
Arthropathy	5	1	1*
Arthralgia	5		
	Placebo		
Arthropathy			1
Arthralgia			1

* three weeks of treatment

Clinical Side Effects

Clinical side effects (Table 5) observed in patients treated did not differ in character, severity and frequency from other reports (3, 12, 16).

Laboratory Findings

There was a statistically significant increase of SGPT values in a group treated with Tigason in comparison with placebo. Increases of SGOT and alkaline phosphatase values were not significant. It is worth noting that in two patients, whose treatment was not discontinued in spite of the abnormal values of SGPT and alkaline phosphatase within the first 4 months of treatment, there was a normalization of those parameters after 6–7 months of therapy. Laboratory findings did not differ from those reported earlier (3, 12, 16). However, in our study they were confirmed by the double-blind test.

Histological, Histochemical and Ultrastructural Findings

In all of the cases, after 10 days of treatment, psoriatic changes were still present, but the horny layer became progressively thinned. At 3 weeks in 3 cases there was an intermittent restoration of the granular layer. At that time an evident increase of PAS and alcian blue-positive substance was seen in all instances within the epidermis and in some specimens at the basement membrane zone. At six weeks of treatment, not infrequently the acanthosis and dermal infiltrates were still present even in cases with no clinical and histological features of psoriasis.

Table 5. Side effects registered during the therapy with Ro 10-9359 (% of patients)

	mild	moderate	severe
Dryness of lips	25	50	20
Dryness of mouth	35	35	25
Dryness of nose	15	30	25
Cheilitis	5	35	15
Thinning of skin	10	10	15
Desquamation of skin		20	15
Alopecia	5	15	

The infiltrates consisted of mononuclear cells. Polymorphonuclears, previously abundant in pustular and erythrodermic forms, were absent.

Examination of healthy skin after 10 days of treatment revealed in 2 of 5 cases a focal parakeratosis, and at 3 and 6 weeks some acanthosis, as noted also by others (4, 19).

Ultrastructural Findings

The characteristic features were widened intercellular spaces, filled with fine and partially coarse granular substance, and vacuolization of cytoplasm of keratinocytes, related in part to degenerated mitochondria and enlarged cytoplasmatic reticulum (Fig. 1). Some vacuoles contained very fine granular alcian blue-positive material, and some cells were so deranged that they were almost about to burst, as reported by Orfanos et al. (15, 19).

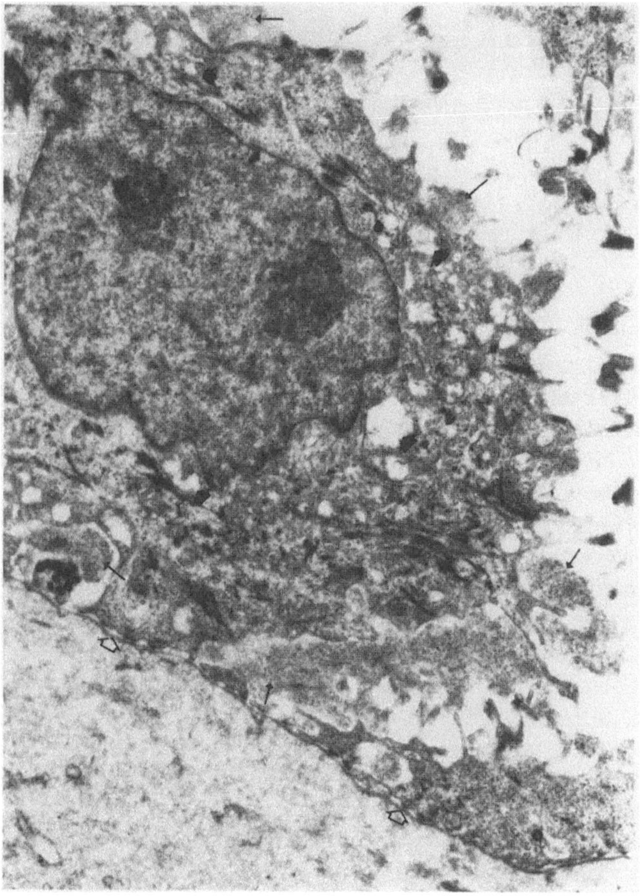

Fig. 1. Case K.S. Widely disseminated lesions, almost erythroderma. Biopsy from psoriatic plaque, which improved considerably, but did not disappear after 6 weeks of treatment with a dose of 1 mg/kg/ weight. Electron microscopy, x 5,400.
Basal lamina (⇔) well preserved. Intercellular spaces considerably widened, partially filled with mainly fine granular material (→).
In the cytoplasm of the basal cell there are numerous vacuoles (↠), some related to enlarged, degenerated mitochondria and/or to enlarged endoplasmatic reticulum. Tonofilaments are visible. The nucleus appears to be unchanged

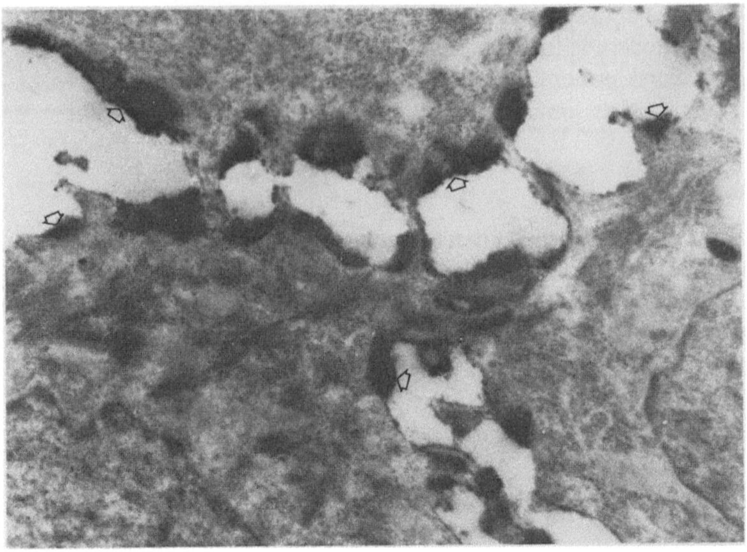

Fig. 2. Case M.K. Widely disseminated, almost erythrodermic lesions. Biopsy from the lesions taken before the treatment. Electron microscopy, x 13,900.
Alcian blue staining. Widened intercellular spaces with alcian blue-positive substance, adhering to the cell membranes (⇔)

The coarse granular substance had some similarity to ribosomes, and in some areas there were traces of cytoplasmic organelles, with no visible remnants of cell membranes.

It should be stressed that in 3 cases studied before the treatment, there were also widened spaces filled with a fine granular, alcian blue-positive substance, more abundant in very early and active lesions of the pin-point type (Fig. 2).

The changes were most pronounced within the first three weeks of treatment; however, in patients in whom the improvement was rather moderate, they persisted up to 6 weeks.

In the upper layers, there was within 3 to 6 weeks a progressive restoration of keratohyalin granules with the reappearance of stratum corneum, which at the beginning was somewhat less compact.

The inflammatory changes in the dermis, pronounced before the treatment and within the first 3 weeks, diminished considerably thereafter, as reported earlier (14). Capillaries were less widened, and the fine mucinous substance, visible around the capillaries and at the basement membrane zone in active lesions, disappeared within the first three weeks. At that time, basal lamina seemed to be almost unchanged, but inflammatory cells were still present in the dermis and occasionally in the epidermis.

In the uninvolved skin at 3 and 6 weeks there were widened intercellular spaces, more pronounced at 6 weeks, some containing fine granular material. The mitochondria of the keratinocytes were abundant, enlarged, and partially deranged (Fig. 3).

Immunofluorescent Studies

Immunoglobulins and C3 deposits, present in virtually all psoriatic lesions before the treatment (9, 10), disappeared very slowly during the therapy. Stratum corneum (SC), although disorganized and even partially destroyed during the first two weeks of treatment, preserved its antigenic properties as a substrate for the reaction of stratum corneum antibodies (pres-

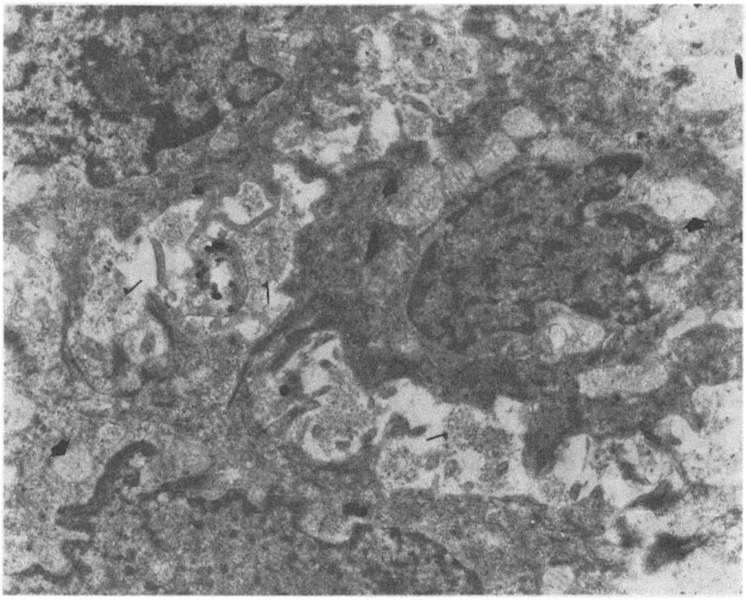

Fig. 3. Case W.K. Psoriasis vulgaris, widely disseminated lesions. Biopsy from the uninvolved skin, taken in the 6th week of treatment in a dose of 1 mg/kg body weight/day. Widened intercellular spaces, filled with mainly fine granular substance (→). In the cytoplasm numerous enlarged, partially deranged mitochondria (⇸). Electron microscopy, x 8,500

ent in normal sera) both in psoriatic lesions and in the seemingly normal skin of the patients (Table 6). The preservation of antigenic properties favours some mechanism of action of retinoids in psoriasis other than through changing of the antigenicity of SC, which could interfere with binding of SC antibodies and the deposition of immune complexes, i.e. with a mechanism presumably involved in self-perpetuation of psoriatic lesions (2).

Summary

A randomized double blind study performed in 40 patients with psoriasis (20 treated with

Table 6. Immunofluorescent studies (direct DIF and indirect IIF) for binding of stratum corneum antibodies in psoriatic plaques and uninvolved skin of psoriatics during the treatment with retinoids

	Skin lesions		Uninvolved skin	
	DIF	IIF	DIF	IIF
	+	+	+	+
Before treatment	11/12	12/12	1/6	5/6*
10–14 days of treatment	4/4	4/4	0/4	3/4**
21–28 days of treatment	5/7	5/7**	0/4	2/4**
42–56 days of treatment	3/7	7/7	0/5	4/5**

* In one case the result was not clear
** In one case there was no stratum corneum

Ro-9359 and 20 with placebo) showed a statistically significant difference in two groups from week 2. Especially good results were obtained in psoriasis pustulosa and psoriatic erythroderma. Further open studies performed in 22 patients with psoriasis, and the maintenance therapy in some patients treated previously in the double-blind study, have shown that maintenance therapy is needed in cases of psoriasis pustulosa and in the majority of patients with erythroderma.

Histological studies confirmed earlier reports on the restoration of normal keratinization in 3–6 weeks of treatment, and the appearance of parakeratosis and acanthosis in the uninvolved skin. Ultrastructural studies have also confirmed previous reports on vacuolization of keratinocytes with the presence of fine granular material in vacuoles and in widened intercellular spaces. Studies performed in the 6th week in flattened psoriatic plaques have disclosed still persistent widened intercellular spaces with less abundant alcian blue-positive material, and numerous keratohyalin granules. In the uninvolved skin, in the 6th week, the intercellular spaces were also considerably widened.

The immunofluorescence studies did show no antigenic changes in the stratum corneum, which in the first weeks of treatment was disorganized and considerably thinned.

References

1. Beutner EH, Jablonska S, Jarząbek-Chorzelska M, Maciejowska E, Rzeşa G, Chorzelski TP (1975) Studies in immunodermatology VI. IF Studies of autoantibodies to the stratum corneum and in vivo fixed IgG in stratum corneum of psoriatic lesions. Int Arch Allergy Appl Immunol 48: 301–323
2. Beutner EH, Jablonska S, Chorzelski T, Binder W (1979) A unified concept of autoimmunity and the nature of stratum corneum antigen conversion phenomenon. In: Immunopathology, Milgrom F, Albini B (eds), Karger, Basel, p 148–153
3. Dahl B, Møllenbach K, Reymann F (1977) Treatment of psoriasis with a new retinoic acid derivative Ro 10-9359: an uncontrolled clinical trial. Dermatologica 154:261–267
4. Dierlich E, Orfanos C, Pullmann H, Steigleder GK (1979) Epidermale Zellproliferation unter oraler Retinoid-Therapie bei Psoriasis. Arch Dermatol Res 264:169–177
5. Dominguez-Soto L, Hojyo-Tomoka M-Th (1978) Ro 10-9359 in the treatment of psoriasis. Dermatologica 157 (Suppl 1):57–59
6. Fredriksson T, Pettersson U (1978) Severe psoriasis - oral therapy with a new retinoid. Dermatologica 157:238–244
7. Goerz G, Orfanos CE (1978) Systemic treatment of psoriasis with a new aromatic retinoid. Dermatologica 157 (Suppl 1):38–44
8. Guilhou JJ, Malbos S, Meynadier J (1978) Traitement oral des psoriasis graves par un nouveau rétinoïde aromatique (Ro 10-9359). Ann Dermatol Venereol 105:813–818
9. Jablonska S, Chorzelski TP, Beutner EH, Maciejowska E, Jarząbek-Chorzelska M, Rzęsa G (1978) Autoimmunity in psoriasis. Relation of disease activity and forms of psoriasis to immunofluorescence findings. Arch Dermatol Res 261:135–146
10. Jablonska S, Jarząbek-Chorzelska M, Beutner EH, Rzęsa G, Maciejowska E, Chorzelski T Clinical relevance of stratum corneum antibodies in psoriasis. In: "Immunopathology of the skin", Beutner EH, Chorzelski T, Bean S (eds), Wiley, New York, 1979, p 427–443
11. Lassus A (1980) Systemic treatment of psoriasis with an oral retinoic acid derivative (Ro 10-9359). Br J Dermatol 102:195–202
12. Mahrle G, Orfanos CE, Ippen H, Hofbauer M (1979) Haarwachstum, Leberwerte und Lichtempfindlichkeit unter oraler Retinoid-Therapie bei Psoriasis. Dtsch Med Wochenschr 104:473–477
13. Orfanos CE, Landes E, Bloch PH (1978) Traitement du psoriasis pustuleux par un nouveau rétinoïde aromatique (Ro 10-9359). Ann Dermatol Venereol 105:807–811
14. Orfanos CE, Goerz G (1978) Orale Psoriasis-Therapie mit einem neuen aromatischen Retinoid. Dtsch med Wochenschr 103:195–199
15. Orfanos CE, Runne U (1978) Tissue changes in psoriasis plaques after oral administration of retinoid. Dermatologica 157 (Suppl 1):19–25

16. Orfanos CE, Mahrle G, Goerz G, Happle R, Landes E, Schimpf A (1979) Laboratory investigations in patients with generalized psoriasis under oral retinoid treatment. Dermatologica 159: 62–70
17. Ott F (1977) Behandlung der Psoriasis mit einem oral wirksamen aromatischen Retinoid. Schweiz Med Wochenschr 107:144–147
18. Ott F, Bollag W (1975) Therapie der Psoriasis mit einem oral wirksamen neuen Vitamin A-Säure-Derivat. Schweiz Med Wochenschr 105:439–441
19. Tsambaos D, Mahrle G, Orfanos CE (1980) Epidermal changes induced by oral excess of aromatic retinoid in guinea pigs. Arch Dermatol Res 267:141–152
20. Viglioglia PA, Barclay CA (1978) Oral retinoids and psoriasis. Dermatologica 157 (Suppl 1):32–37

C.E. Orfanos et al. (eds.)
Retinoids

Intermittent Dose Schedule of Retinoids (Ro 10-9359) for Long-term follow-up on Psoriasis (Preliminary Report)

L. Domínguez-Soto, M.T. Hojyo-Tomoka and J.J. Armas

It has been well established in many publications, that retinoids and especially the one known as Ro 10-9359 (Tigason) are effective in the treatment of psoriasis. Orfanos (3) concludes that its effectiveness may vary according to the different clinical forms of the disease. It is also clear now that the adequate initial dose is 1 mg/kg/day; to be reduced to 0.66 mg/kg/day until an adequate remission is achieved. Patients are then kept on a minimum maintenance dose.

We have given detailed accounts of our observations in previous publications (1, 2), on using this drug for the treatment of severe cases of psoriasis, followed-up for three years, but with a different dose regimen of the retinoid. The long-term results were, generally, good.

With this background, we thought it would be interesting to observe the effects of a two-phase treatment: a continuous dose regimen followed by an intermittent dose phase.

Objectives

The objectives of this study are:

1. To evaluate the effectiveness of this drug over long periods of time - with an initial dose of 1 mg/kg/day, and then alternating a minimum maintenance dose with placebo for one year.

2. To evaluate the tolerance to this drug in both phases (continuous and intermittent).

Table 1. Patients, age and sex

	Sex		
Age (in years)	total	male	female
less than 30	2	1	1
30 to 39	4	4	0
40 to 49	6	4	2
50 to 59	3	3	0
60 to 69	3	1	2
Total	18	13	5

Table 2. Clinical form of psoriasis

Clinical form	No. of patients	Duration (months) Average	Minimum	Maximum
Disseminated (plaques)	16	120	3	456
Localized palms-soles	1	29	0	0
Generalized erythrodermic	1	18	0	0
Total	18	96	3	456

Material and Methods

21 patients with psoriasis were selected, all of them resistant to the usual forms of treatment. This paper concerns only 18 patients. Age and sex as well as the clinical features of the patients are listed in Tables 1 and 2. No patients under 12 years old were included in the study, and women of child-bearing age were given contraceptives parenterally, once a month. Patients' inform consent was obtained prior to therapy.

No patient was given any other concomitant medication, orally or topically, which might mislead information. Every one was only allowed the use of cold cream. Parameters used to evaluate the severity and intensity of the disease before treatment are listed in Table 3. The following laboratory tests were

Table 3. Severity of symptoms in each segment before treatment with Ro 10-9359

Symptoms	Head	Trunk	Extremities	
			Upper	Lower
Erythema				
None	4	2	0	1
Barely detectable pink colour	2	0	0	0
Definite red colour	7	4	6	5
Intense reddening	5	12	12	12
Desquamation				
None	4	2	0	1
Slight scaling	3	0	1	1
Adherent moderately heavy scales	6	7	5	4
Heavily heaped up adherent scales	5	9	12	12
Infiltration				
None	4	2	0	1
Mild	4	1	1	1
Moderate	5	6	5	4
Severe	5	9	12	12
Extension of lesions				
0%	4	2	0	1
1-20%	4	2	2	1
21-40%	3	5	4	2
41-60%	3	2	4	2
61-80%	3	6	6	9
81-100%	1	1	2	3

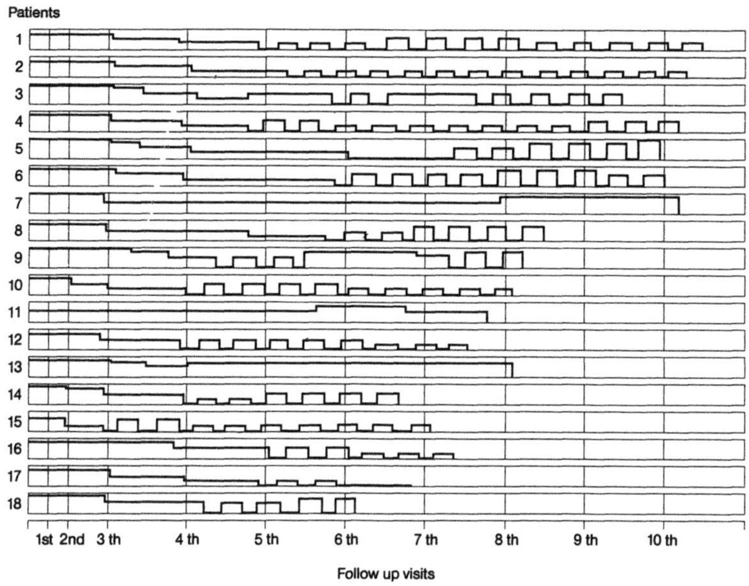

Fig. 1. Graphical dose schedule

performed on all patients: Complete blood count, SGOT and SGOP, DHL and urinalysis. These tests had to be performed prior to inception of treatment, then one, three and six months later, and one year after completion of treatment.

The regimen followed was: 1 mg/kg/day as the initial dose (weeks 1 through 4); 0.66 mg/kg/day (weeks 5 and 6); 0.33 mg/kg/day (weeks 7 and 8). After week 9, the regimen was changed over to the intermittent phase. The patient was given 0.33 mg/kg/day one week, and placebo the next one, alternating in this way until week 52.

This regimen could be modified in the following situations:

1. If we considered that the patient's condition had not improved sufficiently to start with the intermittent regimen, they were to receive a larger dose for 4 weeks or longer.

2. If the patients had a serious relapse during the intermittent phase, they were to return to the continuous regimen until conditions would allow a return to the intermittent phase (Fig. 1).

For evaluation of the effectiveness of the treatment, two criteria were used: the continuous phase was considered successful when there was an improvement in the severity of all symptoms, and a failure if symptoms maintained or went worse. The intermittent phase was considered successful when symptoms improved or maintained, and a failure if patients deteriorated.

The binominal test was used for statistical evaluation with a probability level of 1% ($p < 0.01$) (Tables 4 and 5).

Results

This preliminary report analyzes the results obtained in 18 of 21 patients involved. At this stage they have been followed up for a minimum of three months and for a maximum of eight months.

1. Continuous treatment brought about an overall, statistically significant reduction in the symptomatology in the lower extremities; on the upper extremities and the trunk, only the surface area of the lesions did not improve in any statistically significant way; and on the head, only the intensity of the erythema had a statistically significant improvement.

Table 4. Efficacy evaluation, continuous phase

Results	Erythema				Desquamation				Infiltration				Extension			
	head	trunk	extremities upper	extremities lower	head	trunk	extremities upper	extremities lower	head	trunk	extremities upper	extremities lower	head	trunk	extremities upper	extremities lower
Success	12	14	15	14	11	14	17	15	11	15	15	15	11	12	13	14
Failure	2	2	3	3	3	2	1	2	3	1	3	2	3	4	5	3
Total	14	16	18	17	14	16	18	17	14	16	18	17	14	16	18	17
p <	0.006	0.002	0.003	0.006	0.029	0.002	0.001	0.001	0.029	0.001	0.004	0.001	0.029	0.038	0.048	0.006
Statistical significance	← yes →														no	yes

Table 5. Efficacy evaluation, intermittent phase

Results	Erythema				Desquamation				Infiltration				Extension			
	head	trunk	extremities upper	extremities lower	head	trunk	extremities upper	extremities lower	head	trunk	extremities upper	extremities lower	head	trunk	extremities upper	extremities lower
Success	10	10	12	12	9	10	11	12	10	10	12	12	9	10	11	11
Failure	1	3	3	3	2	3	4	3	1	3	3	3	2	3	4	4
Total	11	13	15	15	11	13	15	15	11	13	15	15	11	13	15	15
p <	0.006	0.046	0.018	0.018	0.033	0.046	0.059	0.018	0.006	0.046	0.018	0.018	0.033	0.046	0.059	0.059
Statistical significance	yes	no	← yes →				no		yes	no	← yes →			← no →		

Table 6. Global clinical evaluation

Results	First visit	Last visit: Continuous	Last visit: Intermittent
Worse	0	0	0
No changes	16	1	2
Minimal improvement	1	4	1
Marked improvement	0	7	2
Almost clear	1	4	5
Complete remission	0	2	5
Total	18	18	15

In general they show that the drug was effective in the continuous phase of the experiment.

2. Intermittent treatment reduced the degree of severity of the erythema and the infiltration on the head. But its statistical significance for other parts of the body still allows the possibility that improvement was in fact due to other factors.
3. However, if we compare the developmental course between the first visit and the end of the continuous phase on one hand, and between the last visit at the end of the continuous and intermittent phases, on the other, we observe statistically significant improvements on the former case, which are not seen in the latter. These results are listed in Tables 6 and 7.
4. Concerning the tolerance to the drug (Table 8) shows that both the number and severity of the side effects are greater at the beginning, and seem to be dose-related; and then there is a gradual decrease, which is dose-dependent (Figs. 2–5).
5. Finally, laboratory tests did not show significant changes using Student's "t test".

Comments

Preliminary observations of our studies had shown that patients should take retinoid (Ro 10-9359) continuously in order to get good results, however, this does not apply to all subjects.

On the other hand, we could not maintain the intermittent dose schedule in all of our patients.

Table 7. Results according to phase

Results	First control vs Last continuous phase	Last control vs Last intermittent phase
Success	17	12
Failure	1	3
Total	18	15
$p <$	0.001	0.018
Statistical significance	yes	no

Table 8. Tolerance evaluation

Adverse effect	Lips		Dryness Mouth		Nose		Rhagades		Healthy skin Thinning		Healthy skin Desquamation		Cheilitis		Loss of hair	
	Conti.	Interm.	Conti.	Interm.	Conti.	Interm.	Conti.	Interm.	Conti.	Interm.	Conti.	Interm.	Conti.	Interm.	Conti.	Interm.
yes	16	7	11	4	7	1	5	0	3	2	8	4	15	2	4	3
no	2	8	7	11	11	14	13	15	15	13	10	11	3	13	14	12
total	18	15	18	15	18	15	18	15	18	15	18	15	18	15	18	15
t	2.68		1.977		2.146		2.224		0.272		1.553		2.04		0.189	
Statistical significance	yes		←						no						→	

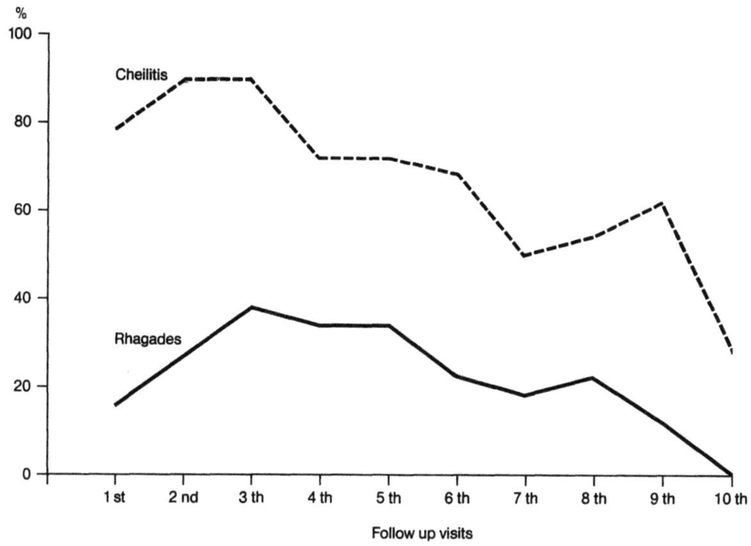

Fig. 2. Cheilitis and rhagades

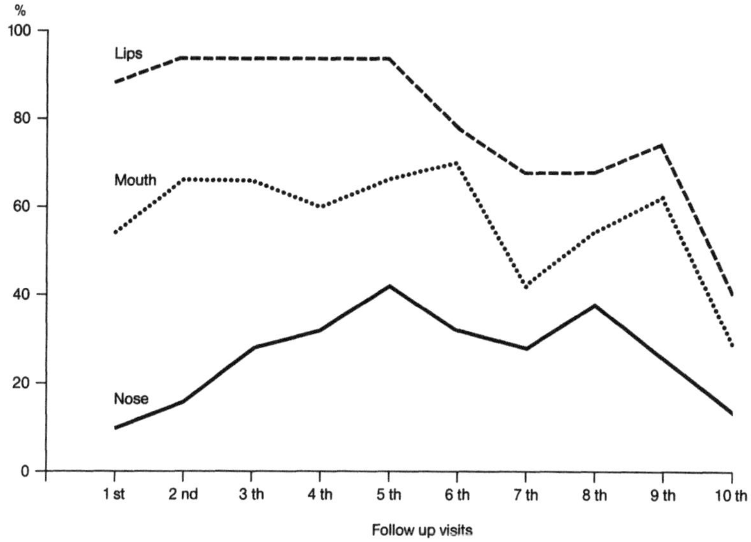

Fig. 3. Dryness

In our past experience, patients were maintained with a dose of 0.66 mg/kg/day for 3 to 4 months, after which the drug is discontinued for a period that varies until a relapse would occur; this regimen has given better results than intermittent dose schedule of treatment.

While these observations are the result of our on-going study, it is only on completion of this trial that we will be in a position to confirm or modify our present opinion.

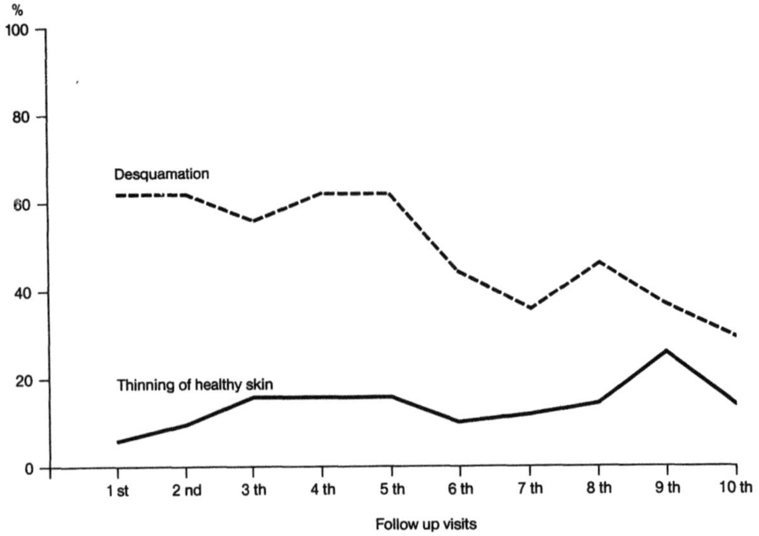

Fig. 4. Thinning of healthy skin and desquamation

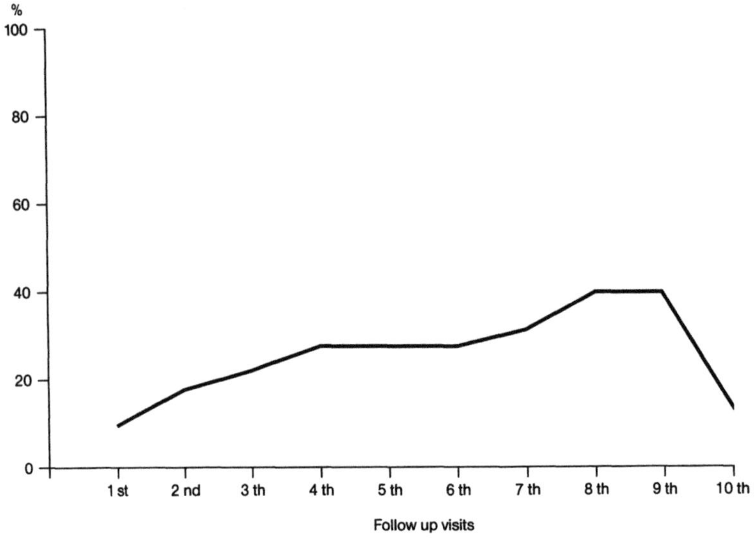

Fig. 5. Loss of hair

Summary

Data from a long-term study of psoriasis patients, treated with Ro 10-9359 in a continuous regimen and alternating placebo with a minimum drug dose, were analyzed.

Results, as listed in this preliminary report, show significant improvements with the continuous dose schedule; the intermittent dose schedule led to a stabilization of the symptomatology, or to a not statistically significant improvement.

There is a large number of adverse effects in the first phase, which decreases significantly with lower doses, although there is no statistical correlation; nor were there noticeable differences in the ratio of patients having adverse effects in both phases.

There were no statistically significant differences in the laboratory tests performed, neither before nor through the study.

References

1. Domínguez-Soto L, Hojyo-Tomoka MT (1978) Aromatic retinoid (Ro 10-9359) in the treatment of psoriasis. Cutis 2:376–379
2. Domínguez-Soto L, Hojyo-Tomoka MT (1978) Ro 10-9359 in the treatment of psoriasis. Dermatologica 157 (Suppl 1):57–59
3. Orfanos CE (1980) Oral retinoids - present status. Br J Dermatol 103:473–481

C.E. Orfanos et al. (eds.)
Retinoids

Treatment of Severe Forms of Psoriasis with a Retinoic Acid Derivative: Ro 10-9359*

J.C. Gatti, J.E. Cardama, M. Gabrielli and H. Cabrera

Ro 10-9359 is an aromatic derivative of retinoic acid which has shown interesting protective properties on the epithelia in animal experiments. Chemically it is the ethyl-all-trans-9-(4-methoxy-2,3,6-trimethylphenyl)-3,7-dimethyl-2,4,6,8-nonatetraenoate. Its therapeutical index is several times more favourable than that of retinoic acid, as has been shown by Bollag (1). This therapeutical index, defined as the ratio between the dose that causes a reduction of 50% of the volume of induced papillomas and that which produces the signs of hypervitaminosis A, is 10 times more favourable than the index of retinoic acid.

Among the different conditions which react to treatment with this drug are bladder papillomas, leukoplakias, ganglionar or hepatic metastasis of epidermoid carcinomas, as well as corneal ulcers and psoriasis.

In the field of dermatology there are several diseases which still raise therapeutical problems that are difficult to solve due to their chronicity and resistance to treatment (2). Among them there are certain severe forms of psoriasis which are undoubtedly important, which we wanted to study for the possible benefits of treatment with the new retinoic acid derivative, Ro 10-9359.

Material and Method

In order to carry out this study we selected 20 patients with severe psoriasis – 17 of the cases generalized, 2 erythrodermic and 1 psoriasis vulgaris with acute outbreak – with periods of evolution between 9 months and 54 years; 4 of them with psoriatic arthropathy.

Twelve of the 20 were outpatients, whereas the other 8 were hospitalized. There were 15 males and 5 females. Table 1 shows the patients' general information.

All of them had received previous treatment with different antipsoriatic agents. In 13 cases, the results were not satisfactory; and in the other 7, the facts reported were insufficient to make an evaluation.

Table 1. Patients' general information

Variable	Arithmetical mean	Standard deviation	Standard error
Age (years)	49.2	12.8	2.9
Weight (kg)	77.5	14.8	3.3
Height (cm)	169	8.7	1.9

* Ro 10-9359 – F. Hoffmann-La Roche & Co. Ltd., Basle, Switzerland

Table 2. Dose by week of treatment[a]

Week	Daily dose (mg)	Cases	Arithmetical mean
1	25 50	1 19	48.8 mg
2	25 50 75	1 18 1	50.0 mg
3	50 75	4 16	70.0 mg
4	50 75	5 15	68.8 mg
5 and 6	50 75 100	4 1 15	88.8 mg
7	50 100 interrupted	13 5 2	63.9 mg
8	50 100	15 3	58.3 mg
9 and 10	50	18	50.0 mg

[a] All the cases continued with 50 mg daily until the end of the study, except one patient who, from the 14th week on, received 25 mg daily for 3 weeks more

A careful study was made before treating in order to have a control and a basis for the conclusions. For this purpose, a score of intensity was assigned to every body region by summing up the scores given to: erythema, scaling, infiltration, ulceration, pustules.

The lowest score was 0 and the highest was 4. Thus, for every body region the sum of the scores varied between a minimum of 0 and maximum of 20. Following this, the mean score of intensity of the lesions was calculated. The intensity of the lesions before treatment was significantly higher on the trunk and upper and lower limbs than on the head and neck.

The dosage of Ro 10-9359 was not the same in all the cases. Table 2 shows the doses given during the different weeks of treatment.

The duration of the treatment was not the same, either. It varied between 6 and 17 weeks; 8 of the 20 cases (40%) were treated for 14 weeks.

It must be stated that the criterion established for adjusting the dose and duration of treatment was based on the seriousness of each particular case.

Laboratory analyses (complete blood count, ESR, blood sugar, urea, creatinine, SGO and SGP transaminases and urine) were carried out before, during and at the end of therapy.

Results

1. Evolution of Signs

Tests of the most important signs (erythema, scaling and infiltration) were performed every two weeks. Figure 1 shows their evolution during treatment. Although the amelioration of erythema was gradual, the most noticeable improvement was seen during the 4th week, when the mean score fell from 3 to 2.

Scaling, which was very striking during the first 2 weeks, was still important up to the 6th week remitting thereafter.

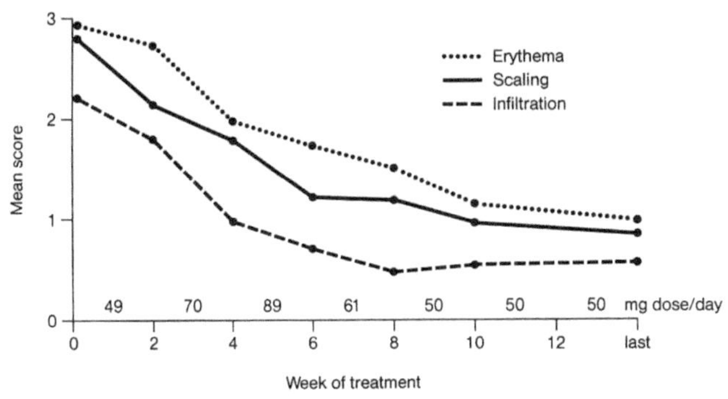

Fig. 1. Evolution of erythema, scaling and infiltration

The improvement of infiltration was evident between the 2nd and 4th weeks of treatment, stabilizing after the 8th. A longer treatment did not result in any greater benefit.

2. Histological Findings

Skin biopsies of typical lesions were taken from 2 patients before and after retinoid administration (Figs. 2–5).

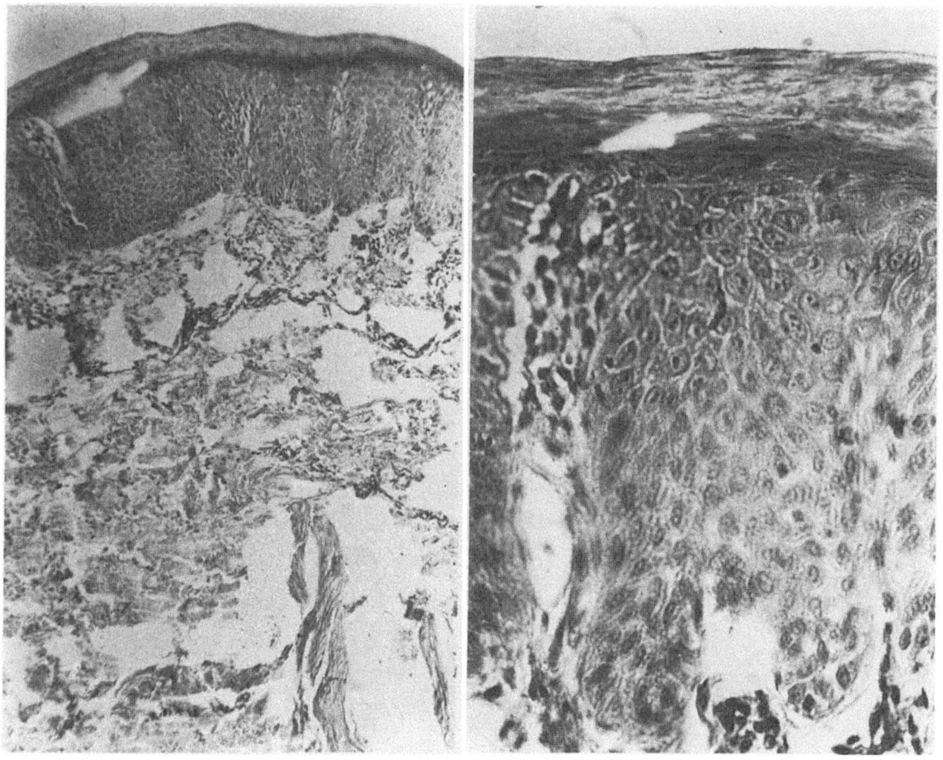

Fig. 2 a, b. Case I. Before treatment

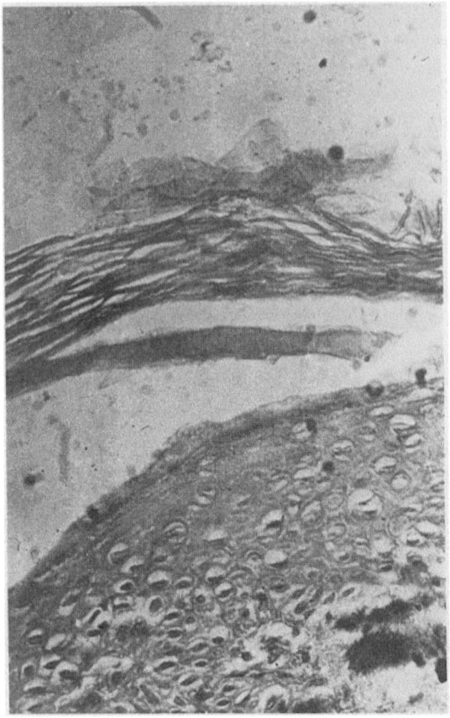

Fig. 3. Case I. After treatment

In 1 case histological findings after 30 days of treatment showed the disappearance of parakeratosis and inflammatory infiltrates, as well as a decrease in acanthosis and a slight orthokeratotic hyperkeratosis.

In the other patient, specimens taken after 50 days of therapy showed normal skin with the reappearance of a granular layer consisting of a single row of cells.

According to these findings, it seems that the systemic administration of the retinoid exerts a well-defined influence on the skin alterations of the disease.

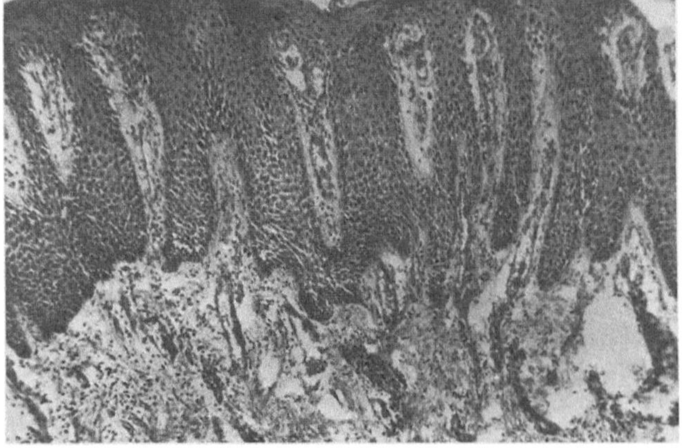

Fig. 4. Case II. Before treatment

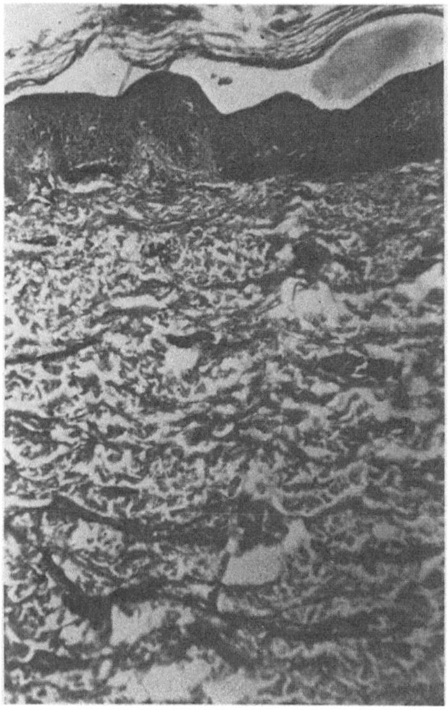

Fig. 5. Case II. After treatment

3. General Evaluation

Treatment with Ro 10-9359 produced a complete remission in 2 patients, excellent results in 12, good in 3 and moderate or insufficient in 3. Compared to previous therapy, the results achieved with the retinoid were considered better in 13 cases, equal in 3 and worse in 4.

4. Side Effects

It is interesting to point out that the side effects were well tolerated by all of the patients. Cheilitis and dryness of nasal and oral mucosae were the most frequently observed side effects. As may be seen on Table 3, these side effects were most significant from the 6th to 8th weeks of treatment, diminishing thereafter. Other symptoms, such as erosion of mucous membranes, perspiration and alopecia, were less frequent.

The humoral parameters, analyzed at the end of the treatment, showed a significant increase in hemoglobin: $0.02 < p < 0.05$.

Discussion

Although the number of patients treated is not large enough to allow definite conclusions as to the therapeutic results, we may point out that the new retinoic acid derivative Ro 10-9359 is an effective drug for the treatment of severe forms of psoriasis. The following considerations support this assertion:

- Rapid clinical improvement was achieved from the beginning of treatment, becoming

Table 3. Side effects by week of treatment[a]

		Cases by week of treatment					
Effect		2	4	6	8	10	Last
Cheilitis	yes	4	5	10	9	9	4
	no	16	15	10	9	9	16
Dryness of	yes	5	7	9	9	9	8
nasal mucosa	no	15	13	11	9	9	12
Buccal dryness	yes	8	10	11	11	10	6
	no	12	10	9	7	8	14
Erosion of	yes	2	3	4	2	2	1
mucosae	no	18	17	16	16	16	19
Perspiration	yes	4	5	3	2	2	1
	no	16	15	17	16	16	19
Alopecia	yes	1	1	2	5	5	3
	no	19	19	18	13	13	17

[a] One patient showed depigmentation of the hair by the 10th week of treatment

especially evident by the 4th week. Psoriatic arthropathy affected 4 patients with one case of complete remission, and 2 others showing slight improvement.

- Histological findings following the administration of the retinoid clearly showed important structural changes in the dermis and epidermis leading to a regression of the psoriatic lesions.
- Two out of 20 cases of severe psoriasis showed complete remission; 12 cases excellent and 3 good results.
- Bearing in mind that the patients had previously undergone different and thorough types of treatment, the results are especially encouraging. In comparison with prior therapies, Ro 10-9359 was considered better in 13 patients, equal in 3 and worse in 4.
- As to the side effects observed, the dryness of mucosae (which is reversible) was the most frequent (11 out of 20 patients).

Referring to humoral parameters, the only significant increase was that of hemoglobin. SGO and SGP transaminases, plasma creatinine and the other routine analyses performed underwent no change.

According to these observations, we may state that Ro 10-9359 is a valuable drug for the oral treatment of severe forms of psoriasis.

We wish to emphasize the importance of adjusting the dosage to the seriousness of the disease, until a maintenance dose able to avoid the frequent relapses of the disease is reached.

Summary

The authors refer to the results of their experience with the use of the new retinoic acid derivative, Ro 10-9359, in 20 patients with severe forms of psoriasis. To evaluate the therapeutic results, a close evolutive control of the lesions was carried out. Each sign of the illness was assigned a score of severity to determine the changes during the course of the treatment. Complete remission of the illness was obtained in 10% of the patients, and results were considered excellent in 60% of the cases, good in 15% and insufficient in 15%. Dryness of mucosae was the most frequent side effect, appearing in 55% of the patients. The histological findings before and after retinoid administration are reported.

References

1. Bollag W (1974) Therapeutic effects of an aromatic retinoic acid analog on chemically induced skin papillomas and carcinomas of mice. Eur J Cancer 10:731–737
2. Orfanos CE (1980) Oral retinoids - present status. Br J Dermatol 103:·473–481

C.E. Orfanos et al. (eds.)
Retinoids

Treatment of Psoriasis Vulgaris with a Low-dosage Ro 10-9359 (Tigason) Orally Combined with Corticosteroids Topically

H.J. van der Rhee and M.K. Polano

Since its introduction in 1975 by Ott and Bollag (7), the use of the new aromatic retinoid Tigason (Ro 10-9359) for the treatment of psoriasis has been well documented. This drug appeared to be highly effective, in the first place against psoriasis pustulosa and erythrodermatic psoriasis (4) and also, although to a lesser degree, against psoriasis vulgaris. In the latter condition the therapeutic ratio of the aromatic retinoid was found to be enhanced by combining the drug with other types of psoriasis therapy such as PUVA (2, 5), dithranol (3, 4), and selective ultraviolet therapy (10).

Tigason, used in the commonly recommended dosage (1 mg/kg body weight = "high dosage"), was also found to have several obnoxious side effects, such as dry mucous membranes, hair loss, and palmo-plantar desquamation. These side effects proved, however, to be closely dose-dependent (1, 2). This finding raised the question of whether additive treatment with topically applied corticosteroids would permit lowering of the oral dose of retinoid to a level at which side effects would be more acceptable (8, 11). We therefore investigated the effect of an *initial treatment* aimed at clearing the psoriasis, i.e., by means of a double-blind trial followed by an open clinical trial (11), and of a *maintenance treatment*, by a follow-up study in patients who could be observed for two years.

Initial Treatment

The first part of this study was designed as a double-blind multi-centre clinical trial with a duration of 6 weeks, and was performed in out-patients with extensive psoriasis vulgaris. Virtually all of them had been treated unsuccessfully with potent corticosteroids, often with occlusive dressings, and 13 had also been treated with PUVA.

Patients were randomly assigned to one of the three following treatment regimens:

1. aromatic retinoid (Ro 10-9359) orally (0.50–0.66 mg/kg body weight) and placebo cream topically (abbreviated as AR/Pl cr);
2. aromatic retinoid (Ro 10-9359) (same dosages) combined with 0.1% triamcinolone acetonide and 5% salicylic acid in lanette wax cream (AR/Tr);
3. placebo capsules with 0.1% triamcinolone acetonide and 5% salicylic acid in lanette wax cream (Pl ca/Tr).

Finally 87 patients were effectively taken into the trial.

At 3 and 6 weeks, the overall improvement (in units of 10%) relative to week 0 was evaluated. The mean overall improvement after 6 weeks, as judged by the physician, was 55.4% for the group treated with the combination therapy (AR/Tr), 40.8% for the group treated

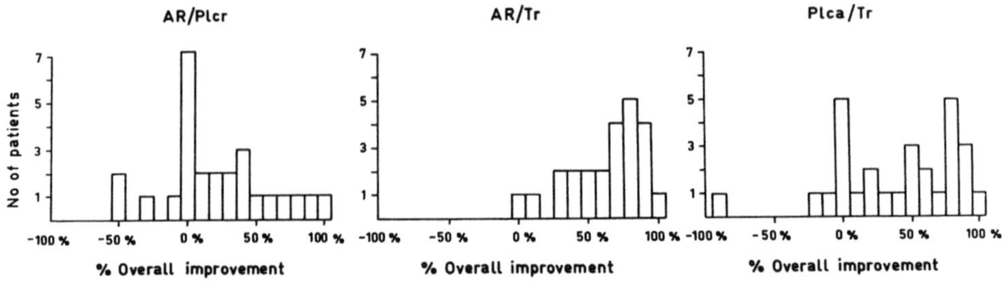

Fig. 1. Histograms representing the overall improvement in percentages 6 weeks after the start of the treatment, for the three treatment groups

with the active cream alone (Pl ca/Tr) and 18.0% for the group given only the aromatic retinoid (AR/Pl cr). Histograms representing the overall improvement of the three treatment groups are given in Fig. 1. Furthermore at 0, 3, and 6 weeks intensity scores were given for the lesions on six body areas separately (scalp, arms, hands, trunk, legs, and feet) according to the grading system used in earlier clinical trials (9). For desquamation the scale was arbitrarily taken from 0 (no desquamation) to 8 (very marked desquamation), for erythema and infiltration from 0 (no erythema) via 4 (moderate infiltration) to 8 (very marked infiltration). The results are given in Table 1. It is evident that the combination therapy was more effective than the aromatic retinoid alone (AR/Pl cr). The AR/Tr regimen was also more effective than the active cream alone (Pl ca/Tr) for all body areas and all symptoms (except desquamation of the scalp and feet), although statistical significance was not found for all parameters. The effect was greater for erythema and infiltration than for desquamation.

After the double-blind study the patients were treated for 12 weeks with regimen 2, i.e., active cream and active capsules in the dosage indicated above (AR/Tr). At the end of this open study, 4 patients had dropped out because of side effects and 8 because of failure to keep appointments.

Fig. 2 shows the course of the mean overall improvement in the three patient groups in the first 8 weeks of the study. For the entire series, the final overall improvement after 18 weeks was as follows: 9 patients were free of lesions, 30 showed 90% improvement; 10 showed 80% improvement; 5 showed 70% improvement; 6 showed 60% improvement; 10 showed 10–50% improvement; 2 patients showed no improvement and in 2 patients the lesions were worse.

The differences in intensity score between the three treatment groups at week 6 disappeared after all patients had been put on the same treatment (AR/Tr). On the whole, the decline of the intensity scores corresponded with the course of the overall improvement. At the end of the study, the average score for all body areas was about 1 for erythema and 1 for desquamation, except for the legs, which on average scored 2 for these symptoms.

These results show that, in the dosage used, retinoid alone has virtually no effect at all. The combined treatment gave better results than the triamcinolone/salicylic acid treatment alone. This effect, which was apparent for almost all variables, was statistically significant for some of them only. Since the active cream alone could be expected to have a considerable impact on desquamation, the absence of a strong effect after the addition of retinoid is not surprising. The effect on erythema and infiltration (see Table 1), which are more difficult to influence, is more striking.

In this trial the effectiveness of the cream containing 0.1% triamcinolone acetonide and 5% salicylic acid is astonishing (mean overall improvement in 6 weeks: 40%), especially since

Table 1. Means of the intensity scores at week 0 and week 6 and P values used to assess improvement after 6 weeks. For week 0 some general data are given too

Treatment	AR/Plcr			AR/Tr			Plca/Tr			Comparison at week 6	
Time	Week 0	Week 6	⊗	Week 0	Week 6	⊗	Week 0	Week 6	⊗	AR/Tr vs AR/Plcr P value*	AR/Tr vs Plca/Tr P value*
Erythema and infiltration											
Scalp	3·4	2·1	1·3	2·6	1·2	1·4	2·8	1·9	0·9	0·05	0·04
Arms	4·1	3·1	1·0	3·9	2·0	1·9	3·7	2·6	1·1	0·01	0·10
Hands	2·6	1·7	0·9	2·8	1·2	1·6	2·2	1·8	0·4	0·009	0·005
Trunk	4·1	3·1	1·0	3·8	2·0	1·8	3·6	2·4	1·2	0·004	0·54
Legs	4·3	3·5	0·8	4·3	2·3	2·0	4·0	2·9	1·1	0·002	0·04
Feet	2·4	1·8	0·6	2·3	1·6	0·7	2·3	1·8	0·5	0·41	0·76
Desquamation											
Scalp	4·3	2·2	2·1	2·7	1·3	1·4	3·5	1·8	1·7	0·52	1·00
Arms	3·2	2·4	0·8	3·5	1·6	1·9	3·3	1·9	1·4	0·09	0·45
Hands	2·1	1·1	1·0	2·1	0·8	1·3	1·8	1·3	0·5	0·21	0·02
Trunk	3·2	2·3	0·9	3·1	1·2	1·9	3·0	1·7	1·3	0·005	0·10
Legs	3·2	2·4	0·8	3·6	1·7	1·9	3·5	2·0	1·5	0·07	0·89
Feet	2·1	1·4	0·7	1·7	1·2	0·5	2·0	1·5	0·5	0·94	0·43
Age (years)	43·7			44·7			43·7				
Weight (kg)	71·2			71·1			72·1				
Duration (years)	20·4			20·8			22·9				
Sex (male/female)	18/11			15/14			15/14				
Prior PUVA (yes/no)	4/25			5/24			4/25				

⊗ improvement at week 6 as compared with week 0
* computed according to the Mantel-Haenszel method
The initial values for the three groups were compared by an analysis of variance. Comparison of the three groups at week 0 yielded, for all items, P values higher thar 0·25 with the exception of desquamation on the scalp, which had a P value of 0·03

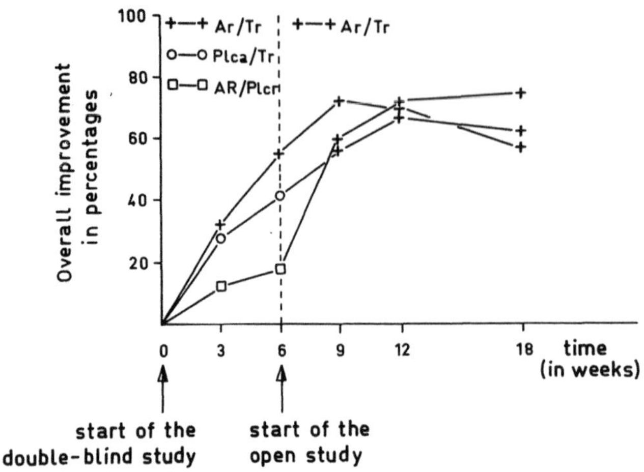

Fig. 2. Course of the overall improvement for the three treatment groups. After 6 weeks all patients were put on the same treatment
(+——+) AR/Tr; (O—O) Pl ca/Tr; (□—□) AR/Pl cr

these patients had previously obtained little or no benefit from various strong corticosteroids applied topically, often in combination with salicylic acid.

As can be concluded from Fig. 2 the maximal results obtained in the three treatment groups could be maintained to varying degrees up to week 18.

Maintenance Treatment

Since long-term ambulatory treatment with topical corticosteroids is often frustrating due to the frequent relapses, we decided to follow the remaining patients for a longer period to find out whether the long-term results of this form of combination therapy are superior to those generally seen after prolonged treatment with topical corticosteroids alone.

After the initial trial, the combination therapy was continued in 75 patients. These patients were followed for up to two years after the start of the double-blind trial. Generally, an attempt was made to lower the dosage of the retinoid after clearance and in a few instances the oral treatment was gradually stopped. The topical corticosteroid therapy was continued and in some patients replaced by stronger corticosteroids, e.g. 0.1% betamethason valerate cream or 0.05% clobetasol propionate cream.

Between the end of the open trial (week 18) and the end of the first year of the treatment, another 16 patients dropped out, 5 of them because of side effects (in 3 cases alopecia, in one case vocal cord nodules, and in one palmo-plantar desquamation and dry. lips), 5 because of unsatisfactory clinical results, and 6 for other reasons (failure to keep appointments, or reason unknown).

Of the remaining 59 patients, 37 were on average in a good clinical condition during this first year, 18 showed only a moderately good response (although their state was considerably better than before the retinoid treatment), and four showed only slight improvement.

Of the 37 patients who responded very well to the treatment, 20 were almost completely clear of lesions throughout the year and 17 had one or two slight exacerbations. In all, there were 20 exacerbations, five of which could be ascribed to lowering of the oral dose, three to interruption of the oral treatment, and for 12 no cause was found. These exacerbations could be corrected by increasing the retinoid dosage (in 5 cases), re-instituting the oral treatment (in 3 cases), or giving a stronger topical corticosteroid (in 5 cases), and in 7 cases remission occurred without a change in the therapy.

In the second year of treatment another 16 patients dropped out, 11 because of unsatisfactory results, five because of side effects (in one case alopecia and cheilitis, and in four gastric complaints). Thus after two years 43 of the 87 patients were still under treatment. Thirty-one of these 43 patients had been almost clear for two years. For most of them, the average dosage was 25 mg/day (range: 0–50 mg). The usual course in these patients is that a few small psoriasis lesions appear of and on, but disappear completely after a few days of topical corticosteroid therapy.

Due to this quick response, only very small amounts of cream were needed, generally not more than 30 g a week.

Of the remaining 12 patients, 10 were in a considerably better state than before the retinoid treatment. In two patients the clinical condition deteriorated, and after 17 and 18 months UVB treatment was successfully substituted for the topical corticosteroid therapy, the retinoid being continued at a dosage of 40 mg/day.

Our long-term results support the view that in this form of combination therapy, both constituents are essential. This refutes the conclusion suggested by the short-term results, i.e., that the topical corticosteroids were mainly responsible for the improvement observed in the double-blind trial.

The sustained good response to the treatment seen in 31 patients and the very rapid clearance of new lesions after the application of corticosteroids in patients who previously had not responded to topical corticosteroid therapy, can hardly be ascribed to the corticosteroids alone.

Side Effects

During the double-blind trial there was, as could be expected, a striking difference in side effects between the two groups receiving active capsules and the group given placebo capsules. As shown in Table 2, 66% of the patients on active capsules had dryness of the lips, albeit generally well tolerated, and the majority of these patients did not show objective signs of cheilitis, such as desquamation and rhagades of the lips. This percentage of patients suffering from dry lips remained unchanged during the first 18 weeks of treatment. A

Table 2. Side effects at the end of the double-blind trial (week 6)*

Side effects	AR/Plcr (n = 29)		AR/Tr (n = 29)		Plca/Tr (n = 29)	
	Mild	Severe	Mild	Severe	Mild	Severe
Dryness of the lips	17	1	21	1	4	0
Rhagades	2	0	3	1	0	0
Dryness of the nose	3	0	8	1	1	0
Dryness of the eyes	2	0	3	0	0	0
Palmo-plantar desquamation	0	0	4	0	0	0
Pruritus	10	3	6	2	0	0
Atrophy of the skin	0	0	3	0	1	0
Alopecia	1	0	0	0	1	0

* All values represent numbers of patients who reported the side effect in question as mild or severe

Table 3. Side effects reported by patients during three treatment periods (6–18 weeks, 18 weeks–1 year, 1-2 years)

Side effect	Number of patients (at * start of period)		
	6–18 weeks (n = 87)*	18 weeks–1 year (n = 75)*	1–2 years (n = 59)*
Dryness of the lips	53	13	9
Rhagades	12	3	
Dryness of the nose	15	2	
Epistaxis	2	1	
Dryness of the eyes	5	1	
Dryness of the throat	0	3	
Palmo-plantar desquamation	3	1	1
Pruritus	17	9	
Atrophy of the skin	2	1	1
Hair loss	3	13	2
Burning sensation on the face	1	1	
Bruises on arms and legs	4	7	1
Paronychia	1	1	
Stomach complaints		4	
Back pain		1	1
Dry skin		2	2
Nail abnormalities		1	1

moderate number of patients suffered from pruritus during the double-blind trial. The side effects reported by patients during the open trial lasting 12 weeks are shown in Table 3. It should, however, be stressed that, with the exception of the alopecia and a few cases of cheilitis, the side effects were well tolerated.

After the first 18 weeks of treatment the dose of the retinoid was gradually lowered whenever possible to 25 mg/day, and the patients who suffered the most severely from side effects dropped out. This led to a considerable decrease in the frequency of side effects. The side effects occurring between week 18 and the end of the first year of treatment are listed in Table 3.

Alopecia occurred mainly in the first six months of treatment, and in three patients was the reason for dropping out. In most of the other patients hair loss stopped after the dose of retinoid was reduced. In the second year of treatment side effects were relatively rare (see Table 3).

The usual laboratory checks were performed frequently (11). Except for one patient who showed pathological liver function in the first three months of treatment, no abnormal values were found during the two-year period. In one patient chronic myeloid leucaemia was discovered at examination of the routine blood smear after 27 months of treatment.

It is clear from Table 3 that the present combination of drugs causes relatively few side effects. The side effects seen during the initial treatment were mild compared with those observed at the currently used dosage of 1 mg/kg, as shown by our earlier results (8) and several reports in the literature (e.g., 2, 4, 7).

Fritsch et al. (2) also found that lowering of the dose led to fewer side effects. During the initial treatment (0–18 weeks) none of the patients showed severe hair loss, the main reason given for the interruption of high-dosage retinoid therapy in other studies.

From the present results it is evident that the gradual decrease in the frequency of side effects continues when the dose is lowered to less than 0.5 mg/kg body weight.

Concluding Remarks

The present results show that the new aromatic retinoid Tigason given in low dosage orally in combination with topically applied corticosteroids offers an effective form of treatment for severe psoriasis vulgaris, side effects being mild. At the end of the open trial (18 weeks) 60% of the patients had attained 80–100% clearance, which is similar to the results obtained with monotherapy with this retinoid in the usual high dosage (4, 6).

For some of our patients the good results could be maintained for up to two years.

In sum, we conclude that:

1. For initial treatment the combination of low doses of the aromatic retinoid Ro 10-9359 with corticosteroids applied topically is just as effective as therapy with the retinoid in high dosage alone and gives markedly fewer side effects.
2. For a proportion of the patients it is possible to find a form of maintenance treatment that will keep them clear of lesions with a minimum of discomfort.

References

1. Fredriksson T, Pettersson U (1978) Severe psoriasis - Oral therapy with a new retinoid. Dermatologica 157:238–244
2. Fritsch P, Hönigsmann H, Jaschke E, Wolff K (1978) Photochemotherapie bei Psoriasis. Steigerung der Wirksamkeit durch ein orales aromatisches Retinoid. Dtsch Med Wochenschr 103: 1731–1736
3. Orfanos CE, Runne U (1976) Systemic use of a new retinoid with and without local dithranol treatment in generalized psoriasis. Br J Dermatol 95:101–103
4. Orfanos CE, Goerz G (1978) Orale Psoriasis-Therapie mit einem neuen aromatischen Retinoid (Ro 10-9359). Dtsch Med Wochenschr 103:195–199
5. Orfanos CE, Pullmann H, Sterry W, Künzig M (1978) Retinoid - PUVA (Re-PUVA): Systemische Kombinations-Behandlung bei Psoriasis. Z Hautkr 53:494–504
6. Ott F (1977) Behandlung der Psoriasis mit einem oral wirksamen aromatischen Retinoid. Schw Med Wochenschr 107:144–147
7. Ott F, Bollag W (1975) Therapie der Psoriasis mit einem oral wirksamen neuen Vitamin-A-Säure-Derivat. Schw Med Wochenschr 105:439–441
8. Polano MK, van der Rhee HJ (1978) Ro 10-9359 and corticosteroids. Intntl Psor Bull 5:1–2
9. Polano MK, Suurmond D, Van der Lely MA, Warnaar P (1970) A clinical trial with hydrocortisone butyrate cream in psoriasis. Br J Dermatol 83:93–97
10. Steigleder GK, Orfanos CE, Pullmann H (1979) Retinoid-SUP-Therapie der Psoriasis. Z Hautkr 54:19–23
11. Van der Rhee HJ, Tijssen JGP, Herrmann WA, Waterman AH, Polano MK (1980) Combined treatment of psoriasis with a new aromatic retinoid (Tigason) in low dosage orally and triamcinolone cream topically: a double-blind trial. Br J Dermatol 102:203–212

C.E. Orfanos et al. (eds.)
Retinoids

Aromatic Retinoid (Ro 10-9359), RePUVA and PUVA in the Treatment of Psoriasis

J. Lauharanta, T. Juvakoski, L. Kanerva and A. Lassus

Oral retinoids - derivatives of vitamin A - have recently been found to be effective in the treatment of dermatoses showing hyperproliferation and disturbed keratinization (6). In previous studies the combination of retinoid and PUVA has given good results in the treatment of psoriasis with reduced UVA doses (3, 4, 9).

The aim of our study was to compare the clinical effects of an aromatic retinoid (Ro 10-9359), combination of retinoid and PUVA (RePUVA), and PUVA alone in the treatment of psoriasis.

Patients and Methods

Eighty ambulatory patients with psoriasis were included in the study; age (yrs): 42.0 ± 3.0 ($\bar{X} \pm$ SEM), weight (kg): 68.6 ± 2.8. The patients were randomly allocated into four different treatment groups, 20 patients in each (Fig. 1).

The retinoid doses in groups I, II and III were initially 50–60 mg/kg/day and after 2 weeks' treatment 30–60 mg/kg/day. In groups I and III the doses were later reduced according to the response, in some cases to 20–30 mg/day.

In PUVA treatment the 8-methoxypsoralen was administered at a dose of approximately 0.6 mg/kg body weight, followed 2 hours later by irradiation in a high intensity cabin (PUVA-22, Airam Ltd, Helsinki, Finland). The initial UVA dose was about the same in all cases (1–1.5 J/cm^2) and increased at

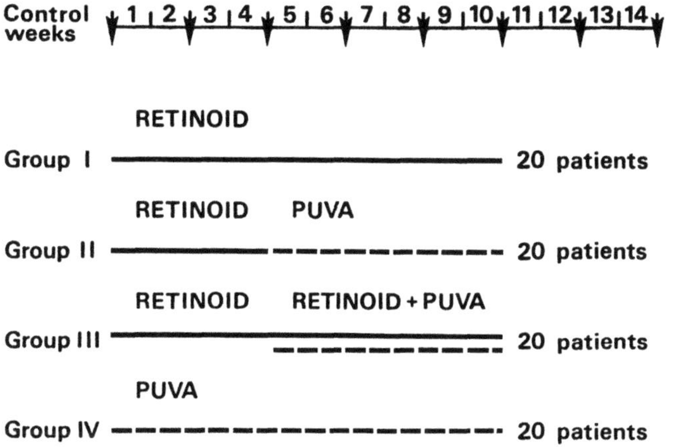

Fig. 1. Treatment regimens and controls

Table 1[1]. Treatment results

	After 4 weeks				After 10 weeks			
Group	I	II	III	IV	I	II	III	IV
Clearing:								
Complete (100%)	0	0	0	0	3	5	13	4
Good (> 75%)	3	3	3	0	10	12	5	15
Moderate (> 50%)	9	7	8	12	5	1	0	1
Slight (> 25%)	6	8	7	6	0	1	0	0
Poor (< 25%)	2	2	2	2	0	1	1	0
Total number of patients	20	20	20	20	18[2,3]	20	19[3]	20

[1] See also Lauharanta et al. (7)
[2] Treatment of one patient discontinued because of paronychia
[3] Treatment of two patients discontinued because of flare-up of the disease

weekly intervals. The maximum single dose used was 12 J/cm^2. PUVA was initially given three times per week; in some cases this fell to 1–2 times per week by the end of the study depending on the treatment response.

Control examinations were made every second week during the ten weeks of active treatment and thereafter during a four weeks' follow-up period. In order to evaluate the overall severity of the disease, the psoriasis area and severity index (PASI) was determined as described by Fredriksson and Pettersson (2). The improvement during treatment was recorded as the percentage of reduction in the PASI score.

At each visit, possible side effects were annotated and serum transaminases and alkaline phosphatase were determined.

Student's t-test and chi-square test with Yates' correction were used in statistical analyses.

Results

Prior to treatment there were no significant differences in the mean PASI scores between the various groups. The results of the four treatment regimens are shown in Table 1. The difference between group III and the other groups was statistically significant as regards complete clearing ($p < 0.01$). Good or complete (75–100%) clearing was seen in 95% of the patients of group IV, in 90% of group III, in 85% of group II and in 65% of group I. In this respect there was no statistically significant difference between groups II, III and IV, but the difference between groups I and IV was significant ($p < 0.02$) in favour of the latter. UVA doses are shown in Table 2.

No real rebound phenomenon was seen after termination of treatment. During the

Table 2. Number of irradiations and total UVA doses given to patients with 75–100% clearing during 10 weeks of treatment. (The figures are mean ± SEM)

Group	Number of irradiations	Total UVA dose (J/cm^2)
II	15.6 ± 0.5	68 ± 5.7*
III	15.9 ± 0.8	67 ± 4.4*
IV	26.5 ± 0.9	200 ± 10.7

* II/IV and III/IV about 1/3 ($p < 0.001$)

four-week follow-up period 20–25% of the patients in every group showed some deterioration.

The side effects during retinoid treatment consisted mostly of dryness of the lips and mucous membranes and of transient erythema and/or desquamation of the healthy skin. In one case the treatment had to be discontinued because of painful paronychia.

Discussion

The antipsoriatic effect of both the PUVA and the retinoid treatment has previously been well documented (2, 5, 8, 10). Therefore, the treatment regimen used in group III could be expected to be the most effective one, since two antipsoriatic modalities were used simultaneously. In RePUVA therapy, pretreatment with retinoid decreases desquamation and, at least to some extent, infiltration. PUVA treatment can then be started at an improved state with less activity of the disease thus resulting in a rapid clearing of the psoriatic lesions at low UVA doses.

The aromatic retinoid Ro 10-9359 has been found to have a distinct normalizing influence on epidermal proliferation, but with a latency of about 3 weeks (1). Because of this lag it is obvious that maximal efficacy with minimal UVA doses can be achieved if the retinoid pretreatment is started at least 3 weeks beforehand. However, shorter periods have also proved to be effective (3, 4, 9). The selection of the type of treatment should, therefore, be based on the individual needs.

Summary

RePUVA proved to be very effective in controlling severe psoriasis. With this regimen the UVA doses were significantly reduced as compared to PUVA treatment.

References

1. Dierlich E, Orfanos CE, Pullmann H, Steigleder GK (1979) Epidermale Zellproliferation unter oraler Retinoid-Therapie bei Psoriasis. Autoradiographische Befunde an befallener und nicht befallener Haut. Arch Dermatol Res 264:169–177
2. Fredriksson T, Pettersson U (1978) Severe psoriasis - oral therapy with a new retinoid. Dermatologica 157:238–244
3. Fritsch PO, Hönigsmann H, Jaschke E, Wolff K (1978) Augmentation of oral methoxalen-photochemotherapy with an oral retinoic acid derivative. J Invest Dermatol 70:178–182
4. Heidbreder G, Christophers E (1979) Therapy of psoriasis with retinoid plus PUVA. Clinical and histological data. Arch Dermatol Res 264:331-337
5. Lassus A (1980) Systemic treatment of psoriasis with an oral retinoic acid derivative (Ro 10-9359). Br J Dermatol 102:195–202
6. Lauharanta J (1980) Retinoids in the treatment and prevention of dermatoses and epithelial neoplasias. Ann Clin Res 12:123–130
7. Lauharanta J, Juvakoski T, Lassus A (1981) A clinical evaluation of the effects of an aromatic retinoid (Tigason), combination of retinoid and PUVA, and PUVA alone in severe psoriasis. Br J Derm (in press)
8. Melski JW, Tanenbaum L, Parrish JA, Fitzpatrick TB, Bleich HL and 28 participating investigators (1977) Oral methoxalen photochemotherapy for the treatment of psoriasis: A cooperative clinical trial. J Invest Dermatol 68:328–335
9. Orfanos CE, Pullmann H, Sterry W, Künzig M (1978) Retinoid-PUVA (RePUVA): Systemische Kombinations-Behandlung bei Psoriasis. Z Hautkr 53:494–504
10. Wolff K, Fitzpatrick TB, Parrish JA, Gschnait F, Gilchrest B, Hönigsmann H, Pathak MA, Tanenbaum L (1976) Photochemotherapy of psoriasis with oral 8-methoxypsoralen. Arch Dermatol 112:943–950

C.E. Orfanos et al. (eds.)
Retinoids

Clinical Observations on Oral Retinoid Therapy of Psoriatic Arthropathy (Ro 10-9359)

R. Stollenwerk, H. Fischer-Hoinkes, K. Komenda and F. Schilling

In recent years, the treatment of retinoid therapy in psoriasis as well as other hyperkeratotic dermatological disorders has attracted increasing attention. On the basis of these rich experiences we decided to use this new vitamin A derivative in the therapy of psoriatic arthritis (5, 6, 11).

We are checking up a group of 24 patients suffering from definite psoriatic arthritis who were treated with retinoid in a long-term study with a range of 6–18 months (average treatment of 9.2 months). The patients' ages ranged between 30–70 years (average 45.6 years). The males dominate the group with 75%. The duration of arthritis was very variable - between 1 and 32 years (mean duration 7.4 years).

Psoriatic arthritis showed, in general, a typical pattern: the distal interphalangeal joints were affected on hands and feet, often in an asymmetric fashion. Dermatological manifestations preceded arthritis in over 50% of the cases and had an average duration of 10.8 years. In an extreme case arthritis did not appear until 36 years following the onset of the skin disorder (Table 1).

We found no correlation between the severity of the dermatological lesions and arthritis. Generally, the dermatological manifestations involved less than 10% of the total body surface area; only two patients showed more extensive lesions - of 30 and 60% of the total skin area, respectively. Approximately one half of the cases showed an arthritis of mild degree and insignificant limitation of joint functions. 40% of the patients had more severe arthritis with distinct reduction of joint functions.

All patients received oral retinoid in 25-mg capsules. Generally an initial dosis of 75 mg daily was given - this amounts to approximately 1 mg/kg body weight. After four weeks the dosis was reduced to 50 mg daily, usually on account of the appearance of retinoid-related side effects. Three months following the start of the therapy, the dosis was reduced by 10 to 25 mg, depending on the individual tolerance of the drug; this was then kept on as maintenance dosage.

Table 1. Patients with psoriatic arthritis on retinoid therapy (n = 24)

Male	18
Female	6
Mean age	45.6 yrs
Duration of arthritis (1–32 y.)	7.5 yrs
Duration of psoriasis (1–55 y.)	10.8 yrs

During our long-term study we instituted monthly follow-up clinical controls of the joint and skin status and, in addition, the following laboratory controls: ESR, CBC, urinalysis, liver and kidney panels, serum protein electrophoresis, immunoglobulin fractions, Fe, potassium, calcium, creatine phosphokinase and glucose levels. At the beginning of the therapy as well as every three-month period thereafter we took X-rays and bone scans, using 99 mTc diphosphonate of hands and feet.

The scans at the start of the therapy showed a more or less accentuated activity in the joints involved, with good correlation to the clinical examination results. At the time of the first control (three months after starting the therapy), eight patients showed increased activity in some of the joints, in contrast to the clinical findings, apparently as an expression of increased bone metabolism in these joints. After three additional months the activity of the scans generally returned to the initial levels or also below these; these results therefore illustrated the clinically evident improvement of arthritis with 16 patients (66.6%) under retinoid. Five patients showed by the scan, at least, no change. Three patients had a

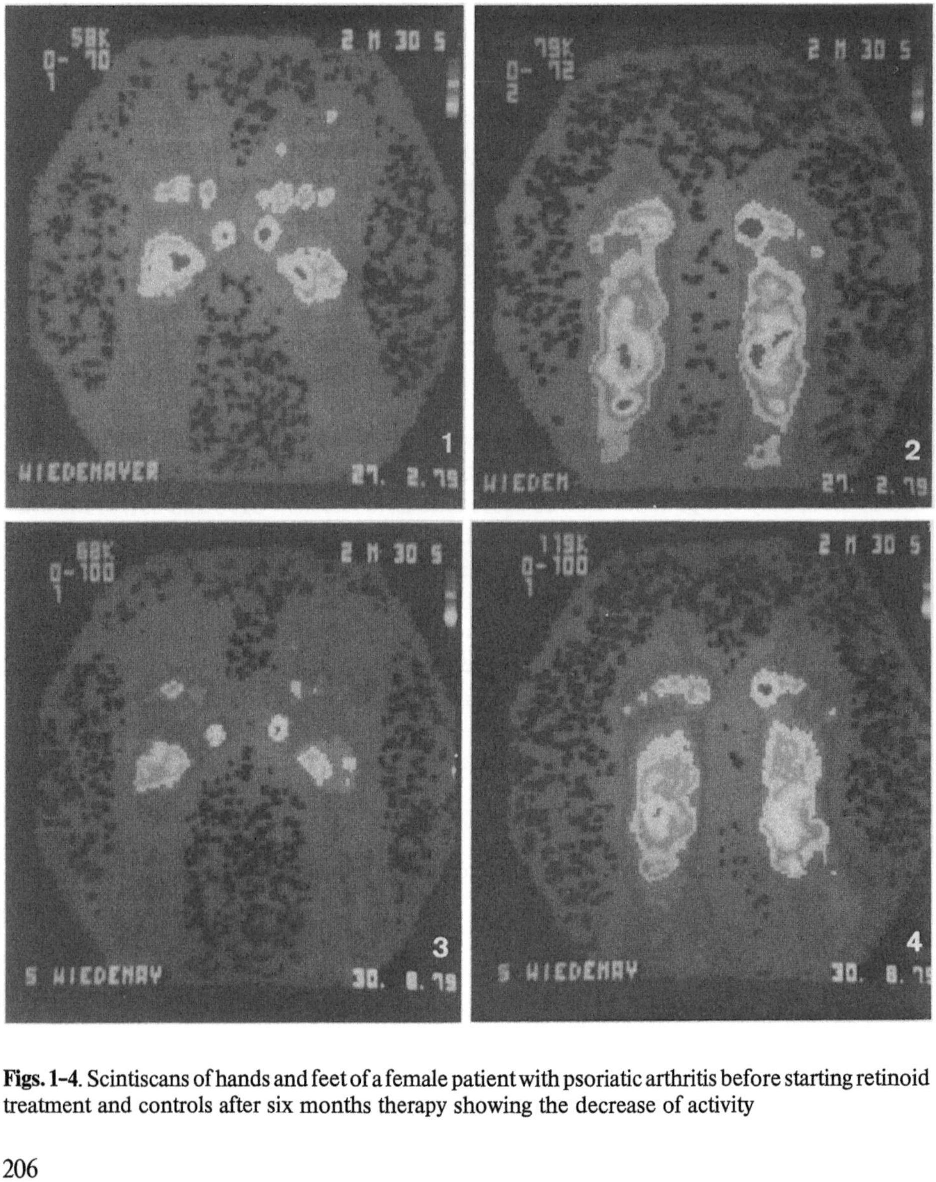

Figs. 1–4. Scintiscans of hands and feet of a female patient with psoriatic arthritis before starting retinoid treatment and controls after six months therapy showing the decrease of activity

definite increase in scan activity, in one case, however, there was no correlation to the clinically evident improvement (Figs. 1–4).

The X-rays showed no progression of the destructive arthritis process in 18 patients (75%), with five patients a slight deterioration being noted, one patient showing a slight sign of improvement.

As far as the *dermatological manifestations* were concerned, 17 patients showed definite improvement under retinoid therapy, some of them with complete cleaning of all skin lesions, three patients showed progression of the skin disease, and four others had no change in their status. Over the long-term study we observed the reappearance of lesions in four to six months under retinoid; this correlates with the observations of other authors (5, 6). We also find it remarkable that skin lesions responded to retinoid therapy generally 2 to 3 weeks following the initiation of therapy; psoriatic arthritis, in contrast, showed improvement, on an average, after two, more often only after three months.

In the opinion of the investigators and also of the patients, a moderate to very good improvement of *arthritis* could be observed in 20 patients (83.3%); a significant decrease in the number of painful and swollen joints and in the duration of morning stiffness was noted, as well as an increase of joint functions and walking time. Almost half of these patients could reduce their anti-inflammatory drugs, three stopped their antirheumatics totally (Table 2).

We had four treatment failures, one of the patients showed even deterioration of the arthritis.

In spite of the improvement of arthritis, two patients had to give up the therapy after four, respectively five months after starting retinoid because of drug-related side effects (such as cheilitis, mouth-dryness, rhagades).

With an additional patient we had to interrupt the therapy on the basis of pathological liver chemistry values (GOT 110, GPT 209, alkal. phosphatase 271 mU). These values returned to normal levels without any specific therapy within three months.

All patients receiving retinoid showed the expected side effects corresponding to a hypervitaminosis A. In general these were tolerable, especially since we had a concurrent improvement of skin and/or joint disease. These mucous membrane side effects, such as chei-

Table 2. Results of the long-term study with retinoid (n = 24)

Scintiscans	
improved	16 (66.6%)
unchanged	5 (20.8%)
deteriorated	3 (12.5%)
X-rays	
improved	1 (4.2%)
unchanged	18 (75.0%)
deteriorated	5 (20.8%)
Skin lesions	
improved	17 (70.8%)
unchanged	4 (16.6%)
deteriorated	3 (12.5%)
Arthritis	
improved (withdrawn for side-effects) 3 (12.5%)	20 (83.3%)
unchanged	3 (12.5%)
deteriorated	1 (4.2%)

litis, mouth-dryness, rhagades, hair loss, atrophy of the skin, desquamation, pruritus, and partially also paronychia could be alleviated significantly by reduction of retinoid dosage. As already mentioned, these symptoms proved to be intolerable in two cases, resulting in the cessation of therapy in these patients.

With the exception of abnormal liver chemistry values in a single patient as mentioned, we had no other abnormal *laboratory parameters*. Uric acid values were slightly elevated, but remained within the normal range.

The suppression of humoral inflammatory activity was surprisingly effective. ESR diminished in 92% of all observations, even in patients who showed no evidence of skin or joint improvement. It is remarkable that retinoid apparently acts as an immunological regulator in metabolic disturbances as seen in the decrease of alpha-2- and gamma-globulins to almost normal levels. Furthermore, the immunoglobulin IgA level reduction amounted to 16%, and the IgG fraction to 10%.

Summary

Retinoid represents a worthful therapeutical possibility in the treatment of psoriatic arthritis. Only 16.6% of the patients did not respond to retinoid and 12.5% had to discontinue the therapy because of drug-related side effects, so that finally 70.8% were considered as able to tolerate retinoid therapy. Also 70.8% showed an improvement of their psoriasis; this correlated - but not in all of the cases - with the improvement of the joint symptoms.

Our experience shows that daily maintenance dosage of 25–50 mg, in some cases even a smaller dose, suffices to stabilize the joint disease. In contrast, despite initial improvement, the skin lesions sometimes show a tendency to return.

We observed recurrence of joint symptoms only following even more pronounced reduction of the retinoid dosage, or following interruption of the therapy after four to six weeks, at the most after three months' time.

Even though our trial group was limited, we feel encouraged to continue with retinoid as a basic therapy in the treatment of psoriatic arthritis.

References

1. Bahous J, Bitter Th, Rosenthal M (1980) Retinoid, Vitamin-A-Säure in der Behandlung der Psoriasis-Arthritis. Report. 19. Tagung d. dtsch. Ges. für Rheumatologie 30.9.–4.10.80, Konstanz
2. Brackertz D, Müller W (1979) Die Beeinflussung der Arthropathia psoriatica und der chronischen Polyarthritis durch ein oral wirksames aromatisches Retinoid. Verh Dtsch Ges Inn Med 85:1343–1346
3. Fassbender H-G, Schilling F (1976) Morphologie der Arthritis psoriatica und deren "pseudoguttöse" Verlaufsform. Verh Dtsch Ges Rheumatol 4:221–228
4. Holzmann H, Hoede N, Eißner D, Hahn K (1979) Die psoriatische Osteoarthropathie. Der Hautarzt 30:343–348
5. Orfanos CE, Goetz G (1978) Orale Psoriasis-Therapie mit einem neuen aromatischen Retinoid (Ro 10-9359). Dtsch Med Wochenschr 103:195–199
6. Ott F (1977) Behandlung der Psoriasis mit einem oral wirksamen aromatischen Retinoid. Schweiz Med Wschr 107:144–147
7. Rosenthal M (1979) Retinoid in der Behandlung von Psoriasis-Arthritis. Schweiz Med Wschr 109:1912–1914
8. Schacherl M, Schilling F (1967) Röntgenbefunde an den Gliedmaßengelenken bei Polyarthritis psoriatica. Z Rheumaforsch 26:442–450

9. Schilling F, Schacherl M (1967) Röntgenbefunde an der Wirbelsäule bei Polyarthritis psoriatica und Reiter-Dermatose: Spondylitis psoriatica. Z Rheumaforsch 26:450–459
10. Stollenwerk R, Fischer-Hoinkes H, Komenda K, Schilling F (1979) Initial experience with a new vitamin A-acid derivative (Retinoid Ro 10-9359) in the treatment of psoriatic arthritis. Report. International Symposium on the Treatment of Psoriasis-Arthritis. Israel Nov. 18–25
11. Viglioglia PA, Barclay A (1978) Oral retinoids and psoriasis. Dermatologica 157 (Suppl 1):32–37
12. Wolf G, Diem E, Czech W, Wickenhauser J (1976) Röntgen- und szintigrafische Befunde bei Psoriasis arthropathica. Fortschr Röntgenstr 125:414–416

Application of Oral Retinoids in Acne

C.E. Orfanos et al. (eds.)
Retinoids

Effect of Retinoids on the Sebaceous Glands of the Hamster Flank Organ*

E.C. Gomez

Derivatives of vitamin A have been shown to have marked effects on cellular differentiation, possess antineoplastic activities *in vivo*, and have therapeutic efficacy in a number of dermatologic diseases (7). In addition to having therapeutic efficacy in several disorders of keratinization, 13-*cis*-retinoic acid has been found to be effective when administered orally to patients with severe cystic acne (7, 8). Such patients have a marked decrease in sebum production (9) as measured by changes in the composition of the surface lipid film. Since this implies an effect upon the sebaceous gland rather than upon follicular keratinization, we studied (5) the effects of 13-*cis*-retinoic acid on the hamster flank organ, an animal model system which has been extensively used for the study of compounds inhibiting the response of sebaceous glands to androgenic hormones (1, 2, 4, 10).

Hamster Flank Organ as an Assay System

1. Anatomy of the Male Flank Organ

The flank organs of the golden or Syrian hamster are paired structures on the back of the animal, near the costovertebral angle. In the immature animal or mature female, the structures are undeveloped and appear as very slightly pigmented, small macules. In the mature male hamster the structures are deeply pigmented areas about 6 millimeters in diameter and have a palpable bulk. The anatomy of these organs has been described (6) and the biodynamics of their response to hormonal influences has been studied (3). The palpable bulk of the flank organs of mature male hamsters is due to the presence of large sebaceous glands which fill the dermis. By comparison, the sebaceous glands of the general body skin of the hamster are tiny structures. In addition to the sebaceous glands, the flank organs have two other components which distinguish them from the adjacent skin of the hamster. There are dermal melanocytes, largely perifollicular in distribution, and large, heavily pigmented hair follicles which extend down into the subcutaneous fat.

2. Hormonal Effects

All three components of the flank organ are dependent upon androgenic stimulation for their growth. Castration of male hamsters while immature prevents the development of the hamster flank organ. Female hamsters likewise do not have well-developed flank organs, the sites being barely visible to the naked eye. On treatment of either castrates or female ham-

* This work was supported by the Medical Research Service of the Veterans Administration

sters with either topical or systemic androgens, there is a rapid growth of the flank organ over a period of approximately three weeks, resulting in large sebaceous glands, large pigmented hair follicles, and dermal pigmentation.

Following castration of mature male hamsters the sebaceous glands of the flank organ show a marked atrophy. The bulk of the gland is replaced by necrotic debris beginning nearest the infundibulum of the hair follicle and proceeding in a wave towards the germinative population of the gland so that after a week or so one sees only a widely dilated infundibulum and a few layers of sebaceous gland cells remaining at the periphery of the gland. It is known that castration results in a marked decrease in the labeling index of the germinative population of the sebaceous gland and it appears that the production of new sebaceous cells is halted, resulting in programmed autolysis of those cells which have begun to differentiate.

Treatment with 13-cis-Retinoic Acid

1. Effect on Flank Organs of Male Hamsters

Treatment of mature male hamsters with 13-*cis*-retinoic acid (24 milligrams of 13-*cis*-retinoic acid per dose administered subcutaneously twice each week as a 25% concentrate in an oil vehicle) resulted in a marked decrease in the palpable bulk of the flank organ without a decrease in pigmentation. Histologic sections showed a marked difference in the flank organ of the 13-*cis*-retinoic acid-treated animals from those of animals treated with the vehicle. As shown in Figure 1, the flank organs of the vehicle-treated hamster show well developed sebaceous glands, pigmented hair follicles and perifollicular dermal pigmentation (Fig. 1a). Animals treated with 13-*cis*-retinoic acid (Fig. 1b) show the presence of perifollicular dermal pigment cells and large pigmented hair follicles but there has been a marked diminution in the size of the sebaceous glands to the point where they are barely visible on low power. The hair follicles show thickening of the follicular wall and atypical configuration. At higher

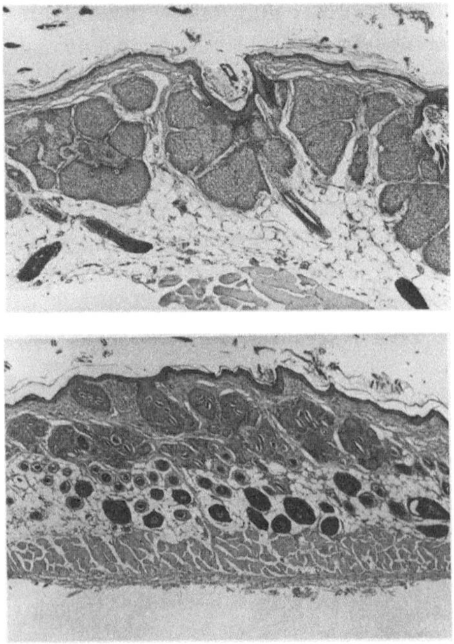

a

b

Fig. 1a. Flank organ of a mature male hamster treated with the oil vehicle. Note large sebaceous glands, perifollicular pigment cells, and large pigmented hair follicles. **b** Flank organ of a mature male hamster treated with 13-*cis*-retinoic acid. Note marked diminution in the size of the gland

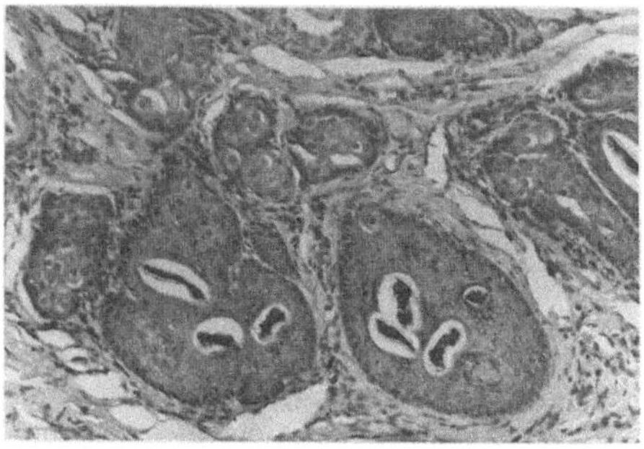

Fig. 2. Higher power view of the flank organ of a mature male hamster treated with 13-*cis*-retinoic acid. Note the tiny sebaceous glands with few lipid filled cells

power (Fig, 2), the sebaceous cells are recognizable in small clusters surrounding the pigmented hair follicles. The cells show little lipid accumulation and in many cases show an accentuation of the basaloid cells at the periphery. Many of the cells in these rudimentary sebaceous glands show eosinophilic cytoplasm.

Treatment with 13-*cis*-retinoic acid for a period of three weeks resulted in a progressive decrease in the size of the sebaceous glands but did not show the rapid changes described previously as occurring following castration. There was no accumulation of eosinophilic cell debris within the body of the gland and the diminution in size of the gland was more gradual. These effects upon the sebaceous glands appear to be reversible. Specimens taken three weeks after the cessation of 13-*cis*-retinoic acid treatment still showed inhibition of the sebaceous glands; however, specimens taken six months after cessation of treatment showed normal flank organs.

Despite this marked effect of 13-*cis*-retinoic acid on the sebaceous glands, there was no discernible diminution of the pigmented hair follicles or of the dermal pigmentation. Since this specificity of effect upon the sebaceous glands might be apparent, resulting from the role of the sebaceous gland as a holocrine gland requiring constant turnover to maintain itself, unlike pigmented hair follicles and pigment cells which would be expected to remain *in situ* if their production was inhibited, sudies were carried out with female hamsters.

2. Effect of Androgen-stimulated Growth of the Female Flank Organ

As indicated previously, flank organs of the female hamster do not develop in the absence of exogenous androgenic stimulation. Histologic examination shows only slight enlargement of a few of the central follicles and the sebaceous gland, probably resulting from endogenous androgen production. Subcutaneous administration of testosterone enanthate or other androgens results in a marked growth of the flank organs including all components, sebaceous glands, large pigmented hair follicles, and dermal pigment cells. This growth occurs within three weeks and the resulting flank organs are indistinguishable from those of the mature male.

By simultaneous administration of both testosterone enanthate and either 13-*cis*-retinoic or the placebo oil vehicle to groups of hamsters, it was shown that, whereas those hamsters treated with testosterone enanthate and the oil vehicle showed normal growth of their flank organs, those animals treated with testosterone enanthate and 13-*cis*-retinoic acid developed flank organs indistinguishable from those of treated males. There was a marked diminution of the sebaceous glands compared to those of the vehicle-treated hamsters but development of the large pigmented hair follicles and pigment cells. The small groups of sebaceous cells present showed little lipid accumulation and many cells showed eosinophilic cy-

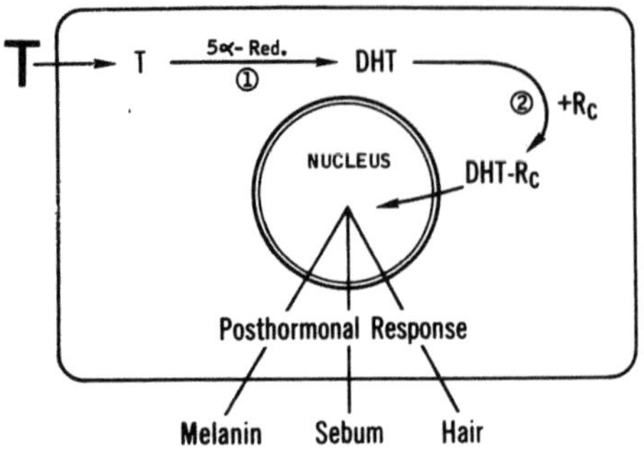

Fig. 3. Compounds interfering with androgen action at sites 1 and 2 affect all androgen dependent cell populations, unlike retinoids which affect only the sebaceous cells

toplasm. The hair follicles showed the same thick walls and atypical configuration as did those of the 13-*cis*-retinoic acid-treated males.

The finding that 13-*cis*-retinoic specifically inhibits one of the androgen-sensitive cell populations of the flank organs without preventing the growth of the other androgen-dependent cell populations strongly suggests that its action is at some extrahormonal site (Fig. 3). Alternative explanations such as concentration of 13-*cis*-retinoic acid within the sebaceous glands or its metabolism to an antiandrogen within the sebaceous gland appear much less likely.

Treatment with an Aromatic Retinoid (Ro 10-9359)

An aromatic retinoid (Ro 10-9359) is known to have significant efficacy in the treatment of keratinizing disorders. Since one of the goals of our model system was to assess the action of retinoids upon sebaceous glands as a means of predicting efficacy in acne, we tested this aromatic retinoid in the same base used for 13-*cis*- retinoic acid. Twice weekly injections of the same dose of the aromatic retinoid for a period of three weeks resulted in no discernible effect upon the flank organ of the hamsters. Unlike the flank organs of positive control animals treated with 13-*cis*-retinoic acid, the aromatic retinoid-treated hamsters had not only large pigmented hair follicles and dermal pigment cells but also large well-developed sebaceous glands. The finding that a potent retinoid failed to inhibit the sebaceous gland growth suggests that there may be some specificity in the action of retinoids on the sebaceous glands and that activity against keratinizing disorders may not be able to be equated with activity in the treatment of acne.

Summary

The hamster flank organ is a specialized, androgen-responsive region of skin that has previously been used as a model system for the study of the effect of antiandrogens on sebaceous glands. 13-*cis* retinoic acid is thought to act in the treatment of acne by the inhibition of sebum production. Utilizing the hamster flank organ as a model for the study of retinoid effects upon sebaceous glands, we attempted to determine whether such effects are mediated by interference with cellular mechanisms for the response to androgenic hormones.

The hamster flank organ contains three populations of androgen-responsive cells, large pigmented hair follicles, dermal pigment cells and sebaceous glands. Subcutaneous injection of 13-*cis* retinoic acid into male hamsters caused a marked diminution in the size of sebaceous glands without noticeable effects upon the large pigmented hair follicles and dermal pigment cells. Stimulation of flank organ growth in female hamsters by the systemic administration of testosterone in the absence of 13-*cis* retinoic acid results in a rapid growth of all of the above components. Female hamsters treated similarly but also receiving 13-*cis* retinoic acid showed growth only of the large pigmented hair follicles and pigment cells but not of the sebaceous glands, which resemble those of the 13-*cis* retinoic acid-treated males. 13-*cis*-Retinoic acid had no effect upon the conversion by hamster flank organ of testosterone to dihydrotestosterone and other 5α-reduced metabolites *in vitro*. Similar studies with hamsters using an aromatic retinoid (Ro 10-9359) showed little or no effect in either male or female hamsters.

References

1. Ferrari RA, Chakrabarty K, Beyler AL, Wiland J (1978) Suppression of sebaceous gland development in laboratory animals by 17α-propyl testosterone. J Invest Dermatol 71:320–323
2. Frost P, Gomez EC (1972) Inhibitors of sex hormones, development of experimental models. In: Advances in Biology of Skin, Vol. XII. Montagna W, Van Scott EJ, Stoughton R (eds). New York, Appleton Century Crofts, pp 403–420
3. Frost P, Giegel JL, Weinstein GD, Gomez EC (1973) Biodynamic studies of hamster flank organ growth. Hormonal influences. J Invest Dermatol 61:159–167
4. Gomez EC, Frost P (1975) Hamster flank organ. Relevance of studies with topically applied antiandrogens. In: Animal Models in Dermatology: Relevance to Human Dermatopharmacology and Dermatotoxicology. Maibach H (ed). New York, Churchill-Livingstone, pp 190–202
5. Gomez EC, Moskowitz RJ (1980) Effect of 13-cis-retinoic acid on the hamster flank organ. J Invest Dermatol 74:392–397
6. Hamilton JB, Montagna W (1950) The sebaceous glands of the hamster. I. Morphologic effect of androgens on integumentary structures. Am J Anat 86:191–233
7. Peck GL, Yoder FW, Olsen TG, Pandya MD, Butkus D (1978) Treatment of Darier's disease, lamellar ichthyosis, pityriasis rubra pilaris, cystic acne, and basal cell carcinoma with oral 13-*cis*-retinoic acid. Dermatologica 157 (Suppl 1):11–12
8. Peck GL, Olsen TG, Yoder FW, Strauss JS, Downing DT, Pandya MD, Butkus D, Arrand-Battandier J (1979) Prolonged remissions of cystic and conglobate acne with 13-*cis*-retinoic acid. N Engl J Med 300:329–333
9. Strauss J, Peck GL, Olsen TG, Downing DT, Windhorst DB (1978) Alteration of skin lipid composition by oral 13-*cis*-retinoic acid: Comparison of pretreatment and treatment values. J Invest Dermatol 70:223
10. Voigt W, Hsia SL (1973) The antiandrogenic action of 4-androsten-3-one-17β-carboxylic acid and its methyl ester on hamster flank organ. Endocrinology 92:1216–1222

C.E. Orfanos et al. (eds.)
Retinoids

Effects of Two Retinoids in Animal Experiments and After Clinical Application in Acne Patients: 13-cis-Retinoic Acid Ro 4-3780 and Aromatic Retinoid Ro 10-9359

G. Plewig, A. Wagner, J. Nikolowski and M. Landthaler

Animal studies with aromatic retinoid Ro 10-9359 and with 13-cis-retinoic acid Ro 4-3780, and clinical studies in acne patients with 13-cis-retinoic acid Ro 4-3780 were performed.

Animal Studies

Systemic Application

The aromatic retinoid and the 13-cis-retinoic acid were fed by gastric tubes to 170 male adult Syrian hamsters, daily for 30 days. A low dose of 1.0–2.0 and a high dose of 20.0 mg/kg bw were used. Oleum arachidis served as vehicle. The daily volume was, depending on bodyweight, 0.5–0.75 mg. Every 3 to 10 days groups of animals were removed from the study. The effects of both retinoids on sebaceous glands were assessed planimetrically (cross sectional surface areas) using the sebaceous follicles on the ventral side of earlobes. Details of this study are reported elsewhere (10, 17).

Topical Treatment

13-cis-retinoic acid was applied daily up to 15 days to ear lobes and flank organs (hairs clipped away) of 31 adult male Syrian hamsters at 3.0; 0.3; 0.05; and 0.01 percent concentrations (in acetone). One or two drops from a Pasteur pipette were evently spread over the skin surface of these two sites. Only the left ears and left flank organs were treated; the right side served as vehicle-treated controls. Another 21 animals served as untreated controls. The effects of the retinoids on sebaceous glands was assessed planimetrically as described above. The cross-sectional areas of sebaceous glands were measured with a projection microscope and a semiautomatic picture analyzer (MOP, model AM 03, Kontron, Munich).

Studies in the Human

13-cis-retinoic acid was given in four different doses to 60 patients with severe ("untreatable") acne as monotherapy for 12 weeks, and in some, for 24 weeks, respectively. All other topical or systemic treatment was stopped at least four weeks prior to entering the study. The procedure was fully explained orally and by a printed hand-out to all patients, and written consent obtained. The study was approved by the ethic committee of the university. Doses were 1.0–2.0 (N = 22); 0.5 (N = 20); 0.2 (N = 10); and 0.05 mg/kg bw (N = 8). All patients were seen before and at weeks 2, 4, 8, 12, 16, 20, 24 and once a month thereafter and are still being seen for long-term follow-ups.

The results to be reported here are not part of the multicenter clinical trial which is presently active in 20 departments in Germany, findings of which are to be described elsewhere.

Laboratory Tests and Clinical Investigations

The following parameters were checked before and at weeks 2, 4, 8, 12, and 24 of treatment: Alcaline phosphatase, SGOT, SGPT, total bilirubin, creatinine, Na, K, Fe, total cholesterol, triglycerides (no diet restriction, blood samples taken 9–11 a.m.), Quick, serum electrophoreses; leukocytes, erythrocytes, differential blood cell count, thrombocytes, reticulocytes, hematocrit, red blood cell sedimentation rate, blood sugar, urin analysis.

Trichograms. Five days after the last scalp shampooing hairs were plugged on a temporal, parietal and occipital area of the scalp. Hair roots were analyzed as anagen, telogen, katagen and dystrophic. The trichograms were performed before and at least twice during treatment at varying intervals between weeks 1–24. Details of this study (in collaboration with Dr. G.P. Heilgemeir) are to be reported elsewhere.

Biopsies. Two excisional biopsies from clinically normal, non-acne involved sites of the upper back between scapula and spine were secured in each subject, one before therapy, and the second at varying intervals during treatment between weeks 1 and 24. The specimens were either paraffin embedded for routine histologic examinations; parts of the tissue were used for an in-vitro-autoradiographic analysis with 3H-thymidine to calculate the labeling index of sebaceous acini; the other parts of the tissue from twelve subjects were used for electron microscopy.

The H&E stained paraffin sections were used for the determination of sebaceous follicles, as 13-cis-retinoic acid is known to affect these structures. Results of this and the autoradiographic analysis are, in part, reported at this Symposium (Landthaler et al. p 259). The date on electron microscopy (in collaboration with H.H. Wolff, Lübeck) are to be reported elsewhere.

Potassium Iodide Patch-Test

On the upper back, a 4 x 4 cm area free from acne-lesions was outlined by tape (Leukosilk $1^1/4$ cm, Beiersdorf, Germany). The area was covered with liberal amounts of 40% KI-ointment (w/w in Unguentum Cordes, Ichthyol Gesellschaft, Germany; KI = Merck No 5044, Darmstadt, Germany). A 5 x 5 cm plastic film covered the site. A woven gauze 4 x 4 cm was placed on top for better adhesion of the patch to the skin, which was itself occluded with impermeable tape (Dermiclear transparent, Johnson & Johnson, USA). The whole patch was finally sealed with a self-adhesive-gauze (Fixomull, Beiersdorf, Germany). The patch was removed at 24 h (13). All subjects received two patch-tests under identical conditions, one before therapy, and the other during the 10th to 24th week of therapy. The second patch was applied while the patients were still on medication.

Scoring: Four qualities were applicable to characterize the inflammation:

Erythema: 0 = none; 1+ = moderate; 2+ = pronounced, filling the 4 x 4 cm area.

Edema: 0 = none; 1+ = moderate, visible and palpable; 2+ = wheal-like elevation of the entire 4 x 4 cm area.

Papules: follicle-bound inflammatory papules, numerical counts.

Pustules: follicle-bound pustules; numerical counts.

For graphic display, the scores for erythema and edema, and for papules and pustules were pooled.

Statistical analysis: Since every patient served as his own control, paired comparisons of the readings were made, using the Student's t-test.

Skin Bacteria

In five patients treated with the 1.0–2.0 mg/kg bw dose, quantitative changes of their bacterial skin flora were investigated. Samples from the forehead and from the skin overlying the fourth thoracic vertebra were obtained with a triton X-100 scrubbing technique before and at 4, 8, 12, and 16 weeks after initiating the treatment regiment. Aerobic cocci and propionibacteria were identified and counted as colony forming units. Details of the study are being reported elsewhere (20).

Spermatological Investigations

Twenty patients, who were treated with varying doses of 0.2 to 2.0 mg/kg bw were selected. Seven analyses were performed before and at several intervals during systemic treatment with 13-cis-retinoic acid. Seven parameters included sperm count, total sperm output, total sperm motility, progressive sperm motility, sperm morphology, ejaculate volume, and seminal plasma fructose. Results of these investigations are reported at this Symposium (p. 389).

Although 60 patients participated and completed the therapeutic trials, some of the figures and tables show results of less than these 60 subjects.

Results

Animal Studies

Systemic Application

Both retinoids, when given in the lower dose of 1.0 or 2.0 mg/kg bw did not affect the size of sebaceous glands. Neither in the ear (Table 1) nor in the flank organ (Table 2) was there a decrease in cross sectional surface areas observed. The animals appeared healthy with a normal looking shiny coat.

In contrast, when the high dose of 20.0 mg/kg bw was given, the sebaceous glands became much smaller (Table 1). Both retinoids were of similar effect. All animals showed signs of systemic toxicity with loss of fur (alopecia), on chest, abdomen and distal extremities. The fur became dry and lost its shiny appearance.

No effects on sebaceous glands or the appearance of the fur was seen from the control feedings.

Table 1. Sebaceous gland cross sectional areas in mm^2 (ventral ear side of Syrian hamsters) following oral treatment with 13-cis-retinoic acid and aromatic retinoid. The 20 mg/kg bw dose caused a significant reduction. Student's t-test. + not done. Modified from (10)

	N animals	9–10 days	20–21 days	30 days
Group I 13-cis-retinoic acid 2.0 mg/kg bw	15	0.0257	0.0394	0.0294
Group II 13-cis-retinoic acid 20.0 mg/kg bw	15	0.0210 $p \leqq .0125$	0.0232 $p \leqq .001$	0.0126 $p \leqq .0005$
Group III aromatic retinoid 1.0 mg/kg bw	100	0.0201	0.0175	0.0197
Group III - A Oleum arachidis control	10	+	+	0.0176
Group IV aromatic retinoid 20.0 mg/kg bw	15	0.0178 $p \leqq .037$	0.0176 $p \leqq .0001$	0.0125 $p \leqq .0005$
Group I-, II-, and IV-A Oleum arachidis controls	15	0.0295	0.0319	0.0436

Table 2. Sebaceous gland cross sectional areas in mm^2 (flank organ) of male Syrian hamsters (N = 30), following oral treatment with aromatic retinoid Ro 10-9359 1 mg/kg bw. No significant change. Modified from (10, 17)

Treatment period in days (gastric tube)	Flank organ mm^2
15	2.05 ± 0.31
30	1.82 ± 0.22
Oleum arachidis control	1.91 ± 0.34

Table 3. 13-cis-Retinoic acid inhibits sebaceous gland cross sectional areas when applied topically. Four different concentrations were compared in the ear, and only one dose (0.01%) in the flank organ. The 3.0% solution caused irritation and had to be discontinued between days 7–10. All other concentrations were applied for 15 days

	13-cis-Retinoic Acid. Syrian Hamsters. Topical Treatment for 15 days (*7–10 days). Per cent Reduction of Sebaceous Glands %				
	3.0 N = 15*	0.3 N = 5	0.05 N = 5	0.01 N = 6	control N = 21
			per cent reduction		
Ears	85	50	0	0	
Flank Organs	x	x	x	40	

x not done

Topical Application

Some evidence is presented that 13-cis-retinoic acid shrinks sebaceous glands when applied topically (Table 3). The highest concentration of 3.0 mg/kg bw caused some irritant dermatitis, which in itself is known to reduce sebaceous glands acini in size. This is unspecific, and a post-inflammatory effect and not related to a true sebum-suppressive action.

Studies in the Humans

13-cis-Retinoic acid led to a quick response in almost every patient. The clinical results were much better than with any other treatment modality known to us. No patient dropped out of

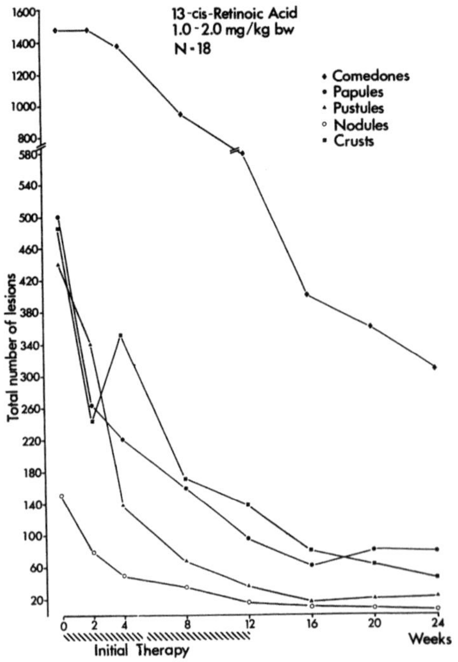

Fig. 1. Regression of total numbers of non-inflammatory lesions (comedones), and inflammatory lesions (papules, pustules, nodules, crusts) in eighteen patients with severe acne. High dose of 1.0–2.0 mg/kg bw

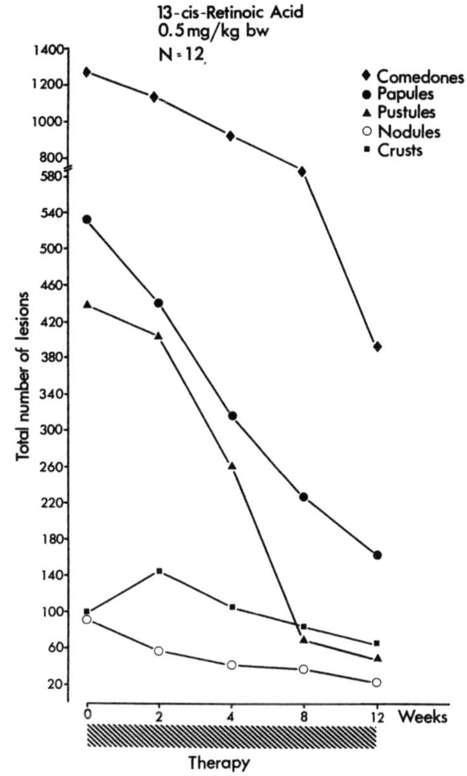

Fig. 2. Similar data as in Fig. 1 for twelve patients being treated with 0.5 mg/kg bw

the study. Patients with acne conglobata and acne fulminans were completely free from all inflammatory lesions and comedones, except for trapped comedo-like material in fistulated comedones (which are actually scars). The higher dose of 13-cis-retinoic acid led to a quicker response than the lower doses. Side effects were minimal in all patients except for saltating myalgia-arthritis in some patients.

Dose-Response

The total number of lesions for the 1.0–2.0, the 0.5, and the 0.2 mg/kg bw doses are shown in Figs. 1–3. There was a steep fall-off of all inflammatory lesions, and also of comedones. The mean number of lesions for these three groups of patients are to be seen in Figs. 4–6.

The longest follow-ups are available for the group of patients being treated with the 1.0–2.0 mg/kg bw dose (Fig. 7). There is no recurrence of inflammatory lesions within 56 weeks (shown), and within 80 weeks at the time of preparing this manuscript.

It is to be noted that Figs. 1–7 show results of only 40 patients, whereas the side effects in Table 4 shows up-dated results of 52 patients for these three groups.

Side Effects

These are compiled in Table 4. Obligatory side effects were cheilitis in every patient, and scaly skin, facial dermatitis, and eye symptoms occurring less frequently. Myalgia and saltating arthralgia, often mild, however, occurred in 7 and 9 patients respectively. It appears that side effects are dose-related.

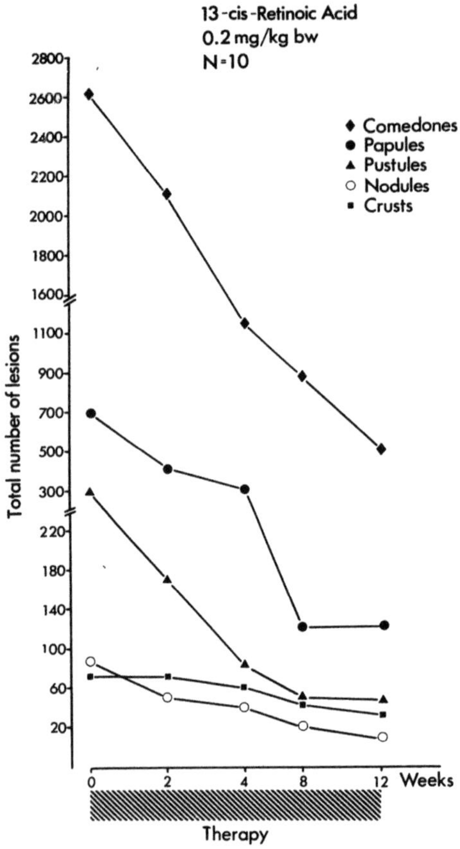

Fig. 3. Similar data as in Figs. 1 and 2 for ten patients being treated with a low dose of 0.2 mg/kg bw. There is a fast improvement with all three doses

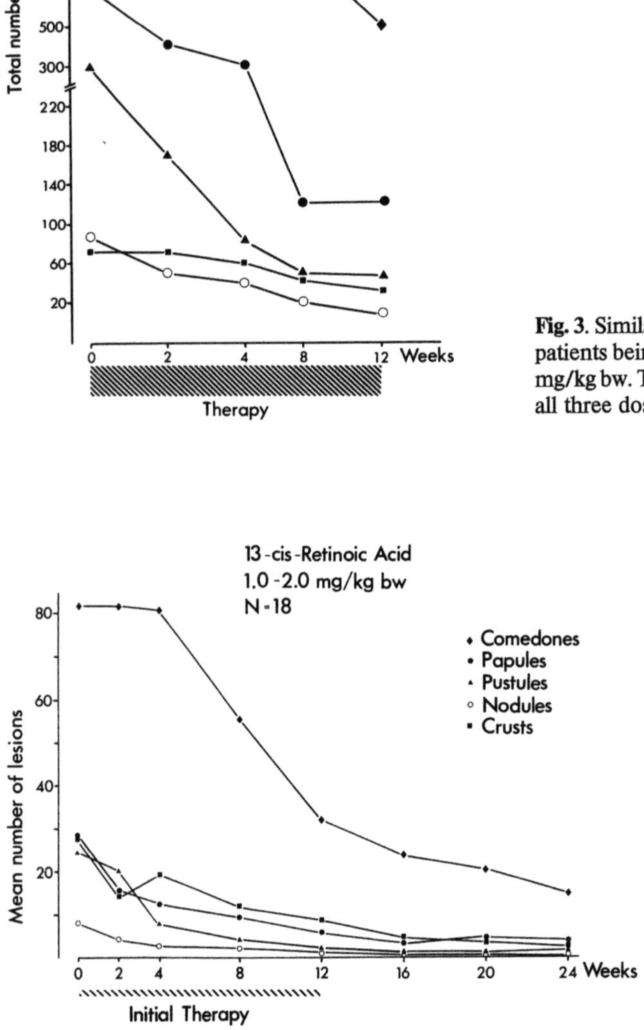

Fig. 4. Regression of mean number of non-inflammatory lesions (comedones) and inflammatory lesion (papules, pustules, nodules, crusts). Same patients as in Fig. 1. The high number of lesions indicate the severity of the disease

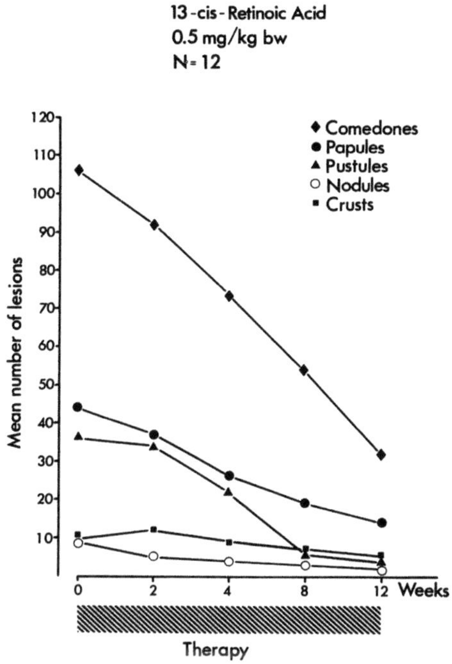

Fig. 5. Similar data as in Fig. 4 for the twelve patients shown in Fig. 2

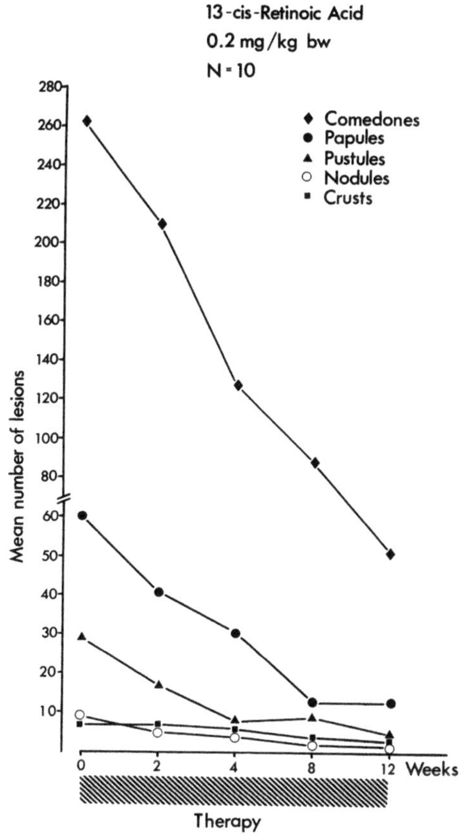

Fig. 6. Similar data as in Figs. 4 and 5 for the ten patients shown in Fig. 3

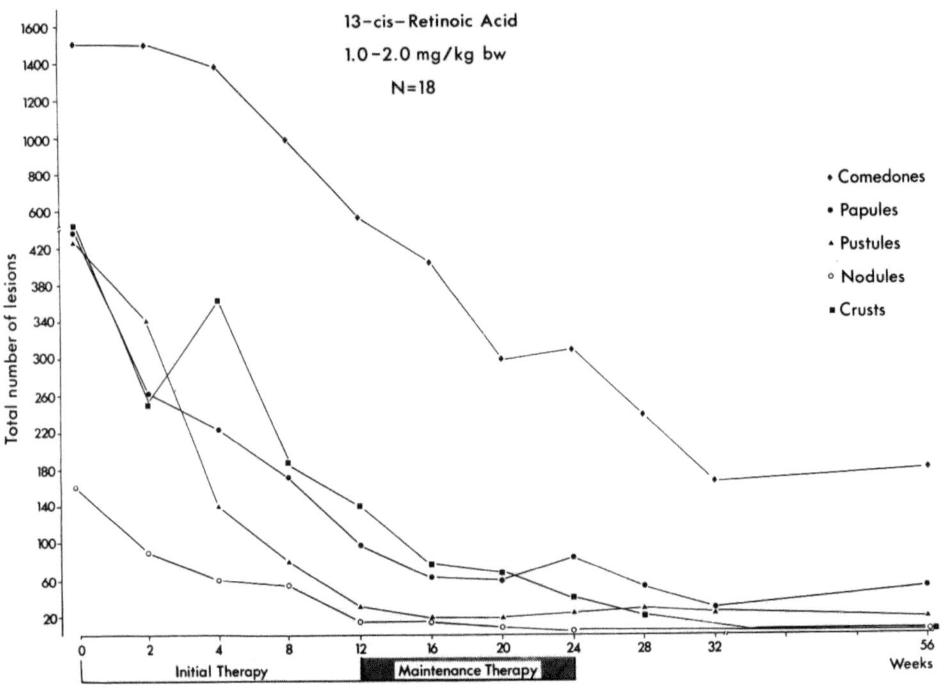

Fig. 7. Initial therapy, maintenance therapy, and follow-up period in the eighteen patients shown in Figs. 1 and 4. There is no recurrence of lesions up to week 56 (and up to week 80 at time of writing)

Table 4. Objective and subjective side effects in 60 patients, being treated with four different doses of 13-cis-retinoic acid for 12 or 24 weeks. More side effects are seen with the highest dose of 1.0–2.0, and almost none with the lowest dose of 0.05 mg/kg bw

	0.05 N = 8	0.2 N = 10	0.5 N = 20	1–2 N = 22	Overall N = 60
Cheilitis	8	10	20	22	60
Scaly skin		9	20	21	50
Facial dermatitis		2	15	20	37
Skin fragility		2	4	5	11
Dry nose		6	19	18	43
Dry mouth		6	4	3	13
Pruritus		2	4	3	9
Myalgia			3	4	7
Arthralgia, Saltating			3	6	9
Epistaxis			7	2	9
Eye symptoms		2	14	16	32
Conjunctivitis					
Blepharitis					
Photophobia					
Epiphora					

Varia X/60
Exsiccated skin 2; Abdominal pain 1; Cough 1; Obstipation 1; Increased appetite 1; Urethritis 1; Warm head 2; Hair loss 4; Heavy feeling 1; Vision obscured 1; Paronychia 1; Hyperhidrosis 1

All side effects disappeared either spontaneously or immediately after cessation of the drug at weeks 12 or 24. None of the patients with arthralgia or myalgia wanted to stop the treatment; all symptoms disappeared despite continuation of the drug at the same dose.

The lowest dose of 0.05 mg/kg bw seems to be less effective than the other three doses used. Clinical improvement is seen, but starts much later. Some patients, however, do not show a satisfactory improvement after 12 weeks of treatment. Increasing the dose to 0.5 mg/kg bw leads to a quick and very satisfactory response.

Laboratory Studies

Triglycerides. There was a dose-related elevation of triglycerides. In Figs. 8–13, the horizontal striped bars indicate conspicuous, but not truly elevated levels of our laboratory. In Fig. 8a comparison between 1.0 and 2.0 mg/kg bw is made. The patients in the higher dose-group were slightly older than in the 1.0 mg dose, as they had very long-lasting severe acne tetrade (16). The effects of initial and maintenance dose are to be seen in Fig. 9. The initial dose of 1.0–2.0 mg/kg bw was given during weeks 1–12, and caused a slight elevation of triglycerides; the triglycerides dropped, when the dose was reduced to 0.5 mg/kg bw for weeks 13 through 24 (solid line in Fig. 9).

Data of all four groups being studied are presented in Fig. 10. In Fig. 11, the triglycerides are recorded for patients with different acne forms and different age-groups. Both groups had base-line triglycerides around 100 mg%. Patients with acne tetrade (mean age 32 years) showed higher elevations than those with acne conglobata or acne fulminans (mean age 19 years). The higher age of the acne tetrade patients appears to be an additional risk factor for elevation of triglycerides.

Cholesterol. Cholesterol levels tended to be less elevated than triglycerides. Representative data for the highest dose of 13-cis-retinoic acid are shown in Figs. 12 and 13. In Fig. 12, combined values of all 18 patients are shown. In Fig. 13, values for initial therapy and maintenance therapy are separated. In Fig. 14, data of all four doses of 13-cis-retinoic acid are compiled. The highest elevation is seen from the 1.0–2.0 mg/kg bw group.

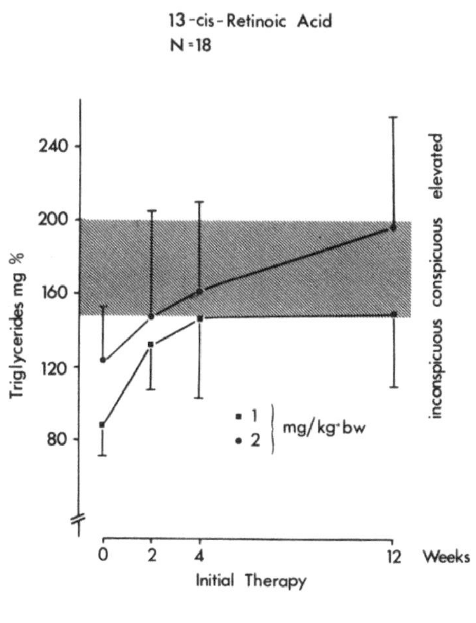

Fig. 8. Effects of 1.0 and 0.2 mg/kg bw 13-cis-retinoic acid on triglycerides. A dose-related elevation into conspicuous but not truely elevated levels. The grey striped horizontal bar in this figure and Figs. 9 through 14 separate normal (inconspicuous) from elevated levels of our laboratory

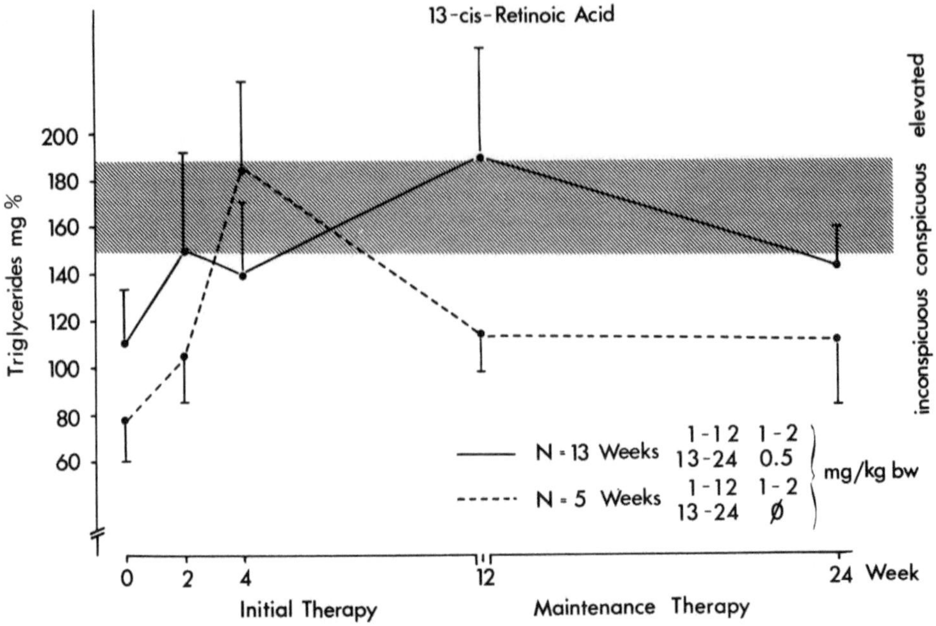

Fig. 9. Effects of various doses of 13-cis-retinoic acid on triglycerides. During the initial therapy thirteen patients received 1.0–2.0 mg/kg bw; this dose was lowered to 0.5 mg/kg bw during maintenance therapy (weeks 13–24). The other group of five patients started with 1.0–2.0 mg/kg bw, but received no maintenance therapy

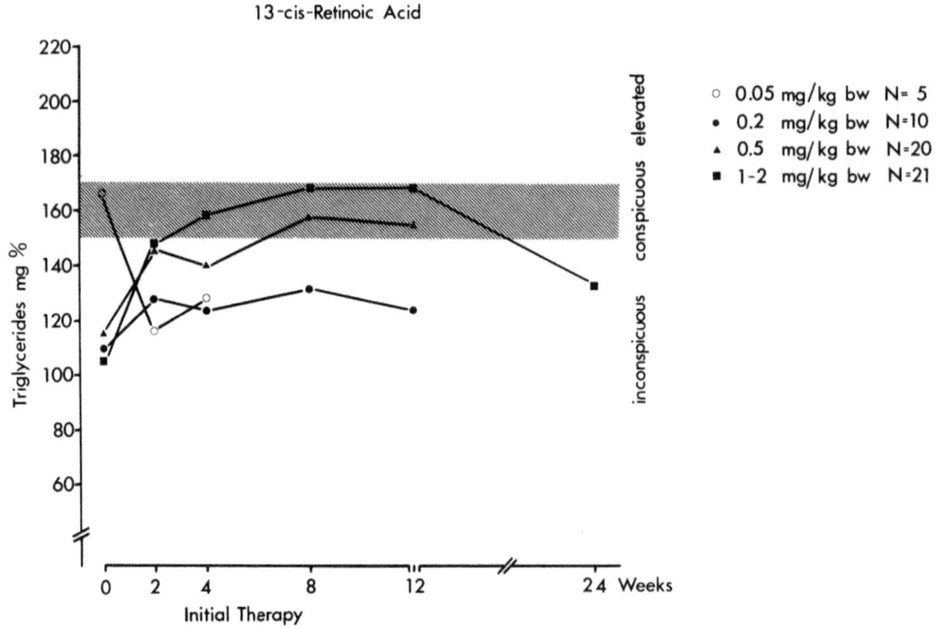

Fig. 10. Effects of four different doses of 13-cis-retinoic acid on triglycerides. Highest elevation with the highest dose. The 0.2 mg/kg bw dose seems to have almost no effect on triglycerides. In the 0.05 mg/kg bw dose group one patient (out of five) had only once high triglyceride levels before entering the study

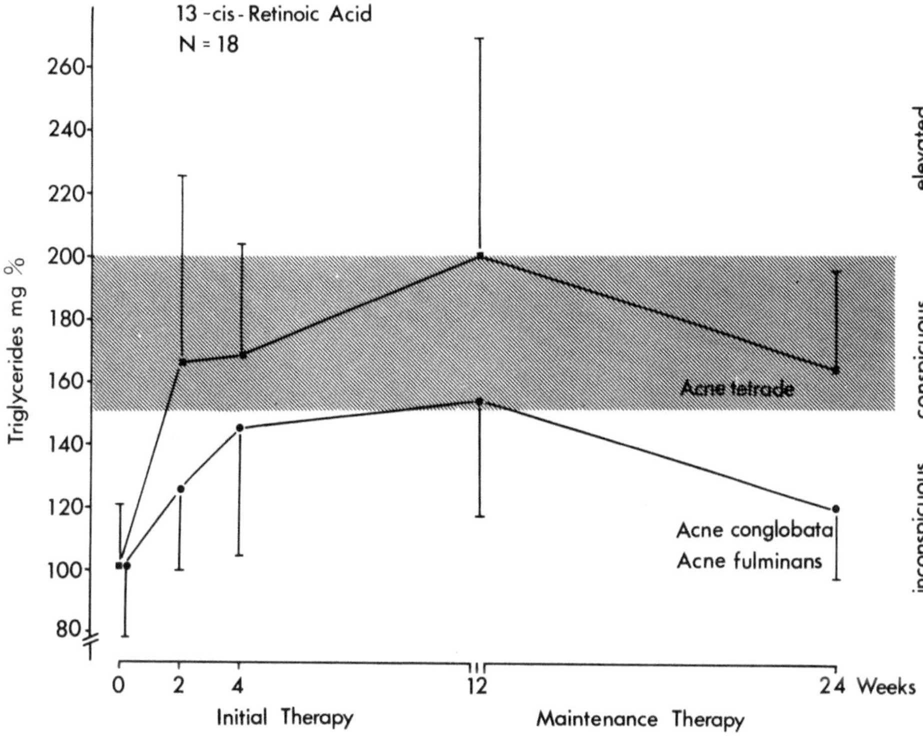

Fig. 11. Triglyceride levels and various types of acne. The patients with acne tetrade tend to have higher triglyceride elevations than patients with acne conglobata and acne fulminans

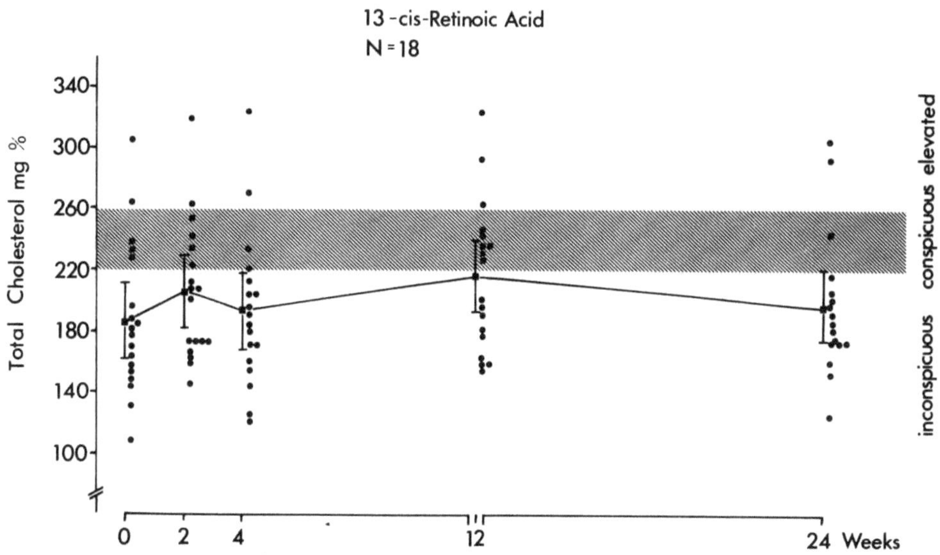

Fig. 12. Effects of 13-cis-retinoic acid on total cholesterol. The eighteen patients received 1.0–2.0 mg/kg bw in the initial therapy period; this was lowered to 0.5 mg/kg bw in the maintenance therapy period, or there was no further medication (compare with Fig. 9). There is no significant change of cholesterol

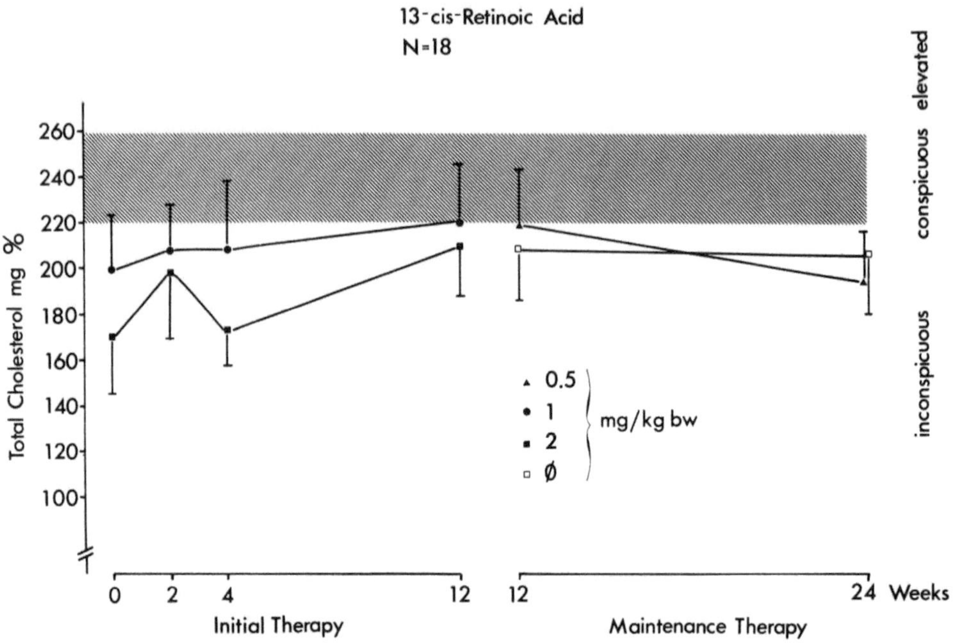

Fig. 13. Effects of various treatment schedules on total cholesterol. Compare with Fig. 9. There is a tendency for elevation without significance

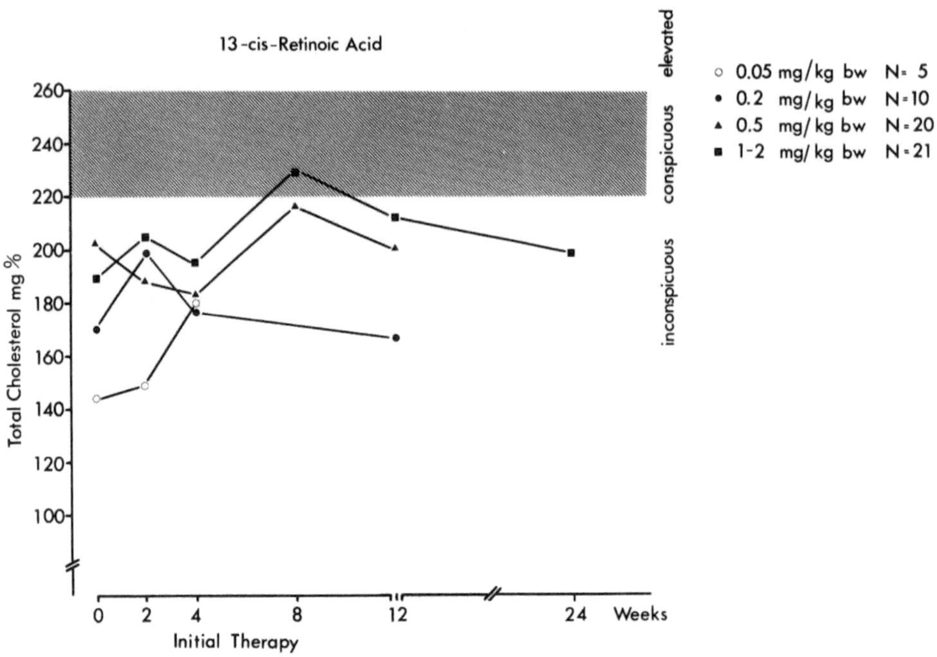

Fig. 14. Effects of four different doses of 13-cis-retinoic acid on total cholesterol. Highest elevation with highest treatment dose

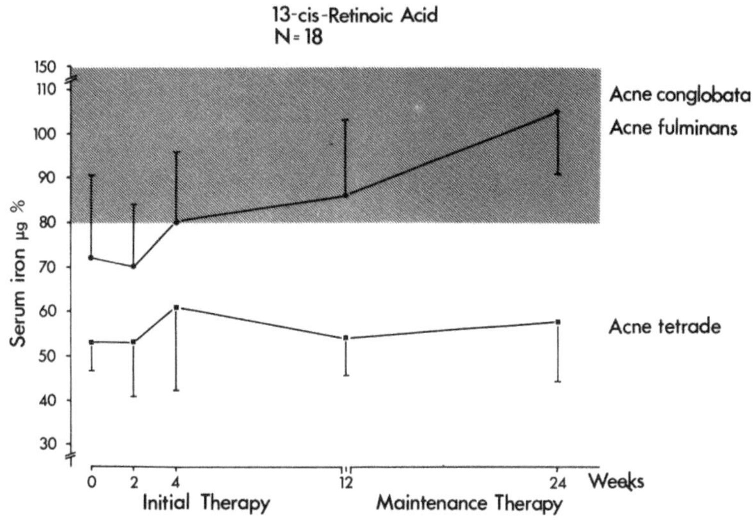

Fig. 15. Effects of 13-cis-retinoic acid on serum iron. Patients with severe acne have low serum iron. Serum iron of patients with acne conglobata and acne fulminans increased into normal levels (normal levels = grey striped horizontal bar) with improvement of inflammatory skin lesions. The patients with acne tetrade showed less improvement of their skin-lesions which consisted of wide-spread abscess formations

Serum iron. Most of the abnormal laboratory data, such as leucocytosis or elevated red blood cell sedimentation rate, returned to normal. Serum iron, low to begin with in patients with severe acne conglobata and acne fulminans (Fig. 15), rose to normal values (striped horizontal bar), but not in patients with acne tetrade.

There were no abnormalities in all other parameter studied, particularly not in alkaline phosphatase, SGOT, SGPT, bilirubin, creatinine or electrolytes.

Potassium Iodide Patch-Test

A marked anti-inflammatory action of 13-cis-retinoic acid appears from the in-vivo inflammatory patch-test model with KI. As was shown in a preliminary study (14) in 16 patients, the inflammatory reaction in all patch-tests was significantly reduced: erythema from 1.13 to 0.34 ($p \leqq 0.01$); edema from 1.06 to 0.25 ($p \leqq 0.0005$); papules from 6.75 to 1.86 ($p \leqq 0.01$); and pustules from 10.44 to 1.54 ($p \leqq 0.0025$).

The KI patch-test was extended to three doses of 13-cis-retinoic acid with a total of 36 patients, results of which are shown in Fig. 16. All inflammatory values regressed between 50 and 80 per cent. A clear dose-response appears for papules and pustules (right side of Fig. 16). The KI-test is mainly designed to study follicular bound papulo-pustules. The erythema-edema scores show also dose-response relations, with the exception that the 0.5 dose leads over the 1.0–2.0 mg/kg bw dose.

Skin Bacteria

There was a steady decrease in the density of propionibacteria during the course of treatment, both on forehead and back. These changes reached levels of statistical significance as compared to pre-treatment values after 12 to 16 weeks (20).

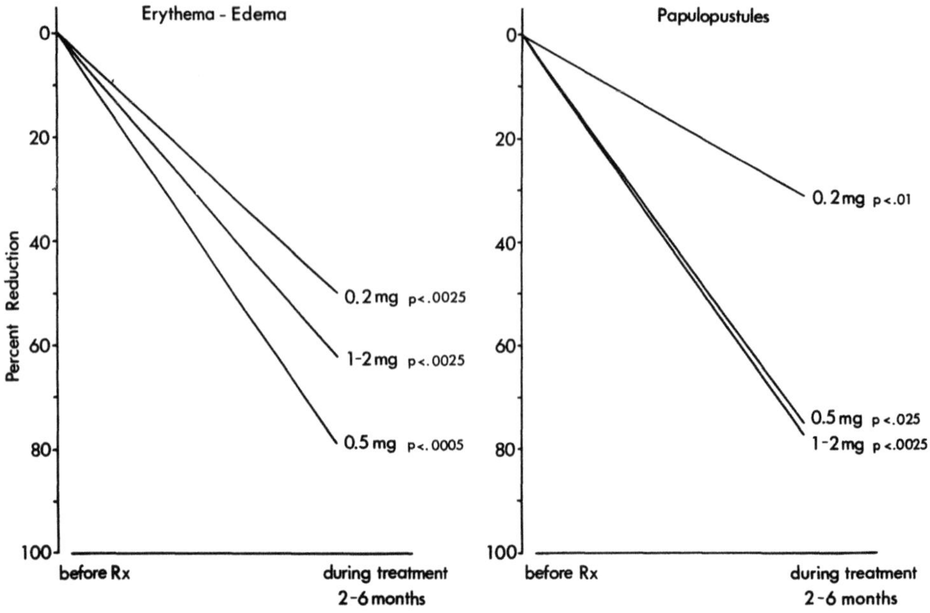

Fig. 16. 13-cis-Retinoic acid acts anti-inflammatory in the KI-patch test model. Three treatment schedules are compared (0.2 mg, N = 9; 0.5 mg, N = 13; 1.0–2.0 mg/kg bw, N = 14). The dose-response is best seen with papulo-pustules

Similar changes were seen in another group of patients studied by us. These were patients with gram-negative folliculitis. Quantitative counts showed a steep decrease of propionibacteria within 12 to 16 weeks of treatment with 13-cis-retinoic acid (6).

Spermatological Investigations

Systemic treatment with 13-cis-retinoic acid does not inhibit spermatogenesis, nor leads to an impairement of sperm motility and sperm morphology.

In contrast, beneficial effects on semen parameters were monitored concerning sperm count, sperm motility and sperm morphology. It is remarkable that 18 out of 20 acne patients had pathologic sperm parameters before treatment (see p. 389).

Comment

With all careful reservation in mind the present information on 13-cis-retinoic acid allows to express enthusiasm. This enthusiasm is shared by patients and physicians. 13-cis-retinoic acid is such a powerful medication that it seems to control even the worst expressions of the acne diseases. Horrendous outbreaks of acne fulminans and severe acne conglobata are improved within 12 to 24 weeks of treatment. This is achieved with monotherapy (11).

Presently we know very little about mechanisms of action of 13-cis-retinoic acid in acne. At least three mechanisms are being discussed.

The sebum-suppressive action is astounding. Up to 90 per cent reduction is being reported (18). Conventional treatment with combined estrogens and chlormadinone acetate or cyproterone acetate reduced skin surface lipids by 25 to 35 per cent (12). The conversion of severe seborrhea into sebostasis was originally seen by Peck et al. (8, 9); skin surface lipids were measured by Strauss et al. (18); and histological evidence that 13-cis-retinoic acid virtually lets sebaceous acini disappear completely was shown by Landthaler et al. (3–5). Presently we are investigating how long the reduction of sebaceous acini lasts after cessation of 13-cis-retinoic acid.

The animal studies in the Syrian hamster disclosed effects of 13-cis-retinoic acid when applied topically. This is the first report of topical effectiveness of this compound on the reduction of sebaceous gland areas. Curiously, the 2.0 mg/kg bw dose of 13-cis-retinoic acid, when given daily by gastric tubes to the Syrian hamster, had no effect on sebaceous glands. This dose is highly effective in the human. With a very high dose of 20.0 mg/kg bw, both, the aromatic retinoid and 13-cis-retinoic acid shrank sebaceous glands; this was accompanied by signs of systemic toxicity (10, 17).

A second mechanism of 13-cis-retinoic acid lies in its anti-inflammatory action. Clinically, all inflammatory lesions regress sharply during treatment (Figs. 1–7), and are abandoned for long periods of remission. In-vivo studies with a standardized model of inflammation (13) underlines this observation. 13-cis-retinoic acid reduces erythema, edema, papules and pustules in the KI-model (15). In accordance is our observation that similar benefits are seen with severe rosacea (7, 15).

A third mechanism is related to keratinization. Acne is primarily a disease of abnormal keratinization (12). Comedones are the hallmark of the disease and are its primary lesions. Unlike any other medication known to us, 13-cis-retinoic acid, when given orally, eliminates comedones, open and closed ones, and prevents new comedo formation (Figs. 1–7) (16). The comedones are unrooted; follicular filaments or casts are removed from normal sebaceous follicles. We have observed finger-like protrusions of follicular filaments from wide facial pores of patients being treated with 13-cis-retinoic acid (15). The diameter of follicular infundibula, wide and spacious in acne patients, is drastically reduced to a third or a fifth of their original size during treatment (5). The number of corneocytes layers in sebaceous filaments, approximately 30–60 in normal follicle (unpublished observation), is reduced to 10 or 15. This leaves less space in cavernous lacunae for propionibacteria, which reside in this location.

Secondary events are also seen in bacteriology. We interprete the significant reduction of propionibacteria (20), or the complete removal of gram-negative bacteria in patients with gram-negative folliculitis (6, 15) as the combined result of reducing the sebum production to minimal amounts, and of reducing the living space in the infundibula (6).

Unlike aromatic retinoid we have not seen any hair loss in our patients. Trichograms revealed no telogen effluvium (Heilgemeir et al.; unpublished observation). Fortunately, headache, associated with vitamin-A toxicity, has not been seen in our patients.

Of concern are the changes in serum lipids. Triglycerides tend to elevate in a clear dose-related fashion. The elevation was not extreme. Patients at risk have to be identified prior to treatment to avoid extreme hypertriglyceridemia (1). The multicenter studies, presently going on in the USA and Germany, and bound to be released in 1981, will elucidate this particular problem. Of highest concern is the fact that 13-cis-retinoic acid is teratogenic like all other retinoids. This applies even to very low doses, such as 0.05 mg/kg bw. All women in childbearing age must be carefully informed about this risk. Reliable contraception is to be followed during treatment, and up to 12 months thereafter, for the metabolic pathways of 13-cis-retinoic acid are partly unknown and seem to be slow.

Summary

Animals

Aromatic retinoid Ro 10-9359 and 13-cis-retinoic acid Ro 4-3780 was fed by gastric tubes in a low dose of 1–2 mg/kg bodyweight and in a high dose of 20 mg/kg bw daily for 30 days to adult male Syrian hamsters. The effects of both retinoids on sebaceous glands on the ventral side of the ear pinna were assessed. 13-cis-retinoic acid was further applied topically in concentrations ranging from 3.0 to 0.01% to ear lobes and flank organs daily up to 15 days.

In animals, the low dose of both retinoids did not affect the size of sebaceous glands. In contrast, the high dose significantly reduced the size; the fur became dry. There was also hair loss.

Topical application of 13-cis-retinoic acid led to a dose-dependent decrease of sebaceous glands.

Humans

13-cis-retinoic acid was given at 1.0, 2.0, 0.5, 0.2, and 0.05 mg/kg bw to 60 patients with severe acne ("therapy resistant") as monotherapy for 12 weeks (initial therapy), or, in some patients for 24 weeks (maintenance therapy) respectively. Numerical counts of acne lesions were recorded biweekly. Laboratory controls included, among others, transaminases, alkaline phosphatase, total cholesterol, triglycerides, serum iron, trichograms, skin biopsies, sperm analyses, and a potassium iodide patch-test (a model for granulocytic inflammation).

All patients responded dramatically to the oral treatment. Within twelve weeks, almost all lesions, inflammatory and the non-inflamed comedones, disappeared. There is almost no recurrence after 80 weeks of observation. The high doses were very effective. The lower doses were also beneficial, with delayed onset of improvement.

Cholesterol levels did not increase significantly; triglycerides were elevated, dose-dependent, but only to minor degrees.

A definite anti-inflammatory effect was demonstrated in the potassium iodide model.

13-cis-retinoic acid has clinical merits in acne, affects abnormal keratinization by eliminating and preventing comedo formation, blocks sebaceous lipid production, and acts anti-inflammatory.

Acknowledgments. Miss A. Ruhfus, medical technician, landed superior help during the study. Dr. H. Schuh assisted with the animal studies. The Deutsche Forschungsgemeinschaft supported this investigation by grant PL 58/6. Dr. W. Bollag, Basle/Switzerland, and Dr. R. Hennes, Grenzach/Germany of Hoffmann-La Roche kindly provided the 13-cis-retinoic acid.

References

1. Dickens CH, Connolly SM (1980) Eruptive xanthomas associated with isotretinoin (13-cis-retinoic acid). Arch Dermatol 116:951–952
2. Gomez EC, Moskowitz RJ (1980) Effect of 13-cis-retinoic acid on the hamster flank organ. J Invest Dermatol 74:392–397
3. Landthaler M, Kummermehr J, Wagner A, Plewig G (1980) Inhibitory effects of 13-cis-retinoic acid on human sebaceous glands. Arch Dermatol Res 269:297–309
4. Landthaler M, Kummermehr J, Wagner A, Plewig G (1980) 13-cis-retinoic acid inhibits sebaceous glands in animals and humans: planimetry and in vitro autoradiography. Eur Soc Dermatol Res Amsterdam, May 12–14, 1980 (abstract). J Invest Dermatol 74:453
5. Landthaler M, Nikolowski J, Plewig G Effekte verschiedener Dosierungen von 13-cis-Retinsäure

auf die Talgdrüsen beim Menschen. Arbeitsgemeinschaft Dermatol Forsch, Innsbruck, Nov 14–16, 1980 (abstract). Arch Dermatol Res, in press
6. Neubert U, Plewig G Gramnegative Follikulitis - Verlaufsbeobachtungen und therapeutische Möglichkeiten. Hautarzt Suppl IV, 1981 (in press)
7. Nikolowski J, Plewig G (1980) Rosazea. Orale Behandlung mit 13-cis-Retinsäure. Hautarzt 31: 660–661
8. Peck GL, Yoder FW, Olsen TG, Pandya MD, Butkus D (1978) Treatment of Darier's disease, lamellar ichthyosis, pityriasis rubra pilaris, cystic acne, and basal cell carcinoma with 13-cis-retinoic acid. Dermatologica 52:1–2
9. Peck GL, Olsen TG, Yoder FW, Strauss JS, Downing DT, Pandya M, Butkus D, Arrand-Battandier J (1979) Prolonged remissions of cystic and conglobate acne with 13-cis-retinoic acid. N Engl J Med 300:329–333
10. Plewig G (1980) Der Einfluß des aromatischen Retinoids Ro 10-9359 und der 13-cis-Retinsäure Ro 4-3780 auf die Talgdrüsen des Syrischen Hamsters. Arch Dermatol Res 268:239–246
11. Plewig G 13-cis-Retinsäure bei schweren Akneformen: Stand der Entwicklung. Hautarzt Suppl IV, 1981 (in press)
12. Plewig G, Kligman A (1975) Acne. Morphogenesis and Treatment. Springer Verlag, Berlin Heidelberg New York
13. Plewig G, Schöpf E (1975) Anti-inflammatory effects of antimicrobial agents: an in vivo study. J Invest Dermatol 65:532–536
14. Plewig G, Wagner A (1981) Anti-inflammatory effects of 13-cis-retinoic acid: An in-vivo study. Arch Dermatol Res 270:89–94
15. Plewig G, Wagner A, Nikolowski J, Landthaler M, Neubert U, Braun-Falco O (1980) Treatment of severe acne, rosacea and gram negative folliculitis with 13-cis-retinoic acid. Scientific Exhibit. Am Acad Dermatol, Dec 6–10, 1980, New York
16. Plewig G, Wagner A, Braun-Falco O (1980) Orale Behandlung schwerster Akneformen mit 13-cis-Retinsäure. Münch med Wschr 122:1287–1293
17. Schuh H (1980) Einfluß des aromatischen Retinoids Ro 10-9359 auf die Talgdrüsengröße beim Syrischen Hamster. Inauguraldissertation. Ludwig-Maximilians-Universität München, München
18. Strauss JS, Stranieri AM, Farrell BS, Downing DT (1980) The effect of marked inhibition of sebum production with 13-cis-retinoic acid on skin surface lipid composition. J Invest Dermatol 74:66–67
19. Wagner A, Plewig G (1980) 13-cis-Retinsäure. Pharmakologische und toxikologische Untersuchungen bei der Behandlung schwerster Akneformen. Münch med Wschr 122:1294–1300
20. Weissmann A, Wagner A, Plewig G (1981) Reduction of bacterial flora during oral treatment of severe acne with 13-cis-retinoic acid. Arch Dermatol Res 270

C.E. Orfanos et al. (eds.)
Retinoids

Oral Retinoids: Effects on Human Sebaceous Glands and Nodulocystic Acne*

J.S. Strauss, R.J. Thomsen, L.N. Farrell and A.M. Stranieri

Some of the most spectacular clinical responses with oral retinoids have been seen in patients with severe nodulocystic acne, as reported by Peck et al. (3). Not only has the short-term clinical improvement been significant, but preliminary results indicate that remissions have lasted for as long as 30 months. We have conducted a dose-response study with 13-cis-retinoic acid (isotretinoin) in which the clinical response and sebaceous gland function have been determined. Some of the patients have been followed now for many months to confirm the long-term improvement. We have also participated in a multicenter study in which the clinical effect and the changes in sebaceous gland function produced by isotretinoin and an aromatic retinoid derivative, Ro 10-9359 (etretinate), have been compared. These studies, which at least in part address the mechanisms by which oral retinoids work in acne, are the subject of this report.

Dose-Response Study

Materials and Methods

Fourteen of 16 male patients with severe nodulocystic acne completed the protocol of this study which involved the administration of isotretinoin in a fixed dose for a total of 12 weeks and a follow-up drug-free period of eight weeks. All systemic medication was discontinued six weeks before entering the patients into the study; topical therapy also was discontinued for at least three weeks. The clinical response was assessed by counting all nodulocystic lesions greater than 4 mm in diameter and measuring the greatest diameters of all of these lesions. Sebum production and skin surface lipid composition, as done routinely in our laboratories, were monitored throughout the study (1, 6). Routine hemograms, urinalyses and clinical chemistries were also done. Three different dosages of isotretinoin (0.1, 0.5, and 1.0 mg/kg/day) were administered in a double-blind fashion. When the code was broken, it was found that five patients had received 0.1 mg/kg/day, five had received 0.5 mg/kg/day, and four patients 1.0 mg/kg/day. One of the two patients who did not complete the protocol received only two weeks of treatment; he discontinued therapy because of perceived hair loss which could not be confirmed by physical examination. The other patient had a marked flare-up of his disease that necessitated breaking the code; he was receiving the smallest

* Supported in part by a grant from Hoffmann-La Roche, Inc., Nutley and by a research grant (Ro-1-AM-22083-02) from the United States Public Health Service

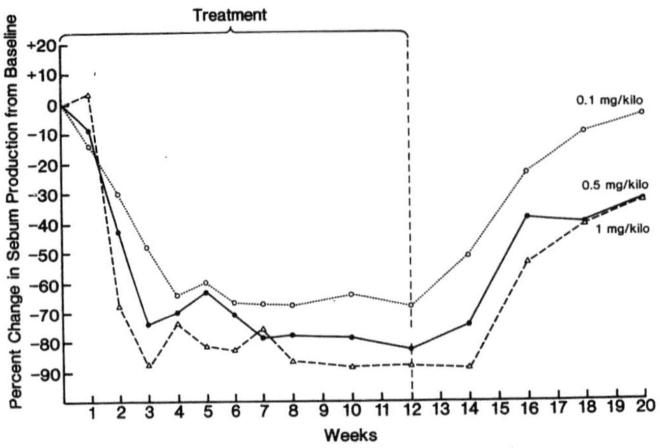

Fig. 1. Summary of changes in sebum production produced by 0.1, 0.5, and 1.0 mg/kg/day of isotretinoin. (Reproduced from Farrell et al. [2] with permission of the publisher and the authors)

dose of 0.1 mg/kg/day. When the drug dosage was increased to 1.5 mg/kg/day, he responded with clearing of his nodulocystic acne.

Changes in Sebum Production

There was a decrease in sebum production in every patient as summarized in Figure 1. More details are published elsewhere (2). The decrease in sebaceous gland activity was rapid, being detectable within two weeks. At this time the percent decrease in sebum production was approximately 30% in patients receiving 0.1 mg/kg/day of isotretinoin, 40% with 0.5 mg/kg/day, and approximately 70% with 1.0 mg/kg/day. By four weeks, near maximum depression of sebum production had occurred with the suppression varying from 65% with the smallest daily dose to close to 90% with the highest daily dose. The suppression of sebaceous gland activity was maintained throughout the next eight weeks of treatment. After treatment was discontinued, sebum production returned rapidly towards normal. This increase in sebaceous gland activity was dose-related; the return to normal was greatest in those patients treated with 0.1 mg/kg/day of isotretinoin.

Changes in Sebum Composition

The first indication that isotretinoin had an effect on sebaceous gland activity was provided by the observation that patients treated with this drug, regardless of their primary disease, showed distinct alterations in skin surface lipid composition (4, 5). The most dramatic change was an increase in the percentage of cholesterol; accompanying this there was a decrease in the percentage of wax esters and squalene. In essence these changes reflected a conversion of the surface skin lipid pattern from that characteristic of an adult to that characteristic of a child. Since approximately 95% of the surface skin lipids in the adult are of sebaceous gland origin, theoretically a change in skin surface lipid composition resulting from inhibition of sebum production would require at least an 85% reduction in sebum production.

In the patients in the present study, skin surface lipid samples were taken at the same time that sebum production was measured. Cholesterol values in excess of 10% have been

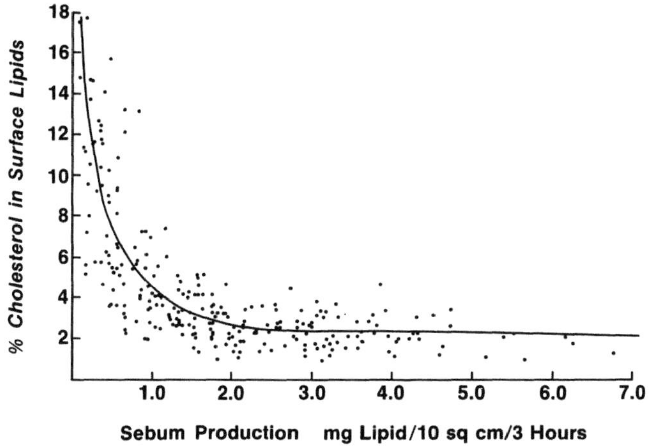

Fig. 2. Comparison of sebum production and cholesterol percentage in skin surface lipids. (Reproduced from Strauss et al. [7] with permission of the publisher and the authors)

observed when sebum production was in general lower than 0.4 mg/10 cm^2/3 h (7) (Fig. 2). Sebum production in normal young adult men is approximately 2.5 mg lipid/10 cm^2/3 h, so that the values of the order of 0.4 mg/10 cm^2/3 h do in fact represent suppression of approximately 85%. Cholesterol percentages greater than 10% were usually only seen in patients receiving 1 mg/kg/day of isotretinoin, since only these patients had sebaceous gland inhibition

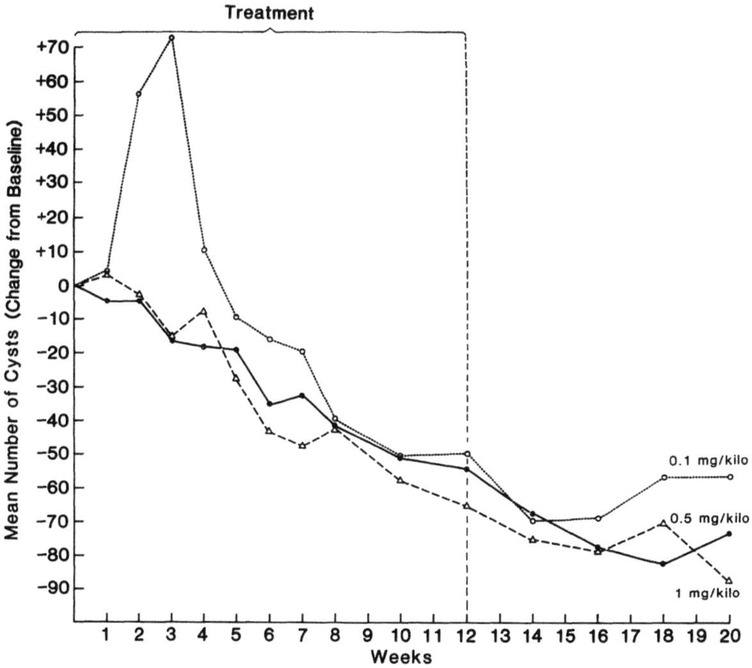

Fig. 3. Summary of the changes in the mean number of cysts produced by 0.1, 0.5, and 1.0 mg/kg/day of isotretinoin. (Reproduced from Farrell et al. [2] with permission of the publisher and the authors)

Table 1. Changes in number of cysts and the sum of their mean diameters during isotretinoin therapy

Daily dose of isotretinoin	0.1 mg	0.5 mg	1.0 mg
	Mean percent change from baseline		
Number of cysts			
12-week treatment	49.1%	54.5%	65.0%
8-week follow-up	56.1%	79.4%	87.5%
Greatest diameter of cysts			
12-week treatment	57.3%	57.2%	75.8%
8-week follow-up	66.8%	80.4%	90.8%

of this degree. It should be emphasized that the change in skin surface lipid composition is not specific; it merely represents a decrease in sebaceous gland activity.

Objective Clinical Response

The clinical response, as stated above, was judged by counting all nodulocystic lesions greater than 4 mm in diameter and measuring the sum of the greatest diameters of these lesions. If there were at least ten nodulocystic lesions on the face, only the lesions on the face were counted. If there were less than the appropriate lesions on the face, then the nodulocystic lesions of the back or chest, or both, were also counted. The data for the number of cysts and the sum of their greatest diameters were roughly the same (2). Initially, there was usually an increase in both the number of lesions and the sums of their greatest diameters, but then there was a steady decrease in both measurements with all three dosage schedules (Fig. 3). Since the effect of isotretinoin is at least in part due to the prevention of the development of new lesions, the clinical response lagged behind that observed for sebum production, and improvement continued throughout the eight-week follow-up period (Fig. 3). The marked increase in the number of lesions early in the treatment period with the 0.1 mg/kg/day dosage is caused by the inclusion of the data from the patient who developed a marked flare-up and who had to be dropped from the protocol after four weeks of therapy. In Table 1, the mean percent change from baseline for both the number of lesions and greatest diameter is presented for two end points, the end of 12 weeks of treatment and the end of the follow-up period. Although there is a greater response with the largest dosage, the differences between dosages are not significant.

Clinical and Laboratory Safety

Clinical side effects were seen in all patients, but the only patient who discontinued therapy was the one individual with hair loss after two weeks; as stated earlier, this was not confirmed by physical examination. Cheilitis was universally present; other mucosal side effects seen in more than 50% of the patients were dry nose and conjunctivitis. Desquamation of the skin was seen in all but one patient and pruritus was reported by more than 50% of the patients. All other observed clinical side effects (excessive thirst, sore mouth, epistaxis, fingertip peeling, loss of hair, insomnia, fatigue, headache and double vision) were far less common.

Many of the patients had white blood cell counts that were near or above the upper limits of normal. The elevated white blood counts decreased during treatment, as would be expected when the inflammatory component of the disease decreased. Transient rises in

SGOT and LDH were observed twice; one patient had an increased total bilirubin. These abnormalities were transient, even though treatment was continued. During treatment one patient receiving 1 mg/kg/day of isotretinoin had an elevation of his serum triglycerides. After treatment was stopped, the serum triglycerides returned to normal.

Long-term Follow-up

The patients in this study were treated with isotretinoin for only 12 weeks, whereas Peck et al. (3) treated their patients for 16 weeks. Furthermore, the dosage used in our study varied from 1/20 to 1/2 of the average dose used in their patients. Many of our patients had not reached maximal improvement at the end of the protocol, and therefore 11 of the patients were re-treated in an open study for additional time periods varying from 12 to 26 weeks. Nine of the 11 of these patients were available for follow-up for at least 12 weeks and for as long as 42 weeks after all therapy was discontinued (Table 2). While three of the nine patients showed essentially complete recovery in sebum production during the final off-treatment period, six patients had at least a 25% reduction of sebum production when last seen, and in three of these six patients there was more than a 50% reduction of sebum production at 21, 27, and 36 weeks, respectively, after all treatment was stopped.

These patients have remained essentially clear clinically except for the occurrence of occasional small acne lesions. There has been no recurrence of the nodulocystic disease for which they were originally treated.

Table 2. Sebum production in patients receiving long-term follow-up

Patient	Percent change in sebum production from baseline			
	End of first treatment period[a]	End of 8-week follow-up[a]	End of extended treatment[a]	Long-term follow-up
S.A.	47.9%	82.1%	22.2%	72.0% (12 weeks)
C.B.	6.1%	53.0%	8.4%	33.3% (13 weeks)
				40.9% (21 weeks)
J.B.[b]	17.3%	92.5%	19.9%	103.5% (17 weeks)
M.D.	19.5%	71.8%	9.5%	86.1% (30 weeks)
				98.8% (42 weeks)
D.F.	43.0%	79.9%	22.5%	79.8% (13 weeks)
				89.8% (17 weeks)
				99.7% (21 weeks)
				97.4% (42 weeks)
J.O.	12.3%	36.3%	9.9%	25.5% (16 weeks)
				28.8% (21 weeks)
				34.2% (27 weeks)
G.P.	7.5%	35.7%	10.4%	64.3% (16 weeks)
B.S.	29.1%	104.5%	11.4%	82.3% (23 weeks)
				62.8% (36 weeks)
J.W.	35.3%	100.5%	4.8%	34.8% (12 weeks)
				46.8% (25 weeks)
				35.3% (36 weeks)

[a] % change expressed as average of last two values obtained during respective period.
[b] Patient received 1.5 mg/kg/day of isotretinoin during the extended treatment period. All other patients received 1.0 mg/kg/day.

Comparison of Isotretinoin and Etretinate

Three groups of investigators (P.E. Pochi, Boston University School of Medicine; A.R. Shalita, SUNY-Downstate Medical Center; J.S. Strauss, University of Iowa College of Medicine) have participated in a double-blind study to compare the effect of isotretinoin and etretinate on sebum production and nodulocystic acne. A total of 29 male patients with nodulocystic acne were treated for eight weeks with 1 mg/kg/day of isotretinoin; 28 patients were treated with etretinate for the same time period. Observations were made after 2, 4, and 8 weeks of treatment. Follow-up observations were made 4 and 8 weeks after treatment was discontinued. The full details of this study will be published elsewhere after all the data have been collected and analyzed. While a small amount of the data from this on-going study is not presently available, it is clear that there are major differences in the effect of the drug on both sebaceous gland function and the course of nodulocystic acne.

As would be expected from our previous study with isotretinoin, there is a marked inhibition of sebaceous gland activity which is evident within two weeks and reaches a maximum of about 85% suppression of sebum production. With etretinate, there is only a slight suppression which at best is on the order of 20%. The clinical response to isotretinoin has been similar to that observed earlier in the dose-response study. The clinical response has lagged behind sebum suppression and has continued during the eight-week follow-up period. There has been only minimal clinical improvement in the etretinate-treated patients, and this improvement is within the range that could occur from placebo therapy.

Discussion

The previously reported effectiveness of isotretinoin in the management of acne has been confirmed in these studies. While a placebo has not been included herein, the patients all had severe treatment-resistant nodulocystic acne. Furthermore, in a sense, the use of etretinate has served as a control in that it was far less effective than isotretinoin in the double-blind study. The oral retinoids represent a new class of drugs for dermatologic treatment. Because of their effectiveness, they undoubtedly will be used therapeutically long before their full mechanism of action is understood. There is no question that a reduction in sebum production is seen promptly when therapy is started and the initial clinical improvement follows shortly thereafter. The decrease in sebaceous gland function and the clinical response occurs with much smaller doses of the drug than those required for a similar therapeutic response in patients with keratinizing disorders. In the dose-response study there was no correlation between the side effects and the dosage used. However, the study was of limited size, and it is possible that with larger groups its side effects might be shown to be dose-related. If this can be shown, the benefit/risk ratio may be increased.

As stated earlier, one of the remarkable observations with isotretinoin therapy has been the protracted remissions produced by the drug. This is unique and has not been as prominent a feature during oral retinoid therapy for other cutaneous disorders. Our initial studies indicated that sebaceous gland function recovered rapidly and, therefore, we suggested that the long-term remissions might be related to an alteration in the pattern of follicular keratinization. It would have to be assumed that the follicular epithelium is more sensitive to the retinoids than the epidermis since, as mentioned above, the dosage of the drug that has been used in acne is considerably less than that used for keratinizing disorders. Our follow-up studies now indicate that, when the course of treatment has been longer, there may be significant inhibition of sebaceous gland activity for over nine months.

We have noted, as have Peck et al. (3), that lesions of the face clear more rapidly than those of the back or chest in these patients. However, the lesions of the back and chest do also respond to oral retinoids.

Etretinate is reported to be very effective in the management of keratinizing disorders, but it is not nearly as effective as isotretinoin in the management of nodulocystic acne. The observed minor effect on sebaceous gland activity and the clinical response in acne is such that, if it is to be further evaluated, a placebo will be required. The difference in the effect of two drugs on the pilosebaceous unit should be a stimulus for further studies to determine if other retinoids can be found which are equally effective in controlling sebaceous gland function and producing clearing of acne but which have less side effects.

Summary

Isotretinoin produces a rapid, marked decrease in sebum production. Inhibition of sebaceous gland activity is close to maximal by four weeks. Dosages of 0.1, 0.5, and 1.0 mg/kg/day all inhibit sebum production, but the degree of inhibition is dose-related. All three dosage levels have resulted in clinical improvement as judged by a decrease in the number of lesions and the sum of their greatest diameters. Long-term therapy may inhibit sebaceous gland activity for long periods of time. Prolonged remission periods have been observed.

Etretinate in a dosage of 1 mg/kg/day produced minimal changes in sebum production. Clinical improvement with etretinate therapy was also minimal.

Isotretinoin is the preferred oral synthetic retinoid for the treatment of acne.

References

1. Downing DT (1968) Photodensitometry in the thin-layer chromatographic analysis of neutral lipids. J Chromatogr 38:91–99
2. Farrell LN, Strauss JS, Stranieri AM (1980) The treatment of severe cystic acne with 13-cis-retinoic acid. J Am Acad Dermatol 3:602–611
3. Peck GL, Olsen TG, Yoder FW, Strauss JS, Downing DT, Pandya M, Butkus D, Arnaud-Battandier J (1979) Prolonged remissions of cystic acne with 13-cis-retinoic acid. N Engl J Med 300:329–333
4. Strauss JS, Peck GL, Olsen TG, Downing DT, Windhorst DB (1978) Alteration of skin lipid composition by oral 13-cis-retinoic acid: Comparison of pretreatment and treatment values. J Invest Dermatol 70:223
5. Strauss JS, Peck GL, Olsen TG, Downing DT, Windhorst DB (1978) Sebum composition during oral 13-cis-retinoic acid administration. J Invest Dermatol 70:228
6. Strauss JS, Pochi PE (1961) The quantitative gravimetric determination of sebum production. J Invest Dermatol 36:293–298
7. Strauss JS, Stranieri AM, Farrell LN, Downing DT (1980) The effect of marked inhibition of sebum production with 13-cis-retinoic acid on skin surface lipid composition. J Invest Dermatol 74:66–67

C.E. Orfanos et al. (eds.)
Retinoids

Oral Vitamin A (Retinol) in Acne Vulgaris

A.M. Kligman, J.J. Leydèn and O. Mills, Jr.

The use of oral vitamin A in the management of acne has been controversial. In 1943, Straumfjord reported that 79 of 100 patients treated with 100,000 I.U. daily were completely cleared or nearly so after six months of therapy (20). Furthermore, only three patients failed to improve. Similar impressive results were reported by Davidson and Sobel (4). Likewise, Germeraad et al. treated 130 cases for 6 to 9 months with 300,000 units daily with significant benefit (7).

In contrast to these enthusiastic reports, there are equally discouraging studies. For example, Lynch and Cook found that approximately 45% of those treated with oral vitamin A or a placebo improved (13). Likewise, Savitt and Obermayer were not impressed with the effect of 100,000 units daily (16). The study which is most frequently quoted to show that oral vitamin A has no effect on acne is that of Anderson and Stokoe (1). On careful scrutiny, however, this study is replete with contradictions in that the physicians who cared for the study patients judged that 75% had improved while those who evaluated pre- and post-photographs labelled them as unchanged or worse. Currently, the present mood, in the USA, is one of dissatisfaction with oral vitamin A in the management of acne. The recent report by Peck et al. that 13-cis-retinoic acid, a stereoisomer of vitamin A acid, is highly effective in severe acne conglobata, has reactivated our long standing interest in oral vitamin A (15).

Materials and Methods

Vitamin A

We used vitamin A dispersed by water (Aquasol A - USV Pharmaceutical co., tuckahoe, N.Y.) throughout. It has been established that vitamin A in suspension is much more readily absorbed than in oily vehicles, furnishing higher blood levels and enhanced biologic activity. Vitamin A contains the physiologic, alcoholic form of vitamin A or retinol.

Study Plan

Two groups of patients were studied. The first consisted of 136 private patients. Every patient had serious, long-standing inflammatory acne with numerous facial lesions, consisting of papules, pustules, and variable nodules. The majority were in the age range from late adolescence to young adulthood; 80 were male and 56 female.

None were new to acne therapy, having usually received oral antibiotics and various topical medicaments, often from two or more physicians. These patients comprise the core group of this investigation. The efficacy data are limited wholly to clinical observations.

Each one received 300,000 I.U. of vitamin A daily for 3 to 4 months. Patients with serious acne are so accustomed to topical treatment that we allowed once daily applications of 5% benzoyl peroxide, a drug that most had used for long periods with questionable benefit. We reasoned that a familiar topical therapy would enhance patient compliance, offsetting the temptation to put something on to "strengthen" the therapy.

Because of the known animal teratogenicity of vitamin A, women were warned not to become pregnant. We prohibited oral contraceptives as a birth control measure, since estrogens suppress sebum and are often helpful in their own right. We were to be notified immediately of a missed menses; happily, this did not occur. The patients were generally seen every 2 weeks for the first month or so and every 3 weeks thereafter. They were told they were receiving vitamin A and were questioned about dietary habits that might be adding to the dose, especially high-potency vitamin pills available in health food stores.

We mentioned that adverse effects could occur but that the symptoms would very quickly disappear after stopping the drug. Beyond this, nothing specific was said regarding side effects. Long experience with drug testing has convinced us that the frequency and severity of symptoms is proportional to the information provided.

The therapeutic response was judged globally as follows: excellent = 75% improved or greater; good = about 50% improved; fair = about 25%; poor = no change or worsening based on a reduction of lesions. SMA-12 evaluations were performed on 26 of these subjects pre and post after 3 months of therapy.

The second portion of the study focused on toxicologic effects and was more closely monitored. The subjects had acne as above but were paid to participate. All were males. The study was conducted in a commercial drug-testing laboratory (Ivy Research Laboratories, Philadelphia, PA). The subjects came daily to receive the drug under supervision. One group of 20 volunteers received 300,000 units daily for 12 weeks. Another group of 10 received 300,000 units daily for the first week, 400,000 for the second and then 500,000 units for another 10 weeks. Serum vitamin A was determined at the start and after 2, 4, 6, 8 and 12 weeks of therapy. SMA-12's were performed at each visit.

Physical examinations were given every other week along with a system review.

Skin Surface Lipids Measurements

The forehead and cheek were prepared by thorough cleansing with 0.1% Triton X-100, followed by wiping with gauze saturated with hexane to remove surface lipids and debris. The areas to be sampled were then protected with plastic weighing boats with numerous perforations to prevent excessive accumulation of moisture. Three hours later, the forehead and cheek were sampled as follows. One ml of hexane was pipetted into a glass cylinder with an area of 3.8 cm^2 agitated for seconds and removed. This procedure was repeated with a second ml of hexane and the two samples pooled. The pooled sample was immediately passed through a 0.22 μ millipore filter to remove bacteria and debris, evaporated under nitrogen and stored at -20 °C. Samples were reconstituted with 0.05 cm^3 of hexane and processed by the thin layer chromatography method of Downing (5). An internal standard of methyl nervonate was added to the scrub fluid, permitting quantification as well as proportional analysis as demonstrated by Green et al. (8).

Results

Clinical Results

Therapeutic responses at the end of 3 to 4 months are summarized in Table 1. About 50% were rated excellent and 35% good. It is immediately apparent that females fared better. There were no poor results in this sex group and the proportion of excellent was considerably greater. Additionally, improvement was noted earlier than in males.

Patients usually noted decreased oiliness in 4 to 5 weeks. Clinical improvement was slow with no changes seen in this first few weeks. Those destined to experience nearly complete clearing were generally somewhat improved in about a month. Thereafter, resolution was more rapid with most of the pustules eliminated by two months. By 3 to 4 months deeper nodules had largely been resorbed. At times, settling of the inflammatory lesions was dramatic, within 5 to 6 weeks. As a rule, the best results were obtained in those with nume-

Table 1. Clinical efficacy of oral Vitamin A

	300,000 units (3 to 4 months)		300,000 units (3 months)	500,000 units (10 weeks)
Clinical Responses	Males (n = 80)	Females (n = 56)	Males (n = 20)	Males (n = 10)
Excellent	34	35	4	5
Good	36	20	14	5
Fair	4	1	2	0
Poor	6	0	0	0

Excellent = 75% or more clearing of inflammatory lesions
Good = 50% to 75% clearing of inflammatory lesions
Fair = 25% to 50% clearing of inflammatory lesions
Poor = less than 25% clearing of inflammatory lesions

rous pustules and papules. Acne conglobata, with its deeper, larger nodules, resolved more slowly. Back lesions were more resistant than facial ones. It was not possible to forecast which persons with acne conglobata would improve the most. Past responsiveness to therapy was not a reliable predictor.

The effect on comedones was uncertain. However, these are not prominent in individuals with severe inflammatory acne. Comedonal acne is now under study.

Of the 20 males receiving 300,000 units daily in the supervised clinicotoxicologic study, only 4 had an excellent response. Still 14 of the 20 were improved by at least 50%. In the second group of ten males who received 500,000 units for 10 weeks, 5 were rated excellent and 5 good, indicating greater benefits with the larger dose. After stopping the vitamin A, most patients showed at least a partial relapse within 3 to 6 weeks.

In the 136 patients receiving 300,000 units daily, side effects were infrequent and of small consequence. Only two patients in the entire series quit, both because of headaches. Another 3 complained of headaches at the start but were persuaded to continue with the help of aspirin. After 2 to 3 weeks the headaches completely disappeared. A sprinkling of other symptoms, tiredness, nausea, difficulty in concentration, were observed in a few patients and are perhaps drug-related.

Mucocutaneous alterations were more frequent and indeed may be regarded as characteristic of vitamin A toxicity. Cheilitis of varying degrees occurred in the majority and xerosis in about 75%, occasionally accompanied by itching. The dryness was readily controlled by lubricating ointments, the greasier ones being best (eucerin, petrolatum). Dryness of the nasal mucosa was a common complaint; about 5% had minor nose bleeds. Nail and hair changes were not noted.

In the closely monitored group receiving 300,000 units daily under supervision, side effects were somewhat more frequent (Table 2). One had headaches which later remitted, and a few had minor nose bleeds. Twelve had xerosis and 10 cheilitis. In those receiving 500,000 units for 10 weeks, 5 developed minor nose bleeds and six had headaches controlled by aspirin. Almost all had cheilitis and xerosis, which was noticeably more intense than at the lower dosage. These studies were carried out in winter time, which aggravated the mucocutaneous symptomatology.

As regards laboratory examination, the SMA-12's were unremarkable. There was little difference between the 300,000- and 500,000-unit groups. A few subjects showed elevated SGOT and SGPT's, but the increases were small. The most consistent finding was a modest

Table 2. Toxicology of oral Vitamin A*

	300,000 units daily (3 to 4 months) (n = 56)	500,000 units (10 weeks) (n = 10)
SGOT	8/56	2/10
SGPT	9/56	4/10
Alk. phosphatase	5/56	1/10
Triglycerides	50/56	10/10
BUN	0	0
Creatine	0	0
Xerosis	53/56	9/10
Cheilitis	54/56	8/10
Nose bleed	27/56	5/10
Headache	38/56	6/10

* Numerator shows number of subjects with abnormal values.

increase in serum triglycerides in a majority of patients. All elevated values invariably returned to normal within two to three weeks after stopping the drug.

Of course, vitamin A levels increased. At the first reading, two weeks after starting the values for the 500,000-unit group were significantly higher than the maximum attained by 4 weeks on the lower dosage. The huge standard errors of the means tellingly reflect the enormous individual differences (Table 3). The blood levels overlapped greatly in both dosage groups. There were some in the 300,000-unit group whose vitamin A levels were higher than with some receiving the larger dose. The reverse situation also was obtained. Some individuals showed only a modest increase in vitamin A levels throughout the entire test period, while in others the levels increased steadily with time. This variability among individuals cannot be too strongly stressed. We searched studiously for correlations between vitamin A levels, therapeutic response and toxicity. No relationships were uncovered. Therapeutic benefits were not greater in those with the highest serum concentration; indeed, dramatic improvement sometimes occurred in patients showing the least elevations. Neither signs nor symptoms could be correlated with serum levels. Headaches did not occur more often in those with the highest levels. Xerosis and dryness also varied independently.

Skin Surface Lipids

The results are summarized in Table 4. In the group treated with 500,000 units for 10 weeks there was an average reduction in the 3-h sebum excretion of 26.2% on the forehead (p

Table 3. Serum Vitamin A levels (µg/dl)

Week	500,000 units (10 weeks) (n = 10)	300,000 units (12 weeks) (n = 20)
0	33.2 ± 13.0	40.5 ± 15.0
2	116.8 ± 95.8	150.4 ± 152.2
4	129.0 ± 180	175.3 ± 204.6
6	193.1 ± 121	174.2 ± 176.5
8	276.5 ± 287	180.1 ± 158.4
12	281 ± 110	184.3 ± 110.2

Table 4. Oral Vitamin A and sebum excretion

	300,000 units (3 to 4 months)		500,000 units (10 weeks)	
	Pre	*Post*	*Pre*	*Post*
Forehead	102.1 ± 52.9	88.1 ± 38.7	110.6 ± 34.7	81.5 ± 32.0
Cheek	98.8 ± 52.5	79.1 ± 47.0	115.7 ± 57.5	81.2 ± 37.6

μg/cm²/3 h

< 0.005) and 29.8% reduction on the cheeks ($p < 0.25$). In the group treated with 300,000 units daily for 12 weeks there was a 14% reduction in the sebum excretion rate on the forehead ($p < 0.05$) and a 19.9% reduction on the cheek ($p < 0.005$).

Discussion

This study has yielded two results which deserve emphasis. Firstly, dosages in the 300,000 I.U. range are efficacious; secondly, the danger of hypervitaminosis A is not great in the time frame of this study.

Perhaps, adverse effects should be discussed first, since this is a sticking point for many physicians. The physiologic requirement for vitamin A is about 5,000 I.U. daily. By using 60 times this amount we have utilized the drug pharmacologically, not physiologically. What constitutes a large dose? The answer has to be relativistic and will depend both on ones' experience and historical perspective. Sulzberger and Witten in 1959 regarded 100,000 I.U. of vitamin A for one month as a large dose (22). Some writers consider 300,000 I.U. daily to be "massive". Yet Kalkoff and Conraths used this dose in 300 patients and barely mentioned adverse effects (10). We cannot vouchsafe that their vitamin A palmitate was the pharmacologic equivalent of 300,000 I.U. of retinol as aquasol A. Nonetheless, we have to agree that the side reactions, though more numerous than in Kalkoff's series, were easily tolerated and mainly limited to the skin and lips.

Our "large" doses pale into insignificance when compared with some of the recent usages of vitamin A. Dosages have taken a quantum leap into the mega-dosage (million units daily) range. Luger and Zip gave psoriatic patients as much as 3 million units daily for 18 days, a total of 54 million in less than 3 weeks, and side effects such as headache and gastrointestinal symptoms were frequent (12). Their boldness was evidently mitigated by the fact that a majority improved greatly. Similarly, in treating psoriasis and mycosis fungoides Schimpf and Jansen started with 600,000 units daily building up in a few days to 3.0–3.5 million units to totals of 30 to 50 million units without severe toxicity (17). Wannenmacher and his colleagues were willing to administer mega-doses for the treatment of leukoplakia of the oral cavity, achieving a total of 30 million units in 10 to 14 days (23). Hoefer-Janker et al. employed what they titled "subtoxic doses" giving 20 million units within 10 days (9). In combination with radiotherapy and a cytostatic drug this enormous dose caused malignant tumors of various kind to disappear. By 1977, cancer therapists were experimenting with 30 million units in three weeks, repeating this to advantage in several courses for hopeless cancer. It is noteworthy that Frey and Schoch much earlier had given 400,000 units daily to psoriatic patients without troublesome side effects, encountering significant toxicity only when the dose was raised to 1 to 2 million units daily (6). It cannot escape attention that practically all these reports using ambitious doses of vitamin A reside in the German literature. Nonetheless, even before the spurt to mega-doses in the seventies, Philadelphia dermatologists had given up to 600,000 units daily for disorders of abnormal keratinization such as Darier's disease and ichthyotic states (3). In their own words, "in spite of large doses of vitamin A, evidences of toxicity were few".

But now does all this fit with the widespread alarms in the medical community concerning the dangers of hypervitaminosis A? Because of the public's access to high-potency vitamin pills, sometimes containing 25,000 units per pill, numerous editorials and lecturers have warned physicians to be on the look-out for vitamin A intoxication. However, the figures on the prevalence of this event betray a great over-reaction. It comes as a surprise that as late as 1971 there were only 17 cases of chronic hypervitaminosis A in the world literature (14). By 1975, the total did not exceed 100 instances (11). Probably the extreme fear can be attributed to the frightening state of acute intoxication of which there were more than 500 cases by 1975. However, most of these were in infants and young children in Latin countries (France, Spain), where astonishingly high prophylactic doses were recommended by physicians. There is evidence that children are far more vulnerable. This practice has stopped and acute intoxication is now a clinical rarity.

The probability of developing chronic hypervitaminosis A is influenced by many factors including age, state of health, body-weight, etc. However, the two most important are dose and duration. Based on the available data, which is handicapped by many deficiencies, curves have been plotted showing the mean times to intoxication for various doses of emulsified forms of vitamin A, now the most frequently prescribed form (19). This works out to be about 7.5 months for doses of 300,000 units daily for a 70 kg person and about 3.5 months for 500,000 units daily. These are but rough estimates.

A thorough reading of the literature on toxicity yields information which is important for the informed use of high doses of vitamin A. Susceptibility varies enormously among individuals. Some persons can take over 500,000 units daily for months without any signs or symptoms while others quickly develop headaches and fatigue. One unusual case showed intoxication within two months after a daily dose of 200,000 to 275,000 units (18). The record consistently shows that the signs and symptoms of intoxication abate with great speed after stopping the vitamin, usually within a matter of weeks. Our experience verifies this. This rapid abatement is also a typical finding in experimental animals receiving mega-doses of vitamin A (2).

The frequency of specific signs and symptoms in chronic hypervitaminosis A is tabulated in several reports (11, 14). Suffice it to say here that the skin and mucous membranes are practically always involved and head the list of adverse effects. Xerosis (dry, peeling skin) variably associated with pruritus and erythema is most frequent. Mucous membrance "dryness" is also very common, particularly cheilitis, variably associated with nose bleeds.

Peck et al., too, in their study of 13-cis-retinoic acid observed that side reactions were mainly limited to the skin and mucous membranes (15). This certainly corresponds to our experience with 300,000 units daily; incidentally, 300,000 I.U. works out to about 90 mg of retinol.

It is noteworthy that the frequency of skin and mucous membrane side effects increased sharply when the dose was increased to 500,000 units daily. Systemic reactions became more evident and more severe, suggesting that doses in this range lie at the beginning of the steep portion of the dosage-response curve.

It is known that hair loss may occur in hypervitaminosis A; the first case, being recorded by Sulzberger and Lazar (21). It is interesting that neither Peck et al. nor ourselves have seen this. However, there is evidence that the proportion of telogen hairs increases with very high doses.

While the literature lists about 20 systemic effects of hypervitaminosis A, some of them uncommon or unusual such as hepato-splenomegaly, edema, and lymphadenopathy, the reactions to look for are as follows: Headaches head the list. These tend to be persistent and are not very responsive to doses of Aspirin. Nausea may occur at the start but usually abates. Other typical signs are fatigue, emotional lability, and muscle and bone pains.

We call particular attention to an observation which recurs repeatedly in the literature, including animal studies, and which corresponds to our own findings. The correlation between toxicity and vitamin A blood levels is rather poor. The serum concentration does not reliably predict adverse effects; serum levels may be just as high in asymptomatic persons. Thus, there is little point in routinely monitoring these patients by determination of serum vitamin A levels. Symptoms may be more closely tied to circulating retinyl esters (19), but this measurement cannot be routinely performed. Elevations in SGOT and SGPT occur erratically and are more likely in symptomatic patients. We do not routinely monitor the blood and depend heavily on clinical judgment. A mild increase in serum triglycerides is to be expected and has been noted previously (2). The significance of this last finding is unknown.

Our experience suggests that an appreciable accomodation to toxic effects can occur. Symptomatology declines with time in the face of continued administration. We, therefore, encourage patients with mild systemic symptoms to carry on. It is particularly noteworthy that the symptoms which may force a temporary halt, headaches particularly, may often not reappear when the drug is restarted at the same dose.

Regarding efficacy, we believe that retinol has a definite place for the treatment of serious inflammatory acne. We emphasize that we use a water-dispersed retinol emulsion. Oily forms prove almost certainly less effective and, of course, less toxic, probably owing to poorer absorption. We cannot give assurance that equivalent doses of vitamin A palmitate will be equally effective.

Our guidelines for administering retinol are as follows:

1. Mild acne is excluded. The best candidates have severe inflammatory acne, including the conglobata form, especially if the response to oral antibiotics and topical medicaments has been unsatisfactory.
2. We start all patients at 300,000 units daily. The majority of females will not require an increase, but we will go to 400,000 if there is no response after one month. Our policy with males is to give 300,000 units the first week and 400,000 units thereafter. We increase to 500,000 units if improvement is insufficient after one month. We know with certainty that this gradual escalation of the dose is far better tolerated. Starting at 500,000 units will frequently precipitate headaches. These can be greatly moderated with the graduated schedule of increases. To date we have paid insufficient attention to body weight. Larger persons should be given larger doses at the start.
3. We will stop the drug if the benefits have not been impressive by 10 weeks. Judgments about the value of the drug should not be made before a trial period of 6 to 8 weeks. Some patients respond very slowly.
4. We do not give retinol indefinitely. As a rule we give the drug for 4 to 5 months and step down thereafter if clearing has been achieved. We do not hesitate to extend full doses for 6 months provided that improvement is steady and satisfying. Currently, this is our maximum. The step-down procedure is to decrease the dose by 100,000 units weekly. During this time other maintenance drugs are vigorously used, viz., topical vitamin A acid, benzoyl peroxide, and especially oral antibiotics. We are convinced that once severe acne is brought under control, the tamed disease can be kept at bay with conventional drugs.
5. Except at the start, we see patients about every three weeks and take detailed histories. No laboratory studies are done unless persistent symptoms emerge. Liver function

studies are the most appropriate. If improvement has been striking in subjects who become intolerant, we will restart the drug after a rest period of a couple of weeks. Systemic side reactions are most frequent at the start of therapy.

6. In cold weather, we forewarn about xerosis and cheilitis. Oily emollients are very helpful; petrolatum is best, especially when accompanied by a warm tub bath. More aggreeable, efficacious moisturizers are aquaphor-water emulsions (eucerin). Chap sticks are useful for cheilitis. Topical steroids are avoided.

7. Our relapse rate stands in sharp contrast to the report of Peck et al., whose patients remained clear for as long as 20 months (dare one say "cured"?). In the absence of other therapy our patients regularly relapse within a few months. We are currently experimenting with finding a lower-limited maintenance dose of retinol. Evidence to date suggests that this cannot be less than 150,000 units daily. We do not know how long such a dose can be given without toxicity.

Summary

Oral vitamin A (retinol) has been studied for therapeutic and toxicologic effects in varying doses in more than 150 patients. Clinical improvement occurred in those treated with doses of 300,000 units or more per day. Sebum excretion rates are suppressed by approximately 30%; no effect in lipid composition or cutaneous bacteriology occurred. Clinical relapse occurred with discontinuation of oral vitamin A. Side effects are mainly limited to the skin and consisted of xerosis of the skin and mucous membranes, epistaxis, increased telogen hairs and occasional headache. Slight but definite increase in serum triglycerides occurred in most patients.

References

1. Anderson JAD, Stokoe IH (1963) Vitamin A in acne vulgaris. Br Med J 2:294–296
2. Bayerle H, Meister P, Wolff H (1973) Serum- und Leberbefunde bei Vitamin A-Megadosen. Arzneim-Forsch 23:1082–1085
3. Burgoon CF, Graham JH, Urbach F, Musgnug R (1963) Effect of vitamin A on epithelial cells of skin. Arch Dermatol 87:63–80
4. Davidson DM, Sobel AE (1949) Aqueous vitamin A in acne vulgaris. J Invest Dermatol 12:221–228
5. Downing DT (1968) Photodensitometry in thin layer chromatographic analysis of neutral lipids. J Chromatogr 38:91–99
6. Frey JR, Schoch MA (1952) Therapeutische Versuche bei Psoriasis mit Vitamin A, zugleich ein Beitrag zur A-Hypervitaminose. Dermatologica 104:80–86
7. Germeraad WF, Vasbinder H, Verbeeck A, Van der Sijde HR (1955) Vitamin A in acne vulgaris. Ned Tijdschr Geneeskd 99:2358–2364
8. Greene RS, Downing DT, Pochi PE, Strauss JS (1970) Anatomical variation in the amount and composition of human skin surface lipid. J Invest Dermatol 54:240–247
9. Hoefer-Janker H, Khazne F, Scheef W (1969) Erste klinische Erfahrungen mit subtoxischen Vitamin-A-Dosen im Rahmen der radiologischen und zytostatischen Tumortherapie. Krebsarzt 24:203–206
10. Kalkoff KW, Conraths H (1956) Zur peroralen Vitamin-A-Therapie von Dermatosen. Münch Med Wochenschr 98:1129–1135
11. Körner WF, Völlm J (1975) New aspects of the tolerance of retinol in humans. Int J Vitam Nutr Res 45:363–372
12. Luger A, Zips IA (1972) Psoriasis-Behandlung mit hohen Dosen von Vitaminen A Palmitat. Arch Dermatol Forsch 244:422–424
13. Lynch FW, Cook CD (1947) Acne vulgaris treated with vitamin A. Arch Dermatol Syph 55: 355–357

14. Muenter MD, Perry HO, Ludwig J (1971) Chronic vitamin A intoxication in adults. Am J Med 50:129–136
15. Peck GL, Olsen, TG, Yoder FW, Strauss JS, Downing DT, Pandya M, Butkus D, Arnaud-Battandier J (1977) Prolonged remissions of cystic and conglobata acne with 13-cis-retinoic acid. N Engl J Med 300:329–333
16. Savitt LE, Obermayer ME (1950) Treatment of acne vulgaris and senile keratosis with vitamin A: results of a clinical experiment. J Invest Dermatol 14:283–289
17. Schimpf A, Jansen KH (1972) Hochdosierte Vitamin A-Therapie bei Psoriasis und Mycosis fungoides. Fortsch Ther 90:635–640
18. Shaw EW, Niccoli JZ (1953) Hypervitaminosis A. Report of a case in an adult male. Ann Int Med 39:131–134
19. Smith FR, Goodman DS (1976) Vitamin A transport in human vitamin A toxicity. N Engl J Med 294:805–808
20. Straumfjord JV (1949) Vitamin A: Its effect on acne. Northwest Med 42:219–225
21. Sulzberger MB, Lazar MP (1955) Hypervitaminosis A. JAMA 146:788–793
22. Sulzberger MB, Witten VH (1959) The management of acne today. Med Clin North Am 43: 887–902
23. Wannenmacher MF, Tetsch P, Esser E (1972) Behandlung der Leukoplakie mit subtoxischen Vitamin-A-Dosen. Dtsch Zahnärztl Z 27:154–158

C.E. Orfanos et al. (eds.)
Retinoids

13-cis-Retinoic Acid in Acne (A Double-blind Study of Dose Response)

D.H. Jones, W.J. Cunliffe and J.H. Cove

Following the work of Peck et al. (5), a double-blind dose response study of the action of 13-cis-retinoic acid in acne has been made.

Patients

One group of 7 males and 1 female with an age of 18–32 years, mean acne grade (4) of 9.0 and mean sebum excretion rate (SER) of 2.0 $\mu g \cdot cm^{-2} \cdot min^{-1}$ were treated as a pilot study. A further group of 12 males and 2 females (aged 14–35 years), mean acne grade of 7.3 and SER of 2.0 $\mu g \cdot cm^{-2} \cdot min^{-1}$, have been treated for 8 weeks.

All patients have a long history of severe acne unresponsive to conventional antibiotic treatment.

Treatment

The patients were divided into three groups, and allocated a daily dose regime of 1.0, 0.5 or 0.1 mg/kg. Treatment was given for 16 weeks, and follow-up of the first group has been for 16 weeks.

Methods

Patients were seen prior to treatment and at 2 and 4 weeks on therapy. Thereafter, assessment was at monthly intervals. At each visit, the following data were collected:

1. Acne grade and individual acne lesions (4)
2. Sebum excretion rate
   - gravimetric method (2)
   - lipometric method (3)
3. Quantitative bacteriology and free fatty acid content of sebum (1). (First group only)
4. Clinical side effects noted
5. Estimations of full blood count - sedimentation rate (ESR), renal and liver function
6. Fasting triglycerides

Results

On Therapy

The SER was reduced overall by 75% in four weeks with a significant reduction even being seen at two weeks. Thereafter, the inhibition was maintained whilst on treatment. The reduction is dose-dependent (Fig. 1) being 55% with 0.1 mg/kg and 85% with 1 mg/kg.

The acne grade (Fig. 2) is more gradually reduced though with an exacerbation in some

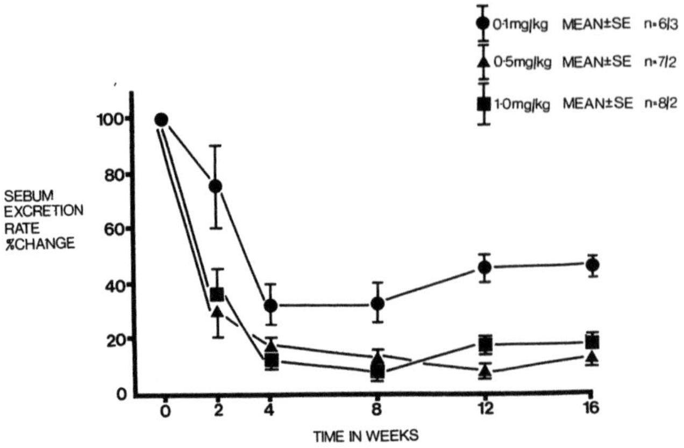

Fig. 1. Sebum excretion rate (% change) vs time (weeks). Different dose regimes

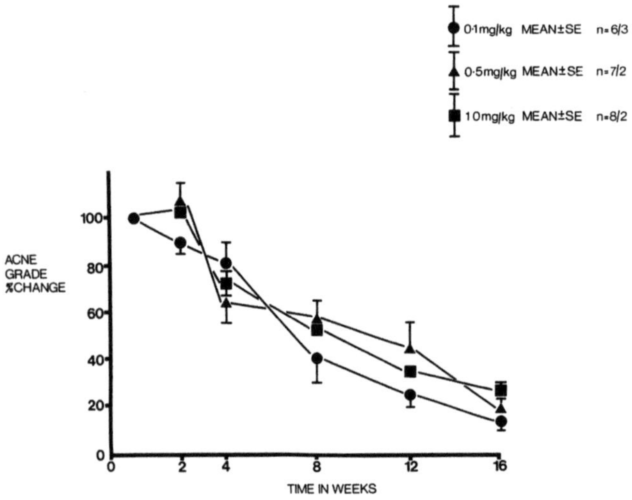

Fig. 2. Acne grade (% change) vs time (weeks). Different dose regimes

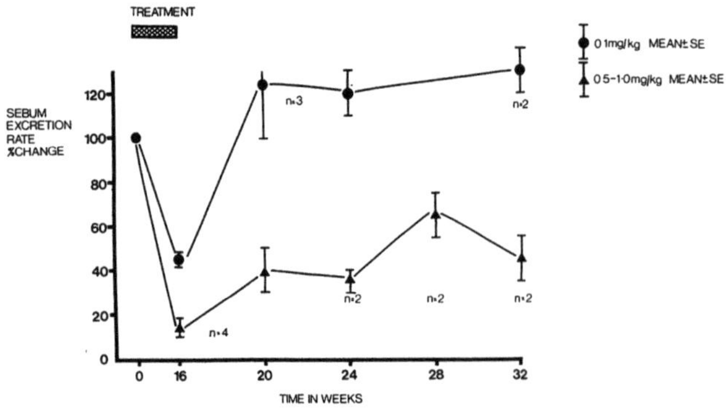

Fig. 3. Sebum excretion rate (% change) vs time (weeks). Off therapy

individuals on the higher doses at two weeks. The difference in response between the dose groups is not marked, but the drug side effect of erythema was more intense in the higher dose groups leading to an overestimation of their grade.

The individual acne lesions disappear gradually in a similar manner throughout the study. It is not only the deep-inflamed lesions of the nodules and cysts which disappear, but also the non-inflamed. One patient had a count of over 100 blackheads on his face at the beginning, but by the end only 10 were to be seen. The different dose response is not great, there being an 80% improvement in the 0.1 mg/kg group, and a 90%-response in the other two groups.

Off Therapy

The response on cessation of therapy seems to have been more individual. In the 0.1-mg/kg group, the SER (Fig. 3) was back to its pretreatment value within four weeks. The acne relapsed in two of these patients, and required antibiotic treatment. One of these patients failed to respond and is back on 13-cis-retinoic acid. The third patient was much older (32 years), and though his SER has increased, there has been no relapse of acne, and he is well satisfied with his treatment.

In the higher-dose group, the SER (Fig. 3) is gradually increasing though still only 50% of the pre-treatment value at 16 weeks follow-up. In only one out of the five patients has the acne recurred, and this was at 12 weeks follow-up. He was happier at the next visit, having improved on only one month's antibiotic treatment.

The patients with relapses were quite intolerant of the return of the acne, as they asked for further therapy when their acne had deteriorated by only 12–20%.

Bacteriology

The only change in terms of bacterial numbers was a fall in the propionobacteria acnes (anaerobes) at 8 and 16 weeks in the high-dose group. The numbers are too small to know if this is significant, but the fall was associated with a decrease in the percentage of free fatty acid in sebum, which represents a decrease in bacterial activity.

Side Effects

These were troublesome, but in only one patient was the dose not tolerated. Angular cheilitis caused the most difficulty, and its severity was dose-related. Other side effects were as recorded before by Peck et al. (5).

There was a rise of serum γ-glutamyl o-transferase on seven occasions out of 60 estimations, and only one rise in fasting triglycerides.

Discussion

13-cis-retinoic acid has been a very successful form of therapy in these patients with severe resistant acne. Though there was a difference in dose response in terms of inhibition of SER, this was not so noticeable in the clinical response. 13-cis-retinoic acid may be acting primarily through its inhibition of sebaceous gland function, but other actions such as on the mediation of inflammation also need to be explored. Side effects in these low doses have not been too troublesome and are, as yet, not a contra-indication to its use. Certainly these low doses are an acceptable form of the therapy, though the lowest (0.1 mg/kg) is associated with a rapid relapse of the acne.

Summary

13-cis-retinoic acid has been used in a double-blind study of 22 severely affected acne patients. Three different dose regimes were used. Though there was a difference in the degree of inhibition of the sebum excretion rate between doses, the clinical response was satisfactory with all regimes. However, the lowest dose (0.1 mg/kg) was associated with a rapid relapse off treatment.

Acknowledgments. We feel indebted to Mr. R.A. Forster for his continual support and technical advice, and to Dr. D. Blanc for his help in the practical work of the pilot study.

References

1. Cove J, Holland K, Cunliffe WJ (1980) An analysis of sebum excretion rate, bacterial population and the production of free fatty acids on human skin. E.S.D.R. May 1980 (Abstract)
2. Cunliffe WJ, Shuster S (1971) The rate of sebum excretion in man. Br J Dermatol 85:119–126
3. Cunliffe WJ, Kearney JN, Simpson NB (1980) A modified photometric technique for measuring sebum excretion rate. J Invest Dermatol, in press
4. Cunliffe WJ, Gould D, Clayden AD, Burke B Acne quantified. In preparation
5. Peck GL, Olsen TG, Yoder FW, Strauss JS, Downing DT, Pandya M, Butkus D, Arnaud-Battandier J (1979) Prolonged remissions of cystic and conglobate acne with 13-cis-retinoic acid. N Engl J Med 300:329–333

C.E. Orfanos et al. (eds.)
Retinoids

Effects of 13-cis-Retinoic Acid on Sebaceous Glands in Humans

M. Landthaler, J. Kummermehr, A. Wagner, J. Nikolowski and G. Plewig

The beneficial effects of 13-cis-retinoic acid in acne patients (5, 8, 10), its effects on sebaceous glands of the hamster flank organ (1) and the ear lobes (6), and sebum production in humans (9) are well documented.

Aim of our histological, planimetric and autoradiographic studies was to proof the effects of 13-cis-retinoic acid on the sebaceous glands of acne patients, treated with this compound (4).

Material and Methods

In the first part of the study 13-cis-retinoic acid was given to 18 male patients (ages 15–41, mean age 23.7 years) with acne conglobata (N = 11), acne tetrade (N = 5), and acne fulminans (N = 2). The dose was 1 (N = 9) or 2 (N = 9) mg/kg bodyweight, daily for twelve weeks. In these patients 36 biopsies from the upper back were obtained, one before the start of therapy, and a second at varying intervals during treatment, from weeks one to twelve. Half of the biopsy material was prepared in a routine fashion using paraffin-embedding and hematoxylin-eosin staining. The other half served as substrate for in vitro autoradiography using a previously described technique (2).

In the second part of the study 22 additional patients with severe acne, rosacea or gram negative folliculitis were treated with different doses of 13-cis-retinoic acid (1.0 mg/kg, N = 4; 0.5 mg/kg, N = 9; 0.2 mg/kg, N = 7; and 0.05 mg/kg bw, N = 2). Also two biopsies were obtained in these patients. The material was processed using paraffin-embedding and hematoxylin-eosin staining for planimetric analysis only, but not for in vitro autoradiography.

Analysis

The mean sagittal surface areas of sebaceous glands before and during therapy were measured planimetrically. Serial cuts were done, but only the largest cross-sectional surfaces from each follicle were evaluated, and only the sebaceous acini were measured. The labelling index (LI) in per cent was determined by counts of basement membrane-bound labelled germinative cells and unlabelled germinative cells in 29 biopsies. In 7 biopsies the evaluation was technically impossible.

In 9 cases the ratio of "differentiating" to "undifferentiating" cells was measured before and during therapy. The "differentiating cell pool" (DCP) are basement membrane-bound cells, and lipid cells (sebocytes) containing lipid droplets at the light microscopic level in their cytoplasm. The "undifferentiating cell pool" (UCP) are sebocytes, which rarely produce lipid droplets at the light microscopic level; they form a sponge-like skeleton throughout the sebaceous gland (7).

For statistical analysis the paired comparison test and the H-test of Kruskal and Wallis were used.

Results

Size of Sebaceous Glands

All doses of 13-cis-retinoic acid led to a significant reduction in size of sebaceous acini (Fig. 1).

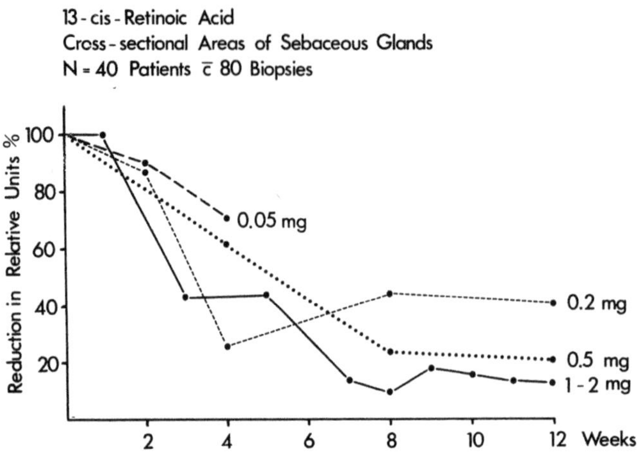

Fig. 1. Effects of 13-cis-retinoic acid on sebaceous glands in humans. Reduction of cross-sectional areas of sebaceous glands by different doses of 13-cis-retinoic acid

After three to four weeks of treatment with the 1–2 mg/kg bw dose a steep reduction in size of up to 50 per cent of the pretreatment value could be seen, and a further decrease with continued therapy. Details of the 1–2 mg/kg bw dose are reported elsewhere (2, 3). After 12 weeks of treatment the reduction of cross sectional areas of sebaceous acini by the 1–2 mg/kg bw dose was up to 12.5 ± 13 per cent of the pretreatment value ($N = 6$), by the 0.5 mg dose to 20.1 ± 11.3 per cent ($N = 6$) and the 0.2 mg dose to 40 ± 31.1 per cent ($N = 2$) (Fig. 2). The differences between pretreatment values and values after 12 weeks of treatment were

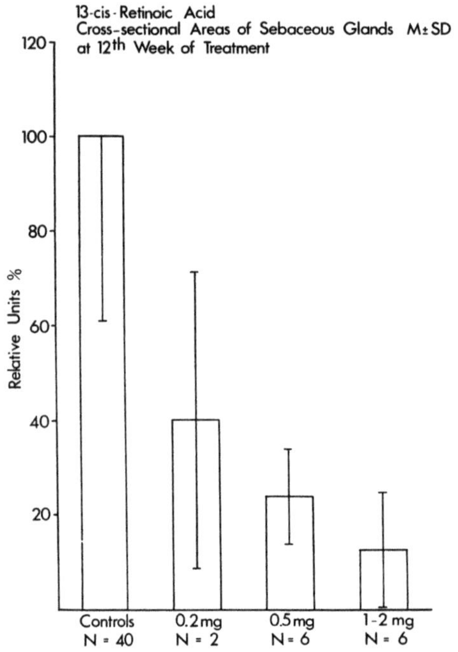

Fig. 2. Effects of 13-cis-retinoic acid on sebaceous glands in humans. Reduction of cross-sectional areas of sebaceous glands by different doses of 13-cis-retinoic acid after 12 weeks of treatment

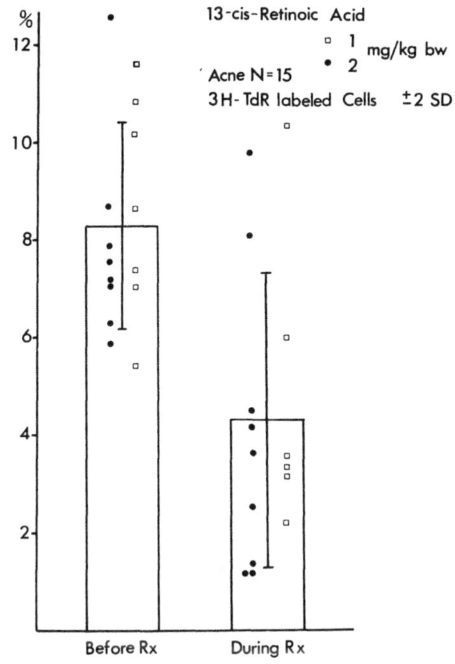

Fig 3. Effects of 13-cis-retinoic acid on sebaceous glands in humans. Reduction of 3H-TdR-labelled cells (adapted from 2)

statistically significant for the different doses ($p \leqq 0.005$). But there was no significant difference in the reduction in size, attained by the different doses after 12 weeks of treatment.

Labelling Index

Before therapy it was 8.3 ± 2.1 per cent; during therapy it receded significantly to 4.3 ± 3.1 per cent (Fig. 3).

Histology

Histologically, the baloon-shaped, large sebaceous lobules seemed to collapse, becoming elongated. In extreme cases sebaceous follicles were reduced to a mere wick-like structure, consisting only of the pilary unit. There was a marked perifollicular fibrosis with many fibroblasts (Fig. 4A–C, 5). Another early phenomenon was that the boundaries of the acini were completely replaced by small "undifferentiating cells". Prior to therapy there had been a ratio of "differentiating" to "undifferentiating cells" of 2:1. Therapy brought about a change to 1:7 (Fig. 6A–C, 7).

Discussion

13-cis-retinoic acid dramatically shrank sebaceous glands in humans. The histological changes in humans were similiar to those found in the hamster flank organ (1). The reduction of size of sebaceous glands of up to 90 per cent of the pretreatment value after twelve weeks of treatment with the 1.0–2.0 mg/kg bw dose agrees well with the results concerning the influence of 13-cis-retinoic acid on sebum production (9). The reduction of size attained with the 0.2, 0.5 and 1.0–2.0 mg/kg bw dose did not differ significantly after twelve weeks of treatment, but there was a tendency for a more pronounced reduction by the higher doses. Though the number of patients is small, it demonstrates that even with low doses of 13-cis-

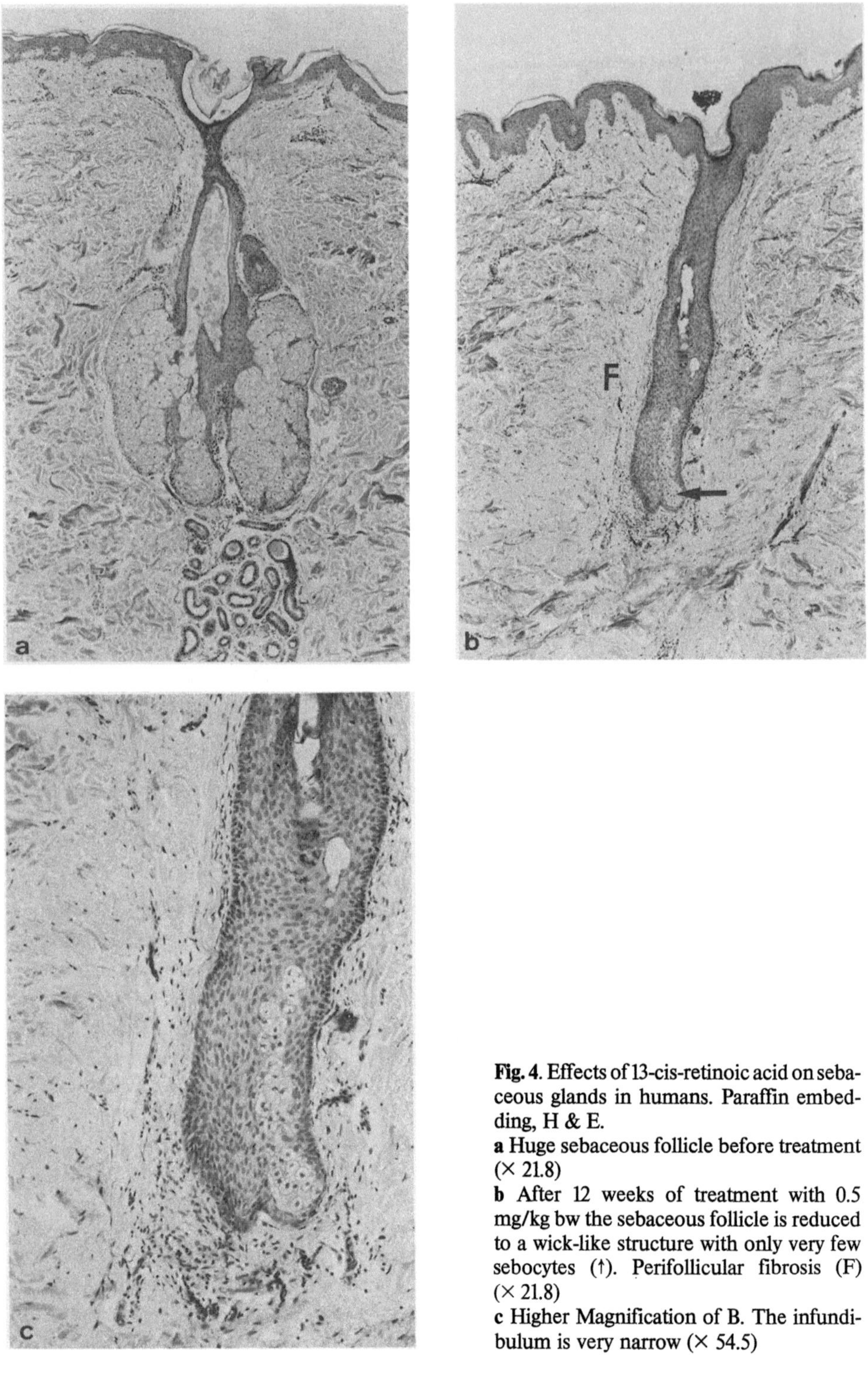

Fig. 4. Effects of 13-cis-retinoic acid on sebaceous glands in humans. Paraffin embedding, H & E.

a Huge sebaceous follicle before treatment (× 21.8)

b After 12 weeks of treatment with 0.5 mg/kg bw the sebaceous follicle is reduced to a wick-like structure with only very few sebocytes (↑). Perifollicular fibrosis (F) (× 21.8)

c Higher Magnification of B. The infundibulum is very narrow (× 54.5)

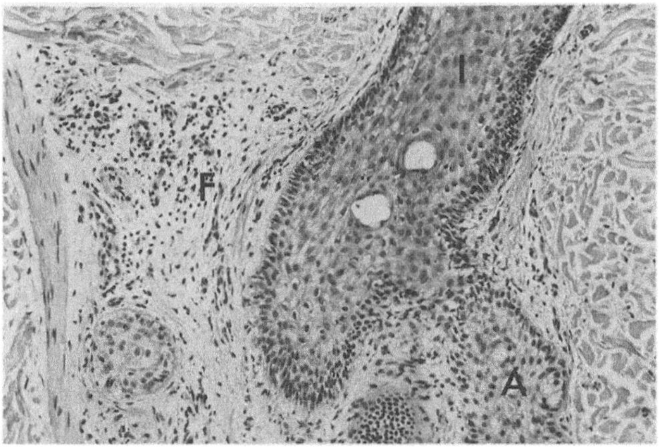

Fig. 5. Effects of 13-cis-retinoic acid on sebaceous glands in humans. 4th week of treatment with 0.2 mg/kg bw. The lower portion of a sebaceous follicle is shown. Tangential cut of the infundibulum (I). A is a remnant of a sebaceous acinus. Perifollicular fibrosis (F). Paraffin embedding, H & E (× 50)

retinoic acid a marked reduction in size of sebaceous glands can be obtained, if duration of treatment is sufficient.

It should be emphasized that there may be an additional individual factor for the patient's response to the compound. In some patients low cumulative doses led to a dramatic reduction in size of sebaceous glands within a few weeks, whereas in other patients a longer time of treatment was necessary. There was a good correlation between clinical and histological response in most of the patients. The reduction of labelling index of sebocytes during therapy may indicate an inhibitory effect of 13-cis-retinoic acid on proliferation of sebocytes and a slowed down turnover. The changing ratio of the "differentiating" cells to the "undifferentiating" cells probably implies a disturbance of differentiation (lipid production) of sebocytes. The clinically highly beneficial effects of 13-cis-retinoic acid in the treatment of severe acne can, at least partially be explained by this effect on the sebaceous glands.

Summary

13-cis-retinoic acid was given to 18 patients with extensive acne conglobata, acne fulminans and acne tetrade, 1–2 mg/kg bw/day for up to 90 days. Two biopsies were obtained from each subject, before and at varying intervals between 8 to 90 days of treatment. In vitro autoradiography with ^{3}H-TdR was performed and 5 µm sections cut from acrylate-embedded specimens. The sagittal section areas of sebaceous follicles as well as the labelling index of sebocytes were determined.

13-cis-retinoic acid led to a significant decrease of sagittal section areas. This started within 4 weeks of treatment. At 90 days sebaceous lobules were reduced to minute buds. The reduction in sagittal section area was up to 90 per cent. Labelled sebocytes were also reduced. The nuclei of differentiating sebocytes were retained longer than in controls, possibly indicating a disturbance of differentiation.

The reduction in sebaceous acini size, and the regression of labelled sebocytes may explain the improvement of severe seborrhea clinically seen in all patients and the prolonged remission (up to 14 months so far) in our patients.

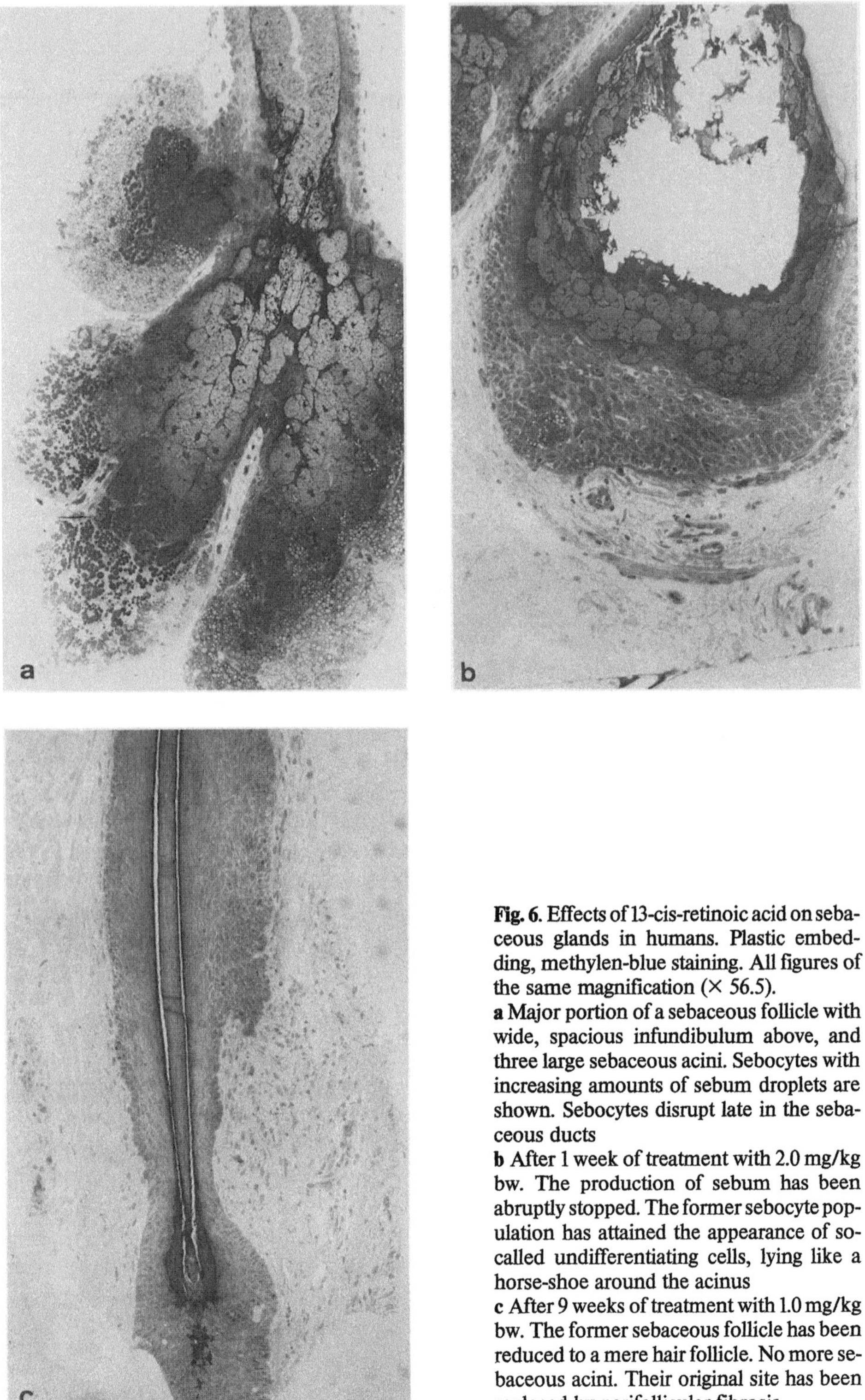

Fig. 6. Effects of 13-cis-retinoic acid on sebaceous glands in humans. Plastic embedding, methylen-blue staining. All figures of the same magnification (× 56.5).

a Major portion of a sebaceous follicle with wide, spacious infundibulum above, and three large sebaceous acini. Sebocytes with increasing amounts of sebum droplets are shown. Sebocytes disrupt late in the sebaceous ducts

b After 1 week of treatment with 2.0 mg/kg bw. The production of sebum has been abruptly stopped. The former sebocyte population has attained the appearance of so-called undifferentiating cells, lying like a horse-shoe around the acinus

c After 9 weeks of treatment with 1.0 mg/kg bw. The former sebaceous follicle has been reduced to a mere hair follicle. No more sebaceous acini. Their original site has been replaced by perifollicular fibrosis

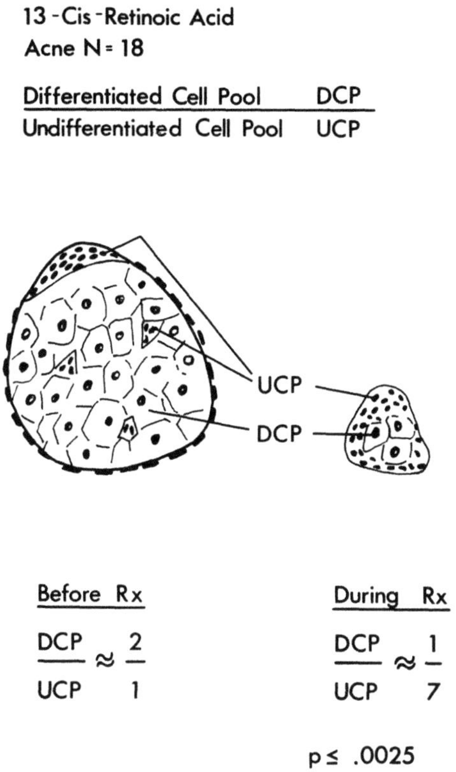

Fig. 7. Effects of 13-cis-retinoic acid on sebaceous glands in humans. Changing ratio of differentiated cell pool (DCP) versus undifferentiated cell pool (UCP)

Acknowledgment. The technical assistance of Miss H. Pfeiffer and Miss A. Ruhfus is gratefully appreciated.
Supported in form of a grant by the Deutsche Forschungsgemeinschaft PL 58/6.
Dr. R. Hennes, Hoffmann-La Roche, Grenzach/Germany provided the 13-cis-retinoic acid.

References

1. Gomez EC, Moskowitz RJ (1980) Effect of 13-cis-retinoic acid on the hamster flank organ. J Invest Dermatol 74:392–397
2. Landthaler M, Kummermehr J, Wagner A, Plewig G (1980) Inhibitory effects of 13-cis-retinoic acid on human sebaceous glands. Arch Dermatol Res 269:297–309
3. Landthaler M, Kummermehr J, Wagner A, Plewig G (1980) 13-cis-retinoic acid inhibits sebaceous glands in animals and humans: planimetry and in vitro autoradiography. Eur Soc Dermato Res, Amsterdam, May 12–14, 1980 (abstract). J Invest Dermatol 74:453
4. Landthaler M, Nikolowski J, Plewig G Effekte verschiedener Dosierungen von 13-cis Retinsäure auf die Talgdrüsen beim Menschen. Arbeitsgem Dermatol Forsch, Innsbruck, Nov 14–16, 1980 (abstract). Arch Dermatol Res (in press)
5. Peck GL, Olsen TG, Yoder FW, Strauss JS, Downing DT, Pandya M, Butkus D, Arnaud-Battandier J (1979) Prolonged remission of cystic and conglobate acne with 13-cis-retinoic acid. New Engl J Med 300:329–333
6. Plewig G (1980) Der Einfluß des aromatischen Retinoids Ro 10-9359 und der 13-cis-Retinsäure Ro 4-3780 auf die Talgdrüsen des Syrischen Hamsters. Arch Dermatol Res 268:239–246
7. Plewig G, Christophers E, Braun-Falco O (1971) Proliferative cells in the human sebaceous gland. Labeling index and regional variations. Acta Dermatovener (Stockholm) 51:413–422
8. Plewig G, Wagner A, Braun-Falco O (1980) Orale Behandlung schwerster Akneformen mit 13-cis-Retinsäure. Klinische Ergebnisse. Münch Med Wochenschr 122:1287–1293

9. Strauss JS, Stranieri AM, Farell LN, Downing DT (1980) The effect of marked inhibition of sebum production with 13-cis-retinoic acid on skin surface lipid composition. J Invest Dermatol 74:66–67
10. Wagner A, Plewig G (1980) 13-cis-Retinsäure. Pharmakologische und toxikologische Untersuchung bei der Behandlung schwerster Akneformen. Münch Med Wochenschr 122:1294–1300

C.E. Orfanos et al. (eds.)
Retinoids

A Clinical Trial of the Use of Tigason (Ro 10-9359) in Male Patients with Severe Acne Vulgaris

R.M. MacKie and D.C. Dick

Many patients with severe acne do not respond satisfactorily to current conventional treatment with systemic antibiotics and topical preparations usually based on benzoyl peroxide. For such patients the preliminary results of treatment of severe acne with oral 13-cis-retinoic acid (3) suggested the prospect of a major advance in therapy. Later work (4) has shown that 13-cis-retinoic acid profoundly reduces sebaceous gland activity and this seems the likely mechanism of the drug's affect in acne.

As 13-cis-retinoic acid is not generally available in the U.K. we report here a study of ten male patients who had severe acne treated with Tigason (Ro 10-9359) with the object of comparing the results to those reported by Peck (2).

Patients and Methods

Ten male patients were selected on the basis of an unsatisfactory response to conventional acne therapy. Their ages ranged from 16 to 26 years (mean 20 years) and the duration of acne varied from 2 to 11 years (mean 5 years). Six of the patients had large nodules or cysts and all of them had a large number of inflammatory lesions and were judged to suffer from severe acne.

For the duration of the trial and for a period of at least two weeks beforehand all other systemic and topical treatment for acne was discontinued. Tigason was administered orally for 2 months in a dose of 1 mg/kg/day. Before and after treatment patients had the severity of their acne assessed on a I-to-V scale (1), as well as by recording the number of lesions, and from clinical photographs. In addition to physical examination and urinanalysis, sedimentation rate, full blood count, urea and electrolytes, and liver function tests were measured regularly throughout the study.

Results

Seven patients completed the full two-month treatment and assessment period. One patient had his treatment discontinued after one month because of marked deterioration of his acne and generalised desquamation. Two other patients failed to attend for final assessment.

No change was observed in the grade of severity of acne in any of the seven patients who completed the trial. However, on counting lesions there was an average reduction in number of 30% from a total of 276 lesions before treatment to 185 afterwards (Table 1). While both comedones and superficial inflammatory lesions were significantly reduced in number, there was a slight increase overall in the number of deep inflammatory lesions (Table 1).

Five of the seven patients showed an individual overall decrease in the number of lesions.

On photographic assessment, which was carried out by comparing three pairs of photographs for each patient without knowledge of whether the photograph was taken before or after treatment, six of the seven patients were judged to be improved.

Table 1. Lesion count before and after treatment with Tigason. Cumulative total for 7 patients

	Comedones	Superficial inflammatory	Deep inflammatory	Total
Before	96	140	40	276
After	76	62	47	185

All patients had dryness or fissuring of the lips; five showed desquamation of palms (particularly finger tips) or soles; one patient developed extensive erythema and scaling affecting the axillae and trunk as well as the hands and feet; one patient noticed a slight degree of hair loss. Only one patient had his treatment discontinued because of side effects, and no unexpected side effects of therapy were noted.

Discussion

The results of treatment of our patients' acne with Tigason look disappointing. Although 6 of the 10 patients who began treatment were improved on photographic assessment and 5 showed a reduction in the number of lesions, none showed a dramatic improvement. We conclude that, although Tigason does appear to have a marginally beneficial effect in acne, the potential value of the drug is not comparable with that of 13-cis-retinoic acid as a single agent in some patients. The reasons for such a marked difference in effect of these two synthetic retinoids require to be investigated. Both drugs modify the differentiation of epithelial tissues but there appears to be a degree of specificity in the direction of differentiation or in the degree to which the epidermal adnexae are affected. Elucidation of the reasons for this difference should help not only in the development of new precisely tailored retinoids with enhanced potency and refined specificity but, perhaps, also in defining the control mechanisms which govern the ultimate phenotypic variation of epithelial cells.

Summary

Ten male patients between the ages of 15 and 25 with severe facial acne vulgaris have taken part in a study of systemic Tigason administered in a dose of 1 mg/kg/day. Patients were selected on the basis of non-response to conventional systemic antibiotic and topical benzoyl peroxide preparations. All other treatment was discontinued at least 2 weeks before commencing Tigason but Patients were seen fortnightly and assessed for positive response to therapy by grading severity of acne vulgaris and also for side effects including cheilitis, desquamation and alopecia. Tigason therapy was continued for 8 weeks and in no patient was any significant improvement in acne lesions observed. Cheilitis was seen in all of the patients in the study but no other side effects were noted.

In view of the similar beneficial response noted in dyskeratotic conditions when either Tigason or 13-cis-retinoic acid are used, it is concluded from this study that the reported benefit to acne vulgaris patients from systemic 13-cis-retinoic acid administration is unlikely to be related to a direct effect on keratinisation.

References

1. Burton JL, Cunliffe WJ, Stafford I, Shuster S (1971) The prevalence of acne vulgaris in adolescence. Br J Dermatol 85:119–126
2. Peck GL, Olsen TG, Yoder FW, Strauss JS, Downing DT, Pandya M, Butkus D, Arnaud-Battandier J (1979) Prolonged remissions of cystic and conglobate acne with 13-cis-retinoic acid. N Engl J Med 300:329–333
3. Peck GL (1980) Retinoids in dermatology. Arch Dermatol 116:283–284
4. Strauss JS, Stranieri AM, Farrell LN, Downing DT (1980) The effect of marked inhibition of sebum production with 13-cis-retinoic acid on skin surface lipid composition. J Invest Dermatol 74:66–67

Oral Retinoid Therapy of Miscellaneous Disorders of Skin and Oral Mucosa

C.E. Orfanos et al. (eds.)
Retinoids

Treatment of Lichen Planus and Leukoplakia with the Oral Retinoid Ro 10-9359*

A.A. Cordero, M.A.J. Allevato, C.A. Barclay, C.A. Traballi and L.B. Donatti

The usefulness of vitamin A in the treatment of skin diseases has been limited by the inconsistency of the therapeutical response and by the toxicity at pharmacological concentrations. The search of more suitable compounds has lead to the synthesis of structural analogs of retinol or retinoic acid with increased effectiveness and specificity, combined with lower levels of toxicity. Since 1977 the oral retinoic acid derivative ethyl all-trans-9-(4-methoxy-2,3,6-trimethylphenyl)-3,7-dimethyl-2,4,6,8-nonatetraenoate = Ro 10-9359, has been investigated by us in several dermatoses such as psoriasis, ichthyosis, Darier's disease, acne, keratodermias, erythrokeratodermia variabilis, pityriasis rubra pilaris, leukoplakia, lichen planus, hypertrophic naevus, monilethrix, congenital pachyonychia, basal cell naevus syndrome and lichen sclerosus et atrophicus vulvae. Based on the excellent results obtained in nearly all disorders of keratinization, the present study is focused on two dermatological conditions - lichen planus and leukoplakia - the treatment of which has been disappointing so far.

Material and Method

A total of 14 outpatients, 10 male and 4 female, with an average age of 45 years (range 18–69 years) were treated with the oral derivative of retinoic acid, Ro 10-9359. Eleven of them suffered from cutaneous lichen planus (LP) and/or LP of the oral mucosa and 3 from leukoplakia of the oral cavity. Out of the 11 patients with LP, 7 showed only a mucous lesion (5 an erosive form of LP mucosae and 2 an oral typical form).

Typical oral LP lesions were localized in the jugal mucosa. Two patients suffering from an erosive form showed lesions in the mucous membranes only, 1 in the jugal mucosa, lower lip and tongue, 1 in the jugal mucosa and tongue, and 1 in the tongue only.

The average evolution period for typical oral LP was 18 months; for the atypical disease, 16.2 months, and for cutaneous LP 25 months.

Two out of the three patients suffering from leukoplakia showed a IInd-grade lesion, localized on the tongue and the third one an erosive form on the lower lip. The evolution period of such lesions was 2, 10 and 1 years, respectively.

Ro 10-9359 was administered orally in 10-mg and 25-mg capsules. Subject to the research schedule, the initial dose was 1 mg per kg body weight a day, being reduced to 0.66 mg/kg and to 0.33 mg/kg daily during the maintenance period. Weekly clinical evaluations and monthly intratherapeutic follow-up controls to explore hepatic, hematic and renal functions were performed.

Results

Table 1 shows the results of the treatment in LP. An excellent response was obtained in 4 out

* Tigason, F. Hoffmann-La Roche & Co. Ltd., Basle, Switzerland

Table 1. Results of treatment in lichen planus

Type	Sex	Age	Site	Duration	Result
Erosive	M	65	Oral mucosa	1 y.	Excellent
n = 5	M	58	Oral mucosa	7 ms	Excellent
	F	64	Oral mucosa, tongue, lower lip	4 ys	Excellent
	M	41	Oral mucosa and lower lip	2 ms	Moderate
	M	34	Tongue	1 y.	Excellent
Typical	F	61	Oral mucosa	3 ys	Good
n = 2	M	24	Oral mucosa	1 y.	Moderate
Cutaneous	M	40	Generalized and oral mucosa	6 ms	Good
n = 4	M	19	Foot	18 ms	Good
	F	53	Generalized	6 ys	Worsening
	F	18	Generalized	6 ms	Worsening

of 5 patients suffering from an oral erosive form. In 2 patients with the typical form of the disease, results were good in 1 and moderate in the other. Two of the 4 patients with cutaneous LP showed a good response, while the lesions of the other 2 aggravated.

Four of the 5 patients with erosive oral LP being administered an initial dose of 1 mg/kg a day, experienced a complete remission of the erosion after 2 to 10 weeks' therapy. The remaining patient required a longer treatment course. Subjective symptoms (burning sensation, pain), present in all cases, improved dramatically from the first days of treatment and disappeared completely when the erosion was cured. The evolution of leukokeratosis, erosion and subjective symptoms is shown on Fig. 1.

In a female patient with an atypical (crusty and vegetating) LP on the lower lip, the involution of it enabled the identification of a lesion, the histopathological diagnosis of which was squamous cell carcinoma. The good condition of the rest of the mucosa and semimucosa achieved through treatment, allowed the surgical ablation, as well as a good postoperative evolution.

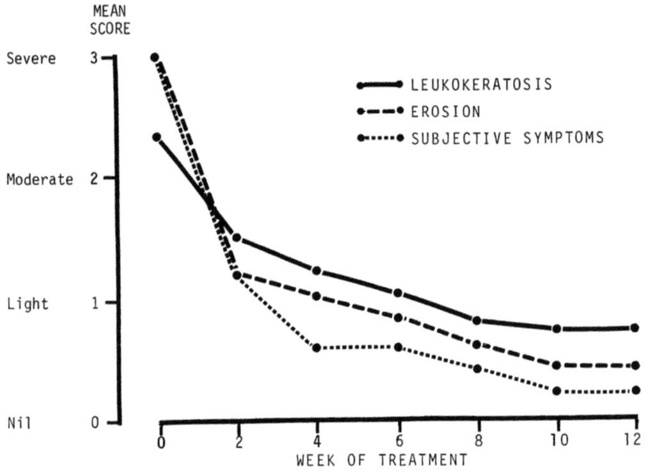

Fig. 1. Evolution of signs and symptoms in 8 patients with lichen planus of the oral mucosa

Table 2. Results of treatment in leukoplakia

Type	Nr. of cases	Sex	Age	Site	Duration	Result
Grade II	2	M	42	Tongue	2 ys	Good
		M	43	Tongue	10 ys	Good
Erosive	1	M	69	Lower lip	1 y.	Excellent

The same intial dose in one of the patients suffering from typical LP produced a total remission of the lesion at the sixth week, whilst in the other, the remission was not complete.

While the maintenance dose of 0.66 mg/kg a day was being administered, no relapse was observed, either in the erosive or in the typical form, but it was noted in one of the 2 patients with the typical oral form of the disease, when the dose was reduced to 0.33 mg/kg a day. Once treatment was discontinued, 2 of the 5 patients with erosive LP relapsed after 1 and 2 months, respectively. The patient with the erosive form and the squamous cell carcinoma did not relapse after 2 years from completion of the treatment. In 1 of the 2 patients with typical LP the lesions relapsed completely after 2 months.

Cutaneous LP responded quite differently. In 2 patients an important clinical improvement was observed after 10 weeks of treatment; in the other 2, therapy had to be discontinued due to aggravation after the third and fifth week of treatment, respectively.

The beneficial effects of the treatment were first noted on the scaling and then on the infiltration and erythema. These changes became evident between the second and the third weeks. Pruritus also responded to the treatment, but improvement of this symptom was achieved later.

Table 2 shows the results obtained in leukoplakia. A partial involution of the leukokeratotic plaques in 2 patients with a IInd-grade lesion localized on the tongue was obtained after 7 and 31 weeks of treatment, respectively. A remarkable fact was the excellent response in an erosive form localized on the lower lip. In this patient, after a 7-week therapy, a total remission of the lesion was observed. The average dose was 0.66 mg/kg a day.

Side effects appeared in 11 out of the 14 patients (Table 3). The most frequent were dryness of lips, dryness of mouth, scaling of palms and soles, rhagades, diffuse hair loss, thinning of the skin and pruritus. The intensity of these effects was directly proportional to the dosage and the time of administration of the treatment; this was clear enough with a daily dosage of 1 mg/kg and 0.66 mg/kg. Severe side effects in the skin and mucosa, as well as an aggravation of the dermatosis forced a patient suffering from cutaneous LP to discontinue treatment. The laboratory tests performed during therapy showed no abnormalities.

Table 3. Side effects

Type	Nr. of cases	%
Dryness of lips	9	64
Dryness of mouth	7	50
Scaling of palms and soles	5	36
Rhagades	2	14
Diffuse hair loss	1	7
Thinning of skin	1	7
Pruritus	1	7

Comments and Conclusions

Although the number of cases of LP and leukoplakia studied is not significant, they have enabled us to enhance our experience on these dermatoses, for which no ideal effective treatment is so far available.

The mechanism of action of vitamin A acid and its derivatives has not yet been made clear. It is known that they influence the growth and differentiation of keratinizing and non-keratinizing epithelia, and for this reason are used in those diseases showing disorders in keratinization. Therefore, a good therapeutical result in LP was to be expected, inasmuch as the disease is commonly included among the dermatoses with disorders of the keratinization. Since the first attempts made by Günther (7–10) to treat this skin condition with retinoic acid, many publications have mentioned its use, either locally or systemically. For the sake of obtaining a wider therapeutical effect together with a lower intensity of side effects, oral derivatives - aromatic and non-aromatic - have been used lately (2, 12–18).

Therapeutic results vary significantly in the different clinical forms of LP mucosae. There is an immediate response in the erosive form both in the subjective and in the objective signs. Even though the typical form improves with systemic treatment, the therapeutic response is slower and relapses are frequent when reducing the dosage or discontinuing therapy.

The topological localization of the oral LP seems to be relevant in the therapeutic result (8). We believe that the presence of aggravating factors (traumatical dental prosthesis, nicotinism, inadequate nutrition, diabetes, hypertension and others) delays therapeutic effects and accelerates relapses.

In our opinion, oral retinoids are the drugs of first choice in the treatment of the erosive form of LP due to their high effectiveness on erosion and the rapid elimination of the subjective signs which nearly always exist, and with a view to avoid a possible malignant transformation. this is not the case in the typical form of the disease, where non of the factors mentioned for the erosive condition exists. We are persuaded that in this clinical form it is more convenient to use retinoic acid topically because this one has proved effective and lacks systemic effects (5, 6, 8–10).

Not only retinoic acid but also its derivatives have been used in patients with LP. The reported results, though generally good, are rather contradictory (2–5, 7, 10, 16, 18). We could verify a good but incomplete therapeutic effect in 2 of our patients with cutaneous LP. Perhaps a combined treatment (glycocorticoids, PUVA) would be most advisable. As observed by us in psoriasis (1) the two patients whose state aggravated, initiated their treatment at the full outbreak of the disease. We think it advisable not to start treatment during the acute stage of the dermatosis or, if doing so, to begin with low doses and increase them gradually. We have observed that the drug is unable to modify the eruption and we consider that it may even aggravate it, whilst increasing inflammatory symptoms.

Particularly regarding cutaneous LP a significant number of treated patients would be necessary to achieve a clearer understanding of the therapeutical efficacy.

There are numerous and relevant reports published on leukoplakia of the oral cavity, which mention the use of retinoic acid and its derivatives topically as well as systemically. In this indication the aromatic retinoid has proved therapeutically more effective than the 13-cis-β-retinoic acid and the all-trans-retinoic acid (1–6, 11–18). Two of our patients showed a partial involution of the leukokeratotic plaques. The remaining one, suffering from an erosive form of the disease, experienced a total response. Histological and ultramicroscopical tests in a significant number of patients would be necessary in order to evaluate whether the changes produced are more relevant for the prognosis than those clinically determined.

We conclude that the aromatic derivative Ro 10-9359 has a remarkable therapeutic action in LP as well as in leukoplakia. Based on the excellent results obtained in the erosive form of LP, we feel justified to state that this retinoid derivative is the drug of choice for this condition. The same cannot be said for the other clinical forms of LP and leukoplakia, on which more experience is required to establish clearly the usefulness of this therapy.

Summary

Since 1977, 66 patients with several skin diseases have been treated in our hospital with the oral retinoid Ro 10-9359. The patient material comprised psoriasis, ichthyosis, Darier's disease, etc., but the aim of this paper is focused on the results obtained in 2 entities, the first one concerning the treatment of 11 cases of lichen planus (LP) and the other of 3 leukoplakias.

In most of the patients, treatment was started with 1 mg/kg a day. A change in dosage to 0.66 and even 0.33 mg/kg daily depended upon severe side effects and/or efficacy.

Results indicated that in the erosive form of LP mucosae the improvement achieved was much better than that obtained in the typical form of the disease, especially with regard to local pain and burning, both of which having disappeared within 1–2 days. A complete remission of the erosion was observed after 1 week of therapy.

Leukokeratosis of the typical forms of LP showed only partial response even after 2 months' treatment.

In 3 patients with leukoplakia (2 on the tongue and the other on the lower lip) good results were obtained, although a total remission of the lesion could only be achieved in the third case.

Side effects were usually moderate and did not compel discontinuation of therapy.

References

1. Cordero AA, Allevato MA, Barclay CA, Traballi CA (1978) Tratamiento oral de diversas dermatosis con el derivado aromático del ácido retinoico, Ro 10-9359. Med Cut ILA 6:243–251
2. Domínguez Soto L, Hotyo MT Retinoides en el tratamiento de diversas dermatosis. XI° Congreso Centroamericano de Dermatología, San José, Costa Rica, 24–29 de noviembre de 1978
3. Ebner H (1978) System retinoid treatment of lichen planus. Simposion of the International Society of Tropical Dermatology, Jerusalem, November 6–12
4. Ebner H (1979) Erfahrungen mit der systemischen Retinoidbehandlung (Ro 10-9359) bei Lichen ruber planus. Wien Klin Wochenschr 91:161–164
5. Ebner H, Mischer P (1972) Lokale Vitamin-A-Säure-Behandlung des Lichen ruber planus. Z Haut Geschlkr 47:773–778
6. Ebner H, Mischer P, Raff M (1973) Lokalbehandlung des Lichen ruber planus der Mundschleimhaut mit Vitamin-A-Säure. Z Hautkr 48:735–740
7. Günther S (1971) Retinoic acid in the treatment of lichen planus. Dermatologica 143:315–318
8. Günther S (1973) The therapeutic value of retinoic acid (vitamin A acid) in lichen planus of the oral mucous membrane. Dermatologica 147:130–136
9. Günther S (1973) Vitamin A acid in treatment of oral lichen planus. Arch Derm 107:277
10. Günther S (1975) Lichen ruber planus und Lichen ruber verrucosus der Haut. Behandlungsergebnisse mit Vitamin-A-Säure bei 98 Patienten. Z Hautkr 50:59–68
11. Koch HF (1978) Leukoplakia of oral mucosa: late results after treatment with derivatives of retinoic acid. Current Chemotherapy, Proceedings of the 10th International Congress of Chemotherapy, 2:1298–1299, Washington, D.C.
12. Maidhof R Tratamiento sistémico del liquen plano oral con un retinoide aromático (Ro 10-9359). (In press)
13. Orfanos CE (1978) Oral administration of retinoids. Dermatologica 157 (Suppl 1):2–4
14. Samman P (1956) A note on the natural history of lichen planus. Br J Dermatol 68:175–181

15. Scheiber W, Plewig G (1978) Behandlung des Lichen ruber mucosae mit Vitamin-A-Säure-Derivaten. Dermatologica 157 (Suppl 1):171–180
16. Schuppli R (1978) The efficacy of a new retinoid (Ro 10-9359) in Lichen planus. Dermatologica 157 (Suppl 1):60–63
17. Shklar G (1968) Erosive and bullous oral lesions of lichen planus. Arch Dermatol 97:411–416
18. Viglioglia PA, Traballi CA (1979) Retinoidi per via orale e dermatopatie non psoriatiche. Chron Derm, Anno X, N° 1, 5–11

C.E. Orfanos et al. (eds.)
Retinoids

Comparative Analysis of Two Retinoids in the Treatment of Disorders of Keratinization

G.L. Peck, E.G. Gross and D. Butkus

During the past decade synthetic derivatives of vitamin A have been introduced into dermatology for study of their therapeutic potential in cutaneous disorders of keratinization, cystic acne, and basal cell carcinoma. Initial emphasis has been placed on the treatment of psoriasis with an aromatic retinoid, the trimethylmethoxyphenyl derivative of ethyl retinoate (Ro 10-9359), either alone or in combination with other active agents (2, 4, 5, 12). In 1976, 13-cis-retinoic acid, the first synthetic retinoid available for clinical testing in the United States, was found to be highly effective in the treatment of cystic acne, Darier's disease, lamellar ichthyosis, chronic pityriasis rubra pilaris (PRP) and, to a lesser extent, psoriasis (7–9). It also had some therapeutic effects in basal cell carcinoma (10, 11). In 1978, Ro 10-9359 became available for testing in the United States and patients who initially were treated with oral 13-cis retinoic acid were subsequently treated with the aromatic retinoid. In this report a retrospective comparative analysis of therapeutic and toxic effects of these two retinoids is made using data from 26 patients.

Materials and Methods

Drugs

13-cis-retinoic acid (Ro 4-3780, isotretinoin) was administered in 10-, 20-, and 40-mg capsules. Ro 10-9359 (etretinate) was administered in 10-, 25-, and 50-mg capsules in a subsequent protocol. Both drugs were obtained from Hoffmann-La Roche Inc., Nutley, N.J. (USA).

Patients

Twenty-six adult patients with chronic cutaneous disorders of keratinization were included in these studies. The diagnoses were based on typical clinical histories, physical examinations, and biopsies of diseased skin.

Concerning Darier's disease, patients 4 and 6 (Table 1) has intense inflammation with erythema and widespread infection, while the other patients had the more typical involvement with brown, hyperkeratotic papules and limited areas of infection.

Patient 9 (Table 1) had psoriatic erythroderma and was photosensitive prior to therapy. Liver biopsy prior to retinoid therapy but after 16 years of methotrexate therapy revealed cirrhosis.

All other psoriatic patients had chronic plaques. The 3 patients with lamellar ichthyosis had typical generalized involvement with thick, brown, centrally adherent, polygonal scales. All had marked hair thinning prior to therapy. The two patients with chronic PRP were females who have had their disease for 7 and 8 years beginning at ages 14 and 17. Clinically, they had myriads of follicular papules. They, therefore, differ from the typical self-limited PRP which is more common in middle-age and in our experience has comparatively few follicular papules.

Table 1. Maximum therapeutic response

Disease	13-cis-retinoic acid	Ro 10-9359
1. Darier's disease	3+	4+
2. Darier's disease	4+	5+
3. Darier's disease	2+	3+
4. Darier's disease	3+	3+
5. Darier's disease	3+	4+
6. Darier's disease	3+	3+
7. Darier's disease	4+	5+
8. Psoriasis	3+	5+
9. Psoriasis	1+	3+
10. Psoriasis	3+	-2 (a)
11. Psoriasis	0	1+
12. Psoriasis	0	3+
13. Lamellar Ichthyosis	4+	4+
14. Lamellar Ichthyosis	3+	4+
15. Lamellar Ichthyosis	3+	4+
16. EHK (b)	1+	3+
17. EHK (b)	2+	3+
18. Chronic PRP (c)	4+	4+
19. Chronic PRP (c)	3+	4+
20. NBCIE (d)	4+	5+
21. Variant form-NBCIE	1+	2+
22. Keratoses, palms and soles	2+	2+
23. Hailey-Hailey disease	-2	-2
24. KPP (e)	1+	3+
25. Pachyonychia congenita	1+	1+
26. Ichthyosis vulgaris	2+	5+

a: patient cleared within 8 weeks of discontinuing therapy (5+)
b: Epidermolytic hyperkeratosis (bullous congenital ichthyosiform erythroderma)
c: Pityriasis rubra pilaris
d: Non-bullous congenital ichthyosiform erythroderma
e: Keratoderma palmo-plantaris
5+: totally clear, 4+: almost clear, 3+: marked improvement, 2+: definite improvement, 1+: slight improvement, 0: no improvement
-1: slight worsening, -2: definite worsening

Patient 20 (Table 1) was diagnosed as non-bullous congenital ichthyosiform erythoderma (NB-CIE) and is distinguished from lamellar ichthyosis by: 1) being primarily an erythroderma, 2) having branny, white, loosely adherent scale instead of the thick lamellar scales and 3) having marked parakeratosis histologically.

Patient 21 is considered a variant form of NBCIE in that her erythroderma was more intense clinically, her skin biopsy was more psoriasiform, and prior to puberty she developed numerous small white islands within the erythroderma. She and 2 similar patients will be described in detail elsewhere.

Patient 22 had acquired palmar and plantar keratoses of unknown etiology. Chronic arsenicism was suspected but could not be proved by history or by blood, hair and skin analysis for arsenic.

Patient 24 had the autosomal dominant, Unna-Thost type of keratoderma palmaris et plantaris. All patients had either partial or no beneficial therapeutic response to prior therapy including in many cases high-dose oral vitamin A and chemotherapeutic agents.

Dosage

Treatment with 13-cis-retinoic acid was usually begun at 1 mg drug/kg bodyweight/day and increased gradually to maximum therapeutic effect or to dose-limiting toxicity and then lowered to a maintenance dose. The average maximum dosage administered in this study was 3.1 mg/kg/day or 213 mg/-day. Similarly, treatment with Ro 10-9359 was initially begun at 1 mg/kg/day. However, particularly in psoriasis, it was subsequently found that lower initial dose schedules were better tolerated and they are now being used. The average maximum dosage of Ro 10-9359 administered was 1.2 mg/kg/day or 87 mg/day. The maintenance doses, however, were never higher than 1 mg/kg/day and were usually between 0.5 and 1 mg/kg/day.

Initially, treatment was given for 4-month periods followed by 2-month treatment-free intervals which were designed into the protocol in order to minimize the possibility of chronic toxicity. Now treatment is given for 6-month periods with intervening 2- to 4-week treatment-free intervals as no chronic toxicity has been observed.

No other active therapeutic agents were used during the periods of treatment with the retinoids. Bland emollients were permitted for relief of the drying and chapping of skin and mucous membranes seen as side effects of the retinoids. Hydroxyzine hydrochloride was given for control of pruritus. Oral antibiotics were used in the two patients with severely infected Darier's disease. Fertile women were required to use effective birth control measures in order to participate in these studies.

Data Collection

Hematologic, hepatic and renal laboratory tests were monitored at baseline and at monthly intervals during and after treatment. These procedures included a complete blood count, platelet count, erythrocyte sedimentation rate, prothrombin time, partial thromboplastin time, serum aspartate and alanine aminotransferases (SGOT, SGPT), alkaline phosphatase, lactic dehydrogenase, total bilirubin, total protein, albumin, glucose, uric acid, electrolytes, blood urea nitrogen, creatinine, calcium, phosphorus, carotene and vitamin A, and urinalysis. Blood for assay of thyrotropin, thyroxine, triiodothyronine, immunoglobulins, triglycerides, and cholesterol was obtained later in the study.

Disease status was scored at each visit on a scale of −2 (definite worsening) to +5 (totally clear) (See Table 1).

Results

Clinical Results

Ro 10-9359 was more effective than 13-cis-retinoic acid in 18 patients; seven patients responded equally and one patient responded better to 13-cis-retinoic acid. Excellent responses were seen with both retinoids in Darier's disease, lamellar ichthyosis, chronic PRP, and in non-bullous congenital ichthyosiform erythroderma (Table 1). Ro 10-9359 was only slightly better than 13-cis-retinoic acid in the treatment of these conditions.

Two patients with psoriasis also had good responses to 13-cis-retinoic acid, whereas the remainder of patients had fair, minimal, or no response to this retinoid. Ro 10-9359 was clearly superior to 13-cis-retinoic acid in the treatment of psoriasis, epidermolytic hyperkeratosis (bullous congenital ichthyosiform erythroderma), keratoderma palmo-plantaris, and ichthyosis vulgaris.

Concerning psoriasis, the superiority of Ro 10-9359 was especially evident in patient 9 with psoriatic erythroderma. Patient 10, however, had a superior response to 13-cis-retinoic acid, if one compares responses on the date at which therapy with each retinoid was discontinued. In his case, the psoriasis had worsened at the time of discontinuing the aromatic retinoid. This may have been due to having increased his dose to 1.5 mg/kg/day, although the psoriasis had already begun to worsen at lower dosages (0.4 mg/kg/day). However, the patient rather suddenly and dramatically cleared completely (5+) within 8 weeks of stopping therapy. During that 8-week period only topical emollients and no active therapy was used. No other patient had a superior therapeutic response to 13-cis-retinoic acid, and furthermore it is possible that the delayed response of patient 10 was a beneficial response to Ro 10-9359.

Patients 11 and 12 also had temporary flares of their psoriasis shortly after beginning treatment with the aromatic retinoid, while patients 8 and 9 did not. This initial temporary worsening of psoriasis in these 3 patients was a consistent finding with each new course of therapy. The severity of the flare seemed to be diminished and of shorter duration if the initial dose was low. We are currently using doses as low as 10 mg/day when initiating therapy in psoriatic patients who experience these initial flares. Once this initial reaction has subsided, the dosage is then increased to more therapeutic levels. The patient with Hailey-Hailey disease worsened with both retinoids and could only tolerate 10 days of treatment with either drug.

The intervals between stopping treatment with 13-cis-retinoic acid and beginning treatment with Ro 10-9359 varied between one month and 21 months with an average time of 8 months. Consequently, it is unlikely that the therapeutic superiority of the aromatic retinoid was due to any continuing partial therapeutic response to 13-cis-retinoic acid. Similarly, it is unlikely that the side effects of Ro 10-9359 were affected by the patients having been pretreated 8 months previously with 13-cis-retinoic acid.

Side Effects

Clinical. Toxicities varied considerably between the two retinoids. The characteristic toxicities that occurred either more frequently or more severely with 13-cis-retinoic acid were those resulting from a drying and chapping of skin and mucous membranes and included cheilitis, conjunctivitis, facial dermatitis, dryness of the nasal mucosa, minor nosebleeds, xerosis with itching, and inflammation of the urethral meatus. The side effects seen more frequently with Ro 10-9359 (Table 2) were palmo-plantar desquamation, hair loss, dry

Table 2. Toxicity

Side effect	13-cis-retinoic acid	Ro 10–9359
1. Cheilitis	26	26
2. Conjunctivitis	20	19
3. Facial dermatitis	16	11
4. Dry nasal mucosa	13	18
5. Minor nosebleeds	9	12
6. Xerosis with itching	15	12
7. Stratum corneum fragility	11	16
8. Palmo-plantar peeling	0	16
9. Hair loss	4	10
10. Dry mouth with thirst	3	7
11. Paronychia	0	6
12. Arthralgias	3	5
13. Stickiness of skin	2	5
14. Chills	0	5
15. Inflamed urethral meatus	4	2
16. Itching	3	3
17. Nail abnormalities	0	5
18. Gingivitis	0	1
19. Fatigue	0	1
20. Transient elevations: SGOT	3	5
21. Transient elevations: SGPT	3	5
22. Transient elevations: LDH	0	1
23. Triglyceride elevations	1	2

mouth with thirst, stratum corneum fragility, chills, paronychia, and nail abnormalities. Arthralgias were seen in both retinoids in almost equal incidence. The three patients who developed arthralgias on 13-cis-retinoic acid also developed arthralgias with the aromatic retinoid. Two of the four men who developed inflammation of the urethral meatus on 13-cis-retinoic acid also developed this side effect with Ro 10-9359.

The 5 patients who complained of a sticky feeling of their skin particularly when the skin was wet all also noted chills while on the aromatic retinoid. Subjective complaints during therapy with both retinoids were thought not to be drug-related and included: 1) headache, during the first 2 weeks of therapy in 2 patients, 2) appetite changes (either increased or decreased) in 5 patients. Similarly sunburn in 1 patient was not considered drug-related.

Two patients with lamellar ichthyosis who had hair loss prior to treatment noted that their hair seemed thicker during therapy. One patient with psoriasis discontinued therapy with Ro 10-9359 because of fatigue and arthralgias, and chose to resume 13-cis-retinoic acid. No other patient is currently receiving 13-cis-retinoic acid.

In spite of the above toxicities, all 12 patients with Darier's disease, lamellar ichthyosis, and chronic PRP have chosen to continue therapy with the aromatic retinoid, while 8 other patients have ceased participation either due to inadequate therapeutic response or to the toxicities.

The 4 patients who had had an inadequate therapeutic response had psoriasis, pachyonychia congenita, Hailey-Hailey disease, or the variant form of NBCIE. The 4 patients who discontinued Ro 10-9359 because of toxicity did so because of hair loss in 3 cases and excessive palmar desquamation in one case.

Laboratory. Abnormal laboratory tests were limited to 3 elevations each of SGOT and SGPT and one elevation of serum triglycerides due to 13-cis-retinoic acid. Ro 10-9359 led to 5 elevations of SGOT and SGPT, one elevation of lactic dehydrogenase, and 2 elevations of serum triglycerides, primarily VLDL. The transaminase elevations were transient, low-grade, then returned to normal and remained normal without discontinuing therapy. These elevations were not associated with signs or symptoms of acute hepatitis and are similar to those reported with other drugs (13). Three patients with elevated transaminases had abnormal tests prior to therapy; these returned to normal prior to the elevations observed during therapy. Therefore, it is unclear in these 3 patients whether the elevations observed during therapy were due entirely to the retinoids. The patient with methotrexate-induced cirrhosis, diagnosed by liver biopsy prior to therapy, did not develop further hepatotoxicity, as measured by liver function tests, during therapy with the retinoids. The observed incidence of serum triglyceride elevations due to 13-cis-retinoic acid is certainly less than the true incidence, since we did not begin analyzing fasting sera until June, 1979. By that time most patients had been switched to the aromatic retinoid. Of the 3 patients demonstrating elevated triglycerides 2 were obese female psoriatics, one of whom had a hyperlipidemia (Type IIb) diagnosed prior to therapy. The third patient had difficulty providing fasting specimens particularly due to his ethanol intake the night prior to the clinic visits. Therefore, analysis of a drug effect in this patient is difficult. These mild to moderate elevations in triglycerides were induced by 0.7 mg/kg/day 13-cis-retinoic acid and by 0.6 and 1.0 mg/kg/day Ro 10-9359 and were controllable by manipulations of diet, ethanol intake, exercise, and by adjusting the dosage of the retinoid.

Discussion

These data indicate that Ro 10-9359 is more effective than 13-cis-retinoic acid in the treatment of certain cutaneous disorders of keratinization. However, certain diseases such as Darier's disease, chronic PRP, lamellar ichthyosis, and NBCIE respond almost equally well to both retinoids. In these diseases the decision to use either 13-cis-retinoic acid or Ro 10-9359, therefore, may depend more on the observed toxicities characteristic of each retinoid and an individual patient's ability to tolerate these toxicities. For instance, a patient may be more distressed by hair loss and palmo-plantar desquamation as seen with Ro 10-9359 than with the more intense cheilitis and facial dermatitis as seen with 13-cis-retinoic acid. In our experience, however, other diseases such as psoriasis, epidermolytic hyperkeratosis, ichthyosis vulgaris, and keratoderma palmo-plantaris, respond better to Ro 10-9359. Although other treatment modalities are available for psoriasis, some patients with severe Darier's disease and epidermolytic hyperkeratosis have become dependent solely on the synthetic retinoids for a more normal life-style. Prior reports describing combination therapy of psoriasis with Ro 10-9359 and other active agents are encouraging in that greater therapeutic efficacy and decreased toxicity were noted. Combination therapy of other disorders of keratinization should similarly be attempted not only with Ro 10-9359 but also with 13-cis-retinoic acid.

Concerning toxicity, there are differences between the results observed with 13-cis-retinoic acid and those of Ro 10-9359 that may be based either on their intrinsic structural differences or on likely differences in their metabolic disposition. This indicates that each new synthetic retinoid should be considered a unique drug based on the observed therapeutic and toxicologic differences already seen between the first two agents tested.

The acute toxicities observed to date with these two retinoids are well tolerated by the patients, are not life-threatening, are dose-dependent in incidence and severity, are treatable with bland therapies, and are reversible on discontinuation of treatment with the retinoids. No chronic toxicities have been observed in any of these 26 patients after more than four years of therapy with the retinoids.

Aside from the transient elevations in liver function tests the two systemic toxicities of the retinoids are arthralgias and hypertriglyceridemia. Arthralgias have been seen in only a minority of patients, none of whom have shown roentgenographic evidence of arthritis. Furthermore, all arthralgias have disappeared after discontinuation of therapy. The question remains, however, whether those patients requiring chronic therapy will experience bony changes after five to ten year's or more exposure to retinoids.

The observed elevations of plasma triglyceride and VLDL levels have been dose-dependent and reversible on discontinuation of therapy. In rats it has recently been found that tretinoin produces an eightfold greater increase in plasma triglyceride levels than does 13-cis-retinoic acid (3). In man, dosages of 13-cis-retinoic acid above 1 mg/kg/day appear to be needed to elevate triglyceride levels markedly beyond the normal range except for very susceptible patients (1). The mild to moderate deviations of triglycerides seen with Ro 10-9359 in this study occurred at dosages of 0.6 to 1.0 mg/kg/day. Certainly, if patients with pretreatment elevations in the level of plasma triglycerides are to be treated with retinoids, their condition must be monitored very closely. The long-term importance of this observation and the effect of dietary management on plasma triglyceride levels during therapy with retinoids remains to be determined.

One potential toxic effect shared by both retinoids is teratogenicity. Specifically, Ro 10-9359 is teratogenic in both rats and rabbits at 2 mg/kg/day; 13-cis-retinoic acid, on the other hand, is not teratogenic in rabbits at doses of 3 mg/kg/day or in rats at 50 mg/kg/day. Ro 10-

9359, furthermore, is excreted much more slowly than 13-cis-retinoic acid, as substantial blood levels of Ro 10-9359 in psoriatic patients have been observed up to 140 days after cessation of therapy (6). Therefore, the duration of the potential of Ro 10-9359 to induce teratogenic effects is still unknown. Consequently, until more information becomes available, females of child-bearing potential are excluded from new protocols using Ro 10-9359 in the United States.

The mechanism of action of the retinoids in the disorders of keratinization is unclear. Any theory will have to take into consideration the apparent drug specificity. This variability of response, such as that observed between Darier's disease and Hailey-Haily disease, indicates that the mechanism of action is more complex than a simple keratolytic effect.

The variation in the therapeutic spectrum between the two retinoids merits continuing investigation, which should help in defining the further development of the retinoids. For instance retinoids with a higher therapeutic index and a decreased potential for teratogenicity would be highly desirable.

Already, in many diseases, the retinoids are more effective and less toxic than alternative therapies. Accordingly, ultimate introduction of these compounds into the dermatologic formulary will probably depend far more on continuing freedom from chronic toxicity than on further proof of therapeutic efficacy or acceptability of acute toxicities.

Summary

Twenty-six adult patients with cutaneous disorders of keratinization were treated initially with oral 13-cis-retinoic acid and subsequently with the aromatic retinoid Ro 10-9359. Diseases included Darier's disease (7 patients), psoriasis (5), lamellar ichthyosis (3), epidermolytic hyperkeratosis (2), chronic pityriasis rubra pilaris (2), and 7 other disorders (1 patient each). The average maximum dosage of 13-cis-retinoic acid was 3.1 mg/kg/day and of Ro 10-9359 was 1.2 mg/kg/day.

Results indicated that Ro 10-9359 was more effective than 13-cis-retinoic acid in 18 patients; 7 patients responded equally, and one patient responded better to 13-cis-retinoic acid. A better response to Ro 10-9359 was especially apparent in patients with epidermolytic hyperkeratosis, psoriatic erythroderma, ichthyosis vulgaris, and keratoderma palmo-plantaris. However, the aromatic retinoid was only slightly more effective than 13-cis-retinoic acid in the treatment of Darier's disease, lamellar ichthyosis, chronic pityriasis rubra pilaris, and non-bullous congenital ichthyosiform erythroderma.

Toxicities vary considerably between the two retinoids. The characteristic clinical toxicities of 13-cis-retinoic acid were those resulting from a drying effect on skin and mucous membranes. On the other hand, among the side effects more commonly seen with the aromatic retinoid were palmo-plantar desquamation, hair loss, dry mouth with thirst, stratum corneum fragility, paronychia, and nail abnormalities. Arthralgias were seen with both retinoids in almost equal incidence. These differences between 13-cis-retinoic acid and Ro 10-9359 may influence drug selection, particularly for patients with Darier's disease, lamellar ichthyosis, chronic pityriasis rubra pilaris, and non-bullous congenital ichthyosiform erythroderma. Other factors, such as differences in the ability of the two retinoids to induce teratogenic effects, may also affect drug selection.

References

1. Dicken CH, Connolly SM (1980) Eruptive xanthomas associated with isotretinoin (13-cis-Retinoic Acid). Arch Dermatol 116:951–952
2. Fritsch PO, Honigsmann H, Jaschke E, Wolff K (1978) Augmentation of oral methoxsalen-photochemotherapy with an oral retinoic acid derivative. J Invest Dermatol 70:178–182
3. Gerber LE, Erdman JW Jr (1979) Hypertriglyceridemia in rats administered all-trans or 13-cis retinoic acid. Fed Proc 38:761
4. Goerz G, Orfanos CE (1978) Systemic treatment of psoriasis with a new aromatic retinoid. Dermatologica 157 (Suppl 1):38–44
5. Orfanos CE, Runne U (1976) Systemic use of a new retinoid with and without local dithranol treatment in generalized psoriasis. Br J Dermatol 95:101–103
6. Pravicini U, Stockel K, MacNamara PJ, Hanni R, Busslinger A (1981) On metabolism and pharmacokinetics of an aromatic retinoid. Ann NY Acad Sci 359:54–67. In: DeLuca LM, Shapiro SS (eds) Modulation of Cellular Interactions by Vitamin A and Derivatives (Retinoids). NY Acad Sci, New York
7. Peck GL, Yoder FW (1976) Treatment of lamellar ichthyosis and other keratinising dermatoses with an oral synthetic retinoid. Lancet 2:1172–1174
8. Peck GL, Yoder FW (1978) Treatment of disorders of keratinization with an oral stereoisomer of retinoic acid. In: Marks R, Dykes PJ (eds) The Ichthyoses. MTP Press Ltd, Lancaster, pp 193–201
9. Peck GL, Olsen TG, Yoder FW, Strauss JS, Downing DT, Pandya M, Butkus D, Arnaud-Battandier J (1979) Prolonged remissions of cystic and conglobate acne with 13-cis-retinoic acid. N Engl J Med 300:329–333
10. Peck GL, Yoder FW, Olsen TG, Pandya MD, Butkus D (1978) Treatment of Darier's disease, lamellar ichthyosis, pityriasis rubra pilaris, cystic acne, and basal cell carcinoma with oral 13-cis retinoic acid. Dermatologica 157 (Suppl 1):11–12
11. Peck GL, Olsen TG, Butkus D, Pandya M, Arnaud-Battandier J, Yoder F, Levis WR (1979) Treatment of basal cell carcinomas with 13-cis retinoic acid. Proc Am Assoc Cancer Res 20:56
12. Van der Rhee HJ, Tijssen JGP, Herrmann WA, Waterman AH, Polano MK (1980) Combined treatment of psoriasis with a new aromatic retinoid (Tigason) in low dosage orally and triamcinolone acetonide cream topically: a double-blind trial. Br J Dermatol 102:203–212
13. Zimmerman HJ (1978) Hepatoxicity. The Adverse Effects of Drugs and Other Chemicals on the Liver. Appleton-Century-Crofts, New York City

C.E. Orfanos et al. (eds.)
Retinoids

Long-Term Follow-up of 30 Children Under Oral Retinoid Ro 10-9359

L. Tamayo and R. Ruíz-Maldonado

Remarkable therapeutic results have been reported during the last decade, with the use of oral synthetic retinoids for the treatment of keratinization disorders (1, 2).

In our opinion, oral retinoids are at present the most effective tool for the control of severe congenital keratinization disorders, viz. lamellar ichthyosis (LI) and epidermolytic hyperkeratosis (EH). Oral retinoids suppress, but do not revert the keratinization defect, therefore they should be given on a long-term basis. Prescription will depend not only on their efficacy, which has already been proven, but on their toxicity after chronic administration. Thus it is mandatory to have an adequate knowledge of their long-term toxicity, particularly in infants and children.

We have previously reported the use of the aromatic oral retinoid Ro 10-9359 in 14 children with severe ichthyotic disorders (3). The results obtained were excellent in 8 children with LI and in 5 with symmetrical progressive erythrokeratodermia (SPE) and mild in one case of EH.

At present, we have 30 children under therapeutic control. They all have shown marked improvement of their skin condition, good tolerance and mild and reversible side effects.

Treatment for those pediatric patients was only initiated after informed witness consent was obtained from the next of kin.

The distribution of the patients according to sex was: 16 female and 14 male. Their age ranged from 7 months up to 15 years, with a mean of 7 years.

The distribution of the various inherited ichthyotic disorders treated, and the number of cases are shown in Table 1.

The retinoid Ro 10-9359 was given orally in a daily dose of 1 to 2 mg/kg/body-weight. When significant improvement or total remission was obtained, the daily dose was decreased and the patients main-

Table 1. Congenital ichthyotic conditions in children treated with Ro 10–9359

Conditions under treatment	Number of patients
Lamellar ichthyosis	16
Epidermolytic hyperkeratosis	5
Symmetrical progressive erythrokeratodermia	5
Palmo-plantar keratoderma	2
Darier's disease	1
Pityriasis rubra pilaris	1
Total	30

Table 2. Time of treatment with Ro 10–9359

Months	Number of patients
1 to 12 months	20
more than 12 months	5
more than 24 months	4
more than 36 months	1

tained under the minimal required dose to remain free of lesions. The minimal required dose for children with LI and for children with EH was of 2 mg/kg/day. Other conditions required 1 mg or less than 1 mg/kg/day.

Ninety to 100% improvement was obtained in LI, SPE, Darier's disease, PRP and palmoplantar keratoderma. This result was considered excellent. In EH a remission of 70 to 80% was obtained, that we considered good.

Time of treatment for this group of patients is shown in Table 2.

Ten out of a total number of 30 patients have been under treatment from 12 to 42 months.

The long-term side effects of the retinoid can be better evaluated in the group of 7 children with LI continuously receiving 2 mg/kg/day for 16 to 42 months (Table 3).

While under treatment, all the seven children have been free of lesions, such as to lead an almost normal life.

Adverse effects related to retinoids such as: cheilitis, mucosal dryness and pruritus were present in all patients during the first months of treatment. They represented a minor inconvenience and tended to disappear spontaneously during the first year of treatment.

Patients 4 and 7 presented two and three episodes, respectively, of nasal bleeding during the 4th and 9th months of treatment. Laboratory tests of these bleedings were found within normal limits.

Case 4, who since the age of 4 years presented esophagostenosis of unknown etiology requiring esophagus dilatations at irregular intervals, remained asymptomatic, during his first year of retinoid treatment; however, the stenosis persisted and he had to be operated on.

Three children suffered from intercurrent conditions, their course was uneventful and the recovery was normal (Table 4).

Control laboratory tests comprised: blood cytology, sedimentation rate, urinalysis, serum transaminases, alkaline phosphatase, calcium, phosphorus and magnesium. They

Table 3. Sex and age of 7 children continously treated with Ro 10–9359

Case No.	Sex	Age of onset	Time of treatment
1	F	7 months	16 months
2	F	9 months	18 months
3	F	3 years	42 months
4	M	8 years	35 months
5	F	8 years	24 months
6	M	9 years	24 months
7	M	11 years	36 months

Table 4. Three cases with complications

Complications	Case No.	Time on retinoid	Course
Chicken-pox	6	3 weeks	uneventful
Bone fracture	3	28 months	uneventful
Bone fracture	3	34 months	uneventful
Tympanotomy	3	39 months	uneventful
Major surgery	4	28 months	uneventful

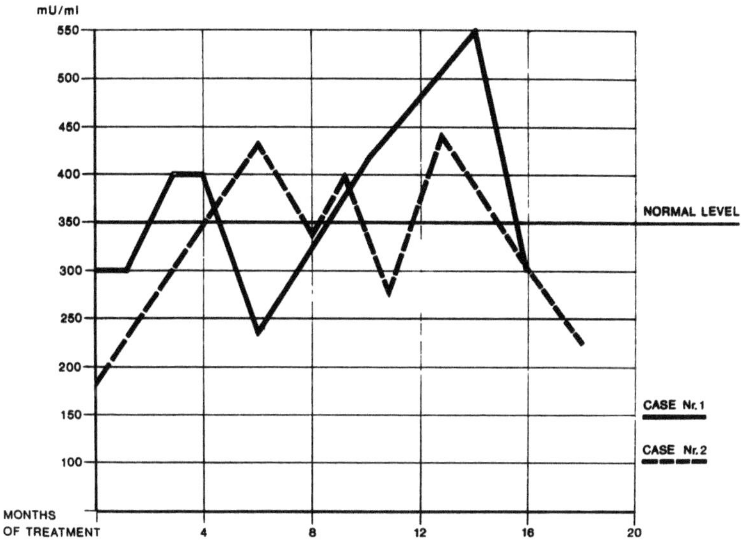

Fig. 1. Serum levels of alkaline phosphatase in cases No 1 and 2

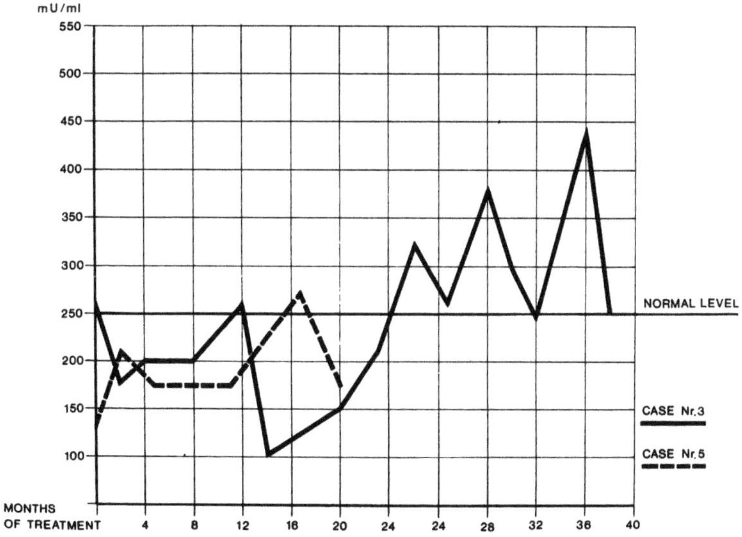

Fig. 2. Serum levels of alkaline phosphatase in cases No 3 and 5

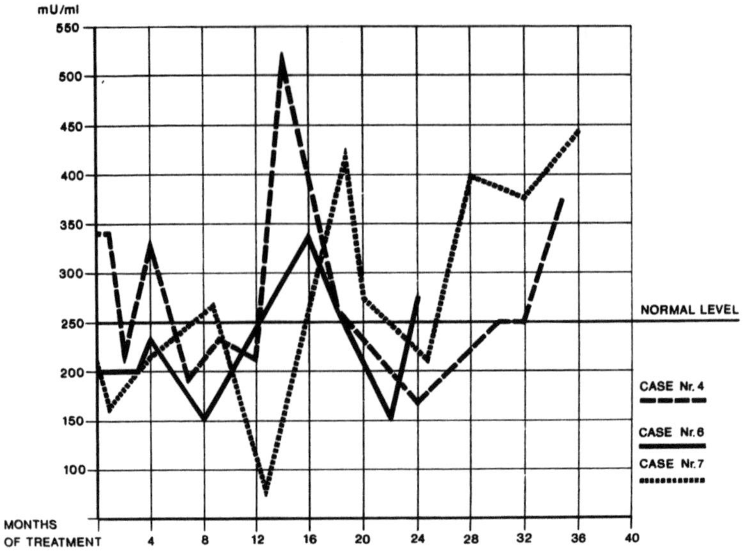

Fig. 3. Serum levels of alkaline phosphatase in cases No 4, 6 and 7

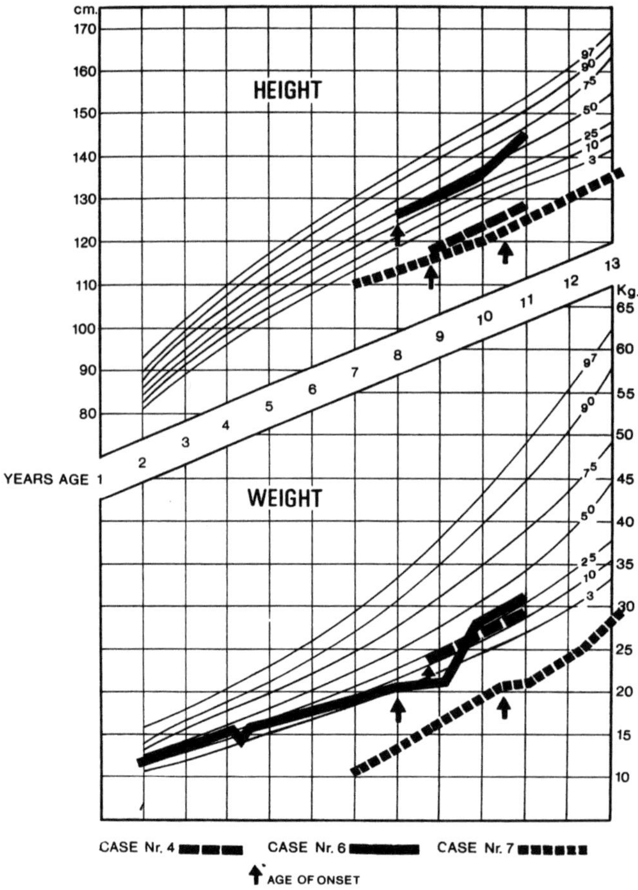

Fig. 4. Physical development of 3 male children (aged 2–13 years) with lamellar ichthyosis

were performed every two weeks during the first month, every month during the first year, and every two or three months thereafter.

In all the cases the laboratory tests remained without significant changes. Occasional slight elevations of either pyruvic or oxalacetic serum transaminases, and exceptionally of both have been observed.

In the 7 patients the serum levels of alkaline phosphatase showed irregular elevations that returned to normal in spite of continued administration of the drug. After the first year of treatment, elevations of alkaline phosphatase were more important and more frequently observed (Figs. 1, 2 and 3). There was no association whats ever with the serum transaminases elevations.

An X-ray study of long bones was done yearly. It has been normal in all children, except in case 3 that will be considered below.

Of particular interest for us has been the long term follow-up of these children with regard to their physical growth and development.

Figures 4, 5 and 6 show the physical growth and development of the patients. The height and weight of the three male patients (cases 4, 6 and 7) have been maintained within the same percentile. Cases 6 and 7 remained as before treatment, under percentile 3.

Two girls (cases 2 and 5) have been within normal limits of weight and height (Figs. 5–6).

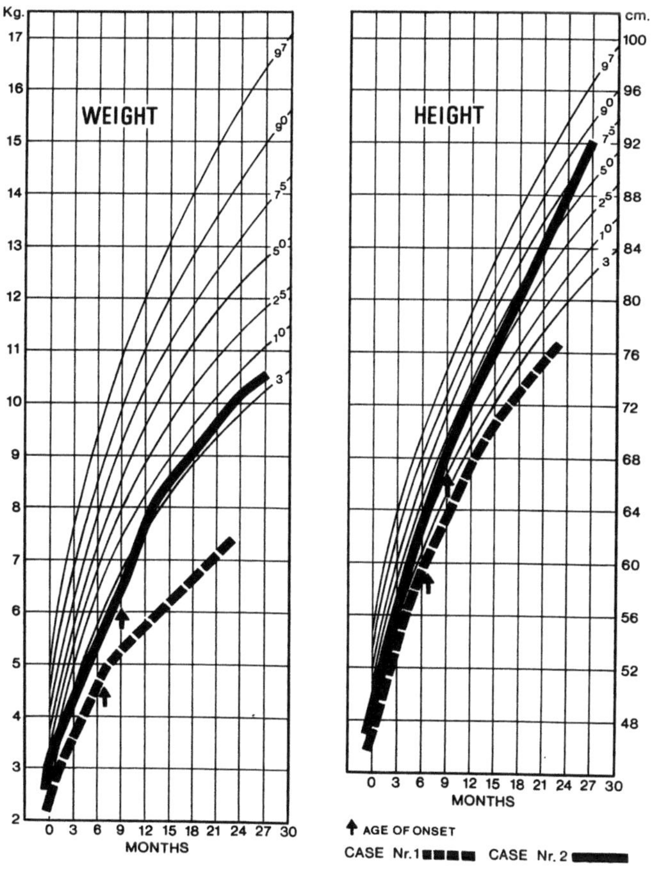

Fig. 5. Physical development of 2 female children (from birth up to 30 months) with lamellar ichthyosis

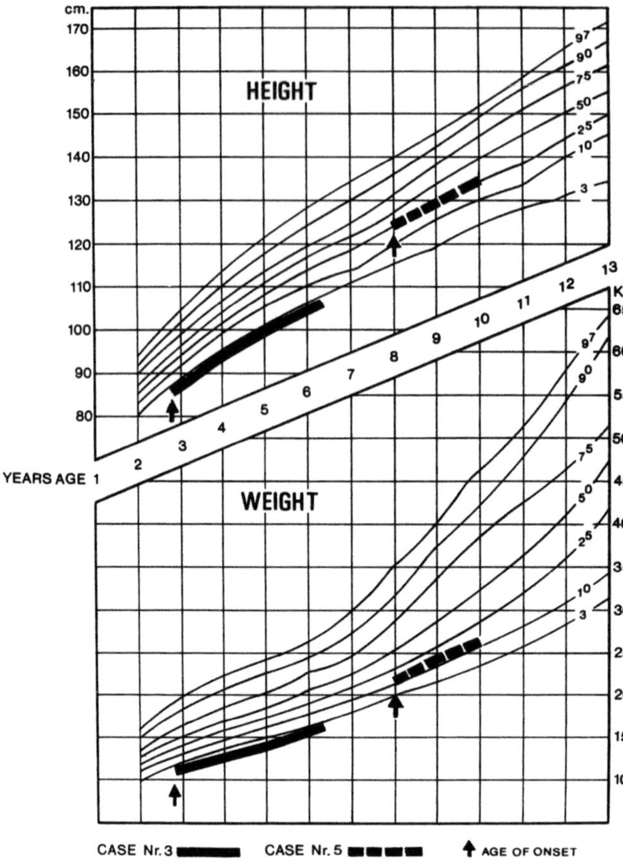

Fig. 6. Physical development of 3 female children (aged 2 to 13 years) with lamellar ichthyosis

Two female patients (cases 1 and 3) deserve special consideration. Both were under percentile 3 before starting the oral retinoid and have remained so, after 16 and 42 months of treatment, respectively (Figs. 5–6).

Case 1, our youngest patient, started treatment at 7 months of age. At birth her weight was 2 kg and her height 44 cm. Her skeletal age corresponds to her chronological age. Her mother is of low height and weight, while data of her father are not available. This patient probably presents familiar short stature. She is slightly mentally retarded.

Case 3 started treatment when 2 years 10 months old. She has been under treatment for $3^1/_2$ years, and she is our patient with the longest time of treatment. She presented a traumatic fracture of the right forearm during the 28th month of treatment and a traumatic fracture of the right clavicle during the 34th month of treatment. Both consolidated in a normal time with a hyperplastic callus. Radiologically her long bones are abnormally slender but without other alterations. As the first X-ray study was done after a year of treatment, the role of the retinoid in this alteration remains unclear. During the 39th month of treatment and under general anesthesia a tympanotomy to remove a polyp was done without any complication.

In order to find an explanation to the irregular high levels of serum alkaline phosphatase, we decided to evaluate the bone condition of 3 selected patients through a

Table 5. Isoenzymes of alkaline phosphatase in 3 selected patients

	Hepatic	Intestinal	Fractions Osseous	Total*
Case 1	41	0	0	41
Case 3	69	0	0	69
Case 7	32	0	0	32

*Normal 38 to 138 mU/ml

bone biopsy of the iliac crest: Case 1, being our youngest patient under treatment and her physical and mental development having remained subnormal; case 3, being the patient with the longest time under treatment and presenting low height, slender bones and history of two traumatic fractures; and case 7, being our oldest patients with 36 months under treatment. - Simultaneously with the bone biopsy we determined the serum isoenzymes of alkaline phosphatase (Table 5).

Light microscopy showed a normal osteoblastic and osteoclastic structure in all three patients. The hepatic intestinal, and osseous fractions, as well as the total amount of alkaline phosphatase were normal. The only detectable fractions was of hepatic origin.

In summary, our results show the therapeutic efficacy and good tolerance of the oral synthetic retinoid Ro 10-9359 in children with severe keratinization disorders.

In our children the long-term administration (up to 42 months) of Ro 10-9359 seems not to interfere with their growth and development. The low height and weight that some children present is not below the ones found before treatment. We feel that the lack of physical and psychological stimulation plays an important role in the deficient development of those patients. While under retinoid, intercurrent conditions and surgical treatment in our patients went on a normal course.

The increased levels of serum alkaline phosphatase are probably not related to osseous pathology since the histological bone structure in three representative patients was normal.

The hepatic tests performed have failed to detect any hepatic alteration.

Up to now, we do not have an adequate explanation for the alkaline phosphatase elevations in our patients.

We think that a larger number of children and a longer follow-up are required to draw definitive conclusions with regard to the influence of the oral retinoids on the growth and development of human beings.

Summary

The oral retinoid Ro 10-9359 (Ethyl-all-trans 9, 3, 7-dimethyl-2, 4, 6, 8-nonatetraenoate) was given to 30 children with diagnosis of lamellar ichthyosis, epidermolytic hyperkeratosis, symmetrical progressive keratodermia, palmo-plantar hyperkeratosis, ichthyosis linearis circumflexa and pityriasis rubra pilaris in order to observe its therapeutic usefulness. Treated children were 7 months to 11 years of age; all of them were hospitalized during the first month of treatment, continuing later as outpatients. The initial dose was between 1 to 2 mg/kg/day, requiring for a greater degree of hyperkeratosis the higher dosage and vice versa. At remission the dosage was reduced by half, or spaced to every 48 or more hours, in order to find the minimal dose necessary to keep the patient's skin free of lesions. Some children have been under continuous treatment up to three years. Control laboratory tests were done every two weeks, during the first month, and every 30 days thereafter. The therapeutic response was similar in each group of children suffering from the same disease, but different for each clinical entity. In lamellar ichthyosis in about one month the patient lost the thick lamellar scales, the ectropion diminished, and patient acquired an appearance never before obtained with other medicines. Epidermolytic hyperkeratosis was modified to the point that the patient was satisfied with the results. Symmetrical progressive erythrokeratodermia, palmo-plantar hyperkeratosis, ichthyosis linearis circumflexa and pityriasis rubra pilaris responded spectacularly, and the required dosage was lower. Pruritus and cutaneous fragility reported as constant symptoms with the use of oral retinoids were occasional in our patients, and never bothersome. Dryness of the lips and other mucous membranes slowly dissappeared after several months of treatment. Laboratory tests remained practically unchanged. Our series shows the therapeutic efficacy and good tolerance of the drug in children.

References

1. Orfanos CE, Schuppli R (1978) Oral retinoids in dermatology. Workshop XV Int. Congr. of Dermatology Mexico, 1977. Dermatologica 157 (Suppl 1)
2. Peck GL (1980) Retinoids in dermatology. Arch Dermatol 116:283–284
3. Tamayo L, Ruíz-Maldonado R (1980) Oral retinoid (Ro 10-9359) in children with lamellar ichthyosis, epidermolytic hyperkeratosis and symmetrical progressive erythrokeratoderma. Dermatologica 161:305–314

C.E. Orfanos et al. (eds.)
Retinoids

Treatment of Erythrokeratodermia Variabilis with Oral Retinoid (Ro 10-9359)

J.G. van der Schroeff and D. Suurmond

Erythrokeratodermia variabilis (EKV) is a rare skin disorder first described by Mendes da Costa in 1925 under this name, which indicates the main clinical features (10). EKV is characterized by erythematous areas and hyperkeratotic patches, both with sharp margins and constantly changing size, shape, and distribution pattern. The erythematous and hyperkeratotic lesions tend to occur independently and usually take bizarre configurations. Compared with the erythemas, the hyperkeratotic patches show less migration. Although the lesions may involve any part of the skin, a symmetrical distribution is found in most cases. The skin lesions may be present at birth, but in the majority of cases they appear during the first three years.

In 1950, Noordhoek (12) established the simple autosomal dominant mode of inheritance which was later confirmed by other authors (6, 16). There is, however, a striking variable expressivity of the trait (12). The treatment of EKV has often been disappointing, but recent reports have described promising results obtained with oral administration of retinoic acid (17) and the aromatic retinoid Tigason (Ro 10-9359) (3–5). This paper reports the results of treatment with Tigason (Ro 10-9359) in ten patients with EKV in whom histological and enzyme-histochemical investigations were performed before and during treatment.

Materials and Methods

Ten patients (7 females and 3 males) were studied between 1977 and 1980 in our outpatient clinic. At the start of therapy the age distribution ranged from 10 to 50 years (mean: 26.2 years). All of these patients showed skin lesions characteristic for EKV, occurring over the entire body, except for nos. 8 and 9, who only showed hyperkeratotic plaques on the face. In all cases variability of the lesions was a common feature. The age at onset of the skin lesions ranged between three months and three years. The patients belong to two families; although both families originate from the same district, no relationship between them could be established (Fig. 1). Family A is related to the predigree described by Noordhoek (12).

All patients were treated with the aromatic retinoid Tigason, kindly supplied by Hoffmann-La Roche, Basel. The therapy was started with a daily dosage ranging from 0.5 to 0.9 mg/kg body weight (mean: 0.78 mg/kg/day). Relevant information about the patients is given in Table 1. Before and during treatment, the following laboratory tests were performed at regular intervals: blood counts, blood glucose, electrolytes, transaminases, lactic dehydrogenase, alkaline phosphatase, urea, creatinine, bilirubine, and serum protein. For children (patients 3, 5, and 7), growth was monitored by regular measurement of height and body weight, evaluation of bone age, and assessment of total 24-h urine hydroxyproline excretion. Histological investigations were carried out in two patients (nos. 4 and 10). Punch biopsy specimens were taken from adjacent sites in hyperkeratotic lesions before treatment and after two, seven, and eight weeks of treatment. These specimens were fixed in formaldehyde and paraffin sections were stained with haematoxilin-eosin. In one of these patients (no. 10), punch biopsies

Table 1. Clinical data on the treatment of erythrokeratodermia variabilis with Tigason, Ro 10-9359

Patient No.	Sex/Age (yrs)	Clinical Features	Initial dosage (mg/kg/day)	Side effects	Maintenance dosage (mg/kg/day)	Clearing of lesions	Duration of treatment (months)
1	F/21	Configurate erythema around eyes and on neck, trunk, arms, and legs; very slight hyperkeratosis	0.5		0.2	100%	6
2	M/24	Erythematous patches and hyperkeratotic plaques on the face, axillae, groins, shoulders, abdomen, elbows, and knees	0.9		0.2	95%	29
3	F/10	Grayish-brown hyperkeratotic patches on neck, groins, axillae, trunk, elbows, dorsa of hands, abdomen, and legs; configurate erythema on the face	0.8	Cheilitis	0.5	90%	33
4	F/25	Reddish-brown hyperkeratotic patches on dorsa of hands and wrists, elbows, hips, knees, ankles, buttocks, and groins; erythema in axillae	0.9	Cheilitis, hair loss, dryness of nasal mucosa	0.4	95%	11
5	M/10	Circinate erythematous and hyperkeratotic patches on the face, trunk, arms and legs	0.9		0.5	90%	31
6	F/20	Hyperkeratotic plaques surrounded by erythema on axillae, groins, elbows, abdomen, and legs	0.9	Cheilitis, hair loss	0.1	95%	35
7	F/12	Except for the face and chest, the entire body is covered with erythematous and hyperkeratotic lesions	0.6	Cheilitis	0.6	90%	36
8	F/50	Grayish-brown hyperkeratotic plaques around the eyes	0.7	Cheilitis, hair loss, dryness of nasal mucosa	0.1	95%	11
9	F/47	Grayish-brown hyperkeratotic plaques around the eyes; brown pigmentation on the chin	0.7	Cheilitis	0.1	95%	11
10	M/43	Grayish-brown plaques on neck, face, chest, abdomen, dorsa of hands, legs, and knees	0.9	Cheilitis, dryness of nasal mucosa	0.3	100%	6

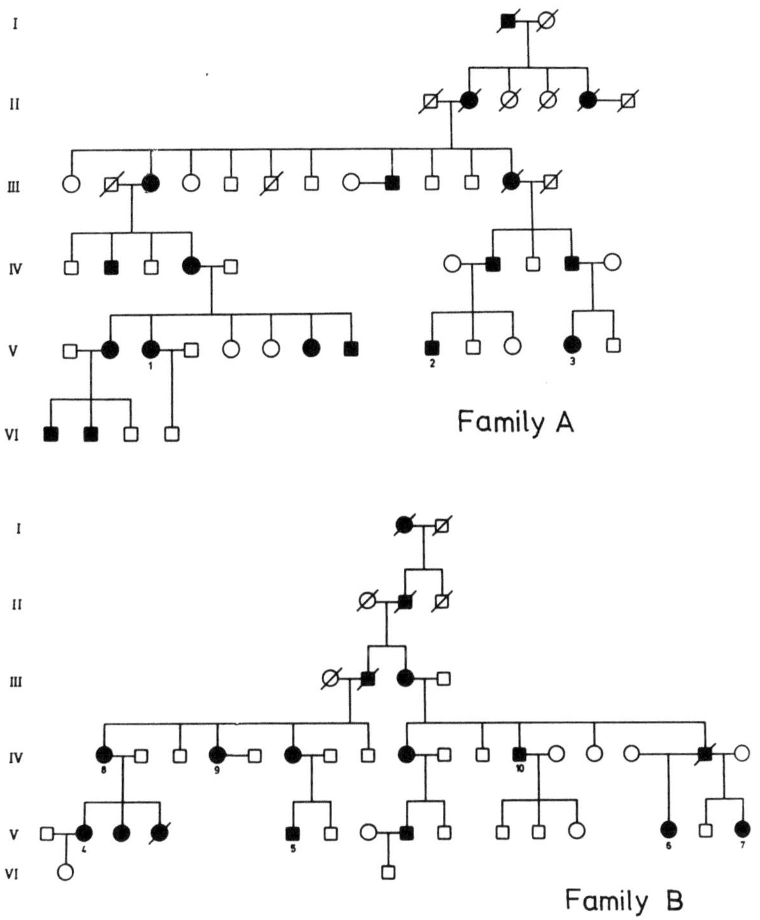

Fig. 1a, b. Pedigrees of two families with erythrokeratodermia variabilis. The patient numbers correspond with those in Table 1. Descendants of uninvolved individuals (the latter indicated by open circles and squares) are not shown because they are not affected

were taken at the same time for enzyme-histochemical investigations. The biopsy specimens were immediately frozen and sectioned on a cryostat. The following staining techniques were used: alkaline phospatase (7), 5-nucleotidase (19), acid phosphatase (7), adenosine triphosphatase (19), leucine aminopeptidase (11), indoxyl esterase (13), and acetylcholin esterase (9). For control studies, a skin biopsy obtained from a healthy volunteer was processed in the same way.

Results of Treatment

After one to two weeks of treatment, all patients noticed increased desquamation of the hyperkeratotic patches. The hyperkeratotic lesions gradually cleared, leaving erythematous or pigmented areas with a normal skin texture. After four to eight weeks of treatment the dosage was decreased stepwise. The erythematous component showed a lower response during the first period of treatment; erythematous areas continued to appear and disappear as before. Two to three months after the start of treatment, the hyperkeratotic lesions and their residual pigmented areas had disappeared completely or almost completely. At this time, erythema either occurred less frequently and less intensely or had also faded. After

Fig. 2 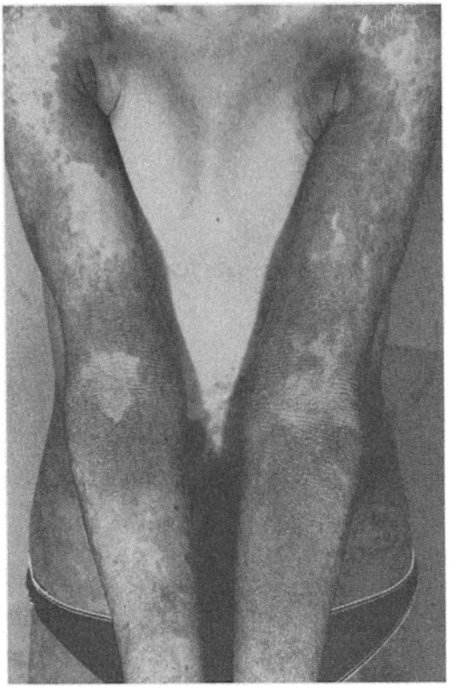 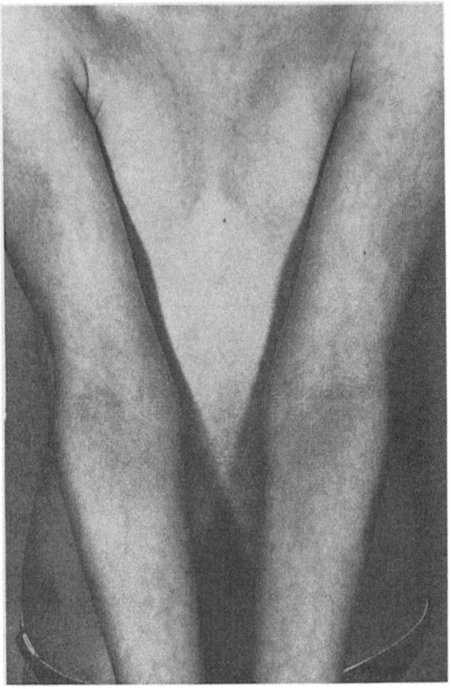 Fig. 3

Fig. 2. Patient 7 before treatment. Sharply outlined erythematous and hyperkeratotic lesions
Fig. 3. Patient 7 after eight weeks of treatment with Tigason (Ro 10-9359), showing almost complete clearing of the skin lesions

four months of treatment, no further clearing was observed. Except for patient 7, the daily dosage could be reduced considerably during the course of treatment (mean maintenance dosage: 0.3 mg/kg/day). The therapeutical results, expressed as percentage of clearing, are presented in Table 1. Figs. 2 and 3 show the results of treatment in patient 7 after eight weeks.

Occasional relapses occurred during therapy in four patients (nos. 2, 3, 5, and 7). These relapses were often induced by external factors such as exposure to cold wind or cold water and friction caused by clothing. Mild topical corticosteroids were prescribed in these cases, but the dosage of Tigason was not increased.

Side Effects

During the initial treatment phase the well-known side effects of retinoids were encountered, such as cheilitis, dryness of the nasal mucosa, and hair loss (see Table 1). After reduction of the dosage, the side effects disappeared.

Laboratory investigations gave no abnormal findings, except a transient rise of the serum alkaline phosphatase level in patient 3 (up to 257 U/L). Additional liver function tests displayed normal values, and no signs of increased bone resorption could be established in this patient.

During a long follow-up period (31–36 months), no growth retardation was observed in the three children. The growth rate lay within the normal ranges in all cases and the hydroxyproline excretion in the urine showed normal values. The bone age remained in accordance with the calendar age.

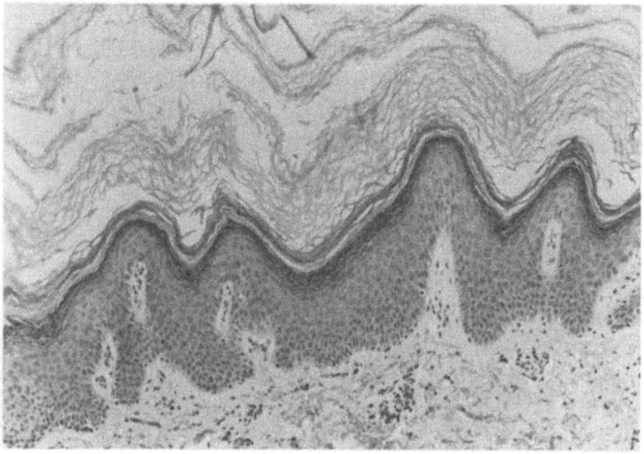

Fig. 4. Pre-treatment biopsy specimen from the groin of patient 4, showing hyperkeratosis, papillomatosis, moderate acanthosis, and a scanty mononuclear infiltrate around the vessels. (Haematoxylin-eosin, × 90)

Histological Findings

Biopsy specimens taken before the administration of Tigason showed striking hyperkeratosis, a granular layer of normal thickness, moderate acanthosis, and papillomatosis. The papillary vessels were surrounded by a scanty mononuclear infiltrate (Fig. 4).

After two weeks of treatment no pronounced histological alterations were observed. However, biopsy specimens taken after 7 and 8 weeks of treatment showed a marked decrease of hyperkeratosis and papillomatosis and thinning of the granular layer (Fig. 5).

Enzyme-histochemical Findings

Most of the applied histochemical procedures disclosed no differences in staining patterns

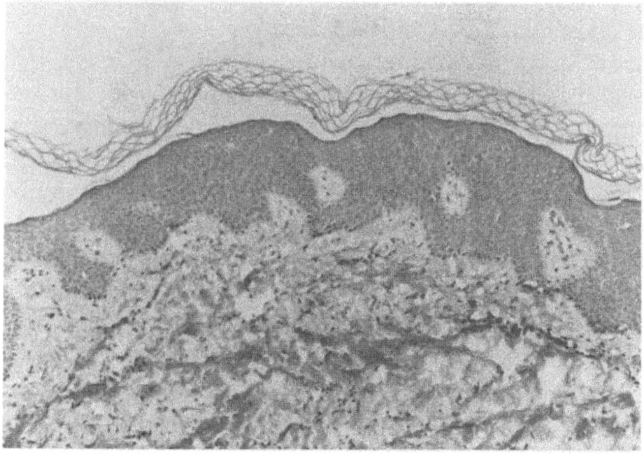

Fig. 5. Biopsy specimen taken from the same lesion as that in Fig. 4 after 8 weeks of treatment with Tigason (Ro 10-9359), showing considerable reduction of the hyperkeratosis and the papillomatosis and thinning of the granular layer. (Haematoxylin-eosin, × 90)

between EKV and normal skin or alterations in these patterns during treatment. However, the following features were observed. In case of EKV, the adenosine triphosphatase technique did not reveal dendritic cells in the epidermis before treatment, but after seven weeks of therapy these cells were numerous in the Malpighian layer.

The papillary vessels stained intensely with both adenosine triphosphatase and alkaline phosphatase, and showed a straight and elongated course. During treatment, the vessels assumed a more tortuous structure, comparable to that in normal skin.

Before treatment a strong acid phosphatase staining reaction was found in the granular layer and throughout the stratum corneum. After seven weeks of treatment, this enzyme activity was localized in the stratum granulosum and only in the basal layer of the stratum corneum.

Discussion

Erythrokeratodermia variabilis is a disorder of keratinization and is usually classified as an ichthyosiform condition. Treatment is mainly aimed at reduction of the hyperkeratosis. The results of local application of keratolytic agents are, however, often unsatisfactory, and the erythematous component remains unaffected. Topical and sublesional administration of corticosteroids has been reported to reduce both erythema and hyperkeratosis (8). Local application of retinoic acid may be of some benefit, but is frequently irritating (6). Improvement of the skin lesions by oral vitamin A therapy has been observed (2, 20) but the toxicity of vitamin A remains a serious problem. Therefore, less toxic retinoids seem more appropriate for long-term treatment.

In our ten patients the treatment of EKV with Tigason gave excellent results. All of these patients responded well, and a striking clinical improvement was obtained. The initial dosage (mean: 0.78 mg/kg/day) could be reduced without loss of therapeutic efficacy. The relatively low maintenance dosage (mean: 0.3 mg/kg/day) diminished the side effects and made the therapy satisfactorily tolerable during a long period of treatment (mean: 20.9 months). Occasional recurrences were usually confined to small areas and were probably caused by environmental factors. In these cases additional treatment with mild topical corticosteroids was sufficient. Laboratory investigations during treatment revealed only a transient rise of the serum alkaline phosphatase level in one patient.

Three children were treated with the aromatic retinoid for more than 2½ years, and careful monitoring failed to reveal growth retardation due to the therapy in any of the cases. This is in agreement with experiences during Tigason treatment of two children with psoriasis vulgaris (14). The histological findings reflect the normalization occurring during treatment, i.e., reduction of hyperkeratosis and papillomatosis and thinning of the granular layer. The strong staining reaction of acid phosphatase in the stratum corneum is in accordance with the results of other investigations (15, 18). In normal human skin the presence of acid phosphatase is confined to the granular layer and a narrow basal layer of the stratum corneum (1). The normalization of acid phosphatase activity during therapy possibly represents one of the modulating effects of the aromatic retinoid on abnormal keratinization.

The absence of dendritic cells in the epidermis in adenosine triphosphatase preparations was mentioned earlier by Vandersteen and Muller (18). The same authors were unable to find Langerhans' cells in skin lesions of EKV at the ultrastructural level either (18). The question remains whether the absence of Langerhans' cells is a characteristic feature of EKV, and further investigations are needed to settle this point.

Summary

Ten patients with erythrokeratodermia variabilis were treated with the aromatic retinoid Ro 10-9359. Excellent therapeutic results were obtained in all cases. The initial dosage could be reduced considerably without loss of therapeutic efficacy.

Side effects were encountered but disappeared during maintenance treatment. No growth retardation was observed in three children during a long follow-up period.

Histological and enzyme-histochemical investigations were performed before and during treatment.

Acknowledgments. The authors wish to thank Mrs. N.J. Dijkshoorn and H. Korff for their excellent technical assistance, and Mrs. G.W. Roest for typing the manuscript.

References

1. Braun-Falco O, Rupec M (1967) Die Verteilung der sauren Phosphatase bei normaler und psoriatischer Verhornung. Dermatologica 134:225–242
2. Carteaud A, Dorfman L (1963) Erythrokératodermie variable de Mendes da Costa. Presse Medicale 55:2685–2687
3. Dinet Y, Achten G, Wanet J, Oleffe J, Uytendaele K, Alexander F (1978) Traitement oral de grands états ichthyosiformes par le rétinoïde éthylester. Ann Dermatol Venerol 105:465–468
4. Fixler ZC (1980) Treatment of erythrokeratodermia variabilis with oral synthetic retinoids. Cutis 25:301–304
5. Fritsch PO (1979) Erythrokeratodermia figurata variabilis Mendes da Costa: erfolgreiche Behandlung mit einem oralen aromatischen Retinoid (Ro 10-9359). Hautarzt 30:161–163
6. Gewirtzman GB, Winkler NW, Dobson RL (1978) Erythrokeratodermia variabilis, a family study. Arch Dermatol 114:259–261
7. Gomori G (1952) Microscopic histochemistry: principles and practice. Chicago: University of Chicago Press
8. Kanaar P (1965) Zur Histochemie und symptomatischen Therapie der Erythro- et Keratodermia variabilis (Mendes da Costa). Hautarzt 16:126–129
9. Karnovsky MJ, Roots L (1964) A direct-coloring thiocholine method for cholinesterases. J Histochem Cytochem 12:219–221
10. Mendes da Costa S (1925) Erythro- et keratodermia variabilis in a mother and daughter. Acta Dermato-Venerol 6:255–261
11. Nachlas MM, Crawford DT, Seligmann AM (1957) The histochemical demonstration of leucine aminopeptidase. J Histochem Cytochem 5:264–278
12. Noordhoek FJ (1950) Over erythro- et keratodermia variabilis. Thesis. Schiedam: De Eendracht
13. Pearson B, Defendi V (1957) A comparison between the histochemical demonstration of nonspecific esterase activity by 5-bromo-indoxyl acetate, α-naphthyl acetate and naphthol as acetate. J Histochem Cytochem 5:72–83
14. Van der Rhee HJ, Van Gelderen HH, Polano MK (1980) Is the use of Ro 10-9359 (Tigason) in children justified? Acta Dermato-Venerol 60:274–275
15. Schellander FG, Fritsch PO (1969) Variable erythrokeratoderma. An unusual case. Arch Dermatol 100:744–748
16. Sommacal-Schopf D, Schnijder UW (1957) Über eine Familie mit 14 Fällen von Erythrokeratodermia figurata variabilis. Hautarzt 8:174–176
17. Van der Wateren AR, Cormane RH (1977) Oral retinoic acid as therapy for erythrokeratoderma variabilis. Brit J Dermatol 97:83–85
18. Vandersteen PR, Muller SA (1971) Erythrokeratodermia variabilis. An enzyme-histochemical and ultrastructural study. Arch Dermatol 103:362–370
19. Wachstein M, Meisel E (1957) Histochemistry of hepatic phosphatases at physiologic pH. Am J Clin Pathol 27:13–23
20. Wulf K, Koch H, Schulz KH (1960) Erythrokeratodermia figurata variabilis vom Typ Mendes da Costa, eine durch Vitamin A beeinflussbare Dermatose. Derm Wochenschr 37:1012–1016

C.E. Orfanos et al. (eds.)
Retinoids

Ultrastructural Study of the Four Main Types of Ichthyosis After One Month's Treatment with Ro 10-9359

C. Blanchet-Bardon and A. Puissant

We have performed electron microscopy on the skin of patients with ichthyosis before and after one month of treatment with 1 mg/kg of body weight/day with Ro 10-9359.

Our cases include:
4 with autosomal dominant ichthyosis vulgaris,
3 with X-linked ichthyosis
2 with érythrodermie congénitale ichthyosiforme sèche
1 with érythrodermie congénitale ichthyosiforme bulleuse of epidermolytic hyperkeratosis
The four types of ichthyoses can be grouped into:
2 recessive types which are characterized by quantitative anomalies of keratinization (1, 3) and into two dominant types marked by structural anomalies of keratinocytes (2, 4).

The recessive types are composed of *érythrodermie congénitale ichthyosiforme sèche* and *X-linked ichthyosis.*

a) Erythrodermie congénitale ichthyosiforme sèche.

The treatment of this type is successful following one month of treatment. Ultrastructurally the keratinocytes remain enlarged as usually seen in this type (1). Perinuclear clear spaces containing fine granules are frequently seen after treatment in the cells of the stratum spinosum (Fig. 1). Sometimes, this space is small but more often is large. Also there is a small amount of mucin-like material in the intercellular space.

One finds membrane bound vacuoles containing fine granular material possibly deriving from smooth endoplasmic reticulum. Also glycogen deposits are seen in the proximity of mucin-like granules. The cells of the granular layer appear edematous and often the keratohyalin granules are diminished in size. There is no change in the basal layer including the number of mitoses. Throughout the epidermis tonofilaments and desmosomes appear decreased; whereas, there are no change in the keratinosome number.

After treatment the lipid-like vacuoles, typical for this disease (1) in the stratum corneum, are no longer seen and the number of layers within the stratum corneum is reduced.

b) X-linked recessive ichthyosis.

As in the previous type the treatment is successful.

The ultrastructural findings in this type of ichthyosis is usually the same as that observed in lamellar ichthyosis except that less edema is seen.

The number and size of keratohyalin granules is reduced as well as the number of tonofilaments and desmosomes. In our observations keratinosomes are somewhat augmented in number. The number of layers within the stratum corneum is again reduced.

The dominant forms of ichthyosis are composed of *epidermolytic hyperkeratosis* and *ichthyosis vulgaris.*

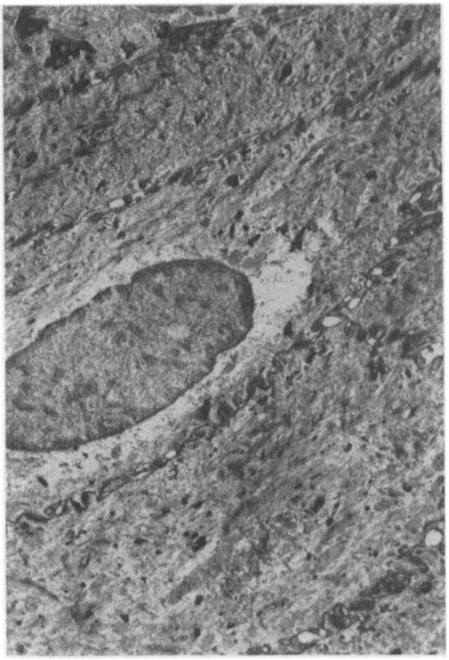

Fig. 1. Perinuclear clear spaces containing fine granules (Erythrodermie congénitale ichtyosiforme sèche). Epon embedded, uranyl and lead stained. Magnification: × 9,700

c) Epidermolytic hyperkeratosis.

Treatment in one particular case was remarkable in that not only did the hyperkeratosis improve, as is usually the case, but augmentation of blisters did not occur; it is more common to observe the augmentation of blisters in this disease following the use of retinoid (5).

After one month's treatment it was noted that the perinuclear tonofilament clumping and cytoplasmic tonofilament clumps remain the same. However the tonofilaments them-

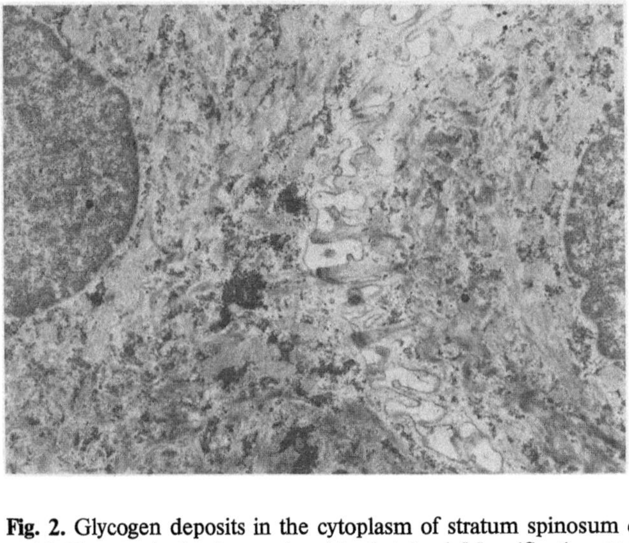

Fig. 2. Glycogen deposits in the cytoplasm of stratum spinosum cells (ichthyosis vulgaris). Epon-embedded, uranyl and lead-stained. Magnification: × 25,000

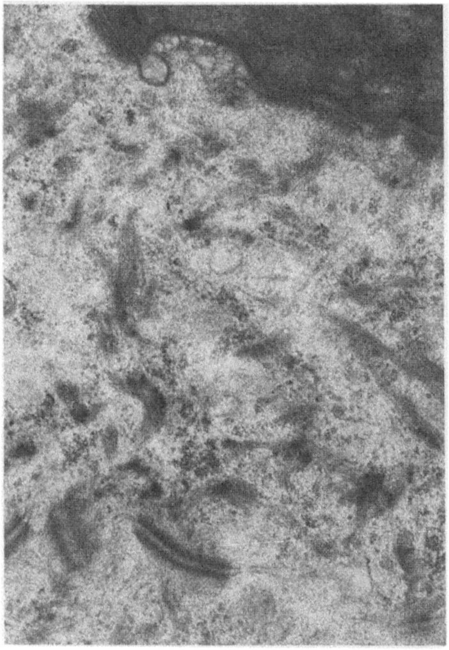

Fig. 3. The specific anomaly of keratohyalin: crumbly granules remain the same after treatment of ichthyosis vulgaris. Epon embedded, uranyl and lead stained. Magnification: × 31,500

selves are reduced in number as in the previous two types. In the stratum granulosum cells, the number of tonofilaments and keratohyalin granules are remarkably reduced following treatment. The cytoplasmic edema and the cytolysis are markedly augmented explaining the increased number of blisters which usually occurs following treatment (5).

d) The second dominant type *ichthyosis vulgaris.* This most common type responds to treatment. However, since the disease is a mild one, often the side effects of the retinoid are worse than the disease itself. In fact, the atopic dermatitis which is known to occur in approximately half of these cases is made worse by retinoid treatment.

Beginning in the basal cell layer, cytoplasmic and extracellular edema are seen; these continue into the stratum spinosum. However, no perinuclear clear spaces are seen.
In these same keratinocytes, glycogen deposits are seen (Fig. 2)
In the stratum granulosum the specific anomaly of the keratohyalin (2), crumbly granules, the marker for this type of ichthyosis, is unchanged (Fig. 3). As in all of the other types the number of stratum corneum cells is reduced.

Conclusion

Following treatment with one month of Ro 10-9359 1 mg/kg of body weight/day the two major ultrastructural, genetically-induced markers of the dominant diseases; namely, the crumbly keratohyalin granules of ichthyosis vulgaris and the clumping of tonofilaments seen in epidermolytic hyperkeratosis, are not changed.

Following treatment, the number of layers of the stratum corneum is reduced in all four types. Tonofilaments, keratohyalin granules and desmosomes are quantitatively diminished. The number of keratinosomes is difficult to evaluate. Edematous changes and mucin-like granules both intra- and extracellular, are common in all the four types, the same changes as has been observed in psoriasis (6).

More cytolysis is produced in epidermolytic hyperkeratosis.

Ro 10-9359 seems to alter some cytoplasmic components of keratinocytes following one month's treatment.

The presence of edema, glycogen deposits and mucin-like granules, the alteration of keratinization and exfoliation of stratum corneum suggest a mucinous "metaplasia" in keeping with current concepts of the mode of action of retinoids (7).

Summary

Ro 10-9359, when used in treatment of the four main types of ichthyosis, produced a quantitative reduction (desmosomes, tonofilaments, keratohyalin granules) as well as a reduction of the number of cornified cells. The qualitative defect of the two autosomal dominant ichthyosis was unchanged. In all four types, retinoid treatment produced after one month extra- and intracellular edema, glycogen deposits and a mucoid appearing substance within the keratinocytes.

References

1. Anton-Lamprecht I (1972) Zur Ultrastruktur hereditärer Verhornungsstörungen I: Ichthyosis congenita. Arch Derm Forsch 243:88–100
2. Anton-Lamprecht I (1973) Zur Ultrastruktur hereditärer Verhornungsstörungen III: Autosomal-dominante ichthyosis vulgaris. Arch Derm Forsch 248:149–172
3. Anton-Lamprecht I (1979) Zur Ultraastruktur hereditärer Verhornungsstörungen IV: X-chromosomal-recessive ichthyosis. Arch Derm Forsch 248:361–378
4. Anton-Lamprecht I, Schnyder UW (1974) Ultrastructure of inborn errors of keratinization VI: Inherited ichthyosis, a model system for heterogeneities in keratinisation disturbances. Arch Derm Forsch 250:207–227
5. Blanchet-Bardon C, Anton-Lamprecht I, Schnyder UW (1977) Erythrodermie congénitale ichtyosiforme bulleuse: Contrôle ultrastructural du traitment par l'éther éthylique d'un dérivé aromatique de l'acide rétinoïque. Ann Derm Vénéréol (Paris) 104:648–653
6. Orfanos CE, Runne U (1978) Tissue changes in psoriatic plaques after oral administration of retinoid. Dermatologica 157 (Suppl I):19–25
7. Tsambaos D, Mahrle G, Orfanos CE (1980) Epidermal changes induced by oral excess of aromatic retinoid in guinea pigs. Arch Dermatol Res 267:141–152

C.E. Orfanos et al. (eds.)
Retinoids

Effect of Retinoids on Precancerous Lesions of Oral Mucosa

H.F. Koch

Leukoplakia ranges among the most frequent precancerous lesions of the oral cavity. In a clinical sense, it is defined as a whitish patch of unknown etiology on the mucous membrane. It neither can be wiped off, nor can it be classified as any other diagnosable disease. The term leukoplakia, however, may represent different histologic changes. The problem resides in correlating the changing histomorphological substrates to the varying clinical manifestations. This inhomogeneous behaviour of leukoplakia substantially complicates diagnosis and treatment, in particular when it appears in the form of wide-spreading and multifocal lesions. According to the law of the series, certain correlations between the clinical type and the histological structure may in fact be deduced (1); however, a safe diagnosis is subject to histologic investigations. As to the therapy, surgical procedures are prevailing. Nevertheless they are of purely symptomatic effect and remain without any consequence on the tendency of impaired cellular differentiation of the mucosa apart from the defects produced. This has repeatedly been proved through relapse and secondary lesions.

Attempts have often been made to provide for a more careful and causal therapy. New possibilities have emerged since the biochemical effectiveness of vitamin A was confirmed experimentally and validated by clinical observations in cases of keratinization of the skin and the mucosa. The first positive results were obtained, however, with systemic application at the expense of considerable side effects in the sense of a hypervitaminosis A. Later on, the adoption of all-trans-retinoic acid has opened up new prospects for the treatment of precancerous states. Along with developing analogues of retinoic acid, the side effects could gradually be reduced while at the same time increasing the therapeutic effectiveness so as to extend the applicational ranges for these substances. We have repeatedly reported on this (3–5, 7). The so far last link in this chain of development is the aromatic retinoid Ro 10-9359 (Tigason).

We have tested this substance since 1974 under different conditions in cases of leukoplakia of the oral mucous membrane. The subject of this study is, first, to investigate the effectiveness of the aromatic retinoid at largely comparable morphologically defined initial criteria, using different dosages and types of application and furthermore to compare the various derivatives of retinoic acid employed so far, concerning their therapeutical results and their side effects.

Patients and Method

The present study includes a total of 48 patients, of whom 31 male and 17 female, with a mean age of 64 years, who have been treated with aromatic retinoid since 1977. Twelve patients of the above total were heavy smokers.

Table 1. Morphological classification

Macroscopic growth pattern	Nr of pat.	Microscopic growth pattern	Nr of pat.	Histol.-cytol. differentiation	Nr of pat.
Homogeneous l. (Leuk. simplex)	9	Flat	9	Dysplasia Grade 0–1	38
Speckled leuk. (Leuk. verrucc. Leuk. erosiva)	39	Papillary-endophytic	31	Dysplasia Grade 2	10
		Papillomatous exophytic	8		

Table 2. Criteria of the two groups

	Group 1	Group 2
Dosage per day	75 mg	50 mg
Total dosage	3150 mg	2100 mg
Form of application	enteral	combined
Period of therapy	6 weeks	6 weeks
Nr of patients	21	24

In each individual case, leukoplakia was classified pretherapeutically and exactly according to the criteria of Burghardt and Seifert (2) and according to the bases of Bánóczy and Csiba (1) (Table 1).

Regarding to the macroscopic growth pattern leukoplakia predominantly belongs to the verrucous type. Microscopically, papillary-endophytic patterns with no or minor grades of dysplasia were prevailing.

Excluded from this study were patients suffering from serious general diseases, in particular hepatic diseases, females in a conceptive age, and all patients with more than moderate epithelial dysplasia. The latter have to be treated surgically according to the rules of tumour therapy.

From the overall number of patients two groups of 24 patients each were formed by randomizing:

Group 1: 21 patients receiving exclusively enteral doses of aromatic retinoid: 75 mg per day within 6 weeks. During the follow-up period, 3 patients were lost of this group. Their data were thus not taken into consideration for evaluation purposes.

Group 2: 24 patients receiving daily doses of 50 mg aromatic retinoid enterally plus 0.1% aromatic retinoid-paste locally (Table 2).

Results

Two weeks after starting the therapy, initial reaction of leukoplakia was almost equally good for both the enteral and the combined form of application (Table 3).

Table 3. Initial reaction under various forms of application

Reaction	Enteral application form	Combined application form
Very good	13	11
Good	6	9
Moderate	2	3
Bad	0	1
Total	21	24

Table 4. Primary results after termination of the therapy

Results	Enteral application form	Combined application form
Remission		
total	5	7
partial	(71.5%)	(83.5%)
> 50%	10	13
< 50%	4	2
Unchanged	2 (28.5%)	2 (16.5%)
Progression	0	0
Total	21	24

After a 6 weeks' treatment, 3.15 g (i.e. 12.6 million I.U.) were administered on an average in group 1 and 2.10 g (i.e. 8.4 million I.U.) were given on an average in group 2. The results obtained at that time are illustrated in Table 4.

When comparing these early results, the combined therapy seems to offer advantages over the purely enteral form of application which manifests – at identical evaluation criteria – in a visibly higher rate of remissions as opposed to the initial findings. Remissions of more than 50% of the lesions are being considered as positive results. This advantage is moreover confirmed in the framework of control results obtained after 24 months on an average for both groups (Table 5).

Relapses mostly occurred 2 months after termination of the therapy. They are, however, frequently less apparent compared to the initial findings. Such relapses can easily be approached with further therapy courses. A regression of over 50% is considered as a permanently favourable effect on the lesion. Such favourable results were obtained with both groups in more than 50% of the cases. A total of 4 from 45 patients with moderate epithelial dysplasia and hyperparakeratosis in the initial findings showed the histologic criteria of a malignant transformation after an average of 2 years: 3 males concerned were heavy smokers and one female diabetic.

Concerning the side effects, a comparison of all retinoic acid derivatives has shown that the combined enteral and local therapy (in group 2) yielded the best of all results obtained so far (Table 6).

Table 5. Long-time results 24 months after therapy

Results	Group 1 Nr. of pat.	Group 2 Nr. of pat.
Remission		
total	5	7
partial	(52.3%)	(58.3%)
> 50%	10	13
Relaps		
partial	5	5
complete	4 (47.7%)	2 (41.7%)
Progression	1	3

Table 6. Side effects of various derivatives of the all-trans retinoic acid

	All-trans-ret. acid	13-cis-ret. acid	Aromat. retinoid enter.	combined
General symptoms	50%	0	0	0
Dermal/mucosal symptoms	79%	83%	72%	46%
Interruption of therapy	11%	4%	0	0

The prevailing individual symptoms stated were dryness of the mucosa, itching of the skin, and desquamation of the epithelium.

Discussion and Conclusions

A decade of experience with all-trans-retinoic acid and analogues made with more than 120 patients with idiopathic oral leukoplakia treated has shown that these drugs may be therapeutically employed. The first tests conducted by systemically applying this biochemically efficient substances entailed, however, a high rate of undesired side effects. Hence consequent further development of new derivatives of retinoic acid aimed, in a first stage at reducing toxicity. Simultaneously it was tried to increase therapeutical effectiveness through precise adjustment of indications, changing of the form of application, and dosage. We have tested the aromatic retinoid clinically with a view to its effectiveness under these conditions. To this end, two groups were formed as per the random principle which differed by the type of application of these substances and the amount of the overall dosage. Though the combined therapy applied in group 2 entailed savings of up to 30% of the overall dosage, the results produced in these cases a more favourable therapeutical effect, i.e. immediately after termination of the therapy and after 2 years as well. To a large extent the lesions showed after a 2 weeks' treatment already some tendencies towards remission, the maximum of which stabilized after roughly 4 weeks. Earlier examinations (3) proved that neither increase of the dosage up to approx. 100 mg per day nor prolongation of the therapy over and above 6 weeks could contribute to further local improvement or prevention of relapses. This is in agreement with the experience of Silverman et al. (8) who failed in proving any direct correlation between serum concentrations of vitamin A and cases of clinical remission. By analog with the results obtained by Bánóczy and Csiba (1), we have likewise succeeded in proving that the reaction of leukoplakia to the therapy is the better, the more homogenous its appearance is, and the more it is marked by orthokeratosis. On the other hand, erosion and dyskeratosis reduce the therapeutical effect. Post-therapeutical biopsy controls show that clinical remission in most cases is accompanied by a reduction of hyper- and dyskeratosis and by normalizing of epithelial standards (Fig. 1a, b). As is generally accepted, vitamin A acts as a regulator to the growth and differentiation of epithelial tissues. Clinical remission reflects, histologically, a keratolytic disintegration of the horny layers, and an acanthosis and diffusion of the proliferation zone. By means of exfoliative cytology, this effect may also be demonstrated after treatment. Proliferation kinetically, an improvement of the epithelium during therapy with retinoic acid is accompanied by an increase in the index of mitosis and a shortening of the various stages of the cell cycle corresponding – as have pointed out Pullmann et al. (6) – to those of normal processes.

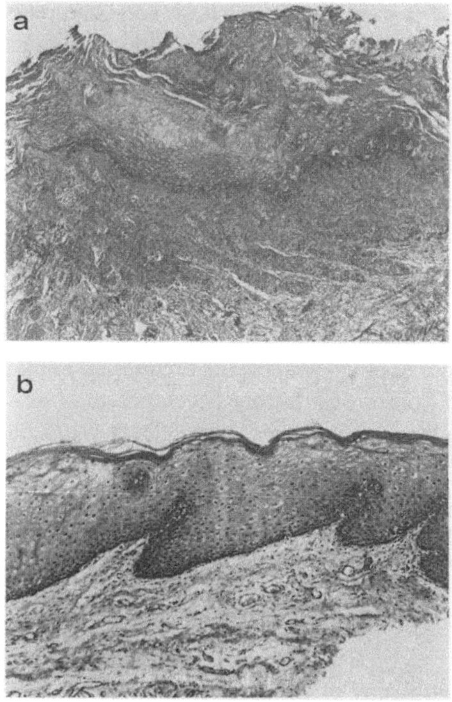

Fig. 1a. Mucosal biopsy before starting treatment. Leukoplakia with severe combined hyperortho- and parakeratosis, and basal papillomatosis. Slide to moderate epithelial dysplasia (H & E, 22.5 ×). **b** Status after six weeks' treatment with Tigason. Oral mucosa with regression of the superficial keratosis and papillomatosis. Normalized epithelial standards with no signs of dysplasia (H & E, 73.5 ×)

The best results of all our clinical test series so far conducted with analogues of retinoic acid were obtained with the aromatic retinoid, which shows the highest therapeutic quotient, i.e. the highest effectiveness, and relatively harmless side effects on the other hand. In our view, the number of 58% of permanently complete or partial remissions would show good promise towards adopting the combined therapy with aromatic acid, allowing precise an adjustment of indication for standard therapy of leukoplakia.

The marked tendency of conservative therapy to relapse has been adversely criticized in all examinations made so far, and has induced many an author to definitely abandon it. In doing so, one has often overlooked, that these relapses while being obviously less apparent gave a much better incent to a further therapy than the initial findings. The combined therapy form seems to offer a possibility to treat even multiple relapses - provided that the morphological criteria do not undergo further impairment - in several repeated courses, as the case may be. The doses required to this end cause only so little side effects that this indication seems advisable even for patients of an advanced age. In the course of therapy with aromatic retinoid, no patient showed the general symptoms of a hyper-vitaminosis A one is in the fear of. While applying severe criteria, 46% of the patients treated with the combined therapy, showed minor side effects on the skin and mucosa which kept, however, within admissible limits even when therapy was continued.

In order to avoid relapses, different ways of treatment with a maintenance dosage of retinoic acid are usually recommended, such as 30 mg or less per day enterally, or by means of a paste as monotherapy. Thus, following our own experience such a maintenance therapy is mostly ineffective such as not to avoid relapses. Instead of this we prefer repeated courses of combined therapy with aromatic retinoid 40 to 50 mg per day plus application of a paste in the way mentioned above. All the same, exact and generally applicable guidelines cannot be laid down, since response to the drug and in particular maintenance dosage is likely to vary from individual to individual.

The further development of analogues of the aromatic acid promises improved therapeutic results in the future. So we are in the point of testing the bichloric aromatic retinoid.

Summary

Leukoplakia is neither a clinical, an etiological nor an histopathological entity. On that basis, treatment is problematic particularly in multifocal and advanced lesions. No kind of therapy is quite satisfying up to now. In the last years attempts were made to provide for a more careful and causal therapy. Adoption of all-trans retinoic acid has opened up new prospects for the treatment of precancerous lesions. A decade of experience with derivatives of the all-trans retinoic acid and analogues made with more than 120 patients has demonstrated that these drugs may be therapeutically employed. Consequent further development of new derivatives with reduced toxicity and increasing therapeutical effectiveness leads to extend the applicational ranges for these substances. 58% of permanent of partial remissions are in our view sufficient to adopt the therapy with analogues of the retinoic acid for standard therapy of oral leukoplakia. The so far best results of our clinical test series were obtained with the aromatic retinoid being the last link in the chain of development up to now.

References

1. Bánóczy J, Csiba A (1972) Comparative study of the clinical picture and histopathologic structure of the oral leukoplakia. Cancer 29:1230–1234
2. Burghardt A, Seifert G (1977) Morphologische Klassifikation der oralen Leukoplakien. Dtsch Med Wochenschr 102:223–229
3. Koch H (1976) Erfahrungsbericht über die klinische Anwendung eines aromatischen Retinoids – Ro 10-9359 bei Präkanzerosen der Mundhöhle. Quintessenz, H 6, 133–136
4. Koch H (1978) Biochemical treatment of precancerous oral lesions: the effectiveness of various analogues of retinoic acid. J max-fac Surg 6:59–63
5. Koch H, Schettler D (1973) Klinische Erfahrungen mit Vitamin A-Säure-Derivaten bei der Behandlung von Leukoplakien der Mundschleimhaut. Dtsch Zahnärztl Z 28:623–627
6. Pullmann H, Lennartz KJ, Steigleder GK (1975) Die Proliferationskinetik normaler Epidermis vor und nach äußerlicher Anwendung einer 1%igen Vitamin-A-Säure-Lösung. Arch Dermatol Res 253:71–76
7. Schettler D, Koch H (1976) Langzeitbeobachtungen nach Vitamin-A-Säure-Therapie bei Leukoplakien der Mundschleimhaut. Fortschr Kiefer- u Gesichtschir 21:179–183
8. Silverman S, Renstrup G, Pindborg JJ (1963) Studies in oral leukoplakias. III. Effects of Vitamin A, a comparing clinical-histopathologic, cytologic and hematologic response. Acta Odont Scand 21:271–292

C.E. Orfanos et al. (eds.)
Retinoids

Treatment of Parapsoriasis en Plaques and Mycosis Fungoides with an Oral Aromatic Retinoid (Ro 10-9359)

P. Souteyrand, J. Thivolet and R. Fulton

Oral aromatic retinoids seem to act principally on the epidermis. They are effective in the treatment of squamous dermatoses such as psoriasis. These are the two main reasons why we have used Ro 10-9359 in the treatment of parapsoriasis en plaques, a squamous dermatosis whose pathogenesis is unknown, and mycosis fungoides, a malignant epidermotropic cutaneous lymphoma of T cell origin in the pathogenesis of which the epidermis seems to play an important role.

Material

We have given the aromatic retinoid to ten patients including three patients with parapsoriasis en plaques, six patients with mycosis fungoides and one patient with Sézary's syndrome. These ten patients were divided into two groups: the first group received Ro 10-9359 as the sole therapy and the second group were treated by a combination of PUVA and Ro 10-9359.

Group I

These five patients (numbers one to five) had never received any previous treatment with PUVA or systemic corticosteroids. They were all men. Their ages are recorded on Table 1 as well as the disease duration at the beginning of treatment by the retinoid. The following is a brief clinical description of each patient:

1. Patient No. 1, who also suffered from multiple sclerosis, presented 12 years previously with erythemato-squamous lesions of the xantho-erythrodermia-perstans type on the upper limbs and lesions of large plaque parapsoriasis on the lower limbs.
2. Patient No.2, a Turkish Cypriot, presented with well demarcated skin lesions on the trunk, obliquely arranged in the direction of the ribs. This benign type of parapsoriasis (chronic superficial dermatitis or digitate dermatosis) appeared two years previously.

Table 1. Patients treated by Ro 10–9359

Patient No.	Age	Sex	Diagnosis	Disease Duration	Treatment Duration
1 (BEI . . .)	50	M	PPP	12 years	1 month
2 (HEK . . .)	38	M	PPP	2 years	3 months
3 (PIL . . .)	61	M	PPP	3 months	4 months
4 (BOU . . .)	49	M	MF	10 years	1 month
5 (DEC . . .)	54	M	MF	9 years	2 months

3. Patient No. 3 had noticed, three months previously several large oval, rose-coloured plaques with thin, discrete scales on the bathing trunk area, axillae and popliteal fossae. The absence of pruritus and the histology were more in favour of large plaque parapsoriasis than mycosis fungoides.

4. Patient No. 4, an Algerian, presented with mycosis fungoides of ten years duration. Clinically most of the lesions were of the poikiloderma atrophicans vasculare type. The lesions were histologically characteristic of mycosis fungoides. The patient complained of moderately severe pruritus. Investigations showed no extracutaneous extension.

5. Patient No. 5, an alcoholic with chronic pancreatitis, also presented with large plaque parapsoriasis and poikiloderma evolving over a period of more than nine years. The patient was asymptomatic. The histology was diagnostic of mycosis fungoides. There was no palpable lymphadenopathy.

Group II

Five other patients (number six to ten) were treated by PUVA for a cutaneous epidermotropic lymphoma. Their age is recorded in Table 2 as well as the disease duration. The clinical history of these five patients is the following.

1. Patient No. 6, obese, treated by PUVA for two years, had noticed the reappearance of oval lesions in the inguinal regions during the previous three months. These lesions were clinically and histologically typical of plaque stage mycosis fungoides.

2. Patient No. 7, who had been treated by PUVA for more than three years, presented a reoccurrence of the cutaneous lesions for a second time. These plaque lesions were localized on the scalp, face and neck.

3. Patient No. 8, obese and hypertensive, treated by PUVA for two years had noticed a reoccurrence of mycosis fungoides lesions for the third time following withdrawal of PUVA. We had commenced retinoid therapy at a time when she had eleven recurrent nodules on the neck.

4. Patient No. 9 was seen in 1940 by Tsanck who had diagnosed acute pityriasis lichenoides (Mucha-Haberman disease). These papular and necrotic lesions have recurred periodically until present. In addition since 1961 parapsoriasis en plaques with poikiloderma had progressively appeared. In 1975 a diagnosis of mycosis fungoides was made and PUVA therapy commenced. In 1980 while still under PUVA he developed a tumor on the face.

5. Patient No. 10 was treated for two years and ten months by PUVA for Sézary's syndrome which had been transiently associated with a monoclonal dysglobulinemia. PUVA had little effect on the cutaneous symptoms and no effect on the number of circulating Sézary cells.

We have given Ro 10-9359 to three other patients with Sézary's syndrome who were also being treated by cytophoresis. Occurrence of a staphylococcal septicemia in one of these three patients caused us to stop the retinoid in all the cases.

Methods

1. Five patients (numbers one to five) were treated by Ro 10-9359 alone at a dose of 1 mg/kg/day during the first month and then 0.7 mg/kg/day during the following months. The duration of treatment by the retinoid is indicated in Table 1 for each patient.

Skin tests of delayed type hypersensitivity were carried out after one month of treatment by retinoid using dinitrochlorobenzene and seven recall antigens (tetanus, diphteria, streptococcus, proteus, candida, trichophyton and tuberculin).

Table 2. Patients treated by Ro 10-9359 and PUVA.

Patient No.	Age	Sex	Diagnosis	Disease Duration	Treatment Duration
6 (CHA...)	66	F	MF	4 years	22 days
7 (DUR...)	48	F	MF	3 years, 4 months	17 days
8 (RAT...)	70	F	MF	8 years	1 month
9 (TAB...)	71	M	MF	19 years	1 month
10 (DUG...)	59	M	SS	2 years, 10 months	3 months

2. The five other patients (numbers six to ten) were treated with retinoid and PUVA. In the whole group the same frequency and dose of PUVA was continued after adding the retinoid. The retinoid was given at a dose of 1 mg/kg/day during the time shown in Table 2.

Results

Patients Treated by Ro 10-9359 (No. 1–5)

None of the three patients with parapsoriasis en plaques improved after the first month of treatment. Clearing of the lesions was achieved in the two cases where the treatment was continued. In patient No. 2 the disappearance of the lesions was obtained at the end of three months treatment. However this patient had been extensively exposed to the sun during this time. In patient No. 3 the clearing was achieved after four months treatment without exposure to sunlight.

In patient No. 4 there was no improvement after one month of treatment. Patient No. 5 seemed to be clinically improved after one month of treatment. However histologically, the lymphocytic infiltrate remained just as intense. Furthermore the epidermotropism of the cells with convoluted nuclei appeared even more accentuated after one month of treatment.

The DNCB and recall antigen reactions did not differ from controls.

Patients Treated by Ro 10-9359 and PUVA (No. 6–10)

In patient No. 6, we noticed the disappearance of the lesions of the bathing trunk area after twentytwo days of treatment. Histology after these twentytwo days showed persistance of the deep perivascular infiltrate. The cells of the infiltrate seemed to be very modified cytologically with the appearance of large vacuoles and modified nuclei.

In patient No. 7 there was a disappearance of the lesions of mycosis fungoides in exposed areas after seventeen days of treatment. In patients No. 8 and 9 the tumors had disappeared after one month of treatment.

In the patient with Sézary's syndrome, addition of the retinoid did not bring about any improvement except on the palmo-plantar keratodermia.

Comments

Our study shows that retinoid used as the sole therapy does not cure by itself mycosis fungoides and parapsoriasis en plaques. However it is effective when combined with sunlight in parapsoriasis en plaques and with PUVA in mycosis fungoides.

We have no precise explanation for its action, but it is possible that the retinoid increases the penetration of solar radiation and PUVA by causing a thinning of the epidermis.

Other explanations may be considered. It has been suggested that retinoids have an immunomodulating effect which may account for their beneficial action in certain skin diseases. However our in vivo results are not in favour of an immunostimulating effect of Ro 10-9359. A stimulating effect of retinoids on Langerhans' cells has also been suggested. Therefore it would be interesting to count precisely the number of Langerhans' cells before and after treatment by retinoid in patients with mycosis fungoides.

We feel that there is probably not a single specific action of retinoid which could account for its effect in mycosis fungoides.

Summary

An oral aromatic retinoid (Ro 10-9359) was given to 6 patients with mycosis fungoides and to 3 patients with parapsoriasis en plaque.

In 5 patients, 3 with parapsoriasis and 2 with mycosis fungoides, the drug was given as the sole treatment for a month at a dose of 1 mg per kg bodyweight per day with an objective clinical improvement in 2 cases out of 3 parapsoriasis. Mycosis fungoides did not respond favourably.

In 4 cases of mycosis fungoides the retinoid was administered simultaneously with PUVA-therapy because the lesions had relapsed under PUVA-therapy alone. A rapid improvement was then obtained with a complete clearing of the lesions.

A study of delayed hypersensitivity tests (DNCB and intradermal reactions to 7 normal antigens) was carried out in all the patients to evaluate the effect of Ro 10-9359 on cellular immunity.

Acknowledgment. Dr. R. Fulton is supported by a Medical Research Council Exchange Fellowship.

C.E. Orfanos et al. (eds.)
Retinoids

Effects of Retinoid Ro 10-9359 Alone or in Combined Therapy in Several Skin Diseases - Clinical Observations and Biochemical Data

M. Binazzi and M. Papini

We have been experimenting with the aromatic retinoid in its oral and local form about 4 years and, after having carried out a large initial trial, we limited their use to certain skin diseases which were then followed up for a long period.

Ro 10-9359 (Tigason) was administered after meals at a dose of 1–2 mg/kg/day for varying periods from 15–20 days to 3–4 months. When necessary the treatment was repeated after differing time intervals.

Ro 11-1430 (Tasmaderm) was used in 0.1% cream or lotion and applied once or twice daily without dressing. Occlusive dressing was employed only on hyperkeratotic lesions.

Naturally, we tried to improve the Tigason activity, reduce the dosage and, therefore, the side effects and increase the duration of the favourable effects. In order to achieve this, we administered combined therapy with 50,000–150,000 UI/day retinol after meals beginning on the 5th–7th day after the start of Tigason to most patients, and continued even after stopping Tigason. The idea of the association was based on the notion that vitamin-A-aldehyde may be irreversibly transformed into vitamin-A-acid by an oxidase (4). The metabolic pathway of vitamin-A-acid in the body is unknown, but it could lead to the formation of metabolites, either aromatic or non-aromatic, with aromatic retinoid-like activity. Another possibility would be that the simultaneous action of retinol and the aromatic retinoid remove the presumed metabolic block.

In addition, we also gave small doses of fluocortolone in some cases.

Results

We, therefore, report the effects observed in certain skin disorders treated with Tigason alone and in combined therapy.

Our most outstanding results were with *15 Darier's disease* patients, 4 of which were extensive. Administration of Tigason resulted in the rapid reduction of the characteristically unpleasant smell and itching in severe cases. A marked decrease in the hyperkeratosis of the soles and palms was obtained within 2 weeks. After 4 week's treatment there was large scale desquamation of the diseased skin towards the surrounding healthy skin. The pigmentation faded, the skin became smoother and softer and, at the same time, less dry. The effect lasted 40–60 days, but proved to be repeatable with an identical latent period and overall duration.

The association of retinol gave more rapid and complete effects without any unwanted side effects. We were also able to reduce the Tigason doses during the maintenance phase and to continue this for long periods. In 2 patients, the treatment was repeated at intervals for 3 years and to date there have been no important side effects to intervene with the treatment.

When Tasmaderm cream and, particularly, the lotion was applied to the more hypertrophic lesions, the effect was considerably accentuated within a relatively short period of time. We observed that Tasmaderm application alone was sufficient to control mild and circumscribed cases and for maintenance therapy of the more diffuse forms. Side effects and laboratory abnormalities were slight and very limited and did not cause interruption of the therapy.

The effects we report in *100 psoriatics* are somewhat different to those of other investigators. We did not observe an early improvement in lesions on the head and neck or complete effects on pustular psoriasis. Combined retinol therapy gave good results in most cases, but in others which seemed identical it was not advantageous. Combined Tasmaderm therapy lead to an earlier and more prolonged effect and was particularly efficacious in elephantine, hyperkeratotic and infiltrative psoriasis. Although it was equally effective in guttate psoriasis, a marked congestion often remained.

In this series unwanted side effects were rare. In fact, in 3 cases we observed a small rise in SGOT and SGPT between the 1st and 2nd week of treatment; but only in one case was it necessary to interrupt the therapy. Extensive telogen effluvium of the head and body hair, then of the eyebrows, pubic and underarm hair, was observed in 3 patients treated continuously for more than 4 months. The side effect promptly improved and the hair grew naturally when treatment was stopped.

Tigason therapy was not consistently beneficial in *24* cases of varying types and severity of *psoriatic arthropathy.*

The treatment was not decisively effective in psoriatic erythroderma, as it reduced the hyperkeratosis, but did not influence the congestion.

On the whole the activity of Tigason can be equalled or surpassed by PUVA or methotrexate therapy, but Tigason is decidedly more practical and less harmful.

Biochemical investigations on dermatome biopsy samples from diseased and healthy *skin of psoriatics* revealed an increase in phospholipids and bound arachidonic acid and this agrees with the findings of Gerstein (3) and Tsambaos et al. (7).
After 10 day's Tigason at 1 mg/kg/day, although the skin was less hyperkeratotic and congested, there was a significant increase in total and single classes of phospholipids in diseased, but not in healthy, skin. At the same time the diseased skin manifest a significant percentage decrease in arachidonic acid bound to the phospholipids, while in healthy skin it was markedly increased.

The phospholipid behaviour can be explained by a reduction in phospholipidase activity, while the behaviour of the arachidonic acid is difficult to interpret and further research is in progress.

Based on reports in the literature and bearing in mind the known effects of Tigason on mucopolysaccharides and glycoproteins (2, 5) we treated *25 skin, skin-mucous and mucous lichen ruber planus* cases. The effect of Tigason was incomplete and the disease sometimes relapsed during the course of treatment, especially when the patient underwent a new bout of psychic stress. Because of its side effects on the mucosa and on hair, it was not well tolerated. Combined therapy with fluocortolone enhanced the effects and partially avoided relapse. However, long-term treatment had to be undertaken.

The association of Tigason and retinol did not give any better effects. However, an improvement was observed when Tigason, retinol and fluocortolone were used in association. Nevertheless, relapse also occurred easily and, because of the statistically significant LRP-diabetes association, the possible diabetogenic action of fluocortolone limits its use (1, 6). In contrast, hypertrophic, verrucous and infiltrative lesions improved markedly when topical Tasmaderm application was combined with the oral therapy.

There were only limited and transitory effects in the *2 cases of X-linked* and *ichthyosis vulgaris* we treated. However, the doses used were low and the trial was not extended beyond a 30-day period owing to the tender age of the patients. However, with further experience this precaution was found to be unnecessary in a baby girl with congenital ichthyosis erythroderma seen at birth, who was studied biochemically without success. She is now 11 years old and also suffers from deafness and tendon retraction. Treatment with Tigason, retinol, and Tasmaderm gave very favourable effects, especially on the hyperkeratotic areas on the elbows, knees and calves.

In another case, a 27-year-old male, Tigason eliminated the hyperkeratosis and there was softening of the skin, but only slight modification of the congestion. Tolerance was good, even if, after 50 days there was extensive falling of body and head hairs. The addition of retinol did not result in any pronounced improvement of the therapeutic effects and/or tolerance; while medication with Tasmaderm was very efficacious in the hyperkeratotic areas. After 2 months of treatment relapsing pyogenic perionyxis was observed in both these cases of congenital ichthyosis erythroderma.

We treated *3 cases* of *pityriasis rubra pilaris.* One, an 8-year-old girl, also had polymyositis. The skin condition cleared within 6 days of treatment and the result was maintained for one year with Tasmaderm lotion; the polymyositis regressed with cortisone treatment. Another girl of 6 years who had suffered from pityriasis rubra pilaris for 3 years, and in whom the skin disease worsened seriously after oral retinol, manifest the same result after the first doses of Tigason when she was later treated by us. However, we observed a slow resolution of the hyperkeratotic papules when 0.5 mg/kg/day Tigason was combined with 300 mg/day zinc sulphate, but the moderate congestion persisted and there was no change in the hypochromia in the following 3 months. In an 18-year-old girl, Tigason administration provoked side effects, but no beneficial therapeutic results; while a remission was obtained with 200 mg/day zinc sulphate. The retinol binding protein level in this patient was more or less zero.

Associated retinol and Tasmaderm treatment cured *several cases* of *Meleda and Unna-Thost-type palmo-plantar keratoderma,* but there was a tendency to relapse.

The same treatment was useful or very useful in *eczematous and mycotic palmo-plantar keratoderma* cases. On the other hand, transitory or negative effects were observed in leukoplakia, Recklinghausen's disease, tuberous sclerosis, Kaposi's sarcoma (3 cases) and mycosis fungoides (5 cases).

Finally, we treated *10 cases* of *persistent palmo-plantar pustulosis* with Tigason, sometimes combined with low doses of fluocortolone and obtained beneficial but transitory results in some, while 3 cases failed to respond. In the positive cases there was progressive reduction in the number and severity of the pustules followed by desquamation and limited decongestion. However, even in the cases where improvement was encouraging, the pustules at times reoccurred during treatment. Furthermore, when the dose was reduced, relapse was frequent.

Maybe persistent palmo-plantar pustulosis could be identified on the basis of its response to treatment with Tigason. Considering the difficulty of interpreting the effects obtained in this disorder and bearing in mind the effects at the cellular level in other conditions, it could be suggested that the persistent palmo-plantar pustulosis cases which show some degree of responsiveness to Tigason may be associated with psoriasis.

Summary

The results obtained with aromatic retinoid Ro 10-9359 in several skin diseases are briefly reported.

Combined therapy with oral retinol, fluocortolone or 0.1% Ro 11-1430 cream or lotion for the enhancement or maintenance of the activity and reduction of side effects is discussed.

Finally, the results of an investigation on phospholipids in healthy and psoriatic skin before and after Ro 10-9359 revealed modifications that were parallel with the curative effects.

References

1. Binazzi M, Lisi P, Calandra P (1978) Studies on the association between skin disorders and diabetes. Ann Ital Dermatol Clin Sper 32:211–234
2. DeLuca L, Maestri N, Bonanni F, Nelson D (1972) Maintenance of epithelial cell differentiation: The mode of action of vitamin A. Cancer 30:1326–1331
3. Gerstein W (1963) The phospholipids of normal and psoriatic skin. J Invest Derm 40:105–109
4. Isler O (1977) Progress in the field of fat-soluble vitamins and carotenoids. Experientia 33:555–696
5. Levinson SS, Wolf G (1972) The effect of Vitamin A acid on glycoprotein synthesis in skin tumors (Keratoacanthomas). Cancer Res 32:2248–2252
6. Lisi P (1980) Associazione lichen ruber planus – diabete. Ann Ital Dermatol Clin Sper 34:129–134
7. Tsambaos D, Kalofoutis A, Stratigos J, Miras C, Capetanakis J (1977) Thin-layer chromatography of phospholipid components of normal and psoriatic epidermis. Br J Dermatol 97:135–138

C.E. Orfanos et al. (eds.)
Retinoids

Effect of Systemic Ro 10-9359 Treatment on Immunological Parameters in Darier's Disease

A.-M. Soppi, E. Soppi and C.T. Jansén

The cutaneous disturbances of patients suffering from Darier's disease (keratosis follicularis) are well known, and are generally thought to reflect an abnormality in keratinocyte maturation. Recently, data have been presented indicating that Darier patients, in addition, suffer from a dysfunction of the cell-mediated immune system (2, 3, 5). As oral retinoids are known to be effective in reverting the epidermal changes of this disease (6), we thought it to be of interest to analyze, whether retinoids also might affect the immune function of Darier patients. To answer this question, several immunological parameters were tested in 5 Darier patients. Thereafter, 4 of the patients took oral etretinate (Ro 10-9359), 50–70 mg daily for 6–8 weeks, and the immunological tests were repeated. Normal values were obtained from analyzing 5 age- and sex-matched individual controls and an additional group of 12 healthy persons.

In lymphocyte transformation tests, using Ficoll-Hypaque isolated lymphocytes and single concentrations of ConA (40 µg/ml), PHA-M (125 µg/ml), PPD (10 µg/ml) and PWM (1:80), results were roughly within the normal range. After retinoid treatment, however, a marked depression in the lymphocyte stimulation response was seen in most assays (Fig. 1). Using a whole-blood incubation system (8), the dose-response profile over the range of 1–625 µg/ml for ConA and 5–1250 µg/ml for PHA were determined. The pre-treatment results of all 5 patients showed an abnormal dose-response curve for ConA lacking the usual inhibitory effect of supraoptimal lectin concentrations; the same was found for PHA in 1 patient. In 3 cases, a normalized dose-response curve was found after retinoid treatment. These results are compatible with a pre-treatment deficiency in suppressor cell function, and the restoration of suppressor cell function by retinoid therapy.

Our test system included 3 different assays for suppressor cells. As an estimate of suppressor cell number, the ability of theophyllin to inhibit the E-rosette formation of isolated lymphocytes was used. The absolute and relative numbers of theophyllin-sensitive rosettes was normal prior to treatment; after retinoid treatment a slight increase in the relative numbers was seen. As an *indirect* functional test of suppressor cell function, we measured the effect of 1 µg/ml of indomethacin in whole-blood lymphocyte stimulation assays (1). The enhancing effect of indomethacin on ConA responses was greater after retinoid treatment than before therapy (indicating an increased suppressor cell function), whereas the effect of indomethacin on PHA responses diminished during treatments. Some variation in the individual responses of the different patients was, however, seen. As a *direct* functional assay of suppressor cell function, the method of Shou et al. (7) was utilized, using ConA or PHA for suppressor cell activation and ConA, PHA or PWM in the second lymphocyte transformation step. Pre-treatment suppressor cell activities were roughly within the normal range. After retinoid therapy, both ConA and PHA-induced suppressor cell activities showed an increasing tendency.

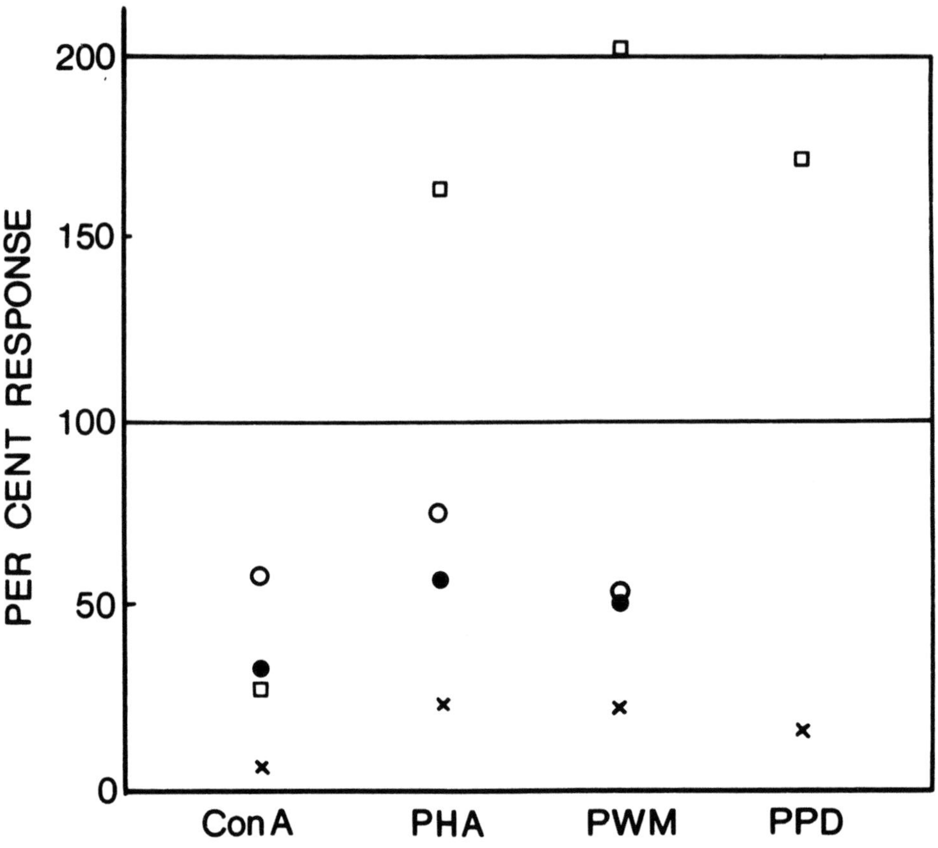

Fig. 1. Effect of systemic etretinate treatment on lymphocyte transformation tests. The results are expressed as the percentage of the response during treatment as compared with pre-treatment values. The different symbols represent different patients

Summary

In conclusion, our studies revealed, in Darier patients, an abnormality in lectin dose response curves, compatible with a deranged suppressor cell function. Systemic etretinate therapy suppressed lymphocyte stimulation tests. Indirect and direct assays for suppressor cell function indicated that this could be due to an activation of suppressor cell function by etretinate.

References

1. Goodwin JS, Bankhurst AD, Messner RP (1977) Suppression of human T-cell mitogenesis by prostaglandin. Existence of a prostaglandin-producing suppressor cell. J Exp Med 146:1719–1734
2. Humeniuk JM, Huwitz W, Jegasothy BV (1979) Immunologic studies in patients with Darier's disease. J Invest Dermatol 73:310
3. Humeniuk JM, Jegasothy BV (1980) Darier's disease: a partially immunodeficient state. J Invest Dermatol 74:260–261

4. Limatibul S, Shore A, Dosch HM, Gelfand EW (1978) Theophylline modulation of E-rosette formation: an indicator of T-cell maturation. Clin Exp Immunol 33:503–513
5. Marks JG, Thor DE, Lowe RS (1978) Darier's disease. An immunologic study. Arch Dermatol 114:1336–1339
6. Orfanos CE, Kurka M, Strunk V (1978) Oral treatment of keratosis follicularis with a new aromatic retinoid. Arch Dermatol 114:1211–1214
7. Shou L, Schwartz SA, Good RA (1976) Suppressor cell activity after concanavalin A treatment of lymphocytes from normal donors. J Exp Med 143:1100–1110
8. Viljanen MK, Eskola J (1977) PPD-induced lymphocyte transformation in vitro using whole blood. Clin Immunol Immunopathol 8:28–33

C.E. Orfanos et al. (eds.)
Retinoids

Freeze-Fracture Study of Psoriatic Lesions After Oral Administration of Retinoid

R. Caputo, G. Gasparini, D. Contini and E. Berti

The ultrastructural investigations carried out up to now with traditional techniques in psoriatic epidermis after oral administration of the aromatic retinoid Ro 10-9359 (7) have shown three prominent fine structural changes: enhanced inflammation with some cell degeneration in the malpighian layer, extracellular accumulation of mucus-like material, reappearance of keratohyalin granules, but they have failed to allow any study of the inner structure of plasma membranes.

Since it is known that vitamin A compounds are able to induce marked modifications of the conformation and distribution of membrane specializations on epithelia in vitro and in vivo (4, 8, 9) we studied epidermis specimens from psoriatic subjects under oral treatment with Ro 10-9359. Our investigations were carried out with the freeze-fracture technique, which is especially suitable for obtaining this kind of information.

This research was obviously preceded by an accurate freeze-fracture study of untreated psoriatic skin (3).

Materials and Methods

Bioptic fragments of affected and unaffected skin were collected from 5 cases of particularly extensive psoriasis, after 10–15 days of oral treatment with 75 mg of Ro 10-9359/day and from further 2 patients, after 30 days of treatment with the same dose of the compound. The specimens were fixed with 3% glutaraldehyde in phosphate buffer 0.12 M, pH 7.3 for 2 to 3 h at 4 °C and then infiltrated with increasing concentrations (10%, 20%, 30%) of glycerol buffered with phosphate 0.12 M, pH 7.3. The samples were frozen by immersion in Freon 22, cooled to -150 °C in liquid nitrogen and freeze-fractured according to the method of Moor et al. (6) in a Balzer freeze-etching device. The fracturing temperature was -115 °C. Platinum carbon replicas were washed in sodium hypochloride to remove the organic material and then in distilled water, and recovered on 200-mesh copper grids. The replicas were examined with an EM 400 electron microscope.

Results

Affected Skin After 10–15 Days of Treatment

The cytoplasm of basal layer cells exhibits a particularly well developed Golgi apparatus, while that of spinous layer cells is rich in particle-free vacuolar formations. Both in the basal and in the spinous layers, intercellular spaces are quite dilated (Fig. 1) and contain a finely granular substance, generally close to the plasma membranes and probably corresponding to the mucus-like substance observed with traditional techniques (7). In addition, the intercellular spaces exhibit particle-free vacuolar formations (Fig. 1).

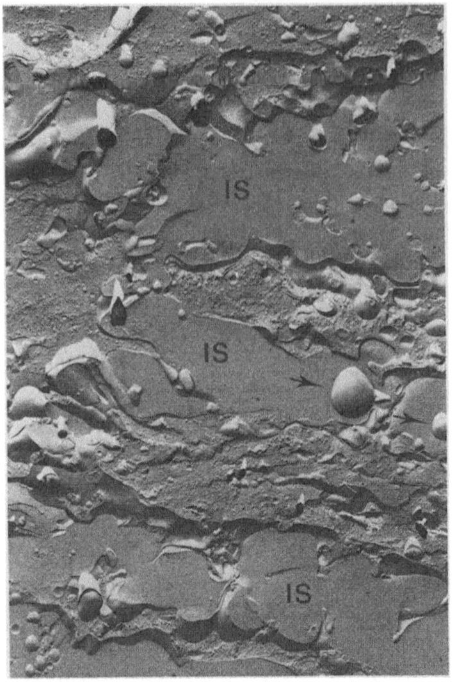

1

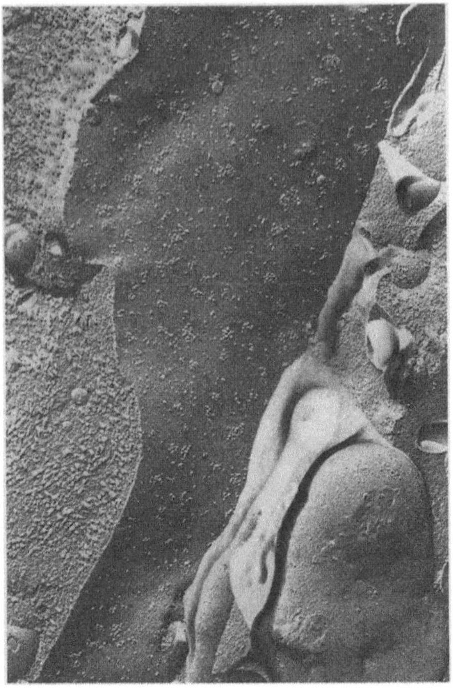

2

Fig. 1. *Affected skin after 10–15 days of oral treatment with 75 mg of Ro 10-9359.* The intercellular spaces of the spinous layer are markedly dilated and contain a finely granular substance and particle-free vacuolar formations (→) IS = intercellular space. × 7,100
Fig. 2. *Affected skin after 10–15 days of oral treatment with 75 mg of Ro 10-9359.* Membrane of a cell of the spinous layer. The membrane particles form small clusters of 10–15 units. No desmosomes are observed. × 28,000

The membranes of many cells show a modified arrangement of particles which, instead of being irregularly distributed, tend to form small clusters of 10–15 units (Fig. 2).

Particle clusters ascribable to desmosomes are rarely observed, while gap junctions are quite frequent and are found also in the cytoplasm (Fig. 3).

In the transition layer, membrane particles are normally distributed and desmosomes tend to be numerous. Gap junctions are always present; tight junction strands are occasionally observed. Intercellular spaces are completely obliterated by keratinosomes (Fig. 3). This technique does not allow keratohyalin granules to be revealed.

The membranes of horny layer cells appear similar to those observed in normal epidermis (2). Only few membrane jumps are observed, in spite of the high amount of keratinosomes present in intercellular spaces.

Affected Skin After 30 Days of Treatment

The cytoplasm of basal and spinous layer cells appears normal, vacuolar formations being only sporadically observed. Intercellular spaces are moderately dilated, but they may contain finely granular material. Membrane particles are irregularly distributed. The number and appearance of desmosomes are normal. Desmosomes centered by a gap junction can occasionally be seen (Fig. 4).

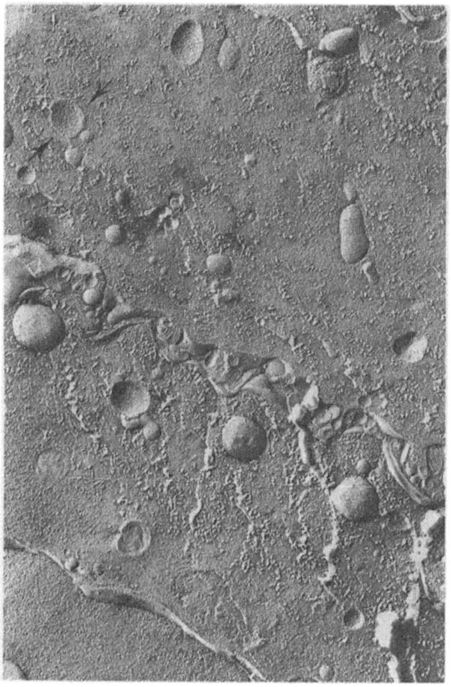

3

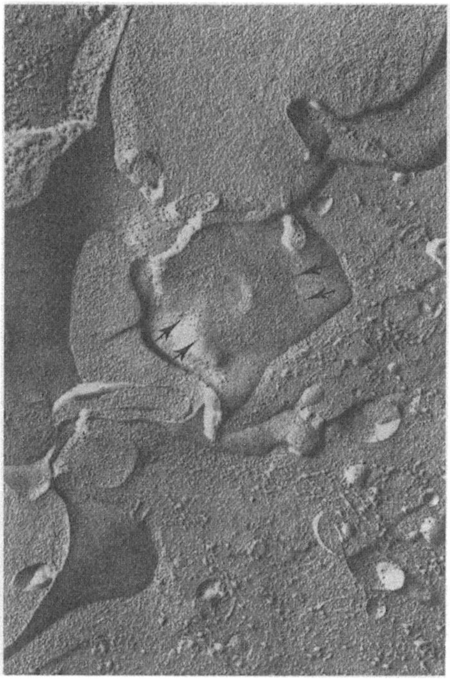

4

Fig. 3. *Affected skin after 10–15 days of oral treatment with 75 mg of Ro 10-9359.* Transition layer. The intercellular space is completely occupied by keratinosomes. Arrows show an intracytoplasmic gap junction. × 21,000

Fig. 4. *Affected skin after 30 days of oral treatment with 75 mg of Ro 10-9359.* Arrows indicate a desmosome centered by a gap junction. × 19,000

Gap junctions are always numerous and keratinosomes occupy the intercellular spaces of the transition layer. The horny layer is unmodified.

Unaffected Skin After 10–15 Days of Treatment

In unaffected skin, the only remarkable modifications are a moderate dilation of intercellular spaces, which however do not contain the finely granular substance, an increase in the number of gap junctions and the presence of many keratinosomes in the intercellular spaces of the transition layer.

Discussion

In untreated psoriatic epidermis (3) the freeze-fracture technique revealed that the plasma membrane changes apparently involved mainly the lower layer where many keratinocytes differed from those of normal epidermis and of unaffected psoriatic skin, because of the higher density of membrane-particles and of the increased number of gap junctions. The increase of membrane associated particles may represent the morphological intramembranous equivalent of changes in the outer cell membrane demonstrated with cytochemical techniques (5), whereas the increase in gap junctions can be interpreted as a phenomenon compensating the uncontrolled cell proliferation.

The freeze-fracture study of affected and unaffected psoriatic skin after oral treatment with Ro 10-9359 showed that drug-induced ultrastructural changes involve mainly the affected epidermis and are particularly evident in the lower layers during the second week of treatment.

An examination of the replicas, in addition to confirming the data obtained up to now with thin sections (7), i.e. an abnormal dilation of intercellular spaces containing a finely granular substance, the peculiar development of the Golgi apparatus and cytoplasmic vacuolization, enabled us to reveal modifications in the inner structure of cell membranes.

Indeed, after 10–15 days of treatment the membranes of many cells of the basal and spinous layers showed a decrease in the number of desmosomes and a modified distribution of membrane particles. The decrease of desmosomes, already reported, and interpreted as a possible effect on epithelial cells by vitamin A compounds (1, 8) might be the consequence of the abnormal dilation of intercellular spaces, or of a reduced availability of particles.

The modified distribution of membrane particles, i.e. the formation of small particle clusters comprising 10–15 units might be:

- an aspecific sign of cell impairment
- the consequence of a modified membrane arrangement, caused by the drug
- the expression of an attempt to form desmosomes (incomplete desmosomes).

In psoriatic skin treated with Ro 10-9359, the increase in the number of gap junctions, which can be induced by vitamin A compounds (4, 9) does not appear to be particularly significative, since these junctions are quite frequent also in psoriatic lesions of untreated subjects.

Finally, the interpretation of the appearance of mixed junctions (desmosomes centered by a gap junction), or of the high amount of keratinosomes in the intercellular spaces of the transition layer still needs to be clarified.

Summary

The freeze-fracture technique was used to study bioptic fragments of affected and unaffected skin from 5 cases of psoriasis, after 10–15 days of oral treatment with 75 mg of Tigason and from 2 cases, after 30 days of treatment at the same dose. This investigation confirmed and extended the data so far obtained with thin sections, namely, the presence of a finely granular substance in the abnormally dilated intercellular spaces of the basal and spinous layers; the peculiar development of the Golgi apparatus; the cytoplasmic vacuolization and the remarkable amount of keratinosomes contained in the intercellular spaces of the transition layer. In addition, it demonstrated that, especially after 10–15 days of treatment, modifications of the inner structure of plasma membranes could be observed. Indeed, the membranes of many cells of the basal and spinous layers showed a decrease in the number of desmosomes and a modified distribution of particles, which were often grouped into small clusters of 10–15 units. The high number of gap junctions did not appear to be particularly significant, since these junctions are quite frequent also in psoriatic lesions of untreated subjects.

References

1. Blanchet-Bardon C, Anton-Lamprecht I, Schnyder UW (1977) Erythrodermie congénitale ichtyosiforme bulleuse. Contrôle ultrastructural du traitement par l'éther éthylique d'un dérivé aromatique de l'acide rétinoïque. Ann Derm Venereol 104:648–653
2. Caputo R, Peluchetti D (1977) The junctions of normal human epidermis. A freeze-fracture study. J Ultrastruct Res 61:44–61

3. Caputo R, Innocenti M, Gasparini G, Peluchetti D (1978) Plasma membranes in psoriatic cells. A freeze-fracture study. J Invest Dermatol 71:245–249
4. Elias PM, Friend DS (1976) Vitamin A-Induced Mucous Metaplasia. An in vitro system for modulating tight and gap junction differentiation. J Cell Biol 68:173–188
5. Mahrle G, Orfanos CE (1975) Ultrastructural localization and differentiation of membrane-bound ATP utilizing enzymes including adenyl cyclase in normal and psoriatic epidermis. Br J Dermatol 93:495–502
6. Moor H, Muhlethaler K, Waldner H, Frey-Wyssling A (1961) A new freezing ultramicrotome. J Biophys Biochem Cytol 10:1–10
7. Orfanos CE, Runne U (1978) Tissue changes in psoriatic plaques after oral administration of retinoid. Dermatologica 157 (Suppl 1):19–25
8. Peck GL, Elias PM, Wetzel B (1977) Effects of retinoic acid on embryonic chick skin. J Invest Dermatol 69:463–476
9. Prutkin L (1975) Mucous metaplasia and gap junctions in the vitamin A acid-treated skin tumor, keratoacanthoma. Cancer Res 35:364–369

C.E. Orfanos et al. (eds.)
Retinoids

Psoriasiform Dermatitis in Patients with Skin Diseases Other than Psoriasis as Side Effect of Ro 10-9359

Th. Rufli

During clinical trials with Ro 10-9359 (Tigason) (aromatic retinoid = AR) in psoriatic patients, we observed for the first time that 9 out of 23 patients developed a dermatitis, occurring as a single event or repeatedly during AR medication. We later termed this eruption retinoid dermatitis (2).

Case 1

A 66-year-old male patient, weighing 78 kg and with a history of extensive psoriasis for 13 years, was given 75 mg AR daily. On the tenth day of medication, he showed a maculo-papular dermatitis extending over the face, the neck, the interscapular region, the exterior surface of the upper arms, the interior surface of the lower arms, the sides of the chest and the abdomen. The patient complained of slight burning and intense itching. After cessation of the AR therapy and the application of topical and systemic corticosteroids, the dermatitis cleared within 10 days.

After 10 days of intermission, the patient was again given AR in a daily dosage of 25 mg. The retinoid dermatitis reappeared immediately and persisted in spite of reduction of the dosage (25 mg every second, then every third day). Only when AR therapy was completely stopped, did it clear.

Five months later, the patient took one capsule of 25 mg of his own accord. Again the dermatitis relapsed, showing papular, partly vesicular lesions with an urticarial component.

A year later, the patient attended a practising dermatologist and was given 50 mg of AR daily. Again, the patient developed a papulovesicular dermatitis with the characteristic distribution after 10 days.

The histological examination of the retinoid dermatitis in psoriatic patients regularly displayed the picture of an acute, unspecific dermatitis with spongiosis, intraepidermal vesicles and distinct intracellular oedema of the surrounding cells. There were perivascular lymphocytic infiltrates extending into the epidermis.

There was no coincidence of this dermatitis with any other known side effects of AR. Pruritus was the only symptom which regularly preceded the appearance of retinoid dermatitis.

The dermatitis did not seem to depend on the absolute daily dose or the total dose received. There was, however, a distinct dose dependence in the individual patient.

In some patients, the retinoid dermatitis caused an outbreak of new psoriasis lesions in sites, which to an experienced psoriatic were unusual, but which coincided with the distribution of the retinoid dermatitis. Early reduction of the dose prevented this reaction regarded as Koebner's isomorphic phenomenon.

By chance we discovered the regression of plantar warts in psoriatics under retinoid therapy. We then tried the effect of AR in selected patients with warts. We found complete

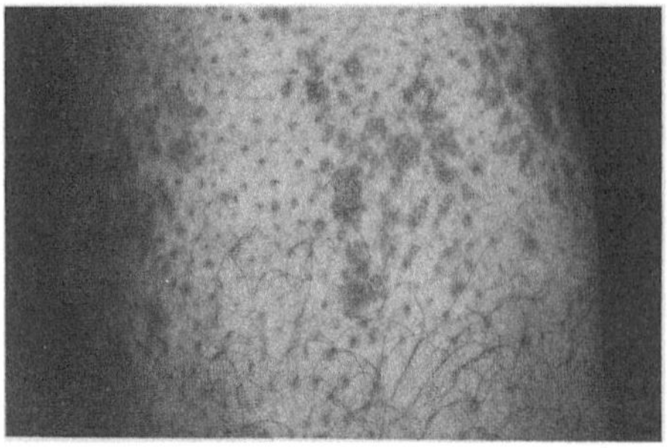

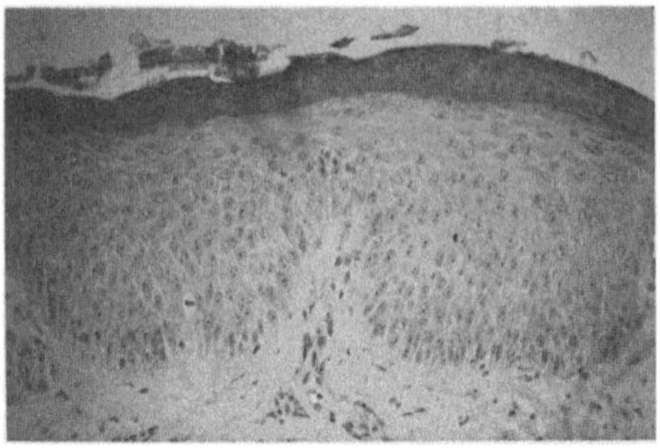

Fig. 1. Case 2. Retinoid dermatitis on the calves in a patient with common warts
Fig. 2. Histological picture of the retinoid dermatitis (case 2): psoriasiform dermatitis

regression in 3 out of 4 patients with plantar warts. AR proved less effective in the treatment of common warts, only 2 out of 12 patients were cured and had no relapse (1).

During this trial, we again observed the occurrence of retinoid dermatitis in 6 out of 18 patients. Sites of election were again the face and neck, the exterior surface of the upper arms, the interior surface of the lower arms, the sides of the chest and abdomen.

Case 2

The 30-year-old male patient with a body weight of 69 kg had multiple common warts on both hands. After an initial medication of 50 mg AR daily during one week and 75 mg during the second and third week, the retinoid dermatitis appeared in the form of a follicular papular exanthema in the popliteal fossa and on the calves (Fig. 1), less pronounced on the neck, and accompanied by severe pruritus.

The histological examination revealed, as in all the other examined patients with warts and retinoid dermatitis, the picture of a psoriasiform dermatitis with a sometimes only focal, sometimes continuous parakeratosis on an acanthotic epidermis with elongated rete ridges. Scanty round cell infiltrates surround the enlarged capillaries in the corium (Fig. 2).

Case 3

A 24-year-old male patient, weighing 79 kg, was given 150 mg AR daily for the treatment of plantar warts. After 6½ weeks of medication, he complained of pruritus at the hair-line, in the intrascapular and praesternal region. A few days later, an erythema developed on these sites with loosely disseminated papules, which were covered with psoriasiform scales. These papules histologically revealed the picture of a psoriasiform dermatitis.

Also in patients suffering from lichen planus, we observed the occurrence of retinoid dermatitis.

Case 4

A 30-year-old male patient, suffering from lichen planus on the oral and genital mucosae and on both wrists, received AR in a daily dosage of 25 mg. After 2 weeks, a micropapular exanthema developed on both sides of the trunk. Flat, grossly scaling papules spread over the exterior surface of the upper arms and the interior surface of the lower arms. After cessation of AR therapy and application of topical corticosteroids, the dermatitis cleared. The lichen planus lesions were unaffected by the short AR medication.

To sum up, it can be said that the retinoid dermatitis occurs as a side effect of the drug in psoriatics as well as in patients with warts and lichen planus. The various case histories do not reveal a dependence on the total dosage or the daily intake of the AR. Nor is there a correlation with other side effects on skin and mucosae.

We make the diagnosis on the basis of the erythematous-papular form of the individual lesion and the characteristic distribution on the head, trunk and upper extremities. The dermatitis is accompanied by a slightly burning, intensely itching sensation. In non-psoriatic patients, the histological examination reveals a psoriasiform dermatitis with characteristics that are not present in the histology of psoriatics with clinically the same retinoid dermatitis. This difference cannot be explained as yet, nor is the pathogenesis of the retinoid dermatitis at all clear.

Summary

Among the cutaneous side effects of the aromatic vitamin A acid derivative Ro 10-9359, we observed a dermatitis which – when fully developed – shows characteristic primary lesions and a characteristic distribution. The lesions favour the face, neck, exterior surface of the upper and interior surface of the lower arms, the back of the hands, the superior thoracic aperture, the sides of the thorax and the flanks.

In psoriatic patients treated with Ro 10-9359, this papulovesicular retinoid dermatitis displayed an unspecific histological picture, later new psoriatic patches developed on these sites.

In patients who received Ro 10-9359 for other skin diseases, the retinoid dermatitis presented clinically and histologically as psoriasis-like lesions with a similar distribution.

The occurrence of retinoid dermatitis is individually dose-dependent and not correlated with other side effects.

References

1. Rüst O, Rufli Th, Forrer J (1979) Erste Erfahrungen mit dem Vitamin-A-Säure-Derivat Ro 10-9359 bei Virusepitheliomen. Schweiz Med Wochenschr 109:1914–1920
2. Rüst O, Rufli Th (1979) Nebenwirkungen des oralen Retinoids Ro 10-9359 in der nicht erkrankten Haut des Psoriatikers: die „Retinoid-Dermatitis". Schweiz Med Wochenschr 109:1921–1925

C.E. Orfanos et al. (eds.)
Retinoids

Immunological Features of Psoriasis: Effects of Ro 10-9359, Concanavalin A (ConA), Pokeweed Mitogen (PWM) and Methotrexate (MTX) on Cultivated Lymphocytes

A.A. Bialasiewicz, D. Lubach and S. Marghescu

The heterogeneous complex of chronic inflammatory diseases with different underlying causes for the initiation of specific lesions seems to be accompanied and perpetuated by antigen-driven production of nonspecific polyclonal antibody formation (3, 6). Hypotheses have been set up involving an impairment of suppressor cells, increase of specific helper cells or an increase in lymphokine secretion. Some of these suggestions have been made for psoriasis as well (4, 5, 9).

Since the drugs Ro 10-9359 and methotrexate (MTX) rapidly normalize clinical as well as immunological parameters, our experiments intend to demonstrate the action of these agents upon nonspecific antibody production.

Methods

Cell Processing

Peripheral blood lymphocytes were obtained from untreated patients with widespread confluent plaque-like lesions, guttata-type, head-localized and erythrodermic psoriasis during acute stages of the disease; for comparison normals' samples were taken as well. Defibrination and Ficoll-Hypaque gradient separation was performed.

Culture Conditions

The cells were cultured at a concentration of 1×10^6/ml in medium RPMI 1640 at 37 °C in a water-saturated atmosphere plus 5% CO_2 and rocked on a rocker platform. 10% fetal calf serum (FCS) was added.

Plaque Forming Assay

The development of antibody forming cells vs the target antigens sheep red blood cells (SRBC) and burro red blood cells (BRBC) as indicators for polyclonality was monitored, applying the technique of Cunningham and Szenberg (2). IgG and IgM class antibody were estimated over the next 6 days. Viability of cells was measured by Trypan Blue exclusion.

Table 1. Plaque forming cells values at day 1, 3, 5

Day of culture	Lymphocytes +AB-serum		+patients' serum		+Pokeweed Mitogen		+FCS +PWM		Kind of disease
	IgM	IgG	IgM	IgG	IgM	IgG	IgM	IgG	PFC/10^6
1	45	11							
3	109	185	215	125	125	137	15600	17800	Healthy individual
5	125	110	155	170	230	205	19500	21350	
1	564	685							Psoriasis patient
3	820	1187	956	1933	14500	16700			
5	1628	3888	2465	4870	20140	22650			

PFC = plaque forming cells vs. SRBC (sheep red blood cells)
FCS = fetal calf serum

Results

Prestudies

On the day of admission, significant differences in the nonspecific immunoglobulin-producing cells vs SRBC and BRBC can be stated. Table 1 demonstrated the plaque forming cells (PFC) values at day 1, 3, 5 of the in vitro culture. Thus the patients' lymphocytes alone develop a high degree of spontaneously IgG-secreting cells. The addition of erythrocyte-absorbed patients' serum, containing an unscreened mass of immune complexes or other humoral "factors" would have no significant proliferative effect on normal lymphocytes; slight augmentation can be stated for the patient's antibody forming cells (AFC) population. Consistent with previous results (8), no activation of healthy individuals' SRBC-responder-cells can be seen, whereas psoriasis-patients' cells react extensively. Pretreatment of normals' cells with FCS (cf method of 7) however, rendering them "immune cells", caused the development of a comparable amount of AFC. The variations in PFC development vs SRBC or BRBC on the first day ranged from 95 IgM-, 100 IgG-PFC for head-localized (close to normal) to 380 IgM-, 884 IgG-PFC for widespread plaque lesions and 180 IgM-, 590 IgG-PFC for erythrodermic psoriasis.

Pokeweed Mitogen (PWM)-incubation

To evaluate the development of PWM-stimulated AFC in a 6 day-culture, PWM was added in varying concentrations up to 100 µg/ml. The disease types varied significantly in the kinetics of the development of AFC whereby the head-localized form again ranged closest to the normals' "immune cells". In each case, however, the first days of culture showed a clear superiority of IgG- over IgM-forming cells.

Concanavalin A (ConA)-incubation

Addition of ConA, a known suppressor-cell recruiting agent, at the concentration of 40 µg/ml would on day 6 result in a reduction of 90% in the IgM and 93% in the IgG class for guttata-type patients' AFC, of 35% in the IgM and 50% in the IgG class for erythrodermic psoriasis patients' AFC, of 41% in the IgM and 54% in the IgG class for confluent plaque-like lesions and of 93% in the IgM and 94% in the IgG class for head-localized patients' AFC. Normals' immune cells were reduced by 93% for IgM- and 94% for IgG-PFC.

Ro 10-9359 Incubation

Addition of Ro 10-9359 at a concentration of 500 ng/ml to the PWM-stimulated culture would after 5 days result in a reduction of 96% IgM-, 98% IgG-PFC in guttata, of 80% IgM-, 97% IgG-PFC in erythrodermic psoriasis, of 97% in IgM-, 99% IgG-PFC in confluent plaque-like lesions, of 99% IgM-, 99% IgG-PFC in head-localized patients' culture as well as normals' immune cells.

In absolute terms, however, the greater reduction of IgG- than IgM-forming cells is highly significant throughout the experiment. At the given concentration of Ro 10-9359, total abolition of any PFC could be achieved in the healthy immune cell population, although the cells were still viable and no cytotoxic effects were detectable. Increase in the concentration up to 200 µg/ml of the drug at the constant concentration of PWM would not alter the experimental data given above significantly. Currently, investigations are under way concerning the influence of other colloidal antigens as a control for this experiment.

Methotrexate Incubation

Addition of MTX at a concentration of 500 ng/ml – 50 µg/ml would result in a 96% IgM-, 85% IgG-PFC decrease for guttata-type, a 90% IgM- and 90% IgG-PFC decrease for erythrodermic psoriasis, a 97% IgM- and 97% IgG-PFC decrease for plaque-like lesions, and 99% IgM- and 99% IgG-PFC decrease for head-localized psoriasis as well as normals' immune cells after a 5-day culture.

In absolute terms, one can note almost equal effects on IgM- and IgG-AFC formation.

Since we were interested in the possible interference of Ro 10-9359 and ConA in the PWM-system, simultaneous addition of those drugs was performed. In brief, one can note a lesser degree of PFC-inhibition than with MTX alone.

Discussion

Lymphocytes from patients with the disease complex psoriasis exhibit differing increases in the in vitro development of PWM-driven anti-SRBC and anti-BRBC formation, depending on the different forms of acuteness, and the extent of involved tissue. Least abnormalities could be stated for head-localized forms, most severe abnormalities in guttata-type and erythrodermic lesions. Addition of Ro 10-9359 was most effective in reducing non-specific polyclonal antibody formation in guttata, head-localized and confluent forms of the disease, least effective in erythrodermia. MTX-application gave best results in plaque-like and erythrodermic, fewest pronounced results in guttata-lesions. The effects of Ro 10-9359 and ConA on non-specific single cell antibody formation can be stated as being at least partially different. ConA-like behaviour of Ro 10-9359 may be responsible for some of the described phenomena in the in vitro system, however, the profound preference of Ro 10-9359 for a most selective reduction of IgG-forming cells cannot yet be explained. The recruitment of suppressor cells and the influence on helper-suppressor-cell imbalances may be one mechanism. On the other hand, Ro 10-9359 does not act at given concentrations like a cytostatic. We therefore speculate on Ro 10-9359 being effective in immunologically relevant intercellular communication (10) as well as blocking of proliferative responses towards mitogens or mitogenic "factors" (1), and consequently, immune surveillance.

Summary

In the course of some chronic inflammatory processes, nonspecific polyclonal activation of lymphocytes associated with even the formation of autoantibodies has been demonstrated.

Isolated peripheral blood lymphocytes from psoriasis patients were compared with controls and their ability to respond to various stimuli in a Mishell-Dutton culture system. PFC were enumerated over 6 days vs. SRBC as indicator for polyclonality, using the Cunningham and Szenberg technique. (1) On the day of admission, patients' PFC consisted mainly of γ-chain production and ranged at about 800, compared to 90 γ-PFC/10^6 cells in normals. (2) Treatment of patients' lymphocytes with their own serum led to an increase mainly in γ-chain production peaking on day 5, ranging from 4,000–6,800 PFC/10^6. Ro 10-9359 application at appropriate concentrations was capable of reducing the increased γ-chain production back to normal. (3) PWM-stimulation was less effective in patients' lymphocytes than in normals, indicating a polyclonal prestimulation. ConA at 40 μg/ml as costimulator could reduce the μ- and γ-chain secretions by more than 50%. Pretreatment with 100–200 μg/ml Ro 10-9359 reduced the polyclonal γ-chain formation up to 95% in this assay system. (4) MTX at appropriate concentration resulted in a 70–90% decrease of both μ-and γ-chains in all stimulation procedures applied. (5) Simultaneous treatment of the cells with Ro 10-9359 and ConA did not result in a more pronounced effect than either of these agents separately.

The experiments indicate that Ro 10-9359 can reduce the expression of PFC of polyclonally activated B-cells during eruptive stages of psoriasis. We postulate that Ro 10-9359 may influence cellular imbalances between T-helpers and T-suppressors. Also, our experiments strongly suggest a regulating function of Ro 10-9359 for immune surveillance.

References

1. Bialasiewicz AA, Lubach D, Marghescu S Effects of Ro 10-9359 and MTX on the polyclonal activation of lymphocytes in an in vitro Balb/c mouse system. Proc. IV. Intern. Congress for Eye-Research, ed. ISER, New York, 1980, pp 8–9
2. Cunningham AJ, Szenberg A (1968) Further improvements in the plaque forming technique. Immunology 14:599
3. Eilat D, Reeves PJ, Steinberg AD, Schechter AN (1978) Measurement of antigen-specific IgG autoantibody production in vitro. J Immunol 121:310–316
4. Glinski W, Haftek M, Obalak S, Jablonska S (1977) Clinical aspects of T- and B-lymphocytes in psoriasis. Arch Dermatol Res 25:89–92
5. Guilhout JJ, Clot J, Meynadier J (1977) T-cell Defect in Psoriasis: Further Studies on membrane markers and T-cell functions from 60 patients. Arch Dermatol Res 26:163–166
6. Moticka EJ, Streilein JW (1976) Nonspecific polyclonal activation of memory B-cells by antigen as a mechanism for the preservation of long-term immunologic anamnesis. Cell Immunol 41: 406–413
7. Pryjma J, Munoz J, Galbraith RM, Fudenberg HH, Virella G (1980) Induction in suppression of immunoglobulin synthesis in cultures of human lymphocytes: effects of PWM and staphylococcus areus cowan I. J. Immunol 124:656–660
8. Ringden O, Rynell-Dall B, Kunori T, Smith CIE, Hammarström L, Freijid A, Möller E (1978) Induction of antibody synthesis in human B-lymphocyte by different polyclonal B-cell activators: evaluation of direct and indirect PFC-assays. Immunol Res 45:115–138
9. Sauder DN, Bailin PL, Sundeen J, Krakauer RS (1980) Suppressor cell function in psoriasis. Arch Dermatol 116:51–55
10. New York Academy of Sciences Publication No. 24: Modulation of cell-interactions by Vitamin A and its analogs (retinoids) (in press)

C.E. Orfanos et al. (eds.)
Retinoids

Prevention of Psoriasiform Reactions After Beta-Receptor Blockers by Retinoid

I. Rácz, M. Berecz and Gy. Soós

Experimental work in psoriasis was hampered till the last year by the fact that analogous skin symptoms could not be produced in experimental animals. Gaylarde et al. reported in 1978 about psoriasiform changes in guinea pig skin from locally applied propranolol (3). The changes were parakeratosis, acanthosis and slight cellular infiltration. The findings seem to be in connection with the beta-adrenergic blocking property of the drug, as other *beta adrenergic blockers* (pindolol, alprenolol) may produce psoriasiform eruptions in patients taking them regularly and the genuine psoriasis may be worsened by them too (1, 2). Although the real connection between these psoriasiform reactions after beta blockers and the true psoriasis is until now uncleared, it seemed to be worth while investigating the effect of aromatic retinoid Ro 10-9359 (Tigason) on these curious reactions.

Material and Method

14 male guinea pigs of about 300 g weight were used. The hair on the back of all has been removed by rasor. 4 control animals were injected always on the same place daily once through 7 days with 0.1 ml of a 10% aqueous solution of pindolol. The 10 test animals have been treated in the same way but they received simultaneously with the injections 1 mg/kg Tigason perorally solved in water through a bougie. On the 8th day the status of the treated skin was registered and a biopsy was done from the lesions.

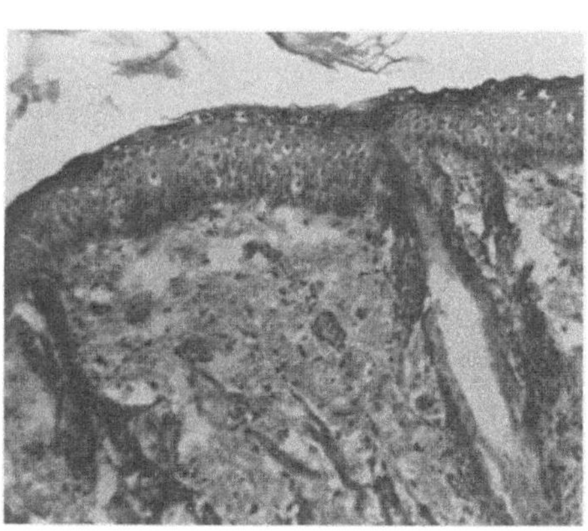

Fig. 1. Skin of guinea pigs treated with pindolol and Tigason. No histological changes

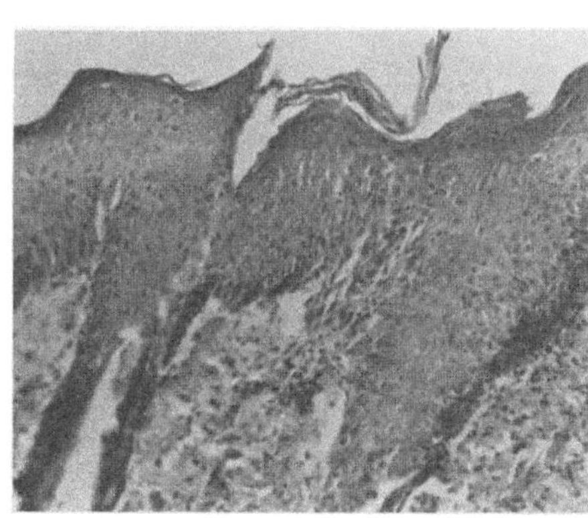

Fig. 2. Skin of guinea pig treated with pindolol only. Parakeratosis, acanthosis and cellular infiltration

Table 1. Prevention of psoriasiform pindolol reaction by Tigason

Applied drug	Number of animals	Psoriasiform reaction
Pindolol	4	4
Pindolol + Tigason	10	0

Results

On the skin of the animals treated by Tigason no clinical changes developed except a pyogenous infiltration in one of the cases. The histological picture showed no significant difference from the normal (Fig. 1). In the control guinea pigs a slight infiltration developed on the place of the injections of pindolol. In two of the four a distinct parakeratotic peeling could also be seen. The histological picture of these lesions exhibited parakeratosis, a distinct acanthosis and a slight cellular infiltration in the dermis (Fig. 2).

Discussion

Gaylarde et al. described the provocation of psoriasiform lesions in guinea pigs by epicutaneous application of propranolol (3). We succeeded to induce the same lesions in guinea pigs by the intracutaneous injection of an other beta adrenergic receptor blocker, pindolol. The simultaneous feeding of the animals with *Tigason inhibits the evolution of these psoriasiform changes* (Table 1). We think to have found in the eruption caused by beta-blockers a *good model* for the experimental investigation in psoriasis.

Summary

In guinea pigs intracutaneous injections of beta-blocker (pindolol) produce a psoriasiform reaction. Simultaneous oral retinoid medication may prevent the appearance of these psoriasiform lesions.

References

1. Brigden WD, Almeyda J (1976) Adverse reaction to β-adrenergic blocking drugs. Br J Dermatol 95:335–338
2. Gaylarde PM, Sarkany I (1975) Side effects of practolol. Br Med J 3:435–438
3. Gaylarde PM, Brock AP, Sarkany I (1978) Psoriasiform changes in guinea pig skin from propranolol. Clin Exp Derm 3:157–160
4. Mikkelsen HI, Erenlund Jensen HA, Wadskov S, Lerche A, Sondergaard J (1976) Aggravation of psoriasis and occurrence of psoriasiform cutaneous eruptions induced by betablocking agents. IRCS Med Sci 3:152–154

C.E. Orfanos et al. (eds.)
Retinoids

Treatment of Psoriasis by Oral PUVA-Therapy Combined with Aromatic Retinoid (Re-PUVA)

Ch. Grupper and B. Berretti

We are presenting here our results on 126 patients suffering from severe psoriasis involving more than 40% of the total body area, some of them representing PUVA-therapy failures, and treated in accordance with 5 different schedules, 3 of which combined aromatic retinoid (AR), with PUVA-therapy.

The best results were obtained with a schedule combining an initial 2-week treatment with AR alone, followed from the 15th day by a combination of classic PUVA-therapy (1, 5, 7, 11, 14, 15, 18), with an immediate and progressive decrease in daily AR dosage (schedule C). This schedule allowed not only a reduction in the number and duration of PUVA treatments and total energy-dose (though the difference was smaller than that reported by other authors), but especially for a given degree of clearing, the duration of remission was far longer than for PUVA-therapy alone. Furthermore this therapeutic association allowed us to salvage 70% of the complete or partial PUVA-therapy failures. We consider that the combination of AR with PUVA-therapy (Re-PUVA) is the most important advance in the treatment of psoriasis since the introduction of simple PUVA.

Materials and Methods

We treated 126 patients (90 males, 36 females; mean age = 40 years, extremes = 20–70) with stable psoriasis involving more than 40% of the total body surface (mean = 60%), evolving over more than 8 years, and refractory to all local treatments. 44 had been complete PUVA failures. The types of psoriasis included:
106 psoriasis vulgaris (plaque type, nummular, a few universalis)
10 psoriasis guttata
9 erythrodermic psoriasis, and 1 case of psoriasis pustulosis (Zumbusch type).

Only localized palmo-plantar psoriasis has been excluded from this study, and results for this type, which were more favourable than for the other types, will be reported upon subsequently.

PUVA was carried out following a standard protocol with Waldmann 6000 light-boxes. In about $^2/_3$ of the patients the photosensitizer used was 0.6 mg/kg 8 MOP, with the remaining $^1/_3$ receiving 5 MOP (Mopalene) at a daily dose of 1.2 mg/kg (1. 5). Aromatic retinoid Ro 10-9359 (AR) (Roche Laboratories) was administered at an initial fractionated daily dosage of 1 mg/kg after fat-containing meals; where necessary, dosage could be increased by 20–30%.

Therapeutic schedules. The 126 patients were divided into 5 groups as shown in Fig. 1.

1. Group A was made up of 32 patients who had never received PUVA and who were treated with Ro 10-9359 at a mean daily dose of 1 mg/kg until clearing (a mean of 4–6 weeks), at which time the daily dosage was reduced to 0.75–0.50 mg/kg. The onset of serious side effects (e.g. alopecia) frequently required an early reduction in dosage, but precocious withdrawal was never necessary.
2. The second group (schedule A') was made up of 25 partial or total PUVA failures. They were treated as per schedule A'.
3. The 10 patients in group B had never received PUVA, and were treated with a combination of Ro 10-9359 as per schedule A, and PUVA as described above (Re-PUVA). Upon clearing, Ro 10-9359 dosage and PUVA frequency were rapidly reduced.

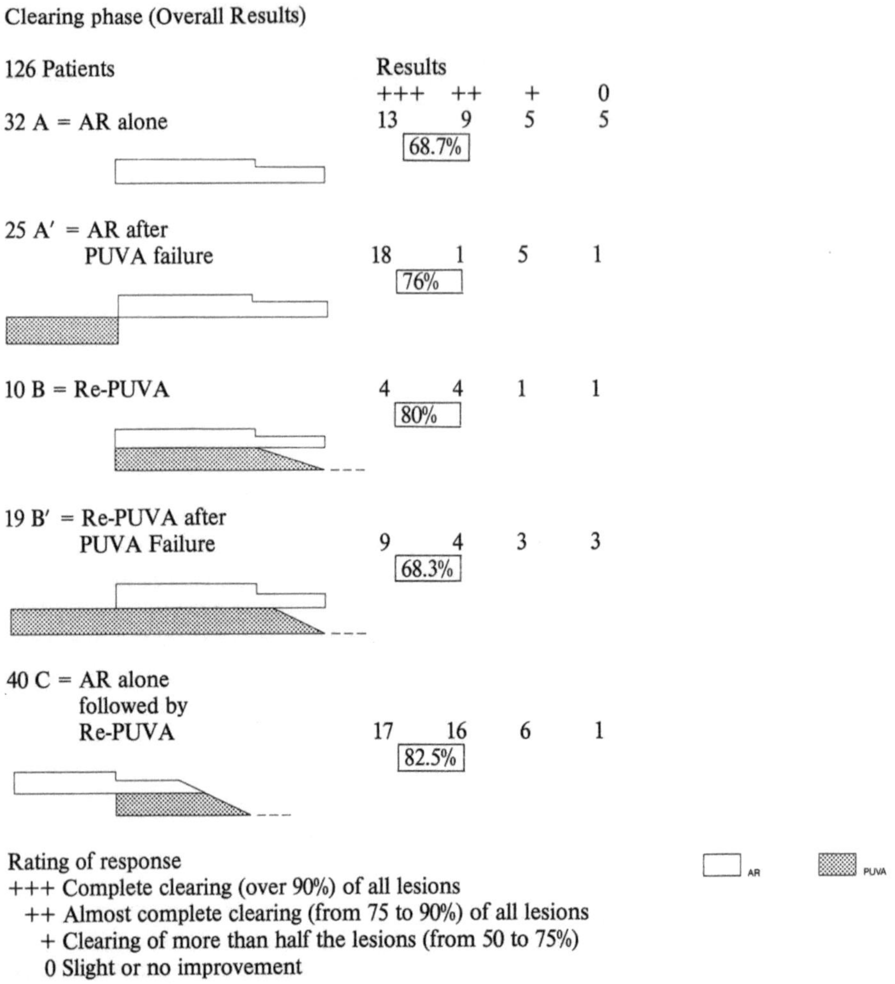

Fig. 1. Initial treatment: protocoles and results

4. The 19 PUVA therapy failures in group B' were treated with Re-PUVA as in group B.
5. The 40 patients in group C received 1 mg/kg Ro 10-9359 alone for 2 weeks. On day 15, standard PUVA was begun simultaneously with a rapid and progressive decrease in AR dosage. Upon clearing, PUVA was reduced to the maintenance regime and Ro 10-9359 was usually withdrawn.

Results

Evaluation of Results

Before and after treatment, all patients underwent a battery of laboratory tests for changes in hematologic, hepatic, renal or lipoprotein status.

Side Effects

With satisfactory absorption of Ro 10-9359, cheilitis with exfoliation, rhagades, stomatitis, glossitis and dryness of the nasal mucosa were noted during the first week; this was the case for 90% of patients. More serious side effects included:

- Palmo-plantar lesions with ragged desquamation, thinning of the skin and hyperhidrosis (approximately 40% of patients).
- Clearly dose-related transitory alopecia requiring early reduction in dosage (approximately 70% of patients).
- Pruritus, generalized erythema, epistaxis and ageusia in a few cases.

Laboratory investigation revealed the following:

- One case of transitory increase in SGOT without clinical repercussion.
- In 7 cases, a transitory increase in triglycerides. In 3 of these patients, there was a concomitant rise in cholesterol and total serum lipids, but no chylomicrons. This may thus have been a function of fat intake and of latent diabetes.

The combination of AR with PUVA increased neither the incidence of side effects nor the degree of photosensitivity.

Discussion

As previously reported (2, 4, 9, 12, 16, 17) AR administered alone shows a clear antipsoriatic effect with 68% positive results and 42% of patients remaining cleared for 6 months, with only minor topical treatment. However, the possibility of delayed relapse raises the question of the necessity for AR maintenance treatment. The treatment type, the dosage, and the duration are still to be determined, both for psoriasis and for other AR sensitive dermatosis such as congenital or acquired dyskeratosis. To date, our experience has supported the notion of a *threshold dosage*, varying both between various dermatoses and between individual patients.

Before discussing our results with Re-PUVA, it is of interest to review our results for 1259 psoriasis patients treated with standard PUVA in a monocentric study, this being the largest statistical analysis available in the literature (5). We found that after a mean of 21 treatments (±8.5) a total UVA energy dose of 131 joules/cm^2 over 42 days (±18), 84% of patients showed clearing. Nevertheless, the majority of patients suffered relapses 4 to 6 months after stopping PUVA; at the 6th month, only 36% of patients were still clear of lesions. While the combined percentage of success for combination Re-PUVA as per schedules B and C was very slightly inferior, with 81% of patients showing clearing, it should be noted that the patients population was here far smaller (50 vs 1259) and with further experience a better success rate may be expected (it should be noted that our *preliminary* study of PUVA yielded only a 75% success rate; also see Roenigk (13, 14)). More significantly, based on our preliminary clinical findings with a 6-month follow-up, we consider that *schedule C Re-PUVA offers several major advantages*:

Table 1. Clearing phase therapy: standard PUVA and Re-PUVA

	Total Joules/cm^2	Treatment	Days	Still cleared at 6 months
PUVA 1259 Pat.	131 ± 75	21 ± 8,5	42 ± 18	36%
Re-PUVA C. Schedule 40 Patients	97	16	38	68%

a) Combining results for schedules A′ and B′, *Re-PUVA retrieved 32 out of 44 previous PUVA failures*, for a *71.5% rate of success.* This was also the case for *generalized pustular* and *erythrodermic psoriasis*, both of which are highly resistant to PUVA therapy.
b) While we cannot be quite as optimistic as certain other authors (3, 6, 8, 10) who have reported a savings of about 50% over standard PUVA therapy in terms of the number of treatments, total energy requirement, and time to reach complete clearing, we did find a *significant reduction in the daily dosage of Ro 10-9359*, the mechanism of action and long-term toxicity of which has not yet been sufficiently studied.
c) Finally, and most important, *6 months after the end of Re-PUVA, 68% of patients remained cleared*, as compared with 36% following PUVA therapy alone.

Conclusions

By comparison with standard PUVA therapy, the combination of Ro 10-9359 with PUVA (Re-PUVA) following schedule C allows a decrease in time-to-clearing, remissions of longer duration, a decrease in all three parameters of PUVA therapy (length of treatment, number of treatments and total energy dose) and a decrease or withdrawal of Ro 10-9359 before the onset of such severe side effects as alopecia. Furthermore, this combination yields remissions lasting more than 6 months in almost twice as many patients as does PUVA alone, i.e. 68% vs 36%.

Summary

We present our results observed in 126 patients affected with severe psoriasis covering more than 40% of the whole body area, some of them representing failures of PUVA-therapy, and treated in accordance with 5 different schedules, 3 of them combining aromatic retinoid (AR) with PUVA-therapy.

The most effective results have been obtained with a schedule involving an initial treatment during a two weeks period with AR only, followed on the 15th day by the adjunction of classic PUVA-therapy combined with an immediate progressive decrease of the AR daily dosage (C schedule).

So, the result was not only a reduction of PUVA-therapy regarding frequency and the length of treatment and to the amount of energy expended (although, less remarkable than that published by the other authors), but also and especially, and even for an identical ratio of clearing, a far longer duration of remissions than after PUVA-therapy used alone. Also, because of this therapeutic association more than 70% of the complete or relative failures of PUVA-therapy can be healed. Thus, the combination of AR with PUVA-therapy (Re-PUVA) in accordance with this schedule appears to be the most important improvement brought to PUVA since its introduction into the therapy of psoriasis.

Abbreviations

AR = Aromatic Retinoid = Ro 10-9359
PUVA-therapy = Oral photochemotherapy
Re-PUVA = AR + PUVA therapy
8 MOP = 8-methoxypsoralen = Meladinine
5 MOP = 5-methoxypsoralen = Mopalene (not yet commercially available)

References

1. Berretti B, Grupper Ch (1979) La photochimiothérapie orale du psoriasis (PUVA). Résultats récents. Gaz Méd Fr 83:3191–3197
2. Dominguez-Soto L, Hojyo-Tomoka, TM (1978) Aromatic retinoid (Ro 10-9359) in the treatment of psoriasis (psoriasis vulgaris). Cutis 22:376–379
3. Fritsch PO, Hönigsmann H, Jaschke E, Wolff K (1978) Augmentation of oral methoxsalen-photochemotherapy with an oral retinoic acid derivate. J Invest Dermatol 70:178–182
4. Guilhou JJ, Malbos S, Meynadier J (1978) Traitement oral des psoriasis graves par un nouveau rétinoide aromatique (Ro 10-9359). Ann Dermatol Vénérol 105:813–818
5. Grupper Ch, Berretti B, Forlot P Bilan de la puvathérapie a propos de 1400 cas personnels. Résultats et progrès récents en 1979. Actes du XVIème Congrès de l'Association des Dermatologistes de langue française. Ichtyoses, peau et lumière, Edition SAGEP, TUNIS 1980
6. Heidbreder G, Christophers E (1979) Therapy of psoriasis with retinoid plus PUVA: clinical and histologic data. Arch Dermatol Res 264:331–337
7. Melski JW, Tanenbaum L, Parrish JA, Fitzpatrick TB, Bleich HL et al (1977) Oral methoxsalen photochemotherapy for the treatment of psoriasis: A cooperative clinical trial. J Invest Dermatol 68:328–335
8. Michaelsson G, Noren P, Vahlquist A (1978) Combined therapy with oral retinoid and PUVA baths in severe psoriasis. Br J Dermatol 99:221–222
9. Orfanos CE, Runne U (1976) Systemic use of a new retinoid with and without local dithranol treatment in generalized psoriasis. Br J Dermatol 95:101–103
10. Orfanos CE, Pullmann H, Sterry W, Künzig M (1978) Retinoid-PUVA = Re-PUVA: Systemische Kombinations-Behandlung bei Psoriasis. Z. Hautkrankh 53:494–504
11. Ortonne JP, Coussa MS, Thivolet J (1977) La photochimiothérapie orale du psoriasis. Résultats chez 100 patients. Ann Dermatol Vénérol 104:635–644
12. Ott F, Bollag W (1975) Therapie der Psoriasis mit einem oral wirksamen neuen Vitamin A-Säure-Derivat. Schweiz med Wochenschr 105:439–441
13. Photochemotherapy for psoriasis. A clinical cooperative study of PUVA-48 and PUVA-64. Arch Dermatol 115:576–579 (1979)
14. Roenigk HH Jr, Martin JS (1977) Photochemotherapy for psoriasis. Arch Dermatol 113:1667–1670
15. Rogers S, Marks J, Shuster S, Vella Briffa D, Warin A, Greaves M (1979) Comparison of photochemotherapy and dithranol in the treatment of chronic plaque psoriasis. Lancet I:455–458
16. Runne U, Orfanos CE, Gartmann H (1973) Perorale Applikation zweier Derivate der Vitamin A-Säure zur internen Psoriasis-Therapie. 13-cis-beta-Vitamin A-Säure und Vitamin A-Säure-aethylamid. Arch Dermatol Forsch 247:171–180
17. Schumacher A, Stüttgen G (1971) Vitamin A-Säure bei Hyperkeratosen, epithelialen Tumoren und Akne. Dt med Wochenschr 96:1547–1551
18. Wolff K, Gschnait F, Hönigsmann H, Konrad K, Parrish JA, Fitzpatrick TB (1977) Phototesting and dosimetry of photochemotherapy. Br J Dermatol 96:1–10

Clinical and Laboratory Monitoring of Oral Retinoid Therapy

C.E. Orfanos et al. (eds.)
Retinoids

The Posology of Oral Retinoids: How Much, How Often, How Long?

T. Fredriksson

When oral retinoids first were used little was known about their pharmacodynamic properties and pharmacokinetics, partly due to analytical difficulties. Since then, our knowledge of single-dose kinetics has increased, while multiple-dose kinetics still are not fully elucidated. The retinoids are extremely lipid soluble, and this property allows them not only to cross cell membranes but to be reabsorbed during their passage through the nephron. Theoretically, they could remain in the body for an indefinite period if they were not metabolized to more water soluble metabolites, active or inactive. Indeed, possible hepatic side effects have been noted in patients even though etretinate had been withdrawn for several weeks, and etretinate has been demonstrated several months after cessation of therapy. This particular retinoid may fullfil the requirements for a three-compartment model, and its pharmacokinetics are thus very complicated.

The posology of the retinoids was more or less empirical when first being used, and still is. In this paper some of these empirically derived experiences will be discussed with the available literature as the main source.

Differences Between Etretinate and Isotretinoin

There are some important differences between etretinate and isotretinoin with regard to clinical effect, toxicity and posology. Etretinate is superior in psoriasis, palmo-plantar pustulosis and possibly in some other indications such as leukoplakia and erosive lichen planus of the oral mucosa, while isotretinoin seems to be the retinoid of choice in the treatment of cystic acne. In most other indications the two retinoids seem to be about equally effective.

Isotretinoin seems to have a wider therapeutic range, being used in doses between 0.5 and 8 mg per kg and day, while it is much narrower in the case of etretinate, 0.5–1.5 mg. Isotretinoin will produce the characteristic acute side effects at a dose level close to 1 mg per kg and day, while etretinate will produce such at about half this dosage. There is also some specificity with regard to the side effects, isotretinoin e.g. produces more dryness of skin and mucous membranes, while etretinate produces more hair loss. The two retinoids have also been administered following different regimens. In the case of isotretinoin usually a low starting dose has been utilized, about 0.5 mg/kg/day, and it has later been increased in increments of 0.5 to 1.0 mg/kg/day at intervals of two to four weeks until either an appreciable therapeutic effect or dose-limiting toxicity has been noted. Such titration of the optimal dose is safe but time-consuming. Etretinate, on the other hand, has usually been given as a comparatively high initial dose, which has been either kept constant or reduced when clinical effect has been ascertained or annoying side effects have appeared. The advantage of the

Table 1. Use of isotretinoin in various dermatoses

Indication	Dose mg/kg/day	Duration in weeks
Acne	0.1–8.0	16
Lamellar ichthyosis	0.5–6.0	2–40
Morbus Darier	0.5–6.0	2–40
Pityriasis rubra pilaris	0.5–6.0	2–40
Keratoderma	0.5–4.0	4–20
Basalioma	1.5–2.0	4–16
Leukoplakia	1.0–2.0	8
Erosive lichen	0.5–1.0	2–20

last mentioned regimen is gain of time, and the major disadvantage loss of patient compliance due to side effects.

Posology

Both drugs have usually been given in divided daily doses, and some investigators have recommended that the drugs should be given during meals with high fat content, since their absorption then might be increased due to their extreme liposolubility. Etretinate has also been given every other day without appreciable loss of efficacy, and at the very extreme, as a high dose twice weekly in palmo-plantar pustulosis. This high twice weekly dose, about 4 mg/kg, was only slightly less effective than a divided daily dose, but the immediate side effects were somewhat more pronounced. In view of this, a single dose given every or every other day during a heavy meal might be the best regimen when combined with dose-titration. Such a posology will probably create optimal patient compliance.

Indications and Dosage

In Table 1 the dosages of isotretinoin used in some of the main indications is shown. Some extremely rare but logical indications have purposely been omitted from this and the following table. It is evident that isotretinoin has been used at most varying dose levels, as mentioned earlier. However, the average dose in most indications has been 2.0 mg/kg/day, except in the treatment of basalioma where the average dose has been significantly higher, and the minimal dose for effect has been around 0.5 mg/kg/day. If the titration method is used, it seems logical to start with 0.5 mg/kg/day.

As seen in Table 2 the therapeutic range for etretinate has been much more narrow. The average dose has been close to 1 mg/kg/day, and the minimal effective dose has been above 0.5 mg/kg/day in most indications. This makes dose-titration more difficult if not impossible.

Table 2. Use of etretinate in various dermatoses

Indication	Dose mg/kg/day	Duration in weeks
Psoriasis	0.7–1.5	24
Palmo-plantar pustulosis	0.5–1.2	8–16
Lichen planus	0.5–1.2	6–26
Morbus Darier	1.0–1.5	6–12
Ichthyosis	1.0	3–12
Leukoplakia	1.0–1.5	8
Psoriatic arthritis	1.0	24

In this connection it might be pertinent to mention that double-blind studies of the oral retinoids at effective dose levels against placebo are close to impossible, since the extremely high frequency of characteristic side effects will unblind every study in a few weeks.

Another problem is to assess the clinical efficacy. It is quite simple in diseases like acne and palmoplantar pustulosis by counting of lesions. It is more difficult in an indication such as psoriasis, since it is essential not to take merely the severity of the individual lesions into account but also the areas involved. A global evaluation of the response as bad, moderate, good and excellent is in this case not subtle enough when limited numbers of patients are used. We therefore constructed a more specific instrument for the evaluation of efficacy: psoriasis area and severity index (PASI). For calculation of this, the four main body areas were assessed: the head (h), the trunk (t), the upper extremities (u) and the lower extremities (l), corresponding to 10, 30, 20 and 40% of the total body area, respectively. The area of psoriatic involvement of these four main areas (A_h, A_t, A_u and A_l) was given a numerical value: 0 = no involvement; 1 = <10%; 2 = 10<30%; 3 = 30<50%; 4 = 50<70%; 5 = 70<90%; 6 = 90–100%. In order to evaluate the severity of the psoriatic lesions three target symptoms, namely erythema (E), infiltration (I) and desquamation (D) were assessed according to a scale 0–4, where 0 means a complete lack of cutaneous involvement and 4 represents the severest possible involvement. In the case of, e.g. erythema, 0 means no erythema at all (not even "macular" psoriasis); 1 = slight erythema; 2 = moderate erythema; 3 = striking erythema, and 4 = exceptionally striking erythema.

In order to calculate the PASI the sum of the severity rating for these three main changes was multiplied with the numerical value of the areas involved and with the various percentages of the four body areas. These values were then added in order to obtain the PASI. This formula can be written as follows:

$$\mathrm{PASI} = \overbrace{0.1\,(E_h + I_h + D_h)\,A_h}^{\text{head}} + \overbrace{0.3\,(E_t + I_t + D_t)\,A_t}^{\text{trunk}} + \overbrace{0.2\,(E_u + I_u + D_u)\,A_u}^{\text{upper extremities}} + \overbrace{0.4\,(E_l + I_l + D_l)\,A_l}^{\text{lower extremities}}.$$

The PASI varies in steps of 0.1 units from 0.0 to 72.0. The last mentioned figure thus represents complete erythroderma of the severest possible degree, while 0.0 means no psoriatic lesions at all. The PASI was found to be a simple and useful tool to assess the effect of retinoids in psoriasis, and it might be as useful in other treatments of this disease, but the PASI score shall not be regarded as an "exact" numerical value, since the severity rating is subjective. However, in our mind it is superior to global evaluation, and one condition for good clinical monitoring is a sensitive test for recording efficacy.

Use in Children and Pregnant Women

There are few reports regarding the use of retinoids in children, but the same posology as in adults has usually been used, i.e. 1–2 mg/kg/day in the case of isotretinoin and 0.5–1 mg in the case of etretinate. On the other hand, both drugs are teratogenic and should not be given to women of childbearing potential without adequate precautions. At least in the case of etretinate it must be remembered that active drug remains in the body for a long time, and pregnancy should not be allowed until many months or possibly a year after withdrawal of therapy.

Duration of Treatment

The duration of treatment involves particular problems except in self-limiting diseases and in cystic acne, where isotretinoin has produced such remarkable long-standing remissions after four months of treatment. In most other indications the retinoids will in general produce maximal effect in about eight weeks on the highest dose tolerated, and continued treatment will usually not result in any further significant improvement. After cessation of therapy slow recurrence is the rule within a few weeks or months. A maintenance dose, about half of the optimal dose, may delay but usually not completely abolish the recurrence.

Table 3. Check-list for oral retinoids

1.	Indication
2.	Contraindications
3.	Specificity of the retinioid choosen
4.	Specificity of side effects
5.	Dosage and dose-titration
6.	Duration of treatment
7.	Maintenance
8.	Combinations
9.	Control of acute side effects
10.	Control of chronic side effects

Intermittent Versus Continuous Treatment

Then, what shall be preferred, intermittent treatment or maintenance dosing? At the present moment, when our knowledge of the chronic toxicity is scant, intermittent treatment seems to offer fewer risks, but whatever regimen used cautious clinical monitoring is mandatory. There are all reasons to follow these patients as closely as those on *e.g.* methotrexate.

Combined Treatment

The retinoids can be successfully combined with other treatments, particularly in psoriasis and palmo-plantar pustulosis, and this has definite advantages. The dosage and duration of treatment may be reduced both for the retinoid and the concomitant treatment with a decrease in dual side effects as a logical result. Also the potency of concomitant topical steroids can be reduced with obvious advantages. Van der Rhee et al. (20) have thus shown that a dose of etretinate that by itself had virtually no effect on psoriasis when combined with a topically applied steroid of intermittent potency, triamcinolone acetonide, had good effect in this condition. Orfanos and Runne (11) found similar results when the retinoid was combined with traditional dithranol treatment.

Of particular interest is the combination of etretinate with phototherapy of psoriasis, utilizing UVA, UVB or PUVA. It has been possible to reduce both the duration of retinoid treatment and the dosage as well as the radiation dose, and the results have been impressive. Various regimens have been used, and it is maybe too early to recommend a particular one. However, I have a feeling that the combination of oral retinoid and phototherapy will be the treatment of choice of suitable cases of severe psoriasis during this decade.

Conclusions

When using oral retinoids we have to be even more cautious than we are when using most other potent drugs. The retinoids *are* very special, and the "check-list" given in Table 3 is an absolute minimum. The posology of oral retinoids is not yet definite: much work remains.

Summary

The dosages used of isotretinoin (13-cis retinoic acid) and the aromatic retinoid, etretinate (Ro 10-9359) have been tabulated with regard to the various indications, based on available data from the literature. The various possibilities to give these drugs are mentioned: single doses, divided doses, and higher doses with longer intervals. The possibilities to reduce the dosage when the disease is under reasonable control is mentioned. The duration of each treatment period for the various indications is discussed with particular regard to side effects. Finally, continuous or intermittent use will be discussed, stressing the importance of cautious clinical monitoring since little is known about the chronic toxicity of the retinoids.

References

1. Beierdorffer H, Wiskemann A (1978) Kombinierte Therapie der Psoriasis mit einem aromatischen Retinoid (Ro 10-9359) und UVB-Bestrahlungen. Akt Dermatol 4:183–187
2. Fredriksson T, Pettersson U (1978) Severe psoriasis - oral therapy with a new retinoid. Dermatologica 157:238–244
3. Fredriksson T, Pettersson U (1979) Oral treatment of pustulosis palmo-plantaris with a new retinoid, Ro 10-9359. Dermatologica 158:60–64
4. Fritsch PO, Honigsmann H, Jaschke E, Wolff K (1978) Augmentation of oral methoxysalen-photochemotherapy with an oral retinoic acid derivative. J Invest Dermatol 70:178–182
5. Heidbreder G, Christophers E (1979) Therapy of psoriasis with retinoid plus PUVA: Clinical and histologic data. Arch Dermatol Res 264:331–337
6. Koch HF (1978) Biochemical treatment of precancerous oral lesions: The effectiveness of various analogues of retinoic acid. J Maxillofacial Surg 6:59–63
7. Lassus A (1980) Systemic treatment of psoriasis with an oral retinoic acid derivative (Ro 10-9359). Br J Dermatol 102:195–202
8. Lauharanta J, Juvakoski T, Lassus A (1980) A clinical evaluation of the effect of an aromatic retinoid (Ro 10-9359), RePUVA and PUVA in severe psoriasis. Paper presented at the Scandinavian Congress of Dermatology, Helsinki
9. Maidhof R (1979) Zur systemischen Behandlung des oralen Lichen planus mit einem aromatischen Retinoid (Ro 10-9359). Z Hautkr 54:873–876
10. Michaëlsson G, Norén P, Wahlquist A (1978) Combined therapy with oral retinoid and PUVA baths in severe psoriasis. Br J Dermatol 99:221–222
11. Orfanos CE, Runne U (1976) Systemic use of a new retinoid with and without local dithranol treatment in generalized psoriasis. Br J Dermatol 95:101–102
12. Orfanos CE, Steigleder GK, Pullman H, Bloch PH (1979) Oral retinoid and UVB radiation: A new alternative treatment for psoriasis on an out-patient basis. Acta Dermatol Venerol 59:241–244
13. Peck GL, Yoder FW (1978) In: The ichthyoses. Marks R, Dykes PJ (eds). 193–210, MTP Press, Lancaster
14. Peck GL, Olsen TG, Yoder FW, Strauss JS, Downing DT, Pandya M, Butkus D, Arnaud-Battandier J (1979) Prolonged remissions of cystic and conglobate acne with 13-cis-retinoic acid. N Engl J Med 300:329–333
15. Peck GL, Olsén TG, Butkus D, Pandya M, Arnaud-Battandier J, Yoder F, Levis WR (1979) Treatment of basal cell carcinomas with 13-cis-retinoic acid. Proc Am Cancer Res 20:56
16. Peck GL (1980) Retinoids in dermatology. Arch Dermatol 116:283–284
17. van der Rhee HJ, Tijssen JGP, Herrman WA, Waterman AH, Polano MK (1980) Combined treatment of psoriasis with a new aromatic retinoid (Tigason) in low dosage orally and triamcinolone acetonide cream topically: A double blind trial. Br J Dermatol 102:203–212
18. Rosenthal M (1079) Retinoid in der Behandlung von Psoriasis-Arthritis. Schweiz med Wochenschr 109:1912–1914
19. Scheiber W, Plewig G (1978) Behandlung des Lichen ruber mucosae mit Vitamin-A-Säure-Derivaten. Dermatologica 157:171–180
20. Steigleder GK, Orfanos CE, Pullman H (1979) Retinoid-SUP-Therapie der Psoriasis. Z Hautkr 54:19–23

C.E. Orfanos et al. (eds.)
Retinoids

Long-term Biological Tolerance of Ro 10-9359

F. Ott

Ro 10-9359 has been proved to be a useful symptomatic treatment for severe psoriasis and other diseases with disorders of keratinization. However, it is not possible to cure the patient and therefore the drug has frequently to be administered on a long term basis. This raises the question of biological tolerance, mainly of possible side effects on liver function, which has been mentioned in several publications (1, 3). We had the opportunity to treat 107 patients for periods of time up to 6 years. We report the results of four laboratory tests, i.e., serum bilirubin, serum transaminases (2) and alkaline phosphatase.

Patients and Methods

107 patients, aged from 8 to 75 years, were treated with Ro 10-9359. 92 were suffering from psoriasis and 15 from various disorders of keratinization. 11 of them were known alcoholics and one had alcoholic liver cirrhosis. Their ages ranged from 8 to 75 years.

The initial daily dosage varied from 25 mg to 100 mg, maintenance daily dosage between 10 and 50 mg.

Duration of observation was 1, 2, 3, 4, 5 and 6 years for 16, 22, 28, 17, 16 and 8 patients respectively.

Laboratory checks were performed before treatment and at various time intervals according to clinical tolerance and patient's convenience.

In 6 patients, baseline values or values during treatment were missing. Thus 101 patients could be evaluated.

Levels of serum bilirubin, SGPT, SGOT and alkaline phosphatase were performed in two different laboratories. The normal values were different in these two laboratories. For this evaluation, all values have been transformed to % of upper normal limit of each laboratory. Only the results obtained on the nearest day to each complete year after entering the trial were used.

The study started in January 1974 and the last examination was done on May 31, 1980.

Results

The results at the end of each year of treatment were compared with baseline values and the statistical significance of differences was calculated using the Wilcoxon matched pair test. The results are shown in Table 1. At end of year 4, there were more patients with elevation of serum bilirubin than patients with diminution of this value. However, all the values were within normal range (15% to 85% of upper normal limit). For the other parameters there was no trend towards increased values. On the contrary, more reduced than increased values were recorded.

As a second step, results for each parameter were classified as normal or abnormal during the whole treatment: normal at start and abnormal during treatment or abnormal at start and normal during treatment. The statistical significance of differences was calculated using the McNemar test. Results of this analysis are shown in Table 2.

Table 1. Comparison of laboratory results with baseline values at each check

Duration of treatment (years)	Bilirubin -	Bilirubin 0	Bilirubin +	Alk. phospha. -	Alk. phospha. 0	Alk. phospha. +	SGPT -	SGPT 0	SGPT +	SGOT -	SGOT 0	SGOT +
1	37	12	34	41	1	39	33	10	38	33	10	38
2	29	4	40	44*	0	21	37*	7	20	36	7	22
3	19	8	28	40*	0	14	32*	4	19	32*	2	16
4	8	3	20*	23*	1	7	20	2	9	19*	1	11
5	6	3	9	14*	0	3	11	2	6	11*	1	4
6	-	-	-	6	0	1	4	0	3	3	1	4

\- = number of patients with decreased values
0 = number of patients without change
\+ = number of patients with increased values
* = $p < 0.05$ (Wilcoxon matched pair test)

There was a trend towards abnormal SGPT values during treatment which was not statistically significant ($p = 0.09$).

Furthermore, it must be pointed out that all the abnormal values registered for patients with normal values at the start were either transitory or not confirmed later on (last value).

As regards the patient with liver cirrhosis, a transitory increase of SGPT was recorded after one year of treatment and SGOT values, increased before treatment, became normal later on.

Discussion

A few cases of hepatitis, possibly related to treatment with Ro 10-9359 have been reported (1, 3). In a multicenter trial, involving 291 patients, a few of whom were treated for more than 210 days, only a few patients showed abnormal SGPT values (2). The results we have found indicate that it is possible to treat patients on a long term basis without inducing liver damage as judged by determination of serum bilirubin, transaminases and alkaline phosphatases.

Summary

107 patients were treated between 1 and 6 years with Ro 10-9359. No disturbance of liver

Table 2. Evolution of laboratory values during treatment with Ro 10-9359

Parameter	Number of patients: Bilirubin	Alkaline phosphatase	SGPT	SGOT
Normal before and during treatment	98	89	79	70
Normal before and abnormal during treatment	1	5	13	16
Abnormal before and normal during treatment	0	6	5	11
Abnormal before and during treatment	2	1	4	4
p (Mc Nemar Test)	NE	> 0.5	0.09	> 0.5

NE = Test not executable (too few patients)

function as judged by evolution of serum level of bilirubin, transaminases and alkaline phosphatase was observed.

References

1. Frederiksson T, Pettersson U (1979) Oral treatment of pustulosis palmo-plantaris with a new retinoid, Ro 10-9359. Dermatologica 158:60–64
2. Mahrle G, Orfanos CE, Ippen H, Hofbauer M (1979) Haarwachstum, Leberwerte und Lichtempfindlichkeit unter oraler Retinoid-Therapie bei Psoriasis. Dtsch med Wochenschr 104:473–477
3. Thune P, Mørk NJ (1980) A case of centrolobular toxic necrosis of the liver due to aromatic retinoid Tigason (Ro 10-9359). Dermatologica 160:405–408

C.E. Orfanos et al. (eds.)
Retinoids

Some Hepatotoxic Side Effects Observed in Patients Treated with Aromatic Retinoid (Ro 10-9359)

H. Schmidt and E. Foged

During recent years we have in our department participated in various double-blind studies of an aromatic retinoid (Ro 10-9359, Tigason). These studies are going to be published in the near future as a result of a multicentre trial. Beside these, we have treated a total of 28 patients with various dermatoses and followed up these patients for a period from 3 to 151 weeks (mean 43.6 weeks). Out of the patients there were 10 males and 18 females. Their ages ranged from 17 to 71 years with a mean of 40.3 years. All the participants were informed of the effects and possible side effects of the drug. The females were instructed to use a secure contraception for at least one year after discontinuation of the drug.

Table 1 visualizes the types of dermatoses and the number of patients in each group. The dosage was given according to the patient's body-weight and was 1 mg/kg. Most of the patients received between 50 and 75 mg daily in one dose. Provided that side effects were present to a large extent, the dose was reduced. In one patient it was necessary to stop treatment due to intolerance. Due to biochemical side effects the treatment was stopped in four patients (see later).

In Table 2, an account is given of the side effects which in type seemingly are identical to the ones mostly described in literature (1). A group of 15 patients (54%) showed these unpleasant but harmless side effects. However, one of the often quoted side effects, viz. fissures on hands and feet, were not observed in our material.

All patients were investigated every 6th week by carrying out the following blood tests: haematology including differential count, haemoglobin, hematocrit, MCV, MCH, MCHC,

Table 1. Indication for treatment with Ro 10–9359

	No. of patients
Pustulosis palmo-plantaris	6
Psoriasis	4
Eczema hyperkeratoticum	4
Darier's disease	4
Pityriasis rubra pilaris	3
Hyperkeratosis palmaris et plantaris	3
Hyperkeratosis palmaris et plantaris hereditaria (Unna-Thost)	2
Keratosis pilaris	1
Acrodermatitis manuum	1
Total	28

Table 2. Side effects in 15 (54%) of the 28 treated patients. In one patient it was necessary to stop treatment

Dryness of mucous membranes	14
Diffuse hair loss	5
Bleeding from nose	1
Conjunctivitis	1

Table 3. Laboratory abnormalities in 8 (35%) out of 28 patients

Transient:	Increased GPT, LDH or alkaline phosphatase . . .	3
	Increased GPT, GOT and LDH which, however, normalized despite treatment was continued . . .	1
Permanent changes:	developed . . . (see Tables 4–7)	4

Table 4. Laboratory findings in a 58-year-old female. Diagnosis: pustulosis palmoplantaris

Parameter	Before treatment	23. 6. 80	8. 8. 80	5. 9. 80
GOT	normal	*44*	31	35
GPT	normal	22	32	24
LDH	normal	*628*	*567*	*508*
Alkaline phosphatase	normal	*478*	*451*	*360*
Bilirubin	normal	–	7.2	6.3
Ro 10–9359:	14. 5. 80 → 50 mg daily			10. 9. 80 0

Table 5. Laboratory findings in an 18 year-old male. Diagnosis: keratosis palmaris et plantaris hereditaria (Unna-Thost)

Parameter	27. 7. 79	30.11.79	18. 1.80	1. 2. 80	22. 2. 80	14. 3. 80	9. 4. 80	4. 9. 80	26. 9. 80
GOT	*54*	*121*	*91*	*91*	*160*	*65*	*136*	19	19
GPT	–	*279*	*217*	*208*	*307*	*135*	*211*	–	18
LDH	204	255	415	–	*476*	406	412	344	342
Alkaline phosphatase	273	245	246	260	*294*	250	244	233	203
Bilirubin	6.9	6.4	5.7	5.0	5.3	6.5	7.9	8.2	6.1
Ro 10–9359:	31. 7. 80 → 50 mg daily			1. 2. 80 → 25 mg daily		14. 3. 80 0			

Table 6. Laboratory findings in a 63-year-old female. Diagnosis: pityriasis rubra pilaris

Parameter	4. 9. 79	27.11.79	4. 12. 79	12.12.79	7. 1. 80	22. 1. 80
GOT	13	*231*	*107*	*59*	43	28
GPT	-	*254*	-	*63*	-	12
LDH	330	*1110*	*927*	*483*	*474*	*548*
Alkaline phosphatase	117	*335*	*379*	*245*	211	139
Bilirubin	62	8.9	6.6	3.4	2.3	2.3
Ro 10-9359:	15.11.79 ⟶ 11.12.79					
	50 mg daily 0					
	20.12.79: Liver Biopsy: Acute hepatitis with small focal liver cell necroses. Inflammatory reaction in portal space and necroses					

Table 7. Laboratory findings in a 40-year-old female. Diagnosis: psoriasis

Parameter	21. 1. 80	17. 6. 80	14. 7. 80	19. 8. 80	25. 8. 80	2. 9. 80	11. 9. 80	18. 9. 80	25. 9. 80
GOT	7	16	*45*	*329*	*272*	*190*	*199*	*245*	*211*
GPT	-	7	*51*	*575*	-	*282*	*313*	*313*	*286*
LDH	351	407	*457*	*555*	*592*	440	325	*475*	399
Alkaline phosphatase	165	185	155	*365*	*335*	263	270	261	228
Bilirubin	6.7	7	9.4	15.9	17.5	19.4	18.2	11.9	16.5
Ro 10-9359:	11. 6. 80 ⟶ 18. 8. 80 ⟶ 8. 9. 80								
	50 mg daily 0								
	Liver Biopsy (Fig. 1): acute hepatitis with confluent bridging and piece-meal necroses. Inflammatory reaction in bile ducts, portal space and necroses								

reticulocytes, thrombocytes, and sedimentation rate. Besides these, also GOT, GPT, LDH, alkaline phosphatase and bilirubin were examined. Triglycerides were not examined routinely.

From Table 3 it follows that 8 patients developed abnormalities in one or more of the parameters as quoted above. However, in 4 of the patients the abnormal value was transient. In 4 other patients permanent changes developed, and in 2 of them liver biopsy was performed, which in both showed acute hepatitis. The abnormal values are italicized in Tables 4–7.

The histopathological results of liver biopsies are shown in Tables 6 and 7.

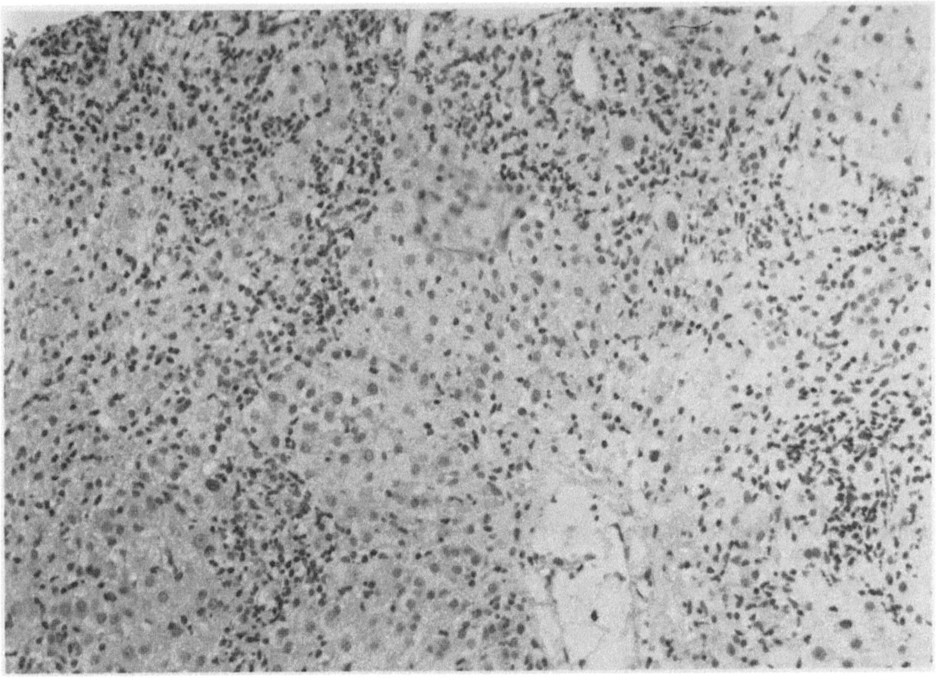

Fig. 1. Liver biopsy from patient in Table 7 showing confluent bridging and piece-meal necroses

Reference

1. Thune P, Mørk NJ (1980) A case of centrolobular toxic necrosis of the liver due to aromatic retinoid - Tigason (Ro 10-9359). Dermatologica 160:405–408

C.E. Orfanos et al. (eds.)
Retinoids

Elevation of Serum Triglyceride Levels from Oral 13-cis-Retinoic Acid

Th.P. Nigra, R.A. Katz and H. Jorgensen

The therapeutic effectiveness of the oral synthetic retinoids has been known since the early seventies as a result of the work done in Europe by Runne et al. (24). It was only after Peck et al. in 1976 published their work on the effectiveness of 13-cis-retinoic acid in the disorders of keratinization and on cystic acne, that widespread interest in the oral synthetic retinoids developed in the United States. Well-controlled clinical studies have now clearly established the effectiveness of the oral synthetic retinoids (19–22).

Thus far, the major adverse effects seen in patients receiving 13-cis-retinoic acid occur in the skin and membranes. These changes, such as cheilitis and conjunctivitis, are dose-related and are reversible when administration of the drug is stopped. Increases in liver enzymes and ESRs have also been observed in a few patients. These, too, are reversible changes, reverting to normal when the drug therapy is discontinued. Serious side effects seen with vitamin A intoxication have not been reported to occur in patients taking the synthetic retinoids (26).

In 1978, we began a clinical trial of 13-cis-retinoic acid on 10 patients with several disorders of keratinization in conjunction with a multi-center investigational protocol. In the course of this study, it was found that seven of our 10 patients developed elevations of serum triglycerides (TG) above the highest normal levels, while maintaining normal levels of serum cholesterol (Chol). To our knowledge, this effect had not been previously reported in humans before we reported it at the Retinoid Workshop in 1979 at the combined meeting of the European Society of Dermatologic Research and the Society of Investigative Dermatology in Amsterdam. Only later did we find that in their original paper in 1973, Runne et al. noted two cases of their 26 patients with increased serum triglycerides (24).

Our clinical studies began in 1978, after a combined meeting of the investigators for the multi-center trial in Nutley, New Jersey. A protocol was established to evaluate the safety and efficacy of 13-cis-retinoic acid in disorders of keratinization. Despite careful consideration by the investigators to evaluate all known toxic side effects of vitamin A, we made no provisions for evaluating serum lipids.

In our institution, serum triglycerides and serum cholesterol were included as part of the blood profile. It was only after the opalescent serum and marked elevation of baseline serum triglycerides of patient No. 4 and their subsequent increase while on the drug, that we began to address the data which, fortunately, had been collected under 12- to 14-hour fasting conditions.

Methods and Results

The 13-cis-retinoic acid was administered to a group of 10 patients. The initial daily dosage of 0.5 mg/kg was increased by 0.5 mg/kg per week until manifestations of the toxic reactions were seen or clinical

Table 1. Disorders of keratinization of patients and baseline and peak serum levels

Patient No.	Age (yrs)	Race	Sex	Height (cm)	Weight (kg)	Primary diagnosis	Baseline TG/Chol. mg/dl	Peak values TG/Chol. mg/dl
1	10	N	M	133	38	Epidermolytic hyperkeratosis	59/159	52/205
2	59	W	M	170	67	Pityriasis rubra pilaris	109/203[a]	350/228
3	46	N	M	173	73	Pityriasis rubra pilaris	93/194	179/227
4	53	W	M	182	71	Ichthyosis vulgaris	357/222	1155/412
5	32	W	F	158	103	Acanthosis nigricans	87/163	560/233
6	11	W	F	140	38	Congenital epidermolytic hyperkeratosis	61/153	180/192
7	48	N	M	174	103	Darier's disease	143/213	488/209
8	13	W	M	151	50	Darier's disease	174/119	436/124
9	30	N	F	166	70	Darier's disease	123/197	161/249
10	20	W	F	160	45	Pustular psoriasis	60/143	138/147

[a] Value obtained after two weeks on the drug. Baseline data not available

improvement was observed, whichever occurred first. The patient then stayed at that dosage level for a total treatment period of 16 weeks, after which the use of the drug was discontinued and the patient was observed at biweekly intervals. If the disease recurred eight weeks or more later, a second course of therapy was initiated at the previous maintenance dosage.

Laboratory studies, obtained before treatment and during the treatment courses, included urinalysis, complete blood cell count, ESR, SGOT and SGPT, alkaline phosphatase, total bilirubin, lactic dehydrogenase, total serum protein and albumin, BUN, creatinine, glucose, electrolytes, calcium, uric acid, platelet count, and prothrombin test. Serum cholesterol level, triglyceride levels, and lipoprotein electrophoresis values were obtained at predetermined intervals after patients had fasted absolutely for 12 to 14 hours (2, 16). No drug was given during this fasting period. None of the patients had unusual dietary habits or a history of excessive alcohol intake. None was receiving estrogen compounds. None of the patients had pre-existing systemic diseases that might predispose to elevated serum triglyceride levels. Six males and four females ranging in age from 10 to 59 years were in this study (Table 1). None were excessively obese, except for patient No. 5. A number of different disorders of keratinization were included suggesting that serum triglyceride elevation was not in relation to a single disease. Peak normal levels of serum triglycerides are generally accepted at 150 mg/dl. Seven of our 10 patients achieved levels in excess of that, while on the drug. Only one patient (No. 4) had a baseline elevation of serum triglycerides of any note. He attained the highest level of serum triglycerides and his cholesterol values nearly doubled; therefore, he had to be terminated from the study. None of the other patients with serum triglyceride elevations had any serum cholesterol elevations above normal.

Dose- and/or time-related elevations of serum triglyceride levels developed in 7 of 10 patients in this study while they were receiving 13-cis-retinoic acid (Fig. 1). Eight weeks after therapy had begun, elevated serum triglyceride levels had developed in five patients. Elevated levels did not develop in two additional patients until 16 weeks after initiating treatment, suggesting that the response might be temporal as well as dose related in some cases. Even some individual patients (Nos. 1, 9, 10) who did not have triglyceride elevations above the highest normal levels, may have shown some dose response increase in triglycerides. Except in patient No. 4, elevation of triglycerides did not occur with doses of drug 1 mg/kg or less. However, in our study, patients did not stay at those levels for greater than two weeks.

After discontinuing use of the drug at 16 weeks or earlier if medically indicated, all patients with elevated serum triglyceride levels showed reversion to baseline levels. This response was slow when the drug was stopped, suggesting perhaps prolonged half-life of the drug. Serum cholesterol levels did not fluctuate substantially during the course of the study

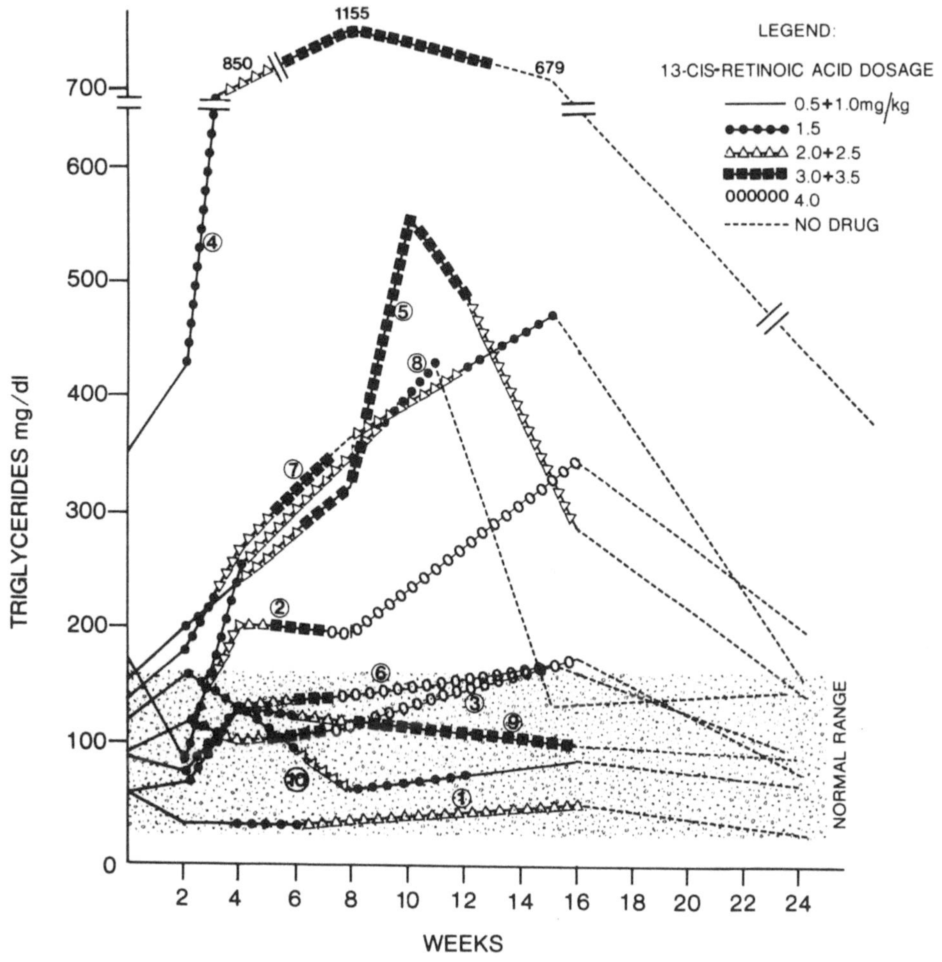

Fig. 1. Dose-response curve with time on various drug dosages

in any of the patients. Serum lipoprotein electrophoresis values obtained in patients at the time that triglyceride levels were raised, showed type-IV patterns with elevated, very-low-density lipoproteins (VLDLs), and no chylomicrons present except in patient No. 2 (Table 2). Two of the patients (Nos. 4 and 8) had type-IV patterns at baseline triglyceride levels. In all other patients, the abnormal patterns disappeared after drug use was discontinued.

Patient No. 4, who was unknown to have type-IV hypertriglyceridemia before receiving the drug, was removed from the study because of increased triglyceride levels greater than 1,000 mg/dl eight weeks after taking the retinoid. Patient No. 5 had an endocrinopathy that included obesity and diabetes mellitus, and was previously reported to have elevated serum triglycerides while on the drug (14). Her triglyceride levels dropped between eight and 16 weeks, due to a decrease in dosage of the retinoid because of cheilitis and conjunctivitis. Patient No. 8 was a 13-year-old boy whose father had died of coronary artery disease at the age of 34 years. He also had a history of hypertriglyceridemia. The child had elevated baseline triglyceride levels that dropped after he began receiving the retinoid, probably as a response to dietary restrictions imposed by the mother. With return to a normal diet, the triglyceride

Table 2. Phenotypes and lipoprotein profiles

Patient No.	Age/ sex		Chol.	TG	VLDL	LDL	HDL	Phenotype
2	59/M	On drug	228[a]	350[a]	-	-	-	
		Off drug for 6 weeks	229	209	29	161	39	Normal
		Off drug for 6 months	208	156	23	142	43	Normal
		Normal range	160–330	10–190	10–40	80–210	30–65	
3	46/M	On drug	206	176	36	139	31	Mild type IV
		Off drug	208	107	24	149	35	Normal
		Normal range	150–310	10–160	5–35	80–190	30–65	
4	53/M	On drug	412[a]	1155[a]	-	-	-	
		Off drug for 7 weeks	270	679	204	52	14	Type IV
		Off drug for 9 months	250	580	173	52	25	Type IV
		Normal range	160–330	10–190	10–40	80–210	30–65	
5	32/F	On drug	189	282	40	132	17	Type IV
		Off drug	196	176	15	149	32	Normal
		Normal range	140–270	10–150	5–35	70–190	35–80	
6	11/F	On drug	194	187	42	141	11	Type IV
		Off drug	136	101	13	95	28	Normal
		Normal range	120–230	10–140	5–25	50–170	30–70	
7	48/M	On drug	210	490	78	112	20	Type IV
		Off drug	208	142	14	174	26	Normal
		Normal range	150–310	10–160	5–35	80–190	30–65	
8	14/M	On drug	60	388	10	40	10	Type IV
		Off drug	111	169	29	72	10	Type IV
		Normal range	120–230	10–140	5–25	50–170	30–65	
9	30/F	On drug	227	130	17	179	31	Normal
		Off drug	182	128	16	122	44	Normal
		Normal range	140–270	10–150	5–35	70–190	35–80	
10	20/F	On drug	185	108	22	133	30	Normal
		Off drug	157	82	17	113	27	Normal
		Normal range	120–240	10–140	5–25	60–170	35–75	

[a] Values obtained at Upjohn Laboratory Procedures South, Inc. All other values Molecular Disease Branch, National Heart, Lung and Blood Institute

levels rose steadily with increased dosage of the drug and dropped toward baseline values when the drug therapy was stopped.

Comment

The oral synthetic retinoids are presently under clinical investigation for use in treatment-resistant dermatologic disorders as well as for their possible application in the chemoprophylaxis of cancer (25). Because of the therapeutic potential of these agents, the spectrum of acute and chronic toxic reactions is of major importance. Elevations of serum triglyceride levels above the highest normal values developed in seven of ten patients in this study treated with 13-cis-retinoic acid while they had normal levels of serum cholesterol. This response seems to be dose-related but may also be time-related in some patients. All blood samples were obtained after patients had fasted 12 to 14 hours so that values were not affected by dietary factors. Since chylomicrons were not present in the samples obtained, it is unlikely that the hypertriglyceridemia is of exogenous origin. Serum lipoprotein electrophoresis values done at the time of elevated triglyceride levels showed type-IV patterns, indicating elevation of VLDLs. These VLDLs are synthesized mainly in the liver and have the function of transporting triglycerides of endogenous origin (8). In contrast to vitamin A, 13-cis-retinoic acid is not stored in the liver; however, it is possible that high doses of the drug may have some toxic effect on the liver that modulates this response (5, 27).

High-density lipoproteins (HDLs) were reduced when there was an elevation of the VLDLs while patients were on the drug. It is possible that mild VLDL elevations may not affect the HDLs and more work in this area is awaited. With the present observations, if elevated or normal HDLs are of protective value in coronary artery disease, then this drug is not helpful (15).

There is considerable evidence that vitamin A and the retinoids affect lipid metabolism in animals. Bring et al. (1) reported that total serum cholesterol levels were inversely related to the dietary vitamin A acetate levels in rats. It was also shown that oral or intramuscular administration of excess vitaminA caused accumulation of triglycerides in the liver and hypertriglyceridemia in rats (17, 18). Erdman and Soloman (7) have reported elevated serum triglyceride levels in cholesterol-fed rats given retinoic acid. This was confirmed by Gerber and Erdman (9), who indicated that this elevation of plasma triglyceride levels from retinoic acid was not related to chylomicrons but to a VLDL-linked elevation. Finally, Gerber and Erdman (10) have shown that dietary administration of all-trans-retinoic acid and 13-cis-retinoic acid given to rats produces hypertriglyceridemia. However, the doses of 13-cis-retinoic acid required to produce this effect were far greater than those needed using the all-trans-retinoic acid derivative. Their studies were short-term and the doses of 13-cis-retinoic acid needed to produce triglyceride elevations in rats were 10x the doses used in humans.

From our study it is clear that patients receiving retinoids must be monitored for triglyceride abnormalities. The importance of serum triglyceride elevations must be considered with respect to short- and long-term effects. The major short-term complication in patients with elevated triglyceride levels is acute pancreatitis. This complication usually occurs when the serum triglyceride levels rise to about 10 times normal (normal, 100 to 200 mg/dl) (3).

Eruptive xanthomas have been reported by Dickens and Connally in a patient on 13-cis-retinoic acid whose levels of triglycerides exceeded 4000 mg/dl (6).

The long-term effects of elevated fasting triglyceride levels are controversial. Some studies have indicated that triglyceride levels are not an important risk factor for coronary artery disease (11). On other studies, an association between elevated serum triglyceride levels and coronary artery disease has been found, but this association may be secondary to the high incidence of diabetes, obesity, and decreased high-density lipoprotein levels (4, 12, 13, 23).

In extensive clinical trials the synthetic Ro 10-9359 has now been recognized to produce triglyceride elevation, but not in such a high proportion of patients on the drug.[1]. Nonetheless, similar precautions must be observed when using all synthetic retinoids.

Patients having elevated fasting serum triglyceride levels before receiving retinoic therapy may be at a greater risk of developing dangerously high levels while receiving the drug, and their condition should be monitored carefully throughout treatment. Individuals with coronary artery disease, diabetes, hypertension, or obesity, or a family history thereof, should be particularly carefully watched. Because of the probable additive effect of diet and

---

[1] Personal communication with Charles Grupper and C.E. Orfanos (see p. 503)

drugs in serum triglyceride levels, all patients being treated with the retinoids who acquire triglyceride abnormalities should have dietary counseling.

Further investigation of the relationship between the retinoids and lipid metabolism is essential because of the vast therapeutic potential of the drug and the necessity of using it effectively but safely.

Conclusions

Seven of 10 patients while on 13-cis-retinoic acid developed serum triglyceride elevations. This phenomena is a result of elevations of very-low-density lipoproteins in their serum. Cholesterol levels did not change and high-density lipoproteins were reduced. When serum triglycerides were elevated, the lipoprotein profiles were type-IV. This phenomenon appears to be a dose response and/or a time response.

Patients receiving synthetic retinoids should be monitored for triglyceride changes, particularly those with obesity, diabetes, exanthema, or a history of coronary artery disease. Sustained elevations of serum triglycerides in light of normal cholesterol has not been established as a predictor of coronary heart disease and should not preclude use of this drug with modest elevations.

Summary

Ten patients with disorders of keratinization were treated with 13-cis-retinoic acid on an investigational protocol to test the efficacy, safety, and optimal dosage schedule for using the drug in these rare disorders. Elevations of serum triglyceride levels above the highest normal levels developed in seven of ten patients, while they maintained normal levels of serum cholesterol. This effect was found to be dose- and/or time-related and reversible. Moderate elevations of serum triglyceride levels have not been clearly established as a risk factor for the development of coronary artery disease. High levels, however, may precipitate acute pancreatitis or eruptive xanthoma. Other synthetic retinoids (Ro 10-9359) have shown to also cause serum triglyceride elevation. Patients receiving retinoids must be carefully monitored for triglyceride abnormalities throughout their course of treatment.

References

1. Bring SV, Ricard CA, Zachringer MV (1965) Relationship between cholesterol and vitamin A metabolism in rats fed at different levels of vitamin A. J Nutr 85:400–406
2. Bucolo G, David H (1973) Quantitative determination of serum triglycerides by use of enzymes. Clin Chem 19:476–482
3. Cameron JL (1977) Lipid abnormalities and acute pancreatitis. Hosp Pract 12:95–101
4. Crepaldi G, Fellin G, Briani G et al (1977) Prevalence of coronary artery disease and peripheral artery disease in patients with different types of primary hyperlipidemia. Arteriosclerosis 26: 593–602
5. DeLuca HF, Roberts AB (1969) Pathways of retinoic acid and retinol metabolism. Am J Clin Nutr 22:945–952
6. Dickens CH, Connolly SM (1980) Eruptive xanthomas associated with isotretinoin (13-cis-retinoid acid). Arch Dermatol 116:951–952
7. Erdman JW, Soloman LW (1977) Effect of retinoic acid feeding on rat serum and liver lipids. Fed Proc 36:1136
8. Fredrickson DS, Levy RI, Lees RS (1967) Fat transport in lipoproteins: An integrated approach to mechanisms and disorders. N Engl J Med 276:34–44, 94–103, 148–156, 215–225, 273–281
9. Gerber LE, Erdman JW (1979) Effect of retinoic acid and retinyl acetate feeding upon lipid metabolism in adrenalectomized rats. J Nutr 109:580–589

10. Gerber LE, Erdman JW (1980) Comparative effects of all-trans- and 13-cis-retinoic acid administration on serum and liver lipids in rats. J Nutr 110:343–351
11. Gordon T, Castelli WP, Hjortland MC et al (1977) Predicting coronary heart disease in middle-aged and older persons: The Framingham study. JAMA 238:497–499
12. Gordon T, Castelli WP, Hjortland MC et al (1977) Diabetes, blood lipids, and the role of obesity in coronary heart disease risk for woman: The Framingham study. Ann Intern Med 87:393–397
13. Hulley SB, Rosenman RH, Bawol RD et al (1980) Epidemiology as a guide to clinical decisions: The association between triglyceride and coronary heart disease. N Engl J Med 302: 1383–1387
14. Katz RA (1980) Treatment of acanthosis nigricans with oral isotretinoin. Arch Dermatol 116: 110–111
15. Keys A (1980) Alpha lipoprotein (HDL) cholesterol in the serum and the risk of coronary heart disease and death. Lancet 2:604–606
16. Lees RS, Hatch FT (1963) Sharper separation of lipoprotein species by paper electrophoresis in albumin-containing buffer. J Lab Clin Med 61:518–528
17. Misra UK (1968) Liver lipids of rats administered excessive amounts of retinol. Can J Biochem 46:697–701
18. Misra UK (1974) Effect of retinol on liver lipid metabolism of rats. Agricultural Biol Chem 38: 247–252
19. Orfanos CE (1978) Oral administration of retinoids. Dermatologica 157 (Suppl 1):2–5
20. Peck GL, Yoder FW (1976) Treatment of lamellar ichthyosis and other keratinizing dermatoses with an oral synthetic retinoid. Lancet 2:1172–1174
21. Peck GL, Yoder FW, Olsen TG et al (1978) Treatment of Darier's disease, lamellar ichthyosis, pityriasis rubra pilaris, cystic acne, and basal cell carcinoma with oral 13-cis-retinoic acid. Dermatologica 157 (Suppl 1):11–12
22. Peck GL, Olsen TG, Yoder FW et al (1979) Prolonged remissions of cystic and conglobate acne with 13-cis-retinoic acid. N Engl J Med 300:329–333
23. Rosenman RH, Brand RJ, Jenkins CD et al (1973) Coronary heart disease in the western collaborative group study: final follow-up experience of 8½ years. JAMA 233:872–877
24. Runne U, Orfanos CE, Gartmann H (1973) Perorale Applikation zweier Derivate der Vitamin A-Säure zur internen Psoriasis-Therapie: 13-cis-beta Vitamin A-Säure und Vitamin A-Säure aethylamid. Arch Dermatol Forsch 247:171–180
25. Sporn MB, Dunlop NM, Newton DL et al (1976) Prevention of chemical carcinogenesis by vitamin A and its synthetic analogs (retinoids). Fed Proc 35:1332–1338
26. Stimson WH (1961) Vitamin A intoxication in adults: Reports of a case with a summary of the literature. N Engl J Med 265:369–373
27. Zile M, DeLuca HF (1968) Retinoic acid: Some aspects of growth-promoting activity in the albino rat. J Nutr 94:302–308

C.E. Orfanos et al. (eds.)
Retinoids

A Proposal for Computing the Dosage of the Aromatic Retinoid Ro 10-9359 in Relation to Skin Surface

S.D. Randazzo, V. Lo Presti and A. Caruso

Pharmacokinetic studies (1, 2) indicate that a single 100-mg dose of Ro 10-9359, administered orally, produces a peak blood level at about 3 h of dosing. About 50% of the administered dose is eliminated into both the urine and feces after 3 h; 90% cumulative is excreted after 96 h; and the remaining 10% is still in the body at 192 h.

Another source (3), however, reports that after several months of continuing treatment with the aromatic retinoid at therapeutic dosages, a plasma residue of 5 to 10% is still detectable as late as 100 days after discontinuation of the treatment, said amount being poured into the blood stream from organs of accumulation such as the liver, adrenal glands, and others (Table 1).

This means that with the daily administration of constant doses for therapeutic purposes there is an accumulation of aromatic retinoid amounting to a situation of overdosing, as indicated by the presence of dose-dependent side effects reflecting hyperactivity of the drug.

Now in view of minimizing side effects (mainly dryness of mucosae, loss of hair, fragility of nails, and pruritus), we (4) have verified the usefulness of administering descending-order doses of the drug (75–50–25 mg) and withdrawing treatment one or two days a week. We found that with this regime the therapeutic effect was somewhat delayed compared to a constant regime of 1 mg/kg daily; but freedom from side effects certainly made ambulatory treatment easier to conduct. One step further, in the hope of arriving at standard dosage cri-

Table 1. Radioactivity per gram of tissue in rats 6 h following oral single dose of radioactively-labelled Ro 10-9359 (Hänni R (1978) Dermatologica 157, Suppl. 1:5)

Tissue	dpm 10^4/g tissue
Liver	370
Adipose tissue	15
Adrenal glands	75
Skin	13
Ovaries	27
Salivary glands	12
Kidneys	28
Lungs	16
Cerebrum	7
Spleen	10
Heart	19
Skeletal muscle	6
Blood, per ml	12

Table 2

Patients	Sex	Age yrs	Height cm	Weight kg	Dosage Ro 10–9359 mg/kg daily	Side effects	Dosage of Ro 10–9359 calculated from skin surface
C.P.	M	51	175	93	90	Yes	79.04
I.C.A.	F	49	155	74	75	Yes	65.74
C.M.	M	65	166	96	95	Yes	77.14
S.G.	M	42	168	80	80	Yes	72.20
D.G.	F	56	160	85	85	Yes	71.44
P.P.	M	64	170	93	100	Yes	77.52
M.M.L.	F	22	166	49	50	No	57.76
A.M.	F	35	168	50	50	No	58.90
A.L.	F	12	155	39	35	No	50.16
O.M.	F	17	160	50	50	No	57.00

teria based on measurable parameters, we now propose to individualize the daily dose relative to each patient's skin surface rather than to body weight. The reason why we propose this change is our observation that daily doses calculated from body weight often proved excessive, and were associated with important side effects, in small-grown and fat patients, whereas the same doses were free of side effects but also less effective therapeutically in tall, lean patients (Table 2).

In normolineal subjects with normal weight-to-height ratio, a daily dose of 1 mg/kg represents 3.8 mg/square decimeter. From the nomogram (Table 3) for determining body surface in adults we read that a subject 173 cm tall, weighing 70 kg, has a skin surface of 1.83 m^2; accordingly, the daily dose of aromatic retinoid should be 1.83 x 38 = 69.54 mg. With the same nomogram, the daily dose in mg is easily calculated for subjects with different weight-to-height ratios (Table 4).

Finally, in order to avoid side effects reflecting the accumulation of aromatic retinoid, we recommend that treatment be discontinued for 1 or 2 days a week in adults and for 2 or 3 days a week in children.

References

1. Hänni R (1978) Pharmacokinetic and metabolic pathways of systemically applied retinoids. Dermatologica 157 (Suppl 1):5–10
2. Hänni R, Bigler F, Vetter W, Englert G, Loelinger P (1975) Der Metabolismus des Retinoids Ro 10-9359. Isolierung und Identifizierung der Hauptmetaboliten aus Plasma, Urin und Faeces des Menschen sowie aus der Galle der Ratte. Synthese von drei Urinmetaboliten. Helv Chim Acta 60:2309
3. Matter A Introductory Report to Giornata di studio sul Retinoide Ro 10-9359 - S.I.D.E.S., Rome, 19 April 1980
4. Randazzo SD, Caruso A, Lo Presti V Effetti terapeutici del retinoide aromatico Ro 10-9359 nella psoriasi grave. Read at S.I.D.E.S. Giornata di studio sul Retinoide Ro 10-9359, Rome, 19 April 1980; Giorn Ital Dermatol in press

Table 3. Nomogram for determining skin surface from height and weight (adults)

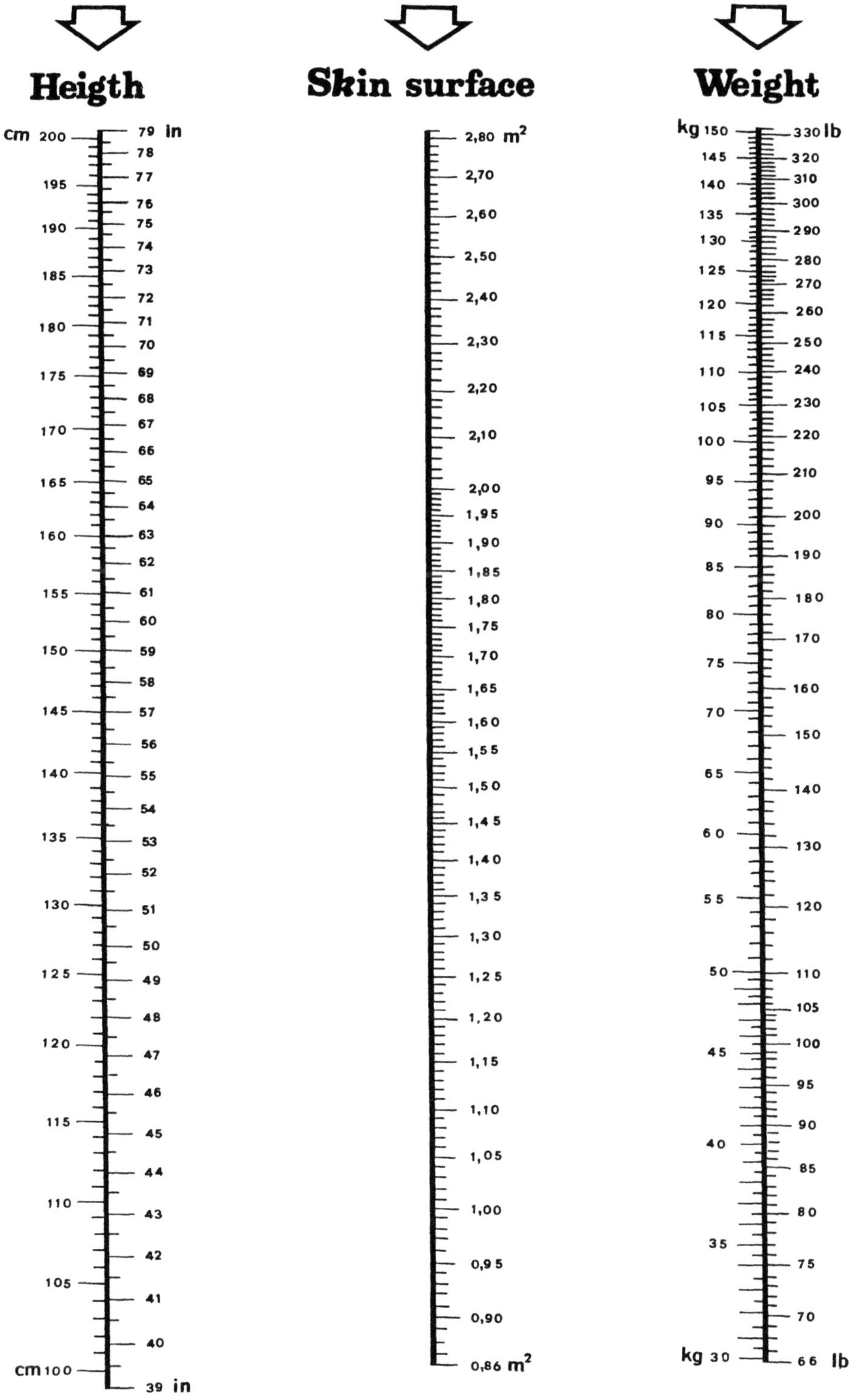

Table 4. Monogram for determining skin surface from height and weight (children)

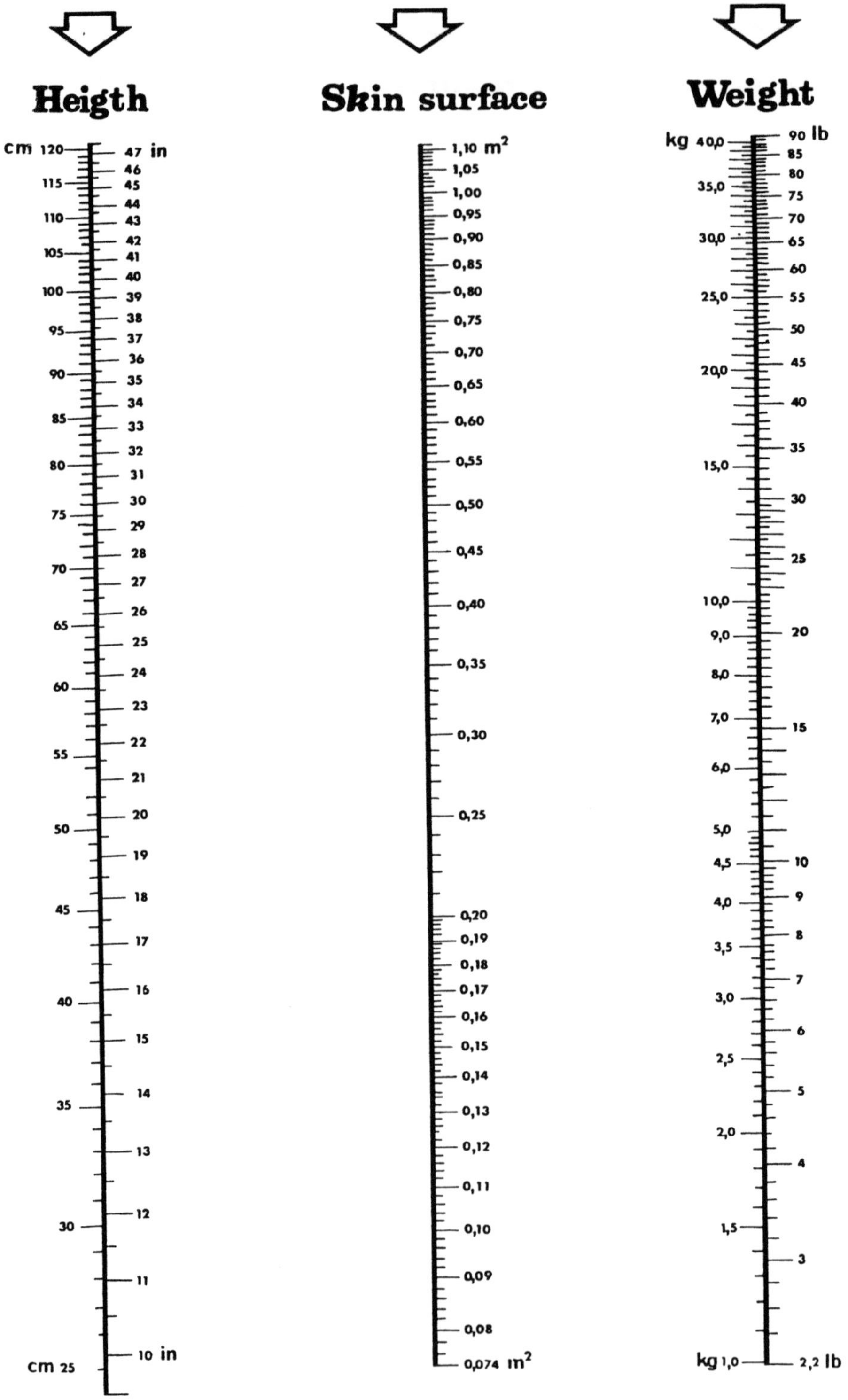

C.E. Orfanos et al. (eds.)
Retinoids

Ro 10-9359 in Psoriasis: Prospective Liver Biopsy Study of Potential Hepatotoxicity

H.H. Roenigk, Jr, M. Sparberg, H. Yokoo and S. Glazer

Psoriasis vulgaris is a chronic recurrent disease of the skin which is frequently disfiguring and emotionally devasting. The etiology of psoriasis is unknown although a genetic predeposition does occur. Many factors such as infection, trauma, climate, emotional upset, alcohol, etc. will precipitate a flare of psoriasis. Systemic therapy to control psoriasis with minimal longterm side effects continues to be a major goal in psoriasis. Systemic corticosteroids will produce remission in psoriasis but the cushingoid side effects and the rebound after discontinuation have made this form of therapy undesirable. Antimetabolite drugs are effective but have significant side effects: azaribine-fatal-thromboembolism; mycophenolic acid-severe diarrhea, increased risk of viral diseases and cancer. Photochemotherapy (PUVA) has become very popular in the past five years with minimal shortterm side effects. However, early aging of the skin and development of skin cancer could limit its use. The search for an ideal and safe systemic therapy continues.

Psoriasis - Liver Diseases?

The skin and the joints are the only organ system known to be affected by psoriasis, but subcellular biochemical and enzyme abnormalities do exist. The liver is frequently abnormal in psoriatic (19, 25) patients but whether these abnormalities are due to psoriasis, abnormal alcohol intake, other diseases, nutritional factors, or systemic therapy for psoriasis, especially methotrexate (MTX) has never been decided.

Methotrexate Hepatotoxicity in Psoriasis

Epidermal cells in psoriasis have a rapid rate of proliferation compared to normal skin. Systemic therapy to control psoriasis has usually attempted to return the rate of cell proliferation to normal by inhibition of the production of DNA. Methotrexate inhibits DNA and for twenty years has been an effective systemic therapy to control psoriasis. Only after years of use in psoriasis, the potential liver toxicity did become apparent.

Retrospective Liver Biopsies - Methotrexate

Possible MTX hepatotoxicity has been reported in malignant and non-malignant disease (3, 17). Coe and Bull (2) reported three non-alcoholic patients with psoriasis who developed post-necrotic cirrhosis of the liver after long term MTX therapy. Most studies were case reports and no pre treatment liver biopsies had been done. A large international study (25) evaluated one or more liver biopsies from about 700 patients with psoriasis who had taken

MTX. Factors such as increased alcohol consumption, age, obesity, diabetes mellitus, duration of treatment with MTX (i.e. cumulative dose) and method of administration (daily versus weekly dosage schedule) may predispose the psoriatic patient to abnormal changes on liver biopsy. A classification of pathological liver biopsy findings and recommendations for the use of MTX were developed (20).

Prospective Liver Biopsies - Methotrexate

Because most studies of MTX hepatotoxicity were retrospective without pretreatment liver biopsies, several prospective projects were started (15, 21, 26). Psoriatics were found to have all degrees of liver pathology including normal livers, fatty metamorphosis, cellular necrosis, periportal inflammation, fibrosis, and cirrhosis. Patients were subsequently placed on MTX or other antimetabolites and yearly follow-up liver biopsies were performed. Roenigk et al. (21) found liver toxicity slightly more often with MTX given orally in divided doses over 36 hours than given as a single weekly dose. Longterm follow-up studies by Zachariae et al. (27) indicate that patients who develop cirrhosis or fibrosis while on MTX do not necessarily progress to rapid hepatic failure and that MTX can be continued for at least a while. The data of Zachariae et al. (27) also support the necessity of liver biopsies in psoriatics controlled with MTX because liver function tests alone are not reliable indicators of fibrosis or cirrhosis (25).

Vitamin A-Hepatotoxicity

Vitamin A is primarily stored in the liver as the biologically inactive palmitate ester. Vitamin A is released to the blood as retinol in association with retinol-binding protein and pre-albumin.

Chronic vitamin A intoxication results in the following clinical features in the skin: dryness, maculopapular rash, fissure, desquamation, pigmentation, and pruritus. Other signs include hair loss, increased intracranial pressure, bone and joint pains, fatigue, and anorexia (14). Since the liver is the major organ for vitamin A storage, hepatomegaly and abnormal liver function studies are often present in chronic intoxication (22, 23).

Animal studies (13) using large doses of vitamin A show lysosomal and mitochondrial damage. Kupfer cells are markedly enlarged and the cytoplasm is filled with fat droplets.

Liver biopsies from humans with chronic vitamin A intoxication show a pattern of perisinusoidal fibrosis, central vein sclerosis, and focal congestion associated with perisinusoidal lipid storage cells (23). The massive accumulation of lipid-storing cells (Ito cells) are found in the network of basement membranes with numerous bundles of collagen, reticulum fibers and lymphocytes (12). Russell et al. (23) suggested that the lesion could result in obstruction of hepatic blood flow, parenchymal cell atrophy, and eventual portal hypertension. Ito cells are considered to be fibroblasts with lipid-storing capacity. They may be transforming into fibroblasts or myoblasts. Vitamin A fluorescence and direct assays of liver revealed substantial increases in vitamin A content.

Retinoids - Ro 10-9359

Metabolism

The retinoid Ro 10-9359 is an analogue of vitamin A acid or retinoic acid. It is absorbed through the portal system, but does not accumulate in the liver in appreciable amounts (9).

The major biliary metabolite is retinoyl-B-glucuronide which is reabsorbed, thereby producing enterohepatic circulation. Retinoic acid is transported in plasma bound to serum albumin. There is also evidence of Ro 10-9359 being excreted unchanged in feces but the conjugation with B-glucuronate in the bile with rapid secretion is thought to protect the liver.

Animal Studies – Liver

Studies in rats indicate the liver retained 16% of the oral dose of Ro 10-9359 while all other tissues had accumulated less than 0.3% of the dose (11). After 8 days the level of Ro 10-9359 in the dog liver was 0.3% of the dose while the level in other tissue was only 0.04%. Toxic doses of Ro 10-9359 given to dogs result in elevation of alkaline phosphatase, SGOT, and SGPT.

Gerber and Erdman (6) found that the all-trans form of retinoic acid induces hypertriglyceridemia in rats. Liver analysis did not reveal fatty liver or alteration in phospholipid, cholesterol, or vitamin A content in any groups. Goerz et al. (8) gave Ro 10-9359 over a thirty-six day period to adult female Wistar rats (5 mg/kg/day) with no histochemically demonstrable changes of the investigated liver enzymes. This may indicate intact function of mitochondria and lysosomes during retinoid treatment. However, a more sensitive method of 0-dealcylation of 7-ethoxycoumarine activity increased significantly beginning at the 8th day of treatment until the end of the study.

Liver Function Study Abnormalities

Several investigators have noted changes in the liver function tests of psoriatic patients treated with Ro 10-9359. Fredriksson (5) commented on two patients with abnormal liver functions and indicated a necessity to follow liver function tests and to exclude patients with liver insufficiency. Guilhou et al. (10) noted that a few psoriatics on Ro 10-9359 showed a slight increase in transaminase and alkaline phosphatase. Goerz and Orfanos (7) in reporting a multicenter controlled study of Ro 10-9359 in psoriasis observed moderate changes only in the serum levels of transaminases – SGOT and SGPT. The serum alkaline phosphatase concentrations showed a slight increase in a few instances. Some of these alterations gradually returned to normal in spite of continued but presumably lower dosage of the drug. Dahl et al. (4) found slightly increased serum alkaline phosphatase and/or SGOT in 6 of 15 patients with psoriasis treated with Ro 10-9359. Orfanos et al. (16) reviewed the laboratory studies of 278 psoriatics in a large multicenter study. They found no significant difference in liver function during or after therapy. Only the serum total bilirubin showed a trend to increase, although SGOT was increased in 14 patients and SGPT in 6 patients. These SGOT and SGPT elevations returned to normal when the drug was stopped, indicating a possible relationship between them. Orfanos indicated that other drugs, alcoholism, preexisting liver damage and muscular activity, etc. needed to be evaluated in these patients.

Liver Biopsies

Few liver biopsies have been performed on humans during Ro 10-9359 therapy. Fredriksson (5) performed a liver biopsy on one patient after Ro 10-9359 which showed chronic aggressive hepatitis. Thune and Mørk (24) reported a 54-year-old female with ichthyosis given Ro 10-9359 at a dose of 75 mg/day and then reduced to 50 mg/day over a three-month period. Laboratory studies showed increases in serum transaminase, bilirubin, and alkaline phosphatase. No pre-treatment liver biopsy was available, but the liver biopsy done one week after Ro 10-9359 was stopped revealed centrolobular necrosis and toxic damage with degeneration of parenchymal cells. Hepatitis B antigens were negative. They suggest a relationship between Ro 10-9359 and the toxic necrosis of the liver cells.

Prospective Study of Liver Biopsies in Psoriatics Treated with Ro 10-9359

Because of the previously recognized liver toxicity from vitamin A, the animal toxicity of Ro 10-9359 in a few studies and the elevation of liver function tests found in a few psoriatics in clinical trials of Ro 10-9359 in Europe over the past three years, it was decided to design a protocol that would demonstrate the safety and effectiveness of Ro 10-9359 and also address the question of hepatotoxicity. Only a few liver biopsies have been done in psoriasis patients receiving Ro 10-9359. Those that were done have been in patients who have demonstrated some toxic effects of Ro 10-9359 based on liver function studies. Since pretreatment liver biopsies in patients receiving Ro 10-9359 have never been performed, this study was designed as a prospective evaluation of liver biopsies during a three year treatment of 20 patients with severe psoriasis given Ro 10-9359.

Patient Selection

Severe psoriatics with or without psoriatic arthritis with at least 20 per cent skin involvement with psoriasis were selected. Most patients had over 50 per cent body coverage and had required previous systemic therapy with either photochemotherapy or methotrexate. Males and females over age 21 could be entered but females with reproductive potential were excluded.

Patients must have had an increased risk of hepatotoxicity defined as presenting with one or more of the following:

1. A history longer than one year of daily alcohol ingestion of three or more equivalent units (one equivalent equaling 12 oz. of beer, 4 oz. of wine, or one mixed drink).
2. A lifetime total use of 2.5 g or greater of methotrexate.
3. Currently with 2 or more persistent abnormalities of liver function tests.
4. Currently with clinical findings of a liver abnormality.
5. A biopsy when last performed with a classification of II or III or a class IV liver biopsy without persistent, significant abnormalities in the liver function tests.

Exclusions

Patients with abnormal kidneys based on renal function studies were excluded. Those with preexisting conditions which may be exacerbated by hypervitaminosis A were excluded. Patients with a liver biopsy finding of cirrhosis were not included although those with fibrosis were allowed. Patients with fasting triglyceride levels more than twice the upper limit of normal or patients on systemic medication for hyperlipidemia were also excluded.

Only bland emollient preparations were used topically except that 1% hydrocortisone cream could be used to limited areas (less than 5% area).

Retinoid Treatment Plan

The initial dose of Ro 10-9359 in all patients was 0.75 mg/kg until the psoriasis was clear and the dose was then reduced to 0.5 mg/kg. Laboratory testing including hemogram, chemistries, liver function studies, and lipid studies were monitored carefully.

The initial treatment trial is scheduled to be 24 weeks (6 months), at which time Ro 10-

9359 will be discontinued for 3 months. The second course of treatment will begin after a 3 month rest period off drug. The chronic three year course of the drug will consist of nine months on drug and three months off drug.

Liver Biopsies

Liver biopsies were done on all patients using the Menghini needle technique and were examined by light microscopy after staining with hematoxylin and eosin and Masson's trichrome stains.

Liver biopsies will be done at the following times:
Pre-treatment
6 months after Ro 10-9359
2 years after Ro 10-9359
3 years after Ro 10-9359

The following is the pathological classification which will be reviewed in a blind fashion by two separate liver pathologists.

Class	Pathologic Changes on Liver Biopsy
I	Normal and no significant changes.
II	Slight-moderate fatty metamorphosis
	Slight nuclear variability
	Mild periportal inflammation
III	Severe fatty metamorphosis
	Moderate-severe nuclear variability
	Moderate-severe periportal inflammation
IV	Fibrosis, mild
V	Moderate-severe fibrosis
	Cirrhosis

Electron microscopic studies of all liver biopsies will also be performed.

Efficacy and Safety

A grading system will be used to judge the efficacy of Ro 10-9359 which will evaluate the extent of disease and estimate extent of scale, erythema, and thickness of lesions. Adverse reactions to the drug will also be noted. Photographs will be used for documentation.

Preliminary Results

Subjects

Thirteen male and 7 female patients have completed their preliminary studies, pretreatment liver biopsy, and started on Ro 10-9359.

Evidence of Previous Hepatotoxicity

Thirteen of the 20 patients have previously received methotrexate therapy for psoriasis.

Eight patients showed abnormalities in at least one liver function test. Moderate to severe history of alcoholism was evident in 3 patients.

Previous Liver Biopsies

Eight patients had previously had liver biopsies (usually because of MTX therapy) prior to being considered for this study. The results of these biopsies were:

Class	Number of patients
I	3
II	1
III	1
IV	2
V	0
Granuloma	1

Pre-Treatment Liver Biopsy

The liver biopsy results of all 20 patients prior to starting Ro 10-9359 are the following:

Class	Number of patients
I	5
II	4
III	0
IV	8
V	0
Non-caseating granuloma (sarcoid)	2
Mild reactive hepatitis	1

Conclusions

There seems to be no question that vitamin A given for long periods of time can result in toxic effects which result in liver damage. These hepatic changes have been demonstrated in both animals and humans. Although Ro 10-9359 is a derivative of vitamin A, most animal studies suggest it is not toxic to the liver. Several preliminary trials with Ro 10-9359 have indicated abnormalities of liver function in some patients. There have been liver biopsies in a few patients who have shown evidence of toxic liver abnormalities due to Ro 10-9359. These biopsies have all been in the posttreatment period. Many other factors such as alcohol, nutrition, and drugs may cause these toxic changes in the liver. A prospective study has been designed involving 20 psoriatic patients with previous liver disease who would be at high risk to develop liver complications from Ro 10-9359. Our preliminary pretreatment liver biopsies have revealed a variety of abnormal pathologic changes. Only 5 biopsies out of 20 were normal. The follow-up liver biopsies which will be done at six months, two and three years after chronic treatment with Ro 10-9359 should answer the question of potential hepatotoxicity from Ro 10-9359.

Summary

Systemic therapy for psoriasis has resulted in severe toxic side effects. Methotrexate produces bone marrow suppression and liver toxicity; azaribine fatal thromboembolism; mycophenolic acid gastrointestinal toxicity and cancer; photochemotherapy skin cancer and cataracts.

Hypervitaminosis A will produce liver damage, and deficiency of vitamin A causes a decrease of cytochrome P-450 content of rat liver. Clinical studies with R 10-9359 show some low incidence of transient changes in serum levels of transaminases (SGOT, SGPT) and alkaline phosphatase. No liver biopsies have been performed.

A prospective study with pretreatment and yearly posttreatment liver biopsies in 20 psoriatics treated with Ro 10-9359 is being studied. Ro 10-9359 is administered at 0.5 mg/kg/day in two divided doses with maximum dose of 1.5 mg/kg/day. Patients with known previous liver disease and no liver disease are included. Liver biopsies are graded I (normal) to V (cirrhosis). Results will give definitive answer to any liver toxicity from Ro 10-9359.

References

1. Babb RR, Kieraldo JH (1978) Cirrhosis due to Hypervitaminosis A. Western J Med 128:244–246
2. Coe RO, Bull FE (1968) Cirrhosis associated with methotrexate treatment of psoriasis. JAMA 206:1515–1520
3. Colsky J, Greenspan EM, Warren TN (1955) Hepatic fibrosis in children with acute leukemia after therapy with folic acid antagonist. Arch Pathol 59:198–206
4. Dahl B, Mollenbach K, Reymann F (1977) Treatment of psoriasis vulgaris with a new retinoid acid derivative Ro 10-9359. Dermatologica 154:261–267
5. Fredriksson T (1978) Oral treatment of psoriasis and pustulosis palmo-plantaris with Ro 10-9359. Dermatologica 157 (Suppl 1):13–18
6. Gerber LE, Erdman JW (1980) Comparative effects of all-trans and 13-cis-retinoic acid administration on serum and liver lipids in rats. J Nutr 110:343–351
7. Goerz G, Orfanos CE (1978) Systemic treatment of psoriasis with a new aromatic retinoid. Dermatologica 157 (Suppl 1):38–44
8. Goerz G, Vizethum W, Kind R, Hornstein M (1978) Influence of a new retinoid (Ro 10-9359) on the cytochrome P-450 system and other enzymes in rats liver. Dermatologica 157 (Suppl 1):26–31
9. Goodman PS (1979) Vitamin A and retinoids: Recent advances - introduction, background and general overview. Fed Proc 38:2501–2503
10. Guilhou JJ, Malbos S, Maznadier J (1978) Oral treatment of severe psoriasis with a new aromatic retinoid (Ro 10-9359). Ann Dermatol Venerol 105:813–818
11. Hänni R (1978) Pharmacokinetic and metabolic pathways of systemically applied retinoids. Dermatologica 157 (Suppl 1):5–10
12. Hruban Z, Russell RM, Boyer JL, Glsgov S, Bagheri SA (1974) Ultrastructural changes in livers of two patients with hypervitaminosis A. Am J Pathol 76:451–461
13. Lane BP (1968) Hepatic microanatomy in hypervitaminosis A in man and rat. Am J Pathol 53: 591–598
14. Muenter MD, Perry HO, Ludwig J (1971) Chronic vitamin A intoxication in adults. Am J Med 50:129–136
15. Nyfors A (1977) Liver biopsies from psoriatics related to methotrexate therapy. Acta Path Microbiol Scand 85:511–518
16. Orfanos CE, Mahrle G, Goerz G, Happle R, Haffauer A, Landes E, Schimpf A (1979) Laboratory investigations in patients with generalized psoriasis under oral retinoid treatment. Dermatologica 159:62–70
17. O'Rourke RA, Eckert GE (1964) Methotrexate-induced hepatic injury in an adult. Arch Intern Med 13:191–194
18. Roenigk Jr HH (1977) Don't give up on the patient with psoriasis. Mod Med, p 59–67, Oct
19. Roenigk Jr HH, Bergfeld WF, St. Jacques R, Owens FJ, Hawk WA (1971) Hepatotoxicity of methotrexate in the treatment of psoriasis. Arch Dermatol 103:250–261

20. Roenigk Jr HH, Maibach HI, Weinstein GD (1972) Use of methotrexate in psoriasis. Arch Dermatol 105:363-365
21. Roenigk Jr HH, Auerbach R, Bergfeld WF, Frost P, Maibach HI, Tindall J, Weinstein GD A cooperative prospective study of the effects of chemotherapy of psoriasis on liver biopsies. Psoriasis: Proceedings of the Second Int. Symposium. Yorke Medical Books, New York, 1976, pp 243-248
22. Rubin E, Florman AL, Degnan T, Diaz J (1970) Hepatic injury in chronic hypervitaminosis A Am J Dis Child 119:132-138
23. Russell RM, Boyer JL, Bagheri SA. Hruban Z: Hepatic injury from chronic hypervitaminosis A resulting in portal hypertension and ascitis. N Engl J Med 291:435-440
24. Thune P, Mørk NJ (1980) A case of centrolobular toxic necrosis of the liver due to aromatic retinoid - Tigason (Ro 10-9359). Dermatologica 160:405-408
25. Weinstein G, Roenigk Jr HH et al. (1973) Psoriasis-liver-methotrexate interactions. Arch Dermatol 108:36-42
26. Werin A, Landells J, Levere G, Baker H (1975) A prospective study of the effects of weekly oral methotrexate on liver biopsy. Br J Dermatol 99:321
27. Zachariae H, Kragballe K, Sagaard H (1980) Methotrexate-induced cirrhosis. Studies including serial liver biopsies during continued treatment. Br J Dermatol 102:407

C.E. Orfanos et al. (eds.)
Retinoids

Polarized Light Examination and Scanning Electron Microscopic Study of Hair, in Patients Treated with Aromatic Retinoids for a Long Time

J.F. Stalder, A. Dupré, P. Litoux, J.L. Bonafé, P. Touron and Ch. Grupper

Existence of alopecia in patients treated with aromatic retinoids (Ro 10-9359, Tigason), justify our study of hair.

Two technics were applied:

1. Polarized-light examination
2. Scanning electron microscopy

Methods

Hair specimens of 27 patients were examined on polarized-light microscopy (Prof. Dupré):

The patients were divided into:

Psoriasis	20
Keratodermia	4
Acroelastopathy	1
Grower's disease	1
Congenital psoriasiform erythroderma	1

The examination of hair was performed after one, two, three, four and six months of treatment.

The scanning electron microscopy was used in 19 cases:

Psoriasis	14
Darier's disease	1
Mycosis fungoides	1
Acroelastopathy	1
Palmo-plantar keratodermia	1

These patients have received aromatic retinoid (1 mg/kg/day) for one to twelve months.

Examination was made systemically, before and after treatment, and by cutting the base of a normal hair. The cutting was done a long time after hair-washing, and the patients always used the same shampoo.

Then sample of hair was dried, metallized with gold, and examined with a scanning electron microscope Jeol (Prof. Litoux).

Results

1. In polarized light:

The results showed no significant abnormalities. We have only noted longitudinal curling, trichorrhexis, which probably existed before treatment.

2. In scanning electron microscopy:

the changes were very small ad had no particular significance:

- in 5 cases: we found many fragments of scales on the hair
- in 2 cases: longitudinal drip

- in 2 cases: there were many spores of yeast
  Often we saw the same nibbled aspect of the edge before and after treatment.
  Horny cells were detached in 7 cases.

Discussion

Neither polarized light examination nor scanning electron microscopy have shown significant changes which would have explained an abnormal fragility of hair.

These techniques fail to explain causes of alopecia in patients who are treated by aromatic retinoids.

Conclusion

We can say that, with our techniques, we could not point out any abnormalities on the hair of patients treated with the aromatic retinoid Ro 10-9359. In the future we will study exfoliated hair rather than cut hair.

Summary

Hair loss observed in patients treated by aromatic retinoid shows that the drug may have side effects on hair development and hair growth (1).

The hair from 10 treated patients was taken on day 0, 30, 60, 90 by cutting the hair at scalp level. This removal was done a long time after hair washing; the patients always used the same scope and with scanning electron microscope. The examination with polarized light microscope showed crystalline appearance of keratin. Scanning electron microscope examination shows the appearance of the cuticule. Alteration of the distal end of cuticular cells was not considered, because it is due to hair combing. On the contrary, proximal alterations of these cells were considered because they possibly represent a side effect of the retinoid acid. Also considered were the ratio height of cuticular cells/hair diameter. The hair examination on day 90 showed that no severe involvement is seen after a long period of treatment.

Reference

1. Mahrle G, Orfanos CE, Ippen H, Hofbauer M (1979) Haarwachstum, Laborwerte und Lichtempfindlichkeit unter oraler Retinoid-Therapie bei Psoriasis. Dtsch Med Wochenschr 104:473–478

C.E. Orfanos et al. (eds.)
Retinoids

Retinoid and Skin Cancer Prevention

L. Schnitzler and J.L. Verret

Relation between vitamin A and cancer is formerly known; the development of synthetic derivatives of vitamin A (synthetic retinoids) as an approach to prophylaxis of neoplasias has been continuing for over ten years (2, 9, 10); the aromatic retinoid has in vitro or in animals an inhibiting action against cutaneous neoplasias (1). It appears therefore very interesting to test this drug in the prevention of cutaneous epitheliomas in human dermatoses with a high risk of cancer.

We started in December 1977 a long prospective study, as comparative as possible, in dermatoses with a high risk of malignant transformation. Preliminary results were given in Tunis (June 1979) (7) and in "Journée dermatologique de Lille" (September 1979). A more detailed issue of this work has been recently published (8).

Material and Methods

1. Aromatic retinoid (etretinate, Ro 10-9359, Roche Laboratories) was used initially at 1 mg/kg/day dose, during meals, once or twice a day. This dose was reduced to 0.75 or 0.50 mg/kg/day when side effects became too marked. Patients were well informed of the experimental nature and inconvenients of this treatment; they were strictly monitored with monthly photographs and biologic controls (plasmatic creatinin, alkalin phosphatase, transaminases and later triglycerids). Teratogenic effects were explained to women able to be pregnant with, if not yet in course, institution of a contraception. Radiographic determination of skeletal development was performed annually in children.

2. Patients. Retinoid activity was studied in patients followed during long periods for cutaneous diseases with high risk of malignant transformation; some were still free of epithelioma; in others one or several epitheliomas had occurred but had been treated and were considered cured when beginning experimentation.

We selected:

- 4 cases of xeroderma pigmentosum (XP) with or without malignant transformation
- 1 case of Mibelli's porokeratosis with multifocal cutaneous carcinoma
- 1 case of basal naevus syndrome (BCNS) with multiple basal cell carcinoma
- 1 case of familial epithelioma of Ferguson-Smith
- 7 actinic keratosis

All these cases except keratosis are detailed elsewhere (3–6).

Results

They were appreciated in each patient by comparsion of the number of epitheliomas occurring in the last two years before and their number since the institution of treatment by retinoid. Furthermore, in two cases (XP and BCNS) we could compare evolution in the treated patient and in an untreated member of the family with the same disease (a twin sister with BCNS and a young brother with XP). In the case of Mibelli's porokeratosis retinoid counterproof of therapy interruption was recently engaged.

Results are summarized in Tables 1 and 2.

1. *Xeroderma pigmentosum.* Four cases were studied: an 11 years boy, a 13 years girl with a

Table 1. Xeroderma pigmentosum – cutaneous lesions before and after retinoid therapy

	1975	1976	1977	1978–1979 Retinoid therapy	Average doses	Duration of retinoid therapy
1 - DUT . . .						
11 years old	Keratosis	Keratosis	Keratosis	–	0,8 mg/kg/day	33 months
2 - RUB . . .						
13 years old	Keratosis	Keratosis	- Keratosis - 1 squamous CC - 2 basal CC	1 basal CC – (recurrence)	0.65mg/kg/day	32 months
3 - CHE . . .						
53 years old	Keratosis M.M.	Keratosis	- Keratosis - 1 squamous CC	M.M. (recurrence)	0,75mg/kg/day	32 months
4 - BOU . . .						
40 years old	–	Keratosis	Keratosis	–	0,75mg/kg/day	20 months

Squamous CC: Squamous cell carcinoma
Basal CC : Basal cell carcinoma
M.M. : Malignant melanoma
F.X.A. : atypical fibroxanthoma
Keratosis : they were always numerous

De Sanctis-Cacchione syndrome, and two adult sisters with variant xeroderma pigmentosum.

In two cases surgical treatment and radiotherapy of several malignant tumors were developed. In these patients photoprotection was effective though not strict enough. Local treatment (mechlorethamine and 5 fluorourazil ointment) had to be stopped because of local irritation. Photoprotection was of course continued during retinoid therapy.

After few months of treatment by retinoid keratoses had almost completely vanished and skin appeared to have recovered its normal softness (as appreciated by patients and their families). Moreover, one epithelioma only was noted (case No. 2) during 32 months of treatment in contrast with multiple keratoses and epitheliomas registered during the previous years. However, this treatment seemed ineffective on pigmentation abnormalities: lentigos

Table 2. Cutaneous lesions before and after retinoid therapy

	1974–1975	1976–1977	1978–1979 Retinoid therapy	Average doses	Duration of Retinoid therapy
Mibelli's porokeratosis	–	3 squamous CC	–	- 0,9 mg/kg/day	28 months
Basal cell naevus syndrome	Numerous Basal CC	Numerous Basal CC	3 Basal CC (basal cell naevus?)	0,5 mg/kg/day	32 months
Ferguson-Smith Epithelioma	Squamous CC Numerous K.A. (5 or 6)	– 2	– 1	0,8 mg/kg/day	21 months

Squamous CC : squamous cell carcinoma
Basal CC : basal cell carcinoma
K.A. : kerato acanthoma

appeared in case No. 2, a Dubreuilh melanosis (lentigo maligna) developed and a malignant melanoma recurred in case No. 3.

2. *Mibelli's porokeratosis.* This case associated generalized eruption of porokeratosis elements with pigmentation disorders and sunlight hypersensitivity.

Over a two years period three epidermoid carcinomas had grown on zosteriform porokeratosis lesions and had been removed surgically without recurrence. During the 1978–1979 treatment period no epithelioma was noticed. Retinoid treatment was then stopped for control in September 1979. Three months later keratosis and verrucous lesions reappeared obviously on lower limb with an histological aspect of Bowen's disease and premalignant keratoses. We think that this sequence of events is clearly in favour of a preventive effect of the treatment.

3. In *Gorlin's disease*, the study was conducted by comparison in identical twins of whom one only was treated by retinoid. Average doses were low (0.6 mg/kg/day) as a consequence of intense side effects (cheilitis); in addition treatment was stopped some weeks because of a severe car's injury with quadriplegia. There was no noticeable diminution of basal cell naevus in number or in size, but the high number of elements initially present impairs counting accuracy. Concerning basal cell carcinomas the treated patient displayed three suspect lesions which were considered as malignant, though they could have been, clinically and histologically, basal cell naevus. In untreated twin sister three typical basal cell carcinomas were noted during the same period.

4. In the case of *Ferguson-Smith disease*, effect of retinoid was difficult to evaluate. A single new lesion, keratoacanthoma-like, was noted during the period of treatment.

5. A particularly good result is to be noticed on *solar keratosis*; regression of keratosis was apparent, beginning from the 2nd month of treatment; stopping of the therapy was followed by partial recurrence three months later.

Toxic Effects

Usual side effects occured but they were reduced or disappeared after reduction of the dose of retinoid; they have never required interruption of the treatment. No biological abnormalities have been noticed.

Efficient Doses

Minimal efficient doses of the drug are not well determined but doses less than 0.75 mg/kg/day seem to have a lower efficiency; a basal cell carcinoma recurrence in a XP and perhaps three basal cell carcinomas in a Gorlin's syndrome were observed; in these two cases the dose of retinoid was lower than 0.75 mg/kg/day.

Conclusion

Oral retinoid therapy seems to prevent or delay development of cutaneous carcinomas in some cutaneous diseases with a high risk of malignancy. Absolute proof cannot by yet given in our cases; of course a longer time, more cases of observation, comparative periods without treatment are needed to confirm our preliminary results.

Summary

The efficacy of oral retinoid in preventing epithelial neoplasias has been demonstrated in animals and by experimental work. In this study, oral retinoid (Ro 10-9359) was used in human skin diseases with high incidence of cutaneous neoplasias: Xeroderma pigmentosum with or without malignant tumors, Mibelli's porokeratosis with multifocal epitheliomas, basal cell naevus syndrome with basal cell carcinomas, familial epithelioma of Ferguson-Smith and actinic keratosis.

This work started in December 1977. Apparent epitheliomas have been treated before trial by surgery, electrocoagulation or radiotherapy. The average dose of retinoid was 0.5 mg to 1 mg/kg daily according to individual tolerance. The number of epitheliomas observed in the years after preceding retinoid therapy was compared to their number appearing during treatment; in two familial cases (basal cell naevus syndrome in twins and xeroderma pigmentosum in two brothers) comparison was made between treated and untreated patients. The first results were very encouraging. An excellent response on solar keratosis is noticed. The occurrence of new epitheliomas seems actually to be prevented or delayed by oral retinoid therapy. In Mibelli's porokeratosis, retinoid was stopped after two years; three months later, keratosis and Bowen' disease had developed. More cases, longer duration of clinical observation and comparative periods without treatment are needed to confirm these preliminary results.

References

1. Bollag W (1974) Therapeutic effects of an aromatic retinoid acid analog on chemically induced skin papillomas and carcinomas of mice. Eur J Cancer 10:731–737
2. Peck LP (1980) Retinoids in dermatology. Arch Dermatol 116:283–284
3. Schnitzler L, Hy R, Schubert B, Eon F, Baudoux C (1976) Xeroderma pigmentosum - présentation clinique de trois familles angevines. Bull Soc Fr Dermatol 4:306–308
4. Schnitzler L, Schubert B, Verret JL, Belperron P, Bernat M (1977) Naevomatose basocellulaire chez deux jumelles. Pédiatrie 1:29–44
5. Schnitzler L, Schubert B, Verret JL, Emeriau M, Brunet A (1977) Epitheliomatose familiale de Ferguson Smith. Ann Dermatol Vénéréol 104:206–216
6. Schubert B, Verret JL, Morer Th, Schnitzler L (1977) Troubles pigmentaires dans un cas de porokératose de Mibelli disséminée. Ann Dermatol Vénéréol. 104:887–892
7. Schnitzler L, Baudoux C, Eon F, Verret JL (1980) Essai de prévention de la dégénérescence épithéliomateuse dans les xeroderma pigmentosum (retinoide aromatique). Résultats dans 5 cas angevins. Congrès des dermatologistes de langue française, Tunis (June 1979). Ed. SAGEP, Tunis
8. Schnitzler L, Schubert B, Verret JL (1980) Essai de prévention des épithéliomas cutanés par le rétinoide aromatique. Ann Dermatol Vénéréol 107:657–663
9. Sporn MB, Newton DL (1979) Chemoprevention of cancer with retinoids. Fed Proc 38:2528–2534
10. Sporn MB (1980) Retinoids and cancer prevention. In: Carcinogenesis, Vol. 5, Slaga TJ (ed), 99–109

C.E. Orfanos et al. (eds.)
Retinoids

Aromatic Retinoid and 13-cis-Retinoic Acid: Spermatological Investigations

W.-B. Schill, A. Wagner, J. Nikolowski and G. Plewig

Investigations using various laboratory tests including semen analyses showed no measurable pharmacological side effects of tretinoin therapy in patients with acne vulgaris treated orally with 20 to 30 mg/day over a period of 90 to 300 days (4). Recently, however, Tsambaos et al. (7) showed a reversible inhibition of spermatogenesis in guinea pigs treated systemically with high doses of aromatic retinoid (Ro 10-9359). This prompted us to study the semen of patients in order to rule out drug-induced inhibition of spermatogenesis or impairment of sperm motility and sperm morphology after systemic treatment with aromatic retinoid or 13-cis-retinoic acid (2).

Aromatic Retinoid (Ro 10-9359)

Materials and Methods

Twelfe men with an everage age of 41.4 ± 13.4 years (range: 23 to 66 years) suffering from exanthematic psoriasis vulgaris were motivated for the study. Semen analyses were performed under standardized conditions with 4 to 5 days of sexual abstinence one week and immediately before treatment. Pretreatment semen analyses showed five men with normozoospermia, three men with asthenozoospermia, three men with oligozoospermia, and one man with teratozoospermia according to the nomenclature of the European Andrology Club (1).

The semen was collected by masturbation within the outpatient clinic of the Department of Dermatology. The following semen parameters were determined according to the methods described by Schirren (6): sperm count (mill/ml), total sperm output (mill/ejaculate), total and progressive motility (%), sperm morphology (% normal shaped spermatozoa), ejaculate volume (ml), and seminal plasma fructose (mg/ml).

In four patients semen analyses were available one month after initiation of therapy, and in twelve patients semen examinations were performed at the end of the three months treatment period. In six patients semen analyses were also available three months after withdrawal of aromatic retinoid.

Statistical analysis was performed by means of the paired Student-t-test. The mean of two pretreatment values was used as baseline to calculate possible differences due to systemic aromatic retinoid therapy.

Aromatic retinoid (Ro 10-9359) was administered orally by a daily dose of 75 mg for a period of one month followed by 50 mg/day for another two months. Thereafter, medication was withdrawn and, if necessary, anti-psoriatic treatment was continued by topical application of dithranol or glucocorticosteroids.

Results

One month after systemic therapy with aromatic retinoid, all semen parameters remained unchanged. Figures 1 and 2 illustrate the results in twelve men obtained at the end of the

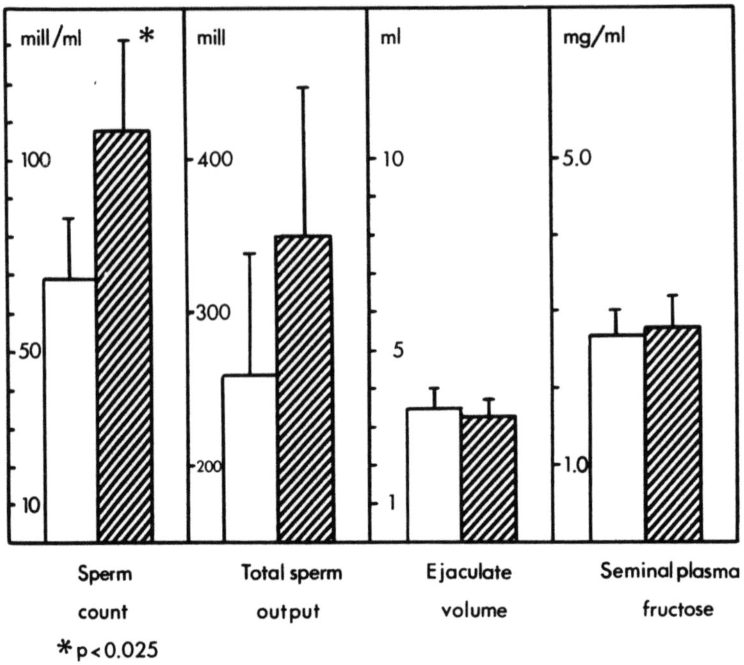

Fig. 1. Treatment of twelve psoriatic men with aromatic retinoid (Ro 10-9359) over a period of three months. For dosage see text. The mean of two pretreatment values (± SEM) is compared with the same value obtained after three months of therapy. Sperm count (mill/ml), total sperm output (mill/ejaculate), ejaculate volume (ml), and seminal plasma fructose (mg/ml) are illustrated

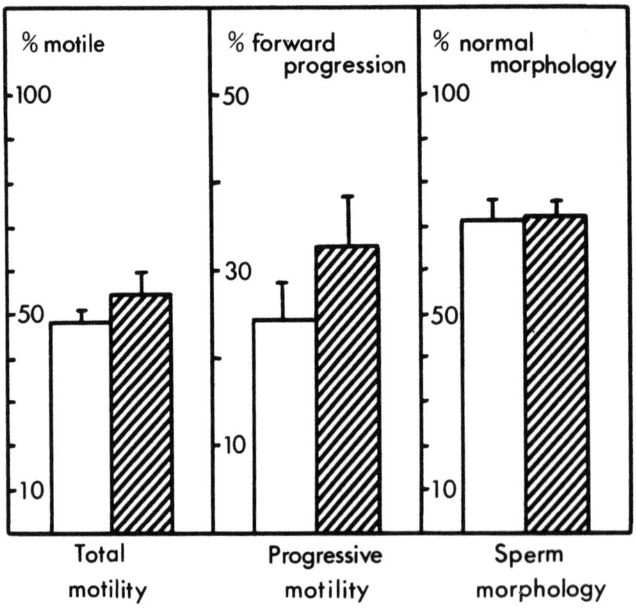

Fig. 2. Total sperm motility (%), progressive sperm motility (%) and sperm morphology (% normal shaped spermatozoa) of the patient material shown in Fig. 1

Table 1. Semen parameters of six men with psoriasis vulgaris treated over a period of three months with aromatic retinoid (Ro 10-9359). Mean values (± SEM) of various semen criteria are shown before, at the end of three months treatment period and three months after withdrawal of the medication

Semen parameters	Treatment with aromatic retinoid		
Mean of six patients	Before	During	After
	Mean of two pretreatment values	End of 3rd month	End of 6th month
Sperm count (mill/ml)	67.8 ± 12.0	127.0* ± 30.0	95.1 ± 18.1
Total sperm output (mill/ejaculate)	204.3 ± 52.1	365.0 ± 120.2	290.9 ± 104.6
Total sperm motility (%)	50.0 ± 5.2	55.0 ± 4.3	61.7** ± 5.4
Progressive sperm motility (%)	32.5 ± 5.4	32.0 ± 8.5	38.3 ± 7.9
Sperm morphology (% normal shaped)	71.8 ± 6.7	70.3 ± 5.2	75.3 ± 4.6
Ejaculate volume (ml)	3.0 ± 0.6	2.9 ± 0.7	2.8 ± 0.7
Seminal plasma fructose (mg/ml)	2.6 ± 0.3	2.6 ± 0.5	2.5 ± 0.3

Student t-test: * $p < 0.05$ ** $p < 0.01$

three months treatment period. A significant increase of the sperm count was observed. In addition, total sperm output increased. Due to greater variations, however, this was statistically not significant. All other semen parameters were not affected, or even showed a tendency towards improved values, as in the case of progressive sperm motility.

Table 1 summarizes the results of six patients in whom semen analyses were available before, at the end of the treatment period, as well as three months later. Again, a significant increase of the sperm count was found at the end of the treatment period. In addition, total sperm motility increased significantly three months after withdrawal of aromatid retinoid. All other semen parameters were not affected during and after therapy.

Comment

In conclusion, the presented spermatological investigations in twelve men subjected to a systemic treatment with aromatic retinoid over a period of three months show that aromatic retinoid in therapeutical doses does not inhibit the spermatogenetic function of the human testis nor leads to an impairment of sperm motility and sperm morphology. The study shows that aromatic retinoid even may have certain beneficial effects on semen parameters.

13-cis-Retinoic Acid (Ro 4-3780)

Materials and Methods

In another study twenty men with an average age of 23.8 ± 7.3 years (range: 15 to 42 years) suffering of acne conglobata (n = 11), acne fulminans (n = 1), acne tetrade (n = 3), acne papulopustulosa (n = 1), gram-negative folliculitis (n = 3) and rosacea (n = 1) were treated orally with 0.2 to 2 mg/kg/day 13-cis-retinoic acid (Ro 4-3780) over a period of three months. Thereafter, 13-cis-retinoic acid was either continued for another three months with a reduced dose of 0.5 mg/kg/day or the medication was withdrawn (5).

Semen analyses were performed before and at several intervals during systemic treatment with 13-cis-retinoic acid as described above.

Results

Remarkably, except for two men with normozoospermia, all other patients showed pathological semen parameters before treatment including ten men with asthenozoospermia, six men with oligozoospermia, and two men with teratozoospermia.

Figure 3 summarizes the results obtained in the total patient group after one, three and six months of treatment with 13-cis-retinoic acid. When compared to the pretreatment values, initial treatment with 13-cis-retinoic acid showed slight changes of the semen parameters after one and three months of observation, but these changes were statistically not significant. At the end of the treatment period, total motility and sperm morphology showed a significant increase, whereas all other semen parameters remained more or less unchanged.

Looking only at those patients who received the highest dose of 1 to 2 mg/kg bodyweight 13-cis-retinoic acid, a similar pattern of the semen parameters was found. Figure 4 shows small changes within the total sperm output, sperm motility and sperm morphology after an observation period of one and three months. At the end of the treatment period, sperm motility and sperm morphology increased significantly. In addition, total sperm output improved, but was statistically not significant. Three months after withdrawal of 13-cis-retinoic acid, all semen parameters reached their initial values.

Comment

From the presented data it is concluded that systemic treatment with 13-cis-retinoic acid in therapeutical doses does not inhibit spematogenesis nor leads to an impairment of sperm

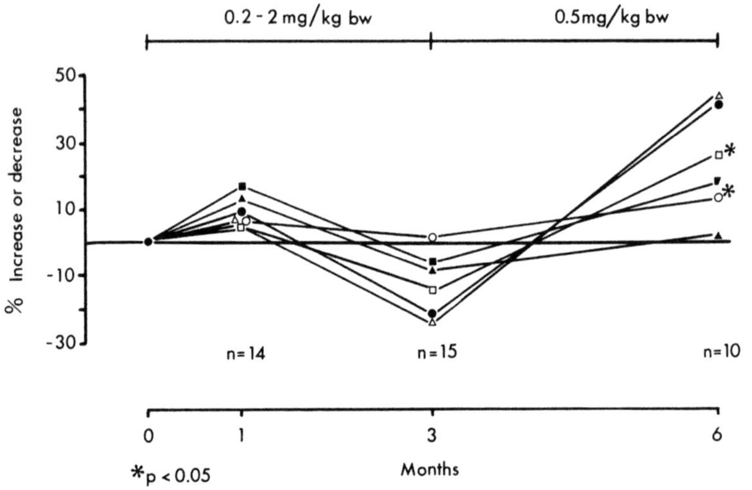

Fig. 3. Semen parameters in twenty patients with acne, gram-negative folliculitis and rosacea treated by various doses of 13-cis-retinoic acid (Ro 4-3780) over a period of six months. The semen parameters obtained after one, three and six months of treatment are compared with those determined before initiation of therapy and expressed in percent increase or decrease. ● = total sperm output, □ = total motility, △ = progressive motility, ○ = sperm morphology, ▲ = ejaculate volume, ■ = seminal plasma fructose

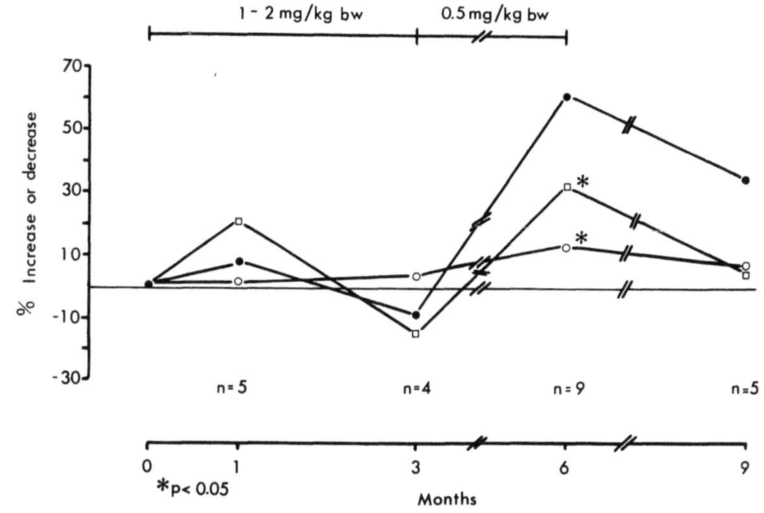

Fig. 4. Semen parameters in patients with acne and rosacea treated with 1–2 mg/kg 13-cis-retinoic acid over a period of three months followed by 0.5 mg/kg for another three months. For details see Figure 3. ● = total sperm output, ○ = sperm morphology, □ = total motility

motility and sperm morphology. In contrast, beneficial effects on semen parameters were monitored concerning sperm count, sperm motility and sperm morphology. The improvement of semen parameters is probably due to the marked anti-inflammatory effect of 13-cis-retinoic acid (3). It is a well-known fact that severe chronic inflammatory processes are able to inhibit spermatogenesis and in addition, may impair maturation and viability of spermatozoa. Thus, parallel to the regression of the severe inflammatory infiltrates and the papulopustular lesions (8) which are found in acne conglobata and acne tetrade, normal functions of the germinal epithelium and the epididymis seem to be restored.

Dramatic improvement of sperm count into the normal range was observed in three men suffering from acne tetrade shown in Fig. 5. The patients received oral treatment with daily 2 mg/kg 13-cis-retinoic acid for three months followed by 0.5 mg/kg for another three months. At the end of the treatment period, a considerable increase of the mean sperm count from 16 mill/ml to 53.5 mill/ml was seen. In addition, sperm morphology increased significantly.

In two of the described men with acne tetrade further semen analyses were available three months after discontinuation of 13-cis-retinoic acid therapy. Total observation period in these two patients was nine months. The individual sperm counts are demonstrated in Fig. 6. Both patients showed different degrees of oligozoospermia before initiation of 13-cis-retinoic acid treatment. After six months of medication, sperm counts were found in the normal range with values above 40 mill spermatozoa/ml. Three months later a further increase of the sperm count was observed. These findings indicate that spermatogenesis was inhibited by the severe chronic inflammation found in acne tetrade. Another possibility is a functional disturbation of the scrotal skin by the inflammatory infiltrates, fistulas, and skin-contractions.

The scrotal skin together with the venous plexus pampiniformis has an important thermoregulatory function in keeping the testicular temperature 1 to 2 °C below the central body temperature which is mandatory to maintain normal spermatogenesis. It is feasable that due to the regression of the horrendous scrotal skin lesions the thermoregulatory func-

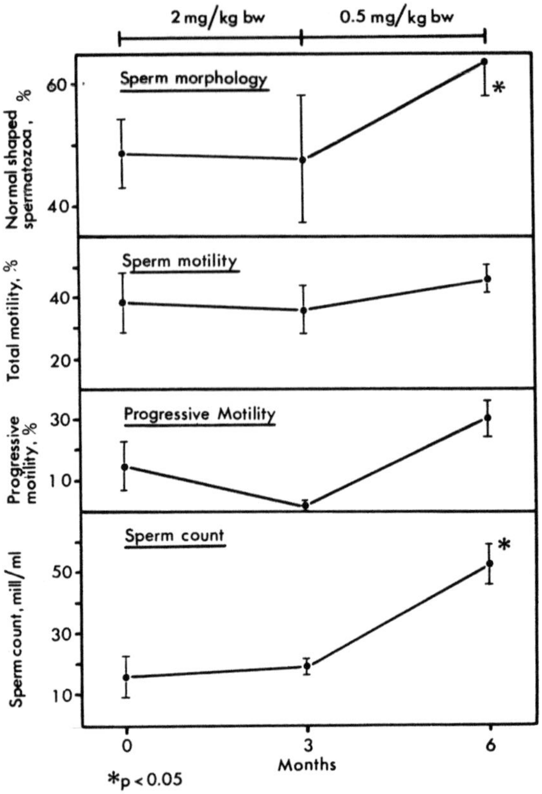

Fig. 5. Semen parameters of three men with severe acne tetrade treated by a daily dose of 2 mg/kg 13-cis-retinoic acid for three months followed by 0.5 mg/kg for another three months. Mean values (± SEM) of semen parameters are plotted before and after three and six months of treatment

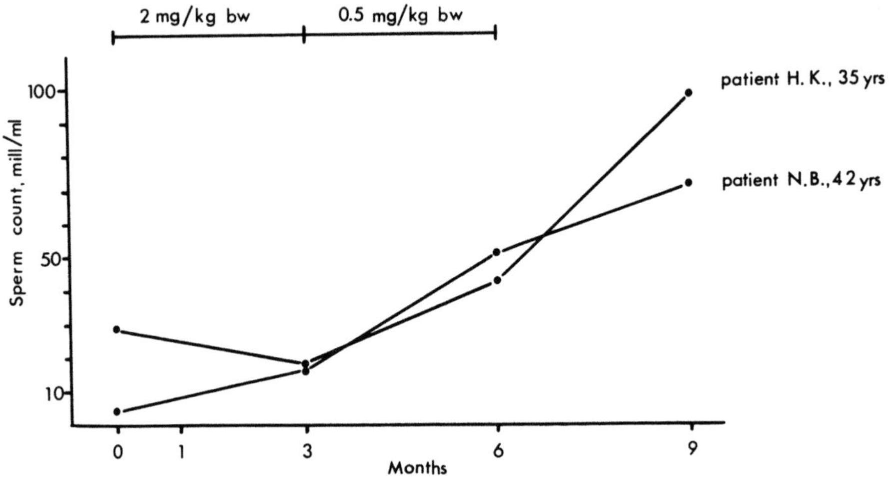

Fig. 6. Individual sperm counts in two men with severe acne tetrade treated with 13-cis-retinoic acid (see Fig. 5) over a period of six months. Semen analyses were available before, one month, three, six and nine months after initiation of therapy

tion of the scrotal skin will be restored in these patients leading to a normalization of spermatogenesis.

In summary, long-term treatment with aromatic retinoid and 13-cis-retinoic acid in therapeutical doses seems not to have any adverse effects in male reproductive functions. In contrast, beneficial effects on semen parameters were observed after treatment with aromatic retinoid and, particularly, with 13-cis-retinoic acid.

Summary

Twelve patients with psoriasis vulgaris were treated orally with 75 mg/day aromatic retinoid Ro 10-9359 for one month, followed with 50 mg for two months. Before and during treatment semen analyses were performed to rule out drug-induced inhibition of spermatogenesis or impairment of sperm maturation. The effects of aromatic retinoid treatment on sperm density, total sperm output, quantitative and qualitative sperm motility, sperm morphology, ejaculate volume and seminal plasma fructose levels are reported and discussed.

In another study twenty patients with acne conglobata, acne fulminans, acne tetrade, ance papulopustulosa, gram-negative folliculitis and rosacea were treated orally with 0,2–2,0 mg/kg/day of 13-cis-retinoic acid Ro 4-3780 for a period of three months. Thereafter, 13-cis-retinoic acid was either continued for another three months (0.5 mg/kg) or the medication was withdrawn. Semen analyses were performed before and at several intervals during systemic treatment with 13-cis-retinoic acid as described above. The results are reported and discussed.

Acknowledgment. The technical assistance of Miss A. Ruhfus and Miss M. Feifel is gratefully appreciated as well as the cooperative help by Drs. C. Hofmann, E. Hölzle, E. Roser-Maaß, G. Wagner and J. Weissmann. Dr. R. Hennes, Hoffmann-La Roche, Grenzach, Germany provided the aromatic retinoid and the 13-cis-retinoic acid.

Supported by grants from the Deutsche Forschungsgemeinschaft Schi 86/7-2 and Pl 58/6.

References

1. European Andrology Club (1970). Andrologie 2:186
2. Mayer H, Bollwag W, Hänni R, Rüegg R (1978) Retinoids, a new class of compounds with prophylactic and therapeutic activities in oncology and dermatology. Experientia 34:1105–1119
3. Plewig G, Wagner A (1980) Anti-inflammatory effects of 13-cis-retinoic acid: an in-vivo study. Arch Dermatol Res 270:89–94
4. Plewig G, Schill W-B, Hofmann C (1979) Orale Behandlung mit Tretinoin. Andrologische, trichologische, ophthalmologische Befunde und Therapieergebnisse bei Akne. Arch Dermatol Res 265:37–47
5. Plewig G, Wagner A, Braun-Falco O (1980) Orale Behandlung schwerster Akneformen mit 13-cis-Retinsäure. Klinische Ergebnisse. Münch med Wochenschr 38:1287–1293
6. Schirren C (1971) Praktische Andrologie. Hartmann, Berlin
7. Tsambaos D, Hundeiker M, Mahrle G, Orfanos CE (1980) Reversible Spermatogenesestörung durch aromatisches Retinoid bei Meerschweinchen. Arch Dermatol Res 267:153–159
8. Wagner A, Plewig G (1980) 13-cis-Retinsäure. Pharmakologische und toxikologische Untersuchungen bei der Behandlung schwerster Akneformen. Münch Med Wochenschr 38:1294–1300

C.E. Orfanos et al. (eds.)
Retinoids

Aromatic Retinoid in the Treatment of Multiple Superficial Basal Cell Carcinoma, Arsenic Keratosis and Kerato-Acanthoma

B. Berretti, Ch. Grupper, Y. Edelson and D. Bermejo

The development of synthetic vitamin A derivatives (synthetic retinoids) as an approach to prophylaxis of neoplasia has been underway for the last ten years (1–5).

Starting in 1971, therapeutic benefits of synthetic retinoids have been reported in some cutaneous non-pigmented premalignant and malignant disorders (1–4).

Since 1977, 36 patients suffering premalignant or malignant skin conditions have been under treatment with aromatic retinoid[1] (Ro 10-9359, Tigason) in our department of dermatology at Aubervilliers.

Patients

36 patients have been treated, 23 males and 13 females with a mean age of 64 years and extremes at 36 and 84 years. 30 patients were of solar type I, 2 of type II, 3 of type III, and 1 of type V.

The following table shows a breakdown of the types of cutaneous disorders represented:

- 2 relapsing multiple basal cell carcinomas
- 2 multiple BCC associated with arsenic intoxication
- 17 multiple BCC associated with multiple actinic keratoses
- 12 multiple actinic keratoses
- 3 keratoacanthomas

Methods

Therapeutic Management

The mean initial daily dosage of Ro 10-9359 (AR) was 1 mg/kg taken in 2 or 3 fractions after fat-enriched meals. This basic dosage was maintained for at least 2 months, at which time the clinical results were evaluated.

The AR dosage was then progressively reduced to 0.75, and then to 0.50 mg/kg/day, and in most cases AR was withdrawn after 4 to 5 months of continuous treatment.

Evaluation of Results

Clinical examinations were performed weekly by the same observer in order to note the clinical results and side effects of initial treatment. Every patient was subjected to a battery of tests before and after the treatment in order to detect not only haematologic, hepatic or renal toxicity, but also to check the lipoprotein status.

[1] The derivative we used was kindly supplied by Roche Laboratories in the form of 10 mg and 25 mg capsules

Table 1. Results of clearing phase therapy[a]

Patients	Results +++	++	+	0
2 Multiple BCC	1	1		
2 Multiple BCC/As		2		
17 Multiple BCC + AK on BCC	1	5	7	1
on AK	10	5		2
12 Actinic keratosis	10	1		1
3 Keratoacanthomas	3			

[a] In some patients treatment had to be withdrawn due to severe side effects; BCC = basal cell carcinoma; AK = actinic keratosis; AS = arsenic

Follow-up

Our patients were evaluated both following the reduction in AR initial dose, and after the drug was withdrawn. We were thus able to check the maintenance of remission, as well as the chronology, incidence and severity of relapses. The follow-up study ranged between 3 and 27 months.

Results

We have classified our results according to our usual rating (Table 1):
+++ = complete clearing
++ = good improvement
+ = limited reduction
0 = failure

Tolerance and Side Effects

Like other authors, we observed a number of clinical side effects attributable to AR treatment. Some were frequent, occurring in about 90% of patients: cheilitis with exfoliation, rhagades, stomatitis, glossitis and dryness of the nasal mucosa. Other effects were seen less frequently, including transitory alopecia, palmo-plantar lesions with ragged desquamation, thinning of the skin with hyperhidrosis, pruritus, and generalized erythema. In a few cases the side effects were severe enough to require early cessation of AR treatment.

No changes were seen in the laboratory parameters studied.

Discussion

In the 3 keratoacanthoma patients complete clearing was obtained after 2 to 3 months of treatment. One patient presented a severe relapsing phagedenic type on the nose; this patient suffered a relapse 27 months after AR was withdrawn.

Of the 29 patients with actinic keratosis, whether or not in association with BCC, complete clearing was obtained in 70%, with a good improvement being seen in an additional 20%. Of the 21 cases of multiple BCC, either isolated or associated with arsenic intoxication or AK, complete clearing was obtained in only 2 patients (or 10%) with a good improvement being seen in 8 others (or 38%). In both conditions relapses occurred at various times after dose reduction or withdrawal of AR. BCC recurrences occurred earlier, more frequently, and with greater severity than did recurrences of actinic keratosis. A maintenance treatment is therefore mandatory, but its accurate dosage and its duration are still to be determined:

our experience supports the notion of a threshold dosage which is both individual and unpredictable.

Conclusions

The aromatic retinoid seems to offer a useful therapeutic approach to the treatment of cutaneous non-pigmented precancerous and cancerous conditions, confirming animal experimental data and some previous clinical reports.

In the treatment of keratoacanthoma and for actinic keratoses the aromatic retinoid appears to offer a promising treatment of first choice. For multiple relapsing BCC it could be of use as an adjuvant before or after conventional destructive methods, especially when these methods are only palliative.

Nevertheless, further multicentre studies are necessary for an accurate evaluation of aromatic retinoid, either as a single agent, or in association with other therapeutic modalities in the treatment of cutaneous malignancies.

Summary

The authors have treated, with aromatic retinoid, 19 cases of multiple superficial BCC, 2 cases of arsenic BCC, 12 cases of disseminated solar keratosis and 3 cases of keratoacanthoma (one giant, phagedenic).

The daily dose was 1 mg–1.5 mg/kg/day, during 4–24 months. For some patients, the follow-up was 3 years.

The initial results were very promising, but further treatments with longer follow-up are mandatory, the daily dose varying from one patient to another.

References

1. Bollag W, Hanck A (1977) From vitamin A to retinoids: Modern trends in the field of oncology and dermatology. Acta Vitaminol Enzymol (Milano) 31:113–123
2. Mayer H, Bollag W, Hänni R, Rüegg R (1978) Retinoids, a new class of compounds with prophylactic and therapeutic activities in oncology and dermatology. Experientia 34:1105–1119
3. Peck GL, Olsentg, Butkus D et al (1979) Treatment of basal cell carcinomas with 13-cis-retinoic acid. Proc Am Ass Cancer Res 20:56
4. Schnitzler L, Schubert B, Verret JL (1980) Essai de prévention des epithéliomas cutanés par le rétinoïde aromatique. Ann Dermatol Vénéréol 107:657–663
5. Sporn MB, Newton DL (1979) Chemoprevention of cancer with retinoids. Fed Proc 38:2528–2534

C.E. Orfanos et al. (eds.)
Retinoids

Ro 10-9359 in Epidermodysplasia Verruciformis. Preliminary Report

S. Jablońska, S. Obalek, H. Wolska and M. Jarząbek-Chorzelska

Ro 10-9359 was shown to have some anti-tumor activity in experimental in vitro studies (4, 15, 17), in chemically induced cancers and papillomas (2, 3, 5) and in multiple keratoacanthomas and epitheliomas in humans (7, 8, 16). There were also some attempts to apply this treatment in cases of epidermodysplasia verruciformis (EV) induced by oncogenic papilloma virus HPV-5 (1, 9, 12).

The aim of our study was to find out whether Ro 10-9359 is effective in EV induced by HPV-3, i.e. in widespread, life-long wart infection induced by non-oncogenic papilloma virus responsible for verrucae planae, as well as in a case of double infection with HPV-3 and with HPV-5 subtype; the latter proved to be highly oncogenic.

Material and Methods

Three patients with EV type 3, and one patient with double HPV-3 and HPV-5 infection were admitted to the trial. In addition, this therapy was applied to a patient with acrokeratosis verruciformis, i.e., cutaneous lesions of verrucae planae type, but not induced by viruses (negative studies for virus DNA, negative electronmicroscopy and immunofluorescence).

In all patients with EV, HPV type was characterized by molecular procedures (molecular hybridization and restriction enzyme analysis) and the clinical, histological and immunological studies of the patients have been reported elsewhere (11, 13, 14). All patients have been previously treated with various methods, with no effect. All had defect of cell mediated immunity (6, 10).

The dosage of Ro 10-9359 was 1 mg/kg/day, the maximum dose 75 mg/kg/day. If side effects occurred, the dosage was reduced to 0.3–0.5 mg/kg/day. No local therapy was applied simultaneously.

Results and Comments

In all three patients with EV induced by HPV-3 there was a very marked improvement after 7 or 8 weeks of treatment with a full dose (Fig. 1a, b). After that, one patient stopped the treatment because of side effects, and in two others the dose was reduced to 50 mg/day. This was sufficient to prevent a relapse, but not sufficient to remove the side effects (moderate to severe dryness of the lips, thinning and desquamation of the skin in both patients and hair loss in one). When the dosage was further reduced to 30 mg/day in one of the patients, there was a relapse of cutaneous lesions, which again improved markedly after the daily dosage was increased. In the second patient the improvement was maintained for several months after the withdrawal of the drug.

In the patient with EV induced by HPV-3 and HPV-5, two types of lesions, due to HPV-3 on the extremities, and to HPV-5 on the face and trunk, improved markedly.

Immunofluorescence studies with the use of specific immune sera against HPV-5 and

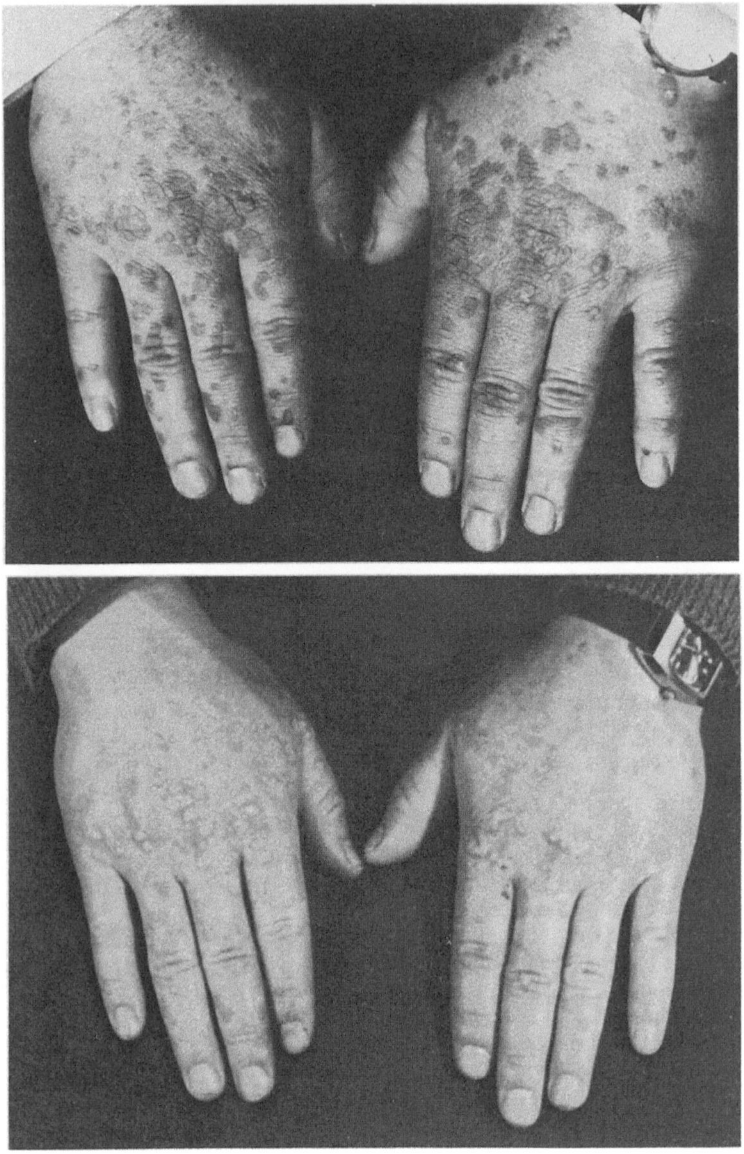

a

b

Fig. 1a, b. Patient M.G. Epidermodysplasia verruciformis induced by HPV-3. **a** before treatment, **b** after 8 weeks of therapy with Ro 10-9359

HPV-3, performed at weeks 3, 6 and 8 in all patients did not disclose viruses (Fig. 2a, b and 3 a, b).

In the patient infected with oncogenic HPV-5 type virus no new cancers and precancerous lesions developed during the therapy.

In the patient with acrokeratosis verruciformis the improvement, although evident after 8 weeks of therapy, was not as remarkable as in patients with EV. After the dose was reduced to 30 mg/day, there was a relapse. The improvement occurred again after the therapy with 60 mg/day on alternate days was installed.

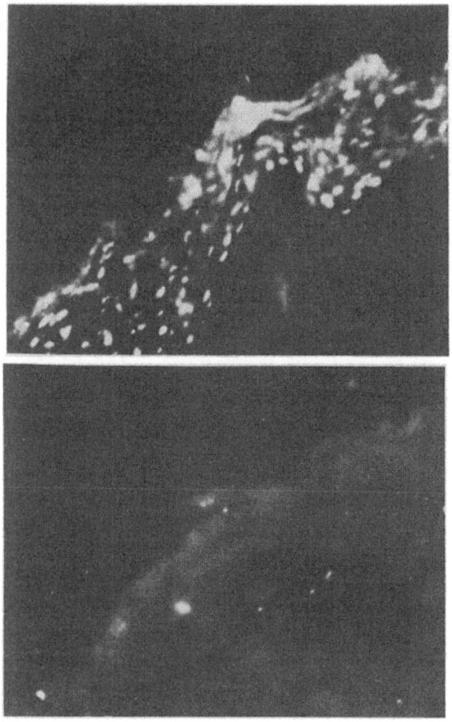

a

b

Fig. 2a, b. Patient P.B. Epidermodysplasia verruciformis induced by HPV-3. Specimens taken from the wart-like lesion on the hands. Immunofluorescence staining with the use of immunserum against HPV-3. **a** before the treatment. Numerous intranuclear viruses present in the stratum granulosum and intermedium (× 440), **b** after 6 weeks of treatment, IF staining does not disclose viruses (× 440)

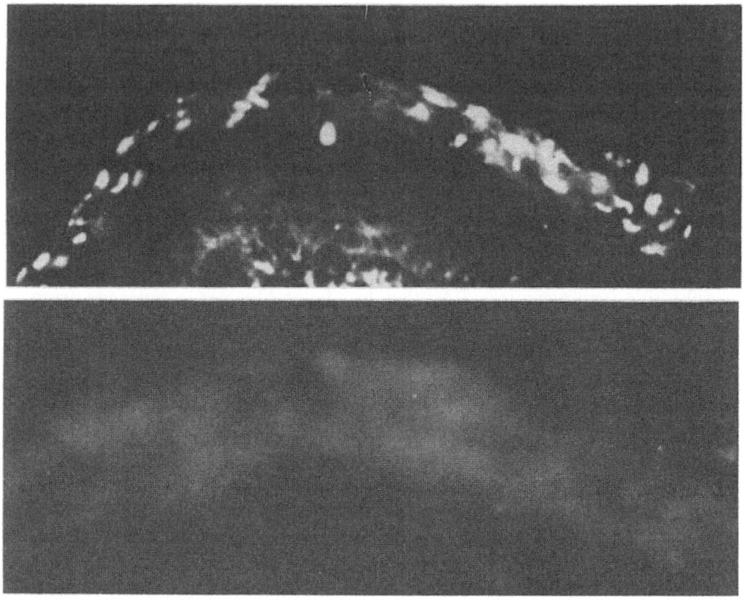

a

b

Fig. 3a, b. Patient J.D. EV induced by HPV-3 and HPV-5. Specimens taken from the red plaques on the trunk (pityriasis versicolor-like lesion). Immunofluorescence staining with the use of immunserum against HPV-5. **a** before the treatment. HPV-5 viruses, usually larger than HPV-3 and of somewhat different morphology, are present in the granular and horny layer (× 490) **b** after 6 weeks of treatment no viruses are disclosed by IF method (× 490)

It is interesting to note, that the improvement in this case was much slower than in patients with EV, and a complete remission was not achieved.

The side effects were mild to severe in all patients treated (see above). In one patient there was a moderate loss of hair when on full dose of drug.

Summary

Preliminary data on the treatment of epidermodysplasia verruciformis, induced by HPV-3 and by both viruses HPV-5 and HPV-3, have shown a high efficacy of Ro 10-9359, which has produced a great improvement in all patients for the first time in this life-long infection. The effects depended on the dose of the drug, since the decrease of the dosage resulted in a relapse of cutaneous lesions. Interestingly, in patients treated with Ro 10-9359 and highly improved, the control immunofluorescence studies did not disclose viruses, present before the treatment, within the granular and horny layers. However, this cannot be regarded as evidence of cure. Side effects occurred in all patients and were mild to severe; in some, prevented further therapy. At the present time, Ro 10-9359 appears to be the only effective, or at least partially effective drug, in EV. Further trials are needed before the full effectiveness of this therapy in both forms of EV could be assessed.

References

1. Blanchet-Bardon Cl, Ghouti C, Bzowski A, Puissant A, Croissant O, Favre M, Lutzner M, Orth G Epidermodysplasie verruciforme de Lutz Lewandowsky (2 cas). Présenté, Journ Dermatol Paris, March 1980
2. Bollag W (1975) Therapeutic effects of an aromatic retinoic acid analog on chemically induced skin papillomas and carcinomas on mice. Eur J Cancer 10:731–737
3. Bollag W (1979) Retinoids and cancer. Cancer Chemother. Pharmacol 3:207–215
4. Chopra DP, Wilkoff LJ (1979) Activity of retinoids against benzo (A) pyrene-induced hyperplasia in mouse prostate organ cultures. Eur J Cancer 15:1417–1423
5. Frigg M, Torhorst J (1977) Autoradiographic and histopathologic studies on the mode of action of an aromatic retinoid (Ro 10-9359) on chemically induced epithelial tumors in Swiss mice. J Natl Cancer Inst 58:1365–1371
6. Gliński W, Jablonska S, Langner A, Obalek S, Haftek M, Proniewska M (1976) Cell-mediated immunity in epidermodysplasia verruciformis. Dermatologica 153:218–227
7. Grupper Ch Keratoacanthomes géantes recidivantes. Exposé, Journ Dermatol, Paris, March 1979
8. Grupper C, Berretti B Polyepitheliomatose superficiale multiple avec keratoses ponctuées palmo-plantaires et dyschromie (arsenicisme?). Résultats très favorables par la rétinoide aromatique. Exposé, Journ Dermatol, Paris, March 1980
9. Grupper C, Bermejo D, Briche R, Rambert A Epidermodysplasie verruciforme ou verrues multiples disséminées: 2 cas. Exposé, Journ Dermatol, Paris, March 1980
10. Jabłońska S, Orth G, Jarząbek-Chorzelska M, Rzęsa G, Obalek S, Gliński W, Favre M, Croissant O (1978) Immunological studies in epidermodysplasia verruciformis. Bull Cancer (Paris) 65:183–190
11. Jabłońska S, Orth G, Jarząbek-Chorzelska M, Rzęsa G, Obalek S, Gliński W, Favre M, Croissant O (1979) Epidermodysplasia verruciformis versus disseminated verrucae planae: Is epidermodysplasia verruciformis a generalized infection with wart virus? J Invest Dermatol 72:114–119
12. Lutzner MA, Blanchet-Bardon Cl (1980) Oral retinoid treatment of human papillomavirus type 5-induced epidermodysplasia verruciformis. N Engl J Med 302:1091
13. Orth G, Jabłońska S, Favre M, Croissant O, Jarząbek-Chorzelska M, Rzęsa G (1978) Characterization of two types of human papillomaviruses in lesions of epidermodysplasia verruciformis. Proc Natl Acad Sci USA 75:1537–1541
14. Orth G, Jabłońska S, Jarząbek-Chorzelska M, Obalek S, Rzęsa G, Favre M, Croissant O (1979) Characteristics of the lesions and risk of malignant conversion as related to the type of the human papillomavirus involved in epidermodysplasia verruciformis. Cancer Res 39:1074–1082

15. Puglisi CV, De Silva JAF (1978) Determination of retinoic acid/13-cis-retinoic and all-trans/ and aromatic retinoic acid analogs possessing anti-tumor activity in biological fluids by high-performance liquid chromatography. J Chromatogr 152:421–430
16. Steigleder GK, Sterry W, Pullmann H Kerato-acanthomes multiples. A propos d'un cas avec examen histologique, ultrastructural, enzyme-histochimique et autoradiographique. Exposé, Journ Dermatol, Paris, March 1980
17. Verma AK, Rice HM, Shapas BG, Boutweel RK (1978) Inhibition of 12-0-Tetradecanoylphorbol-13-acetate-induced ornithine decarboxylase activity in mouse epidermis by vitamin A analogs (retinoids). Cancer Res 38:793–801

C.E. Orfanos et al. (eds.)
Retinoids

Oral Aromatic Retinoid (Ro 10-9359) Treatment of Two Patients Suffering with the Severe Form of Epidermodysplasia Verruciformis

M.A. Lutzner, C. Blanchet-Bardon and A. Puissant

Epidermodysplasia verruciformis (EV) is a disease ordinarily beginning in childhood and characterized by widespread chronic pityriasis versicolor-like lesions (PV-like), multiple bowenoid cancers, and usually depressed cell-mediated immunity (5). It has been shown that benign lesions are induced by human papillomavirus group 5 (HPV-5) (9), and that HPV-5 is potentially oncogenic since most all patients with the severe form of EV have skin cancers and those cancers so far studied contain multiple copies of this viral genome (8).

Our first EV patient is a 32 year old black Congolese male with PV-like lesions present since age two; a younger sister had similar lesions since childhood. Both are the product of a consanguineous marriage, the parents having been distant cousins. There are five other normal siblings. At age 27 he first developed multiple tumors on his buttocks, palms, and inguinal-scrotal region which proved to be bowenoid cancers. These were surgically removed. One large tumor at the base of his thumb, following irradiation therapy, became invasive and proved to be a squamous cell carcinoma, requiring amputation of the thumb. HPV-5 was identified in his benign lesions by recognition of specific cytopathic effect (8), and by specific immunofluorescence (8). Papillomavirus was identified by electron microscopy. Extraction and analysis of viral DNA from his benign lesions indicated infection with HPV-5c (8) (analysis by M. Favre).

Since retinoids are known to alter keratinization (13), we reasoned that Ro 10-9359 might be effective in treating EV, since the papillomaviruses are known to be fastidious in their host specificity, requiring human keratinocytes in an advanced stage of differentiation for their replication and assembly; that is, cells of the granular layer. Thus, we began treatment with Ro 10-9359, 1 mg/kg/day. After two months, we noticed that most of his achromic lesions were repigmenting (Fig. 1), and that his pigmented papular lesions were flatter and less scaly. Two bowenoid tumors, inadvertently missed at the time of surgery, reduced in size following four months of treatment. After three months of retinoids, two skin biopsies and multiple scrapings were taken from residual lesions and examined for the presence of human papillomavirus. No cytopathic evidence for the presence of virus was found histologically, and specific immunofluorescence was now negative. By electron microscopy, the large amount of virus seen prior to treatment was radically reduced and after a long search only one cell could be found with virus particles. Extraction and analysis of viral DNA revealed an approximate reduction of one hundred fold (analysed by W. Jibard). Thus, it appeared that our patient was nearly free of papillomavirus infection and it was hoped that continued treatment would prevent or retard new cancer growth (6).

Because of encouraging results with our first patient, we began treating a second EV patient (7), a 40 year old man with one normal sibling and no parental consanguinity, thus a sporadic case. He had developed widespread PV-like lesions at the age of six, and at age 25 bowenoid cancers began to appear on the left side of his forehead. Following treatment with electrosurgery and irradiation, the lesions became invasive, as in our first patient, requiring excision of his left eye and extensive skin grafting. Unfortunately, new lesions continued to develop adjacent to the graft on the right side of his forehead and proved to be resistant to combined chemotherapy consisting of bleomycin and vinblastine, which had been initiated at the time of surgery. Oral Ro 10-9359, 1 mg/kg/day was begun. PV-like lesions which had been originally scaly, became smoother and more erythematous. But, unfortunately, the forehead cancer worsened. Immunofluorescence specific for group HPV-5, which had been positive

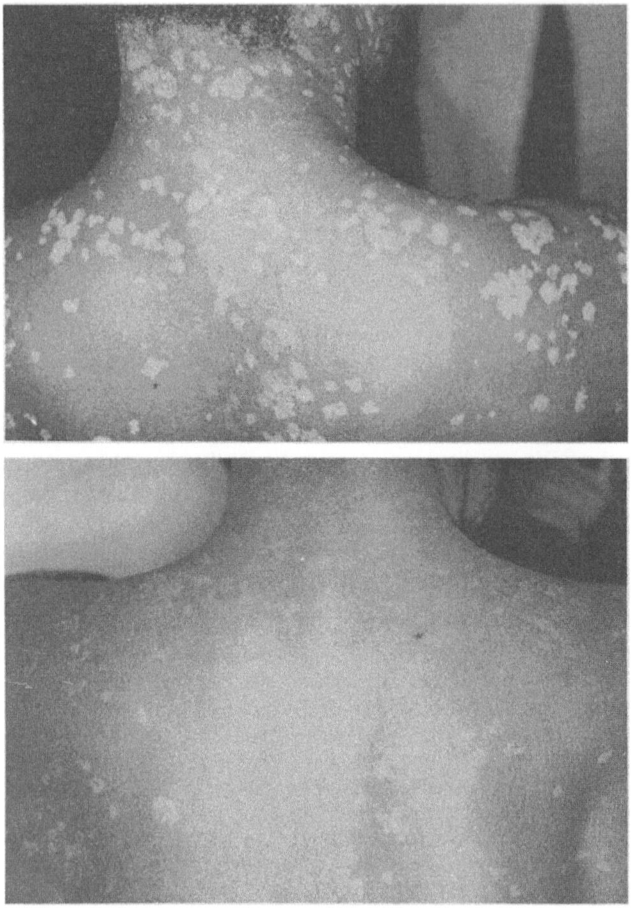

a

b

Fig. 1. a Achromic pityriasis versicolor-like lesions on the back of patient one, prior to retinoid treatment. **b** Repigmentation of achromic lesions following six months of retinoid treatment

prior to therapy, remained strongly positive in spite of three months of treatment with retinoids. Also, papillomavirus seen by electron microscopy previously, was still found in large quantity following three months of treatment. So, unlike our first patient, Ro 10-9359 appeared to have little effect in inhibiting virus production in this second patient, even though there was some clinical improvement.

Post-retinoid structural abnormalities of keratinocytes could be seen in 1 mμ sections from skin biopsies of both patients' residual lesions; that is, multiple cytoplasmic vacuoles, sometimes compressing nuclei to crescents, and in addition a reduction in the number of stratum corneum cells. By electron microscopy, some of the vacuoles were seen to be electron lucid; others contained finely granular material (Fig. 2). No virus particles were found in cells which showed this post-retinoid effect, even in patient two where much virus was seen, suggesting that retinoids might inhibit viral replication and assembly in individual keratinocytes as originally hypothesized.

We are at a loss to explain, at the moment, the differences in the response of these two patients to Ro 10-9359. However, we have recently found patient two to be infected with an unusual subtype of HPV-5 (analysed by M. Favre), differing from the more common HPV-5c of patient one. Perhaps there are differing responses to retinoids according to the virus type or subtype. Another difference is that patient one is a familial case while patient two is a a 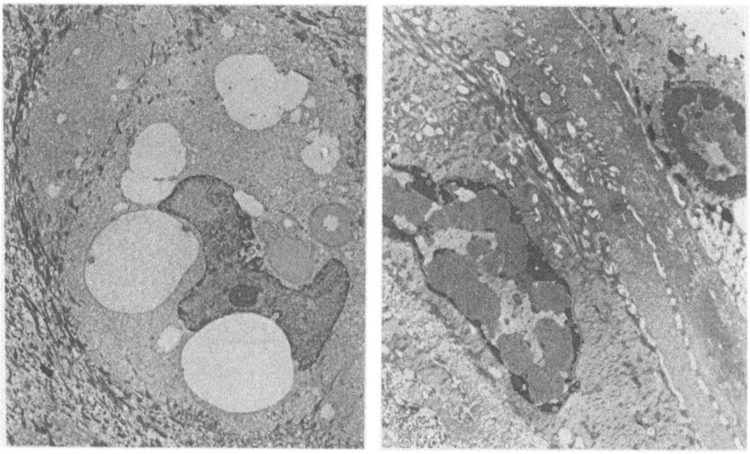 b

Fig. 2. a Electron micrograph showing effect of three months of retinoid treatment on a keratinocyte of patient two. Note the multiple cytoplasmic vacuoles, some electron lucid, others moderately electron dense with fine granular material. No virus particles can be seen in the nucleus. (Epon embedded, Uranyl and lead stained, magnification approximately × 3,000). **b** Electron micrograph of a "post-retinoid" keratinocyte from the same biopsy as Fig. 2a, showing no cytoplasmic abnormalities. Two cells are seen with nuclei filled with virus particles. (Processing same as for Fig. 2a, magnification approximately × 2,500)

sporadic case. Both patients had depressed cell-mediated immunity (CMI) as measured by DNCB sensitization prior to treatment, and both remained negative following treatment. One previously reported EV patient treated with retinoids had shown recovery of CMI as well as some clinical improvement (3). More EV patients must be studied to work out this problem, and longer treatment periods must be used in these EV patients to better evaluate the role of retinoids in retarding or preventing new EV cancers. Also, the effect of retinoids on other types of papillomavirus-induced diseases should be probed, since there already is some evidence that retinoids might be effective in certain other kinds of warts (11).

The mechanism of action of retinoids in EV remains unknown, but in addition to our initial hypothesis of inhibition of replication and assembly of virus resulting from retinoid alteration of keratinization, others could be imagined, such as a direct virucidal effect (4, 10), or enhancement of the immune system (2). The beneficial effect of retinoids on bowenoid cancers is not completely unexpected, because of the known anti-tumor effect of the retinoids (1, 12). Finally, the efficacy and mechanism of action of the retinoids in EV remains to be fully determined.

Summary

We have successfully treated a patient suffering from the severe form of epidermodysplasia verruciformis (EV), using the oral aromatic retinoid Ro 10-9359 (Roche). This form of EV is familial and characterised by widespread, human papillomavirus type 5 (HPV-5). HPV-5 is considered potentially oncogenic since all patients with the severe form of EV, so far reported, have had skin cancers, and since the HPV-5 genome has been found in EV cancers by molecular hybridization.

Since retinoids are known to affect keratinization, we reasoned that retinoids might prove successful in inhibiting the replication of HPV-5; especially since human papillomaviruses are known to be fastidious in their growth needs, requiring for their replication keratinocytes in an advanced stage of development, the formation of keratohyaline granules. After two months treatment with 1 mg/kg/day, we noticed that most of his flat wart-like lesions were gone, and that his plaques were repigmenting and no longer scaly. Two tumors at the inguinal-scrotal margin, inadvertently missed at the time of surgery, had reduced remarkably in size. No evidence for HPV-5 in the remaining benign lesions could be found histologically or by specific immunofluorescence; viral DNA extraction and analysis revealed a 100 fold reduction in HPV-5 viral DNA.

Thus it seems as if, at least for the moment, that our first patient is almost free of HPV-5, but our second patient continued to be infected with HPV-5 in spite of clinical improvement in his benign lesions. It is of interest to consider that the aromatic retinoid Ro-10-9359 might help control the replication of the potentially oncogenic HPV-5.

References

1. Bollag W (1974) Therapeutic effects of an aromatic retinoic acid analog on chemically induced skin papillomas and carcinomas of mice. Eur J Cancer 10:731–737
2. Glazer M, Lotan R (1979) Augmentation of specific tumor immunity against a syngeneic SV-40-induced sarcoma in mice by retinoic acid. Cell Immunol 45:175–181
3. Guilhou JJ, Malbos S, Barnéon S, Habib A, Baldet P, Meynadier J (1980) Epidermodysplasie verruciforme (2 observations). Etude immunologique. Ann Dermatol Venereol 107:611–619
4. Ito Y Effect of an aromatic retinoic acid analog (Ro 10-9359) on growth of virus-induced papillomas (Shope) and related neoplasia of rabbits. Eur J Cancer (in press)
5. Lutzner MA (1978) Epidermodysplasia verruciformis. An autosomal recessive disease characterized by viral warts and skin cancer. A model for viral oncogenesis. Bull Cancer 65:169–182
6. Lutzner MA, Blanchet-Bardon C (1980) Oral retinoid treatment of human papillomavirus type 5-induced epidermodysplasia verruciformis. N Engl J Med 302:1091
7. Migozzi MM, Baréty et al (1965) Epidermodysplasie verruciforme de Lutz-Lewandowsky. Bull Dermatol Syph Fr 72:747–748
8. Orth G, Favre M, Breitburd F, Croissant O, Jablonska S, Obalek S, Jarząbek-Chorzelska M, Rzęsa G Epidermodysplasia verruciformis. A model for the role of papillomaviruses in human cancer. In: Viruses in naturally occurring human cancer. Essex M, Todaro G, Zur Hausen H (eds). Cold Spring Harbor Press, New York (in press)
9. Orth G, Jablonska S, Favre M, Croissant O, Jarząbek-Chorzelska M, Rzęsa G (1978) Characterization of two types of human papillomavirus in lesions of epidermodysplasia verruciformis. Proc Natl Acad Sci USA 75:1537–1541
10. Reinhardt A, Sands JA, Snipes W (1979) Virucidal activity of retinal. Antimicrob Agents Chemother 16:421–423
11. Rüst O, Rufli T, Forrer J (1979) Erste Erfahrungen mit dem Vitamin-A-Säure-Derivat Ro 10-9359 bei Virusepitheliomen. Schweiz med Wochenschr 109:1914–1920
12. Todaro G, Delarco J, Sporn M (1978) Retinoids block phenotypic cell transformation produced by sarcoma growth factor. Nature 276:272–274
13. Tsambaos D, Mahrle G, Orfanos CE (1980) Epidermal changes induced by oral excess of aromatic retinoids in guinea pigs. Arch Dermatol Res 267:141–152

C.E. Orfanos et al. (eds.)
Retinoids

Lack of Enhancement of Experimental Photocarcinogenesis by Retinoic Acid

L.H. Kligman and A.M. Kligman

In the last 10 years, cancer researchers have been excited by vitamin A and its analogs, the retinoids, because of their anti-tumor capabilities. In vitro, retinoids can inhibit carcinogen induced metaplasia in organ culture (5, 10), as well as the growth of many transformed and tumor cell lines (12). In animals, retinoids can prevent chemically induced tumors in various organs including skin (1, 4), lung (15) and mammary gland (13). They can also block the action of promoters of chemical carcinogenesis (16). In human skin, retinoids have been shown to cause regression of pre-malignant actinic keratoses and basal cell carcinomas (2).

Recently, conflicting reports have appeared regarding the enhancement of photocarcinogenesis in albino hairless mice treated topically with retinoic acid (RA). Using a strongly carcinogenic dose of ultraviolet light (UV), Epstein produced more tumors in the animals treated with a toxic dose of RA than in the UV controls (6). In a second experiment, he showed tumor inhibition with 0.05% RA (7). Forbes et al., with a weakly carcinogenic dose of UV showed enhanced tumor formation with low doses of RA (8).

We decided to examine the problem using lightly pigmented hairless mice which, in addition to a dermal melanocytic system, have, like man, epidermal melanocytes. We performed three separate experiments with differing treatment schedules, UV and RA doses.

Materials and Methods

Animals: Lightly pigmented female SKh:hairless--2 mice, age 6–8 weeks were obtained from the Skin and Cancer Hospital, Temple University Health Sciences Center, Philadelphia, Pennsylvania. They were individually housed in special irradiation cages.

Light Source: A bank of 9 Westinghouse FS20 sunlamps were suspended 45 cm above the dorsum of the mice. The emission of the FS20 bulbs ranges from 275 to 400 nm with approximately one-third of the total output as UV-B, one-third as UV-A and one-third as infra-red and visible light. The dose delivered per minute was 0.006 J/cm^2 UV-B and 0.005 J/cm^2 UV-A as measured with an IL-700A Research Radiometer (International Light, Inc., Newburyport, Mass.).

Chemicals: Retinoic acid was supplied by Ortho Pharmaceuticals, Division of Dermatology, Raritan, New Jersey. Topical concentrations were 0.001%, 0.01% and 0.05% applied following irradiation with a 100 μl pipette. The oral concentration was 0.025%, administered with a 100 μl pipette. Vehicles varied in the different experiments.

Treatment Schedules

Experiment 1a: Concomitant UV and RA. Five groups of 24 animals each received, for the first 30 weeks, the following treatment: group 1, UV only; group 2, UV and 0.001% RA; group 3, UV and vehicle (70% ethanol : 30% propylene glycol); group 4, RA only; group 5, vehicle only. From week 31 to 45, group 1 received nothing, while the others continued with RA or vehicle.

Experiment 1b: RA after Tumor Induction. Animals were divided into 4 groups of 24 each. For the first 30 weeks, each received only UV. From week 31 to 45, the treatment was as follows: group 1, nothing; group 2, 0.001% RA; group 3, 0.01% RA; group 4, vehicle. In both 1a and 1b, UV was given 3 times a week at a dose equivalent to 6 human MED. RA or vehicle were applied 5 times a week.

Experiment 2: Oral vs Topical RA. For the first 18 weeks, 3 groups of 20 mice each were treated as follows: group 1, nothing; group 2, 0.05% RA in polyethylene glycol applied 5 times a week to abdominal skin; group 3, 0.025% RA in 8% Cremaphor-el delivered orally 3 times a week. For the next 20 weeks, the same treatments continued except for the oral feeding which was changed to 0.01% five times per week, and all groups were irradiated with approximately 4 human MED 3 times a week. The treatment in the final weeks was the same except irradiation was stopped.

Experiment 3: Two Vehicle Study. Three groups of 24 animals each were irradiated 5 times a week for 6 weeks with approximately ½ human MED daily. Beginning with week 7 the three groups received either nothing, 0.01% RA in polyethylene glycol with BHT, or 0.01% RA in methanol. Treatment was dispensed 3 times a week in 20 µl amounts. Six other groups served as RA and vehicle controls with or without UV.

Tumor Counting: In all experiments, animals were examined and tumors were measured once a week. In experiment 1a and 1b, tumor appearance and growth, as well as disappearance, were followed by careful mapping of all tumors ≧ 1 mm in diameter.

Results

Experiment 1a. Concomitant UV and RA: Animals in the three irradiated groups developed multiple tumors with 100% incidence by the 35th week. Groups 4 and 5 developed no tumors. The average number of tumors per animal was not significantly different in the three irradiated groups. Although the RA treated animals developed a few more tumors than the UV controls, so did the vehicle treated group (Table 1). This data can be analyzed in a straightforward manner only up to week 35 of this 45 week study because of coalescing tumors and animal deaths. The average time of appearance of the first papilloma was also not significantly different: 21.2, 18.8 and 19.1 weeks for group 1, 2 and 3, respectively. Regarding tumor progression, the RA treated animals showed a tendency for more rapid tumor growth, but again, the vehicle group behaved similarly. Thus in this experiment, RA did not affect photocarcinogenesis with respect to tumor yield, latent period or tumor progression.

Experiment 1b. RA after Tumor Induction: Both RA treated groups had more tumors than the two control groups. However, it should be noted that the 2 groups destined to receive RA had more tumors at 20, 25 and 30 weeks while all groups were still receiving only UV (Table 1). The percent increase from week 30 to 35 after 5 weeks of subsequent treatment was similar for all groups. Since this experiment was in the therapeutic mode, we paid particular attention to tumor loss. Statistical analysis of the data revealed a significantly

Table 1. Experiments 1a and 1b: Prevalence of tumors. Total number of tumors/Total number of survivors at intervals of 5 weeks throughout the course of the experiment

	Weeks					
	20	25	30	35	40	45
Exp. 1a: Concomitant RA and UV						
UV only	9/24	48/24	124/23	198/20	215/16	62/5
UV + 0.001% RA	18/23	77/22	176/21	191/17	83/9	0/0
UV + vehicle	18/23	71/22	188/22	238/20	166/12	68/6
Exp. 1b: RA after Tumor Induction						
UV only	9/24	48/24	124/23	198/20	215/16	62/5
UV then 0.001% RA	23/23	74/23	198/23	284/23	229/17	148/13
UV then 0.01% RA	18/23	81/23	173/21	268/19	148/12	20/3
UV then vehicle	7/24	63/23	133/21	176/19	165/16	101/10

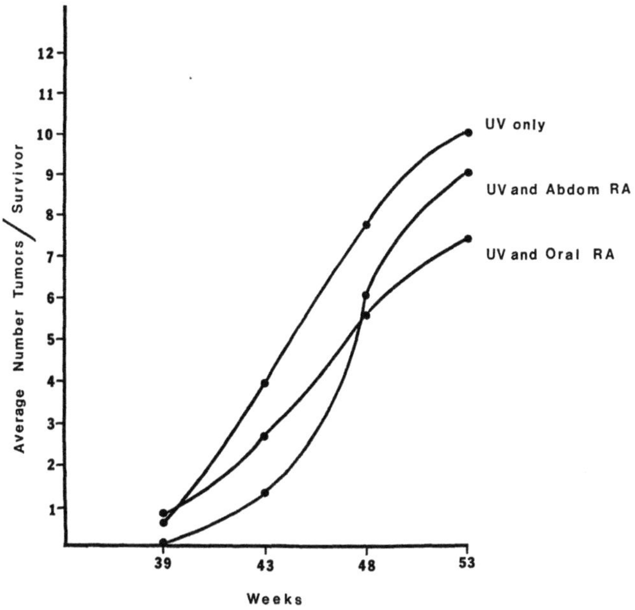

Fig. 1. Experiment 2: Oral versus topical RA. Average number of tumors/survivor

higher rate of regression in the 0.001% RA treated animals than in UV controls. Biopsy of regressed lesions frequently revealed only remnants of the tumor.

Experiment 2. Oral vs Topical RA: Compared to UV controls, tumorigenesis was inhibited by both modes of RA delivery (Fig. 1). The mice pre-treated with RA had received enough of the drug to produce a mild lymphadenopathy indicating a systemic effect by both abdominal painting and oral administration.

Experiment 3. Two Vehicle Study: After 58 weeks, there were no tumors in any of the groups except for two (2) 1 mm papillomas in the UV controls and three (3) 1 mm papillomas in the UV-RA-methanol animals.

Discussion

In three different experiments with lightly pigmented hairless mice, we have failed to show that RA enhances photocarcinogenesis as it appears to in albinos. The hairless mouse has many advantages for studying photocarcinogenesis, not the least of which is the similarity of its neoplasms to those found in irradiated human skin. However, unlike man, the mouse has a poor ability to repair UV-induced pyrimidine dimers in its DNA (11). In humans, this defect is associated with xeroderma pigmentosum with its multiple squamous and basal cell carcinomas (3). Moreover, the albino mouse lacks the small, but measurable protection from melanin. At equal doses of irradiation, the albino hairless is more vulnerable than the pigmented variety. The latent period is shorter, tumors progress to larger sizes more rapidly (9) and the dermis shows greater damage histologically. This vulnerability is demonstrated by experiment 3 where the same UV dose with the same light source produces papillomas in albino mice by week 35.

Extensive use, for a decade, of RA in human facial acne has brought no evidence of photocarcinogenesis. Bollag has reported success in the treatment of basal cell carcinomas which appear mainly on sun exposed skin (2). RA alone and in conjunction with 5-fluorouracil has caused regression of actinic keratoses in badly sun-damaged skin (14). Our animal studies show inhibition of tumor formation when given systemically and significant regression of UV-induced tumors with topical treatment. These and the human studies are in agreement with the abundant literature showing retinoids to be chemopreventive and anticarcinogenic agents.

Summary

Conflicting reports appear in the literature regarding the enhancement, by retinoic acid (RA) of photocarcinogenesis in albino hairless mice. We examined the question with lightly pigmented hairless mice. The first experiment, using a strongly carcinogenic dose, included two designs: 1) ultraviolet light (UV) and RA (0.01% and 0.001%) given concomitantly with the RA continued for many weeks after the irradiation stopped; 2) tumors were first induced by UV light and then treated with RA. In both studies, RA did not enhance photocarcinogenesis with regard to latent period, tumor yield or tumor progression and in the latter study there was significant regression of small tumors. In a second experiment, 20 weeks of concomitant RA and a moderate dose of UV irradiation followed 18 weeks of pre-treatment with RA. Tumorigenesis was inhibited by both oral and topical RA. The third experiment used 6 weeks of a very low dose of UV light which has been shown to be weakly carcinogenic in albino mice, followed by RA in methanol or polyethylene glycol. After 58 weeks, there were no tumors in any of the groups except for three (3) 1 mm papillomas in the RA-methanol animals and two 1 mm papillomas in the UV controls. In conclusion, using various UV doses and schedules, we failed to show that RA enhances photocarcinogenesis.

References

1. Bollag W (1972) Prophylaxis of chemically induced benign and malignant epithelial tumors by vitamin A acid (retinoic acid). Eur J Cancer 8:689–693
2. Bollag W, Ott F (1970) Retinoic acid: topical treatment of senile or actinic keratoses and basal cell carcinomas. Agents and Actions 1:172–175
3. Cleaver JE (1974) Repair processes for photochemical damage in mammalian cells. Adv Radiat Biol 4:1–75
4. Davies RE (1967) Effect of vitamin A on 7, 12-dimethylbenz(a) anthracene-induced papillomas in Rhino mouse skin. Cancer Res 27:237–241
5. Dickens MS, Custer RP, Sorof S (1979) Retinoid prevents mammary gland transformation by carcinogenic hydrocarbon in whole organ culture. Proc Natl Acad Sci USA 76:5891–5895
6. Epstein JH (1977) Chemicals and photocarcinogenesis. Aust J Dermatol 18:57–61
7. Epstein JH, Grekin DA (1979) Topical retinoic acid (R.A.) and ultraviolet (UV) carcinogenesis. J Invest Dermatol 72:272
8. Forbes PD, Urbach F, Davies RE (1979) Enhancement of experimental photocarcinogenesis by topical retinoic acid. Cancer Lett 7:85–90
9. Kligman LH, Akin FJ, Kligman AM (1980) Sunscreens prevent ultraviolet photocarcinogenesis. J Am Acad Dermatol 3:30–35
10. Lasnitski I, Goodman DS (1975) Inhibition of the effects of methylcholanthrene on mouse prostate in organ culture by vitamin A and its analogs. Cancer Res 34:1564–1571
11. Ley RD, Sedita BA, Grubbe DD, Fry RJM (1977) Induction and persistence of pyrimidine dimers in the epidermal DNA of two strains of hairless mice. Cancer Res 37:3243–3248
12. Lotan R, Nicholson GL (1977) Inhibitory effects of retinoic acid or retinyl acetate on the growth of untransformed, transformed and tumor cells in vitro. J Natl Cancer Inst 59:1717–1722

13. Moon RC, Grubb CJ, Sporn MB (1976) Inhibition of 7, 12-dimethylbenz(a) anthracene-induced mammary carcinogenesis by retinyl acetate. Cancer Res 36:2626–2630
14. Robinson TA, Kligman AM (1975) Treatment of solar keratoses of the extremities with retinoic acid and 5-fluorouracil. Br J Dermatol 92:703–706
15. Saffiotti U, Montesano R, Sellakumar R, Borg SA (1967) Experimental cancer of the lung: inhibition by vitamin A of the induction of tracheobronchial squamous metaplasia and squamous cell tumors. Cancer 20:857–864
16. Verma AK, Shapas BG, Rice HM, Boutwell RK (1979) Correlation of the inhibition by retinoids of tumor promotor-induced mouse epidermal ornithine decarboxylase activity and of skin tumor promotion. Cancer Res 39:419–425

C.E. Orfanos et al. (eds.)
Retinoids

Oral Treatment of Psoriasis with the Aromatic Retinoid Ro 10-9359

C.F. Lopes and B.A. Rodrigues

Treatment of psoriasis and other keratinization disorders with the aromatic retinoid Ro 10-9359 has been the subject of many recent publications (1-3, 5, 6).

Our own experience with this new medicament in psoriasis comprises three different studies, envisaged in order to determine the optimal therapeutic regimen and the effects of associating this etretinate to local treatment with steroid preparations. The present paper is a report of these studies.

Casuistics and Methodology

Sixty-eight patients were included, no restrictions being made as to clinical forms, age, sex or race. With regard to clinical forms, 63 had psoriasis vulgaris (47 localized and 16 generalized), 2 were cases of erythrodermic form, 2 had erythrodermic arthropathic psoriasis and 1 was a case of pustulosis palmoplantaris (Barber). Concerning race, 47 patients were white, 14 mestizos and 7 blacks.

Etretinate was given orally in capsules containing 10 and 25 mg of active substance, respectively and the local treatment was carried out with difluocortolone valerate 0.1% ointment (Tables 1 and 2).

The first study, performed in 1976 and 1977, comprised 13 cases (Group A) treated with 25 mg b.i.d. of Ro 10-9359. In 3 cases the daily dose was raised up to 75 mg in view of poor therapeutic response to

Table 1. Oral treatment of psoriasis with Ro 10-9359

	Group "A" (open) Daily dose: 50 mg No local treatment	Group "B" (double-blind) Daily dose: 30 mg Local treatment	Group placebo (double-blind) Local treatment	Group "C" (open) Daily dose: various Local treatment	Total	%
Number of patients	13	19	16	20	68	
Sex: male	9	11	10	10	40	58.8
female	4	8	6	10	28	41.1
Race: white	10	11	12	14	47	69.1
mestizos	3	4	3	4	14	20.5
blacks	-	4	1	2	7	10.2
Age: < 20	2	2	-	1	5	7.3
20–39	7	8	10	10	35	51.4
40–59	3	5	4	7	19	27.9
> 60	1	4	2	2	9	13.2

Table 2. Clinical forms

	Group "A" (open) Daily dose: 50 mg No local treatment	Group "B" (double-blind) Daily dose: 30 mg Local treatment	Group placebo (double-blind) Local treatment	Group "C" (open) Daily dose: various Local treatment	Total	%
Number of patients	13	19	16	20	68	
Vulgar:						
localized	8	11	13	15	47	69.1
generalized	3	6	3	4	16	23.5
Erythrodermic	2	-	-	-	2	2.9
Erythrodermic-arthropathic	-	2	-	-	2	2.9
Pustulosis palmo-plantaris	-	-	-	1	1	1.4
	13	19	16	20	68	99.8

the initial dose, while in another patient the dose had to be reduced to 25 mg daily due to the presence of more severe side effects (cheilitis).

The second trial, performed in the years 1978 and 1979 (Groups B and Placebo) was a double-blind study comparing low doses of etretinate (10 mg t.i.d.) to placebo in two groups of 19 and 16 cases, respectively. All the patients in this study were also treated with local application of difluocortolone valerate in part of the lesions.

The third study was an open trial in 20 patients (Group C) realized between 1978 and 1980, also associating etretinate to local treatment with the steroid ointment referred to in part of the lesions. In this trial the posology of Ro 10-9359 was not fixed, and in many of the patients it was below 30 mg daily due to manufacturing problems. Three patients were given 75 mg/day, 13 cases received 50 mg daily, 3 cases received a daily dose of 40 mg, 14 patients were treated with 30 mg/day, 11 cases received 25 mg daily, 11 cases 20 mg daily, and 11 patients had 10 mg/day. It can be seen that the dose had to be changed frequently, in order to maintain a good degree of improvement and at the same time to treat all the pa-

Table 3. Daily doses

Group "A" (open) 13 Patients No local treatment		Group "B" (double-blind) 19 Patients Local treatment		Group "C" (open) 20 Patients Local treatment	
mg	Patients	mg	Patients	mg	Patients
50	13	30	19	75	3
50 & 75	3	30 & 20	5	50	13
50 & 25	1	30, 20 & 10	3	40	3
				30	14
				25	11
				20	11
				10	11
				(see text)	

Table 4. Duration of treatment

	Group "A" (open)	Group "B" (double-blind)	Group placebo (double-blind)	Group "C" (open)	Total	%
	Daily dose: 50 mg	Daily dose: 30 mg		Daily dose: various		
	No local treatment	Local treatment	Local treatment	Local treatment		
Number of patients	13	19	16	20	68	
Weeks						
8–14	3	6	5	2	16	23.5
16–22	5	7	9	4	25	36.7
24–32	4	6	2	9	21	30.8
40–52	1	–	–	2	3	4.4
56–76	–	–	–	3	3	4.4
	13	19	16	20	68	99.8
Mean weeks	20.7	16.8	17.8	33.6		

tients with a deficient stock of medicament. The doses adopted in the 3 studies are summarized in Table 3.

The length of treatment varied according to the response of each patient (Table 4).

The results were assessed by means of a weekly clinical examination until the sixtieth week, and every fortnight or month afterwards, respectively, and the following parameters were recorded: degrees of erythema, desquamation, infiltration and pustulosis, rated from zero (worsening) to five (complete remission).

Routine laboratory examinations including serum alkaline phosphatase and transaminase levels were performed before and throughout the period of treatment. Women of childbearing age were instructed to use a reliable contraceptive measure.

Results and Comments

As can be seen in Table 5, the best therapeutic results were observed in Group A, whose patients received a daily dose of 50 mg etretinate. In this group the length of treatment averaged 20.7 weeks, and 8 out of 13 patients experienced a complete remission of the lesions. In

Table 5. Results

	Group "A" (open)	Group "B" (double-blind)	Group "C" (open)
	Daily dose: 50 mg No local treatment	Daily dose: 30 mg Local treatment	Daily dose: various Local treatment
Number of patients	13	19	20
Complete remissions			
excellent	8 = 61.5%	10 = 52.6%	10 = 50%
Partial remissions			
good	3 } = 38.5%	4 } = 42.1%	6 } = 45%
moderate	2 }	4 }	3 }
Unaltered			
failure	–	1 = 5.3%	1 = 5%

Table 6. Results of the double-blind study

Patients	Complete remission	Partial remission	Unaltered or aggravated	Number of patients
Group "B" medicated	10	8	1	19
Placebo	1	4	11	16
	x^2 = 16.77 - highly significant			

the groups B and C, treated with smaller doses, results were not so good, in spite of an associated local treatment. The comparatively poor results in Group C can be explained by the lack of medicament during the trial and the consequent use of insufficient doses for various weeks, in many of the cases. Also because of this, the mean length of treatment in Group C was much longer than in the other groups: 33.6 weeks, as compared to 20.7 weeks in Group A and 16.8 weeks in Group B.

The second study, carried out in double-blind fashion, shows a highly significant difference between etretinate and placebo (Table 6), and also indicates that local treatment does not seem to influence the final result. - Interestingly enough, one of the cases under placebo showed a complete remission of the lesions: It was a patient presenting psoriasis vulgaris with slight and localized lesions, and also suffering from diabetes and alopecia areata.

Concerning the effects of local treatment, the results obtained in Groups B and C seem to indicate that it did not improve the final results. On the contrary, in some patients lesions not treated locally regressed quicker than those treated with the ointment. Furthermore, we observed that the concomitant use of etretinate and local corticoid exacerbates the atrophy

Table 7. Side effects

	Group "A" (open) Daily dose: 50 mg No local treatment	Group "B" (double-blind) Daily dose: 30 mg Local treatment	Group "C" (open) Daily dose: various Local treatment	Total	%
Number of patients	13	19	20	52	
Dryness of lips and cheilitis	13	15	17	45	86.5
Dryness of mucosae oral and nasal	11	8	6	25	48.0
Skin thinning	7	7	9	23	44.2
Desquamation palmo-plantaris	6	5	9	20	38.4
Diffuse alopecia	5	4	9	18	34.6
Pruritus	4	-	2	6	11.5
Onychia	-	-	4	4	7.0
Paronychia	-	-	2	2	3.8
Conjunctivitis	-	-	1	1	1.9
Striae	-	-	1	1	1.9
Increase of transaminases	1	-	1	2	3.8
No side effects	-	2	-	2	3.8

of the skin, specially in sensitive areas, as described for the use of steroids alone (4). One of our patients, a white girl aged 19, developed severe striae in the skin of the axillae and groins, under the combined treatment.

With regard to the clinical forms, we have already mentioned that there was no special selection, and most of our cases had localized forms. Results were equally good in these mild cases as in severe ones: complete remission in our patients with erythrodermia and arthropathy and partial remission in the patient with pustulosis palmo-plantaris, after 12 weeks' therapy. This latter patient was seen afterwards, and she presented complete remission of her lesions in the absence of a new treatment.

Side effects observed are those already described in previous reports on etretinate (Table 7). Their intensity is usually related to posology, although some specially sensitive patients are presenting severe side effects with small doses. These adverse reactions subside in many patients at the end of the 6th week, as if the patient's organism became adapted to the drug, and in no instance any side effect persisted after the end of the treatment. It is interesting to notice that thinning of the skin is absent or is of merely mild nature in blacks.

Concerning laboratory parameters, two patients showed elevation of transaminase blood levels, such as their treatment was suspended. Three cases receiving placebo complained of dry mouth (without any conspicuous signs of cheilitis) and two other patients of dryness of the oral or nasal mucosae. - We believe that this can be explained by the psychological influence of neighbour patients which were being treated with the active drug and presented such side effects.

Conclusions

Although our research, considered per se, does not allow definite conclusions, the following facts can be confirmed:

1. Ro 10-9359 (etretinate) is active against psoriasis in daily doses as low as 30 mg, eliciting complete remission of the lesions in more than 50% of the cases.
2. Tolerance to treatment can be considered as good, and eventual side effects are well supported by the patients, disappearing at the end of the treatment.
3. The concomitant use of local steroid ointment is unnecessary and should even be avoided, in view of the risk of an effect of potentiation concerning skin thinning. We are now adopting the use of inert emollient preparations such as vaseline, when local treatment seems necessary.
4. Further studies in psoriasis are needed in order to better define the effect of etretinate, including its influence on the prevention of relapses.

Summary

A total of 68 patients with different forms of psoriasis were treated with Ro 10-9359 or placebo, between 1976 and 1979. A first group of 13 cases received 50 mg of the active drug in an open schedule from periods ranging from 2 to 10 months (median 5 months). The second study comprised the use of smaller doses of Ro 10-9359 in a further 20 cases under an open schedule, associating local treatment with difluocortolone in selected lesions. Finally, a third group of 35 patients received either Ro 10-9359 (19 cases) or placebo (16 cases) in a double-blind schedule, as well as topical treatment with difluocortolone on selected areas. The evaluation of these three subsequent studies indicate that best results were obtained with daily doses of 50 mg Ro 10-9359 (approximately 0.75 to 1 mg/kg). Smaller doses, even with the association of local corticoids, lead to a slower improvement which sometimes causes the patient to abandon therapy. In the double-blind study, the active drug elicited remission or improvement of the lesions in 18 out of 19 cases, whilst in the placebo group just 5 of the 16 patients improved, possibly due to the concomitant use of topical corticoid. Side effects seem to be dose-related, and consist mainly of cheilitis, dryness of the oral and nasal mucosae, alopecia, palmo-plantar exfoliation, thinning of the skin and pruritus. In two patients treatment was suspended because of elevated serum transaminase levels. The judicious use of Ro 10-9359 is probably the best available therapy for psoriasis.

References

1. Chandon JR, Devaux JF, Gamby T, Privat Y (1978) Psoriasis pustuleux generalisé (Zumbusch). Effet remarquable d'un ester de la vitamine A acide administré per os. Nouv Presse Med 7:4234–4235
2. Fredriksson T (1978) Oral treatment of psoriasis and pustulosis palmo-plantaris with Ro 10-9359. Dermatologica 157 (Suppl 1):13–18
3. Goerz G, Orfanos CE (1978) Systemic treatment of psoriasis with a new aromatic retinoid. Dermatologica 157 (Suppl 1):38–44
4. Maibach HI, Stoughton RB (1975) Topical corticosteroids. In: Steroids therapy, Azarnoff D, Saunders WB
5. Pehamberger H, Neumann H, Holubar K (1978) Oral treatment of ichthyosis with an aromatic retinoid. Br J Dermatol 99:319
6. Viglioglia P, Barclay A (1978) Oral retinoids and psoriasis. Dermatologica 157 (Suppl 1):32–37

C.E. Orfanos et al. (eds.)
Retinoids

Treatment of Darier's Disease with Systemic Ro 10-9359 (Tigason) - a Retinoic Acid Derivative

J.V. Christiansen, H. Hino, R. Møller, F. Reymann and H. Schmidt

Darier's disease is an autosomal dominant disorder of keratinization with characteristic clinical manifestations and histopathology.

Until recent years the treatment of Darier's disease has been unsatisfactory, and in severe cases odour and distorted appearance has made normal life impossible. Fortunately the disease is rare. In 1959, Svendsen and Albrectsen examined all known cases of Darier's disease and their relatives and found a total of 37 cases in Denmark, giving them a prevalence of 1:100,000 (6). Introduction of retinoic acid and its less toxic derivatives for systemic use has offered new possibilities in the treatment of Darier's disease and excellent results have been reported during recent years (1–5).

We report the results of systemic long-term treatment of Darier's disease with the retinoic acid derivative Ro 10-9359 from four departments of dermatology in Denmark.

Material and Methods

The material consists of 33 patients (19 women and 14 men) in whom the diagnosis of Darier's disease has been confirmed by histological examinations of skin biopsies. The patients, presenting all types of the disease, were divided into 4 groups according to severity, as judged by the degree of hyperkeratosis, extension, itching, odour, frequency of bacterial infections and so on. The distribution of the patients, their mean age at the inception of treatment and the mean duration of the disease as a function of the severity of the disease are shown in Table 1.

Twenty patients had relatives with Darier's disease and some of the patients were members of the same families. Laboratory investigations, including serum transaminases, alkaline phosphatases and lactic dehydrogenases were normal for all patients before treatment and the values were followed up at monthly intervals together with clinical evaluation of the effect of treatment and the side effects.

The initial dose of Ro 10-9359 was in the range of 0.5 mg/kg body weight and was adjusted to clinical effect and side effects.

Table 1. Distribution of number of patients, sex, mean age at treatment and mean duration of disease according to severity of the disease

Degree of severity	Number and sex of the patients	Mean age at treatment	Mean duration of the disease
I	5 F/ 1 M	34.3	20.8
II	9 F/ 7 M	31.5	16.8
III	3 F/ 4 M	48.6	28.0
IV	2 F/ 2 M	41.5	31.5
Total	19 F/14 M	36.7	22.3

Table 2. Effect of treatment in 30 patients with Darier's disease treated with Ro 10-9359 for more than 2 months

Degree of severity	Effect of treatment			Total number of patients
	+	++	+++	
I		2	4	6
II		8	6	14
III		5	1	6
IV	2	1	1	4
Total number of patients	2	16	12	30

The clinical effect was graded from zero to +++; + meaning 25–50% improvement, ++ 50–75% improvement and +++ 75–100% improvement.

Results

In 12 cases the result must be considered as excellent, and all except 2 patients experienced an improvement of more than 50% (Table 2). Even in the very severe cases of hypertrophic disease, odour, itching and infections diminished and the enormous hyperkeratotic areas cleared to some degree. Three patients were treated for less than 2 months and are not included in the evaluation of the effect. The remaining patients were treated for an average of 16 months (Table 3). In 9 patients the treatment has been stopped, in 2 patients due to excellent result. Two patients had unbearable side effects. One got a severe cheilitis on a very low dose and was treated for less than two months. The other patient was treated for 26 months when itching and desquamation became intolerable. The other reasons for terminating the treatment are indicated in Table 4.

The maintenance dose varied from patient to patient due to individual tolerability, but was on an average higher in the more severe cases. The average maintenance dose was 0.62 mg/kg body weight.

In the initial treatment period side effects were common (Table 5). One patient had to stop treatment due to untolerable cheilitis. One patient, known to abuse alcohol had a transient rise in lactic dehydrogenase. Its value returned to normal in spite of continued treatment.

Table 3. Duration of treatment with Ro 10–9359 in 30 patients with Darier's disease treated for 2 months or more

Degree of severity	Months	Number of patients
I	13 (3–25)	6
II	13 (2–25)	14
III	20 (10–27)	6
IV	22 (14–26)	4
Total	16 (2–27)	30

Table 4. Reasons for terminating the treatment with Ro 10-9359 in 33 patients with Darier's disease. Three patients (a) have been treated for less than 2 months

Excellent result	2
Side effects	
excessive cheilitis[a]	1
itching and desquamation	1
Other reasons	
diagnosis of malignant tumors[a]	2
planning of a pregnancy	1
travel abroad	1
lost to follow-up[a]	1
Total	9

Table 5. Side effects in 33 patients with Darier's disease in the initial treatment period with Ro 10-9359

Side effects	Number of patients
Cheilitis	22 (73%)
Itching	15 (50%)
Dryness of mucous membranes	7 (23%)
Desquamation	6 (20%)
Diffuse hair loss	4 (13%)
Abnormal laboratory tests	1 (3%)
Other side effects	4 (13%)
No side effects	8 (24%)

Loss of hair was slight except in 1 patient where regrowth occurred on a reduced dose. Eight patients had no side effects whatsoever.

At maintenance therapy 16 patients had no side effects at all (Table 6). As already mentioned, one patient had to stop treatment due to severe itching and desquamation after 26 months of an otherwise successful therapy. In an other patient with grade IV disease, systemic steroids were administrated in order to diminish itching, cheilitis and desquamation. On this regimen an improvement of the condition was obtained. In the other patients side effects were mild and well tolerated by them.

Discussion

For the first time we have reached an efficient treatment of Darier's disease. No serious side

Table 6. Side effects in 30 patients with Darier's disease treated with Ro 10-9359 for more than 2 months on maintenance dosage

Side effects	Number of patients
Cheilitis	12 (40%)
Itching	7 (23%)
Desquamation	1 (3%)
Dryness of mucous membranes	1 (3%)
No side effects	16 (53%)

effects could be demonstrated in a long-term treatment of this range. It is still unknown for how long a time it will be possible to continue maintenance therapy, without inducing liver damage or other serious side effects.

Summary

In a multicentre study 33 patients with Darier's disease were treated with retinoic acid derivative Ro 10-9359. The age of the patients ranged from 10 to 80 years. The total spectrum of the disease was represented in extension as well as in severity of the lesions. The dose of Ro 10-9359 was within the range of 0.5 mg/kg body weight. Clinically, there was a marked improvement of skin lesions and symptoms during the treatment. Two patients had to stop treatment due to side effects (exanthema, severe dryness of the lips), but the symptoms subsided as soon as the treatment was discontinued. Further 5 patients had to stop treatment for other reasons. The duration of treatment was in the range of 2–27 months for the rest of the patients. No serious side effects were found.

References

1. Binazzi M, Cicilioni EG (1979) Systemic treatment of Darier's disease with a new retinoid (Ro 10-9359). Arch Dermatol Res 264:365–367
2. Burge S, Wilkinson JD, Miller A, Ryan JT (1980) Darier's disease: Initial results on twenty patients treated with a new aromatic retinoid (Tigason). Br J Derm 103 (Suppl 18):12
3. Orfanos CE, Kurka M, Strunk V (1978) Oral treatment of keratosis follicularis with a new aromatic retinoid. Arch Dermatol 114:1211–1214
4. Peck GL, Yoder FW, Olsen TG, Pandya MD, Butkus D (1978) Treatment of Darier's disease, lamellar ichthyosis, pityriasis rubra pilaris, cystic acne, and basal cell carcinoma with oral 13-cis-retinoic acid. Dermatologica 157 (Suppl 1):11–12
5. Schimpf A (1976) Zur systemischen Anwendung eines aromatischen Vitamin-A-Säure-Derivates (Ro 10-9359) bei Psoriasis und Keratosen. Z Hautkr 51:265–274
6. Svendsen BI, Albrectsen B (1959) The prevalence of dyskeratosis follicularis (Darier's disease) in Denmark. Acta Derm Venerol 39, 256–269

C.E. Orfanos et al. (eds.)
Retinoids

Thermography of Psoriasis. Effects of Retinoids

G. Stüttgen

Distinct psoriatic lesions display a small increase in skin temperature of about 0.5–1.0 °C compared to the surrounding not affected skin. Conventional therapy of psoriasis with dithranol (0.5–1%) or UVB, including photochemotherapy, leads to a remarkable increase anywhere between 1 and 4 °C. These effects can be demonstrated by thermography (AGA-thermovision) which shows the infrared radiation from the skin surface. Thermography can be used to examine the long-term effect of drug therapy because the basic pattern of the thermographic picture of the skin surface remains constant (1–3).

Oral application of 100 mg of the aromatic retinoid Ro 10-9359 leads to a decrease of the skin temperature in *psoriatic skin lesions* within 2–3 days and lowers the temperature to that of non-affected skin. This decrease in skin temperature precedes the improvement of the psoriatic lesions about 2 to 3 days (d). Some hours after the oral uptake of a high dosage of retinoid - 100–200 mg - a small increase in skin temperature can take place (Figs. 1–2, Table 1).

The aromatic retinoid in psoriatics shows a tendency to reduce the infrared radiation of the affected skin with decrease of the heat pattern of the psoriatic lesions. These effects precede the reduction of water evaporation of psoriatic skin lesion which develops parallel to the improvement of the psoriasis.

In *acne conglobata* about 12 h after oral application of 13-cis-retinoic acid 1 mg/kg the infrared temperature of the skin increased about 1 °C beyond the localization of the single efflorescence of the acne conglobata in the whole skin area (Fig. 3). The effect of orally given retinoid depends on the stimulation of the sweat-glands which of course lowered the temperature of the skin surface, yet our investigations have been performed in a climatized room with a constant temperature of 21 °C.

Our results confirm the histological and electron microscopical observation that the signs of superficial inflammation like conditions in distinct lesions of psoriasis are decreased as it concerns the arterial blood supply to the microcirculation. Healed psoriatic lesions show a distinct reduction of the skin temperature about 0.5 °C compared with the surrounding skin.

Summary

Contrary to the effects of dithranol and UVB on the lesions of psoriasis the aromatic retinoid Ro 10-9359 lowers the infrared radiation emitted from the skin surface. Within some days this effect precedes the beginning improvement of the psoriatic lesions and shows no correlation to the water evaporation from the skin.

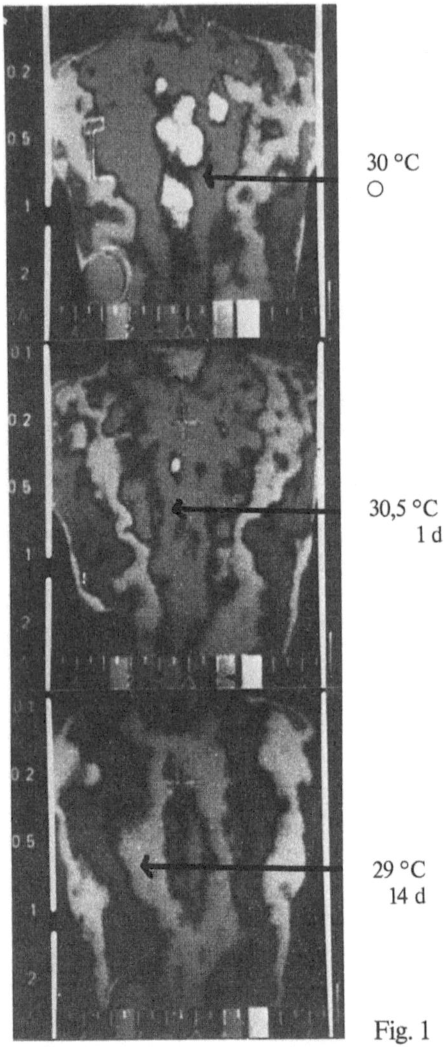

Fig. 1

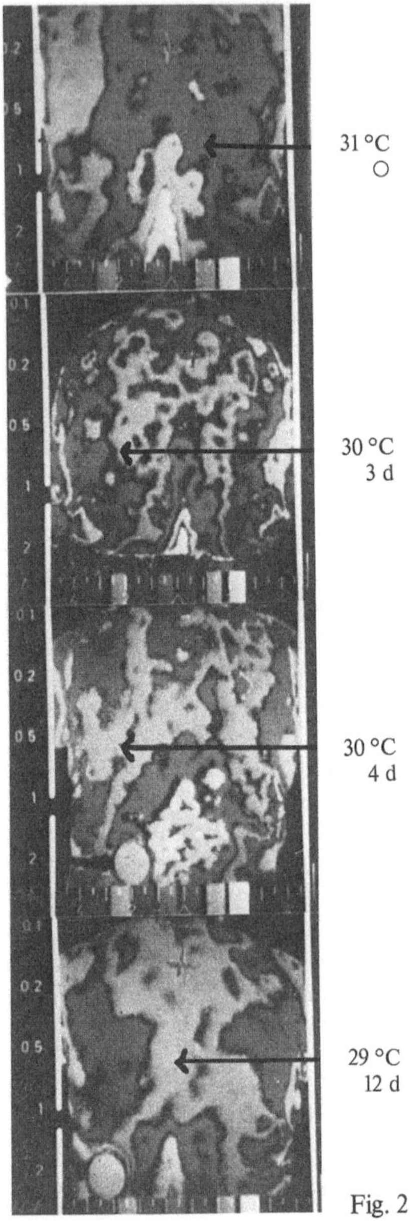

Fig. 2

Fig. 1. Erythrodermic psoriasis 1 day (d) after 100 mg Ro 10-9359, moderate (+ 0.5 °C) short-lasting elevated heat radiation visible by isotherms of the back. After 3 days' reduced heat radiation (–1 °C)

Fig. 2. Generalized psoriasis: 1 day (d) after 100 mg Ro 10-9359, decreased (–1 °C) heat radiation visible by isotherms of the back corresponding to the psoriatic lesions. After a 12-day uptake of 100 mg Ro 10-9359, heat radiation was lower than the controls without psoriasis

Table 1. Heat radiation of skin surface (back) after daily uptake of 100 mg Ro 10-9359. Comparison with the thermographic isotherms before treatment. Psoriasis vulgaris generalisata (n = 10)

Changes of heat radiation	
1st day after aromatic retinoid:	−0.5 °C (+0.5 to −1.5 °C)
2nd day after aromatic retinoid:	−1.0 °C
3rd day after aromatic retinoid:	−1.0 °C

After complete improvement of the lesions this skin area showed a distinct decrease of 1.5 °C as compared with the surrounding, previously not affected skin

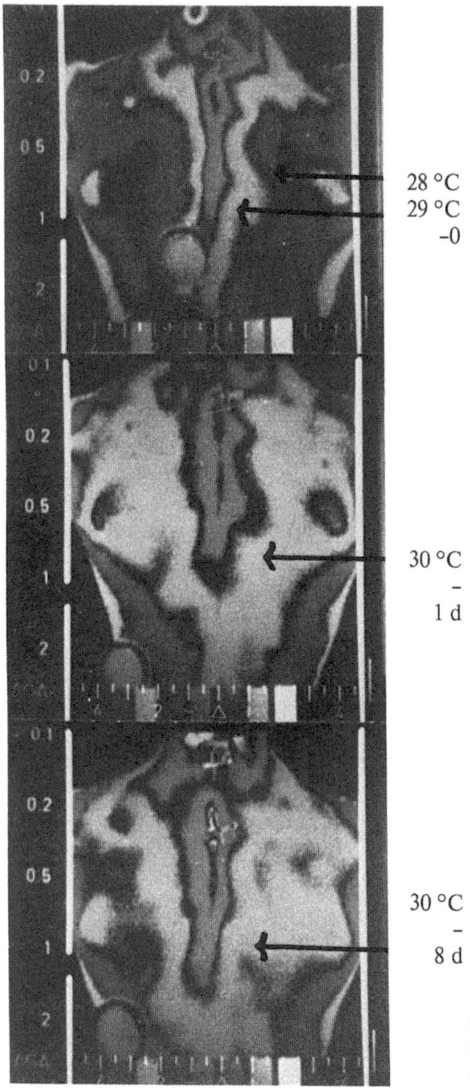

Fig. 3. Acne conglobata: The isotherms including the cystic lesions are about 1 °C below standard values. After 100 mg 13-cis-retinoic acid, the heat radiation is approximately at a normal level (30 °C)

References

1. Herstel W (1969) Fundamental physical aspects of thermography, in: Medical thermography, Bibliotheca Radiologica, No. 5, Herma van Voss SFC, Thomas P (eds). S. Karger, Basel, New York, 22–28
2. Mali JWH (1969) Some physiological aspects of the temperature of the body surface, in: Medical thermography, Bibliotheca Radiologica, No. 5, Herma van Voss SFC, Thomas P (eds). S. Karger, Basel, New York, 8–21
3. Stüttgen G, Flesch U, Witt H, Wendt H (1980) Thermographic analysis of skin test reaction using AGA thermovision. Arch Dermatol Res 268:113–128

Short Clinical and Experimental Reports

C.E. Orfanos et al. (eds.)
Retinoids

Results of Oral Retinoid Therapy in Different Forms of Psoriasis

M. Berecz, I. Rácz and E. Imregh

Efficacy of oral retinoid treatment was examined on various clinical types of psoriasis and according to the degree of heredity. The treatment schedule was approximately 1 mg aromatic retinoid Ro 10-9359 for 1 kg bodyweight daily at least for 6 weeks. The individual dose was never higher than 75 mg/day.

The number of the treated cases was 85. According to the clinical picture and the provocative factors the patients could be divided into 8 groups. The results of the treatment in the different groups are summarized in Table 1.

The results of treatment could be grouped also according to the grade of inheritence. Grade I means at least one other case of the disease among the parents or brothers and sisters, grade II means at least one other case among the secondary relatives. Cases where no family history for psoriasis could be traced can be found in group of grade III (Table 2).

From the data of the investigation the following conclusions can be drawn:

The oral retinoid therapy has guaranteed the best results in the treatment of erythrodermic psoriasis, generalizated pustular psoriasis, and large plaques psoriasis (provoked by a

Table 1. Results of treatment and correspondence between different of psoriasis and provocative factors

Forms of psoriasis	Provocative factors	Improvement						
		100%	90%	80%	50%	30%	0%	worse
1. Localized on scalp and trunk	Seborrhoea	3	-	1	3	1	3	0
2. Disseminated guttate	Bacterial focus, drugs	4	2	2	2	-	1	1
3. Disseminated large plaques	Seborrhoea, bacterial focus, mycosis, contact dermatitis	10	5	8	2	2	3	1
4. Localized on intertriginous and lumbosacral areas	Mycosis, contact dermatitis	1	1	1	-	-	3	2
5. Flexural psoriasis	Mechanic, folliculitis	1	-	-	-	-	2	2
6. Localized pustular psoriasis	Bacterial focus, contact dermatitis mycosis	2	-	-	1	1	-	-
7. Generalized pustular psoriasis	Contact dermatitis Bacterial focus, drugs	2	1	2	-	-	-	-
8. Erythrodermic psoriasis	(Contact dermatitis, Bacterial focus, drugs)	6	-	3	-	-	-	-
		29	9	17	8	4	12	6

Table 2. Connection between therapeutic results (number of patients) and genetic determination

Grade of hereditary taint	Improvement							
	100%	90%	80%	50%	30%	0%	worse	Total
I.	12	4	5	2	–	2	3	28
II.	9	3	2	–	–	1	–	15
III.	8	2	10	6	6	9	1	42
Total	29	9	17	8	6	12	4	85

number of factors), and less excellent results were observed in the treatment of disseminated guttate psoriasis; in the other forms of psoriasis some improvements can be observed as a result of the retinoid therapy. It is important that the retinoid therapy makes a *very good effect* at psoriatic patients with great eruptive and high genetic predisposition. This fact points out that oral retinoids may effect in the substantial phase of the process, which leads to the appearance of psoriasis.

C.E. Orfanos et al. (eds.)
Retinoids

Topical Aromatic Retinoid in the Treatment of Ichthyosis Vulgaris

H. Berger and D. Tsambaos

Previous investigations have shown that a new topical aromatic retinoid (Ro 11-1430) has a distinct influence on the growth and differentiation of epidermal cells.

In recent years the oral application of retinoids such as Ro 10-9359 and 13-cis-retinoic acid, has been established as a successful therapeutic approach in various ichthyotic conditions.

Nevertheless the present oral therapy in high doses - required to prevent recurrences - is often associated with systemic side effects; particularly the risk of retinoid-induced teratogenic effects is high.

Therefore we found it of interest to study the efficacy of the topical aromatic retinoid in the treatment of ichthyosis vulgaris.

Material and Methods

Aromatic retinoid Ro 11-1430 was locally applied once daily in a 0.5% solution in oleyl-alcohol; later we used a 0.25% solution, which was less effective (Fig. 1).

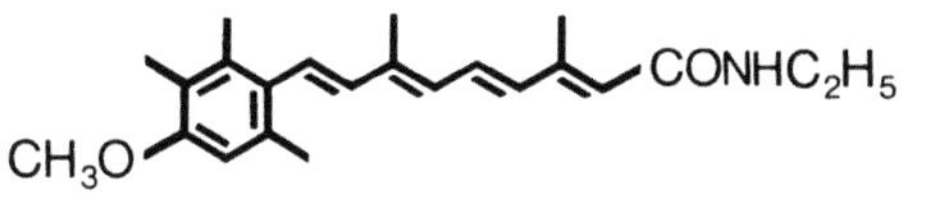

Fig. 1. Structural formula of Ro 11-1430 (Tasmaderm) Ethyl-all-trans-9-(4-methoxy-2,3,6-trimethylphenyl)-3,7-dimethyl-2,4,6,8-nonatetraenoate

Table

Age years	Sex	Clinical diagnosis	Histological findings
19[a]	♂ (brothers)	Ichthyosis vulgaris	Small granular layer, orthohyperkeratosis (retention hyperkeratosis)
11[a]	♂ (brothers)	Ichthyosis vulgaris	Small granular layer, orthohyperkeratosis (retention hyperkeratosis)
69	♀	Ichthyosis simplex	–
11	♂	Ichthyosis simplex	–

[a] Xg-blood groups and steroid-sulphatase activity in cultured skin fibroblasts are under investigation in the patients and the members of their families

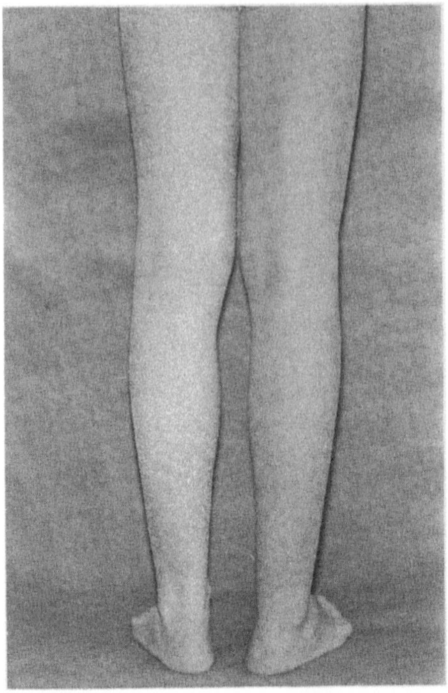

Fig. 2

Fig. 2 and 3. The 11-year-old boy with ichthyosis vulgaris after 2 weeks of local treatment with 0.5% Ro 11-1430 (right)

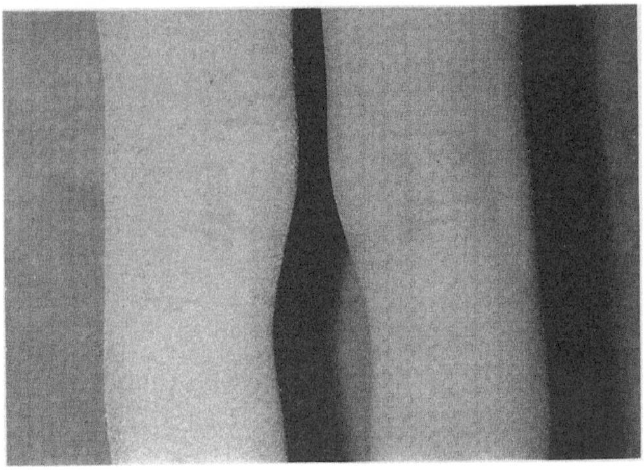

Fig. 3

Results

Complete remission of the hyperkeratotic skin lesions was achieved within 3 weeks in all four patients, moreover under a maintenance of local treatment with 0.5% Ro 11–1430 two or three times weekly no recurrences were observed (Figs. 2–5). In our patients no local irritation was seen.

Conclusion

The treatment of ichthyotic skin conditions has always been a frustrating therapeutic problem.

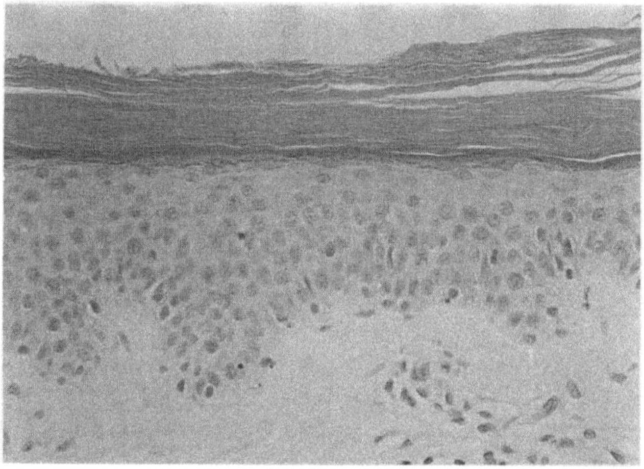

Fig. 4

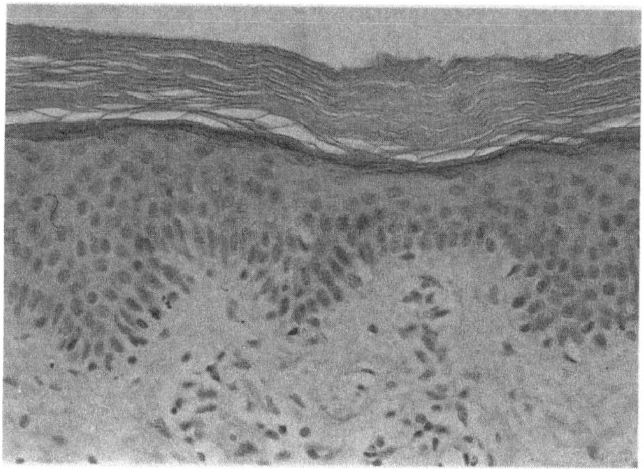

Fig. 5

Fig. 4 and 5. The histology of the 19- and 11-year-old patients with ichthyosis vulgaris before treatment. Hematoxilin and eosine

The results of this preliminary study demonstrate the favourable therapeutic affect of topical aromatic retinoid Ro 11-1430 (0.5%) in ichthyosis.

Unlike retinoic acid, locally applied Ro 11-1430 produced no skin irritation in our patients. Moreover, the low percutaneous absorption of this drug (0.5–3.0%) probably limits the risk of possible systemic side effects and permits a long-term application. However, the chronic toxicity of topical Ro 11-1430 has to be within sight.

Topical aromatic retinoid Ro 11-1430 may represent a new therapeutic approach in ichthyosis, which could displace the oral Ro 10-9359 or 13-cis-retinoic acid.

Although the mechanism of action is unknown, it is conceivable that its effect on the regulation of the keratinization process and possibly the stimulation of proliferation are of importance for the morbidistatic influence on the treated ichthyotic forms.

C.E. Orfanos et al. (eds.)
Retinoids

Combined UVB Phototherapy and Low-dosage Oral Retinoid (Ro 10-9359) for Psoriasis Responding Inadequately to UVB Alone

J. Boer and D. Suurmond

In the past few years good results have been obtained by treating psoriasis with UVB irradiation from artificial light sources (1, 4). In a previous paper on UVB phototherapy for psoriasis we reported 80% or higher therapeutic response in 33 (73.3%) out of 45 patients. During maintenance treatment, irradiation once every 1–5 weeks proved adequate in 64.4% of the patients (1).

The question then arose whether the results in the group in which UVB therapy failed for both clearing and maintenance phase, could be improved by the addition of Ro 10-9359. Orfanos et al. (3) found that simultaneous application of UVB irradiation and Ro 10-9359 orally in a daily dose of 1.0 mg/kg body weigth gave definitely better results than UVB therapy alone. In their study, however, the combination treatment was not applied separately in the group of patients who failed to respond to UV alone.

The usual dosage for the initial treatment with Ro 10-9359 alone or in combination treatments is 1 mg/kg body weight. Recent studies (2, 3) suggest that with this dosage side effects are relatively slight. Nevertheless, the side effects of Ro 10-9359 sometimes make it necessary to discontinue the therapy prematurely. Recently, van der Rhee et al. (5) studied the effect of oral Ro 10-9359 in a lower dose (approximately 0.5 mg/kg body weight) in combination with triamcinolone acetonide cream (0.1%) with 5% salicylic acid. This combination appeared to be as effective as the high-dose retinoid therapy alone, and gave markedly fewer side effects.

The present study represents an attempt to improve the results in the 14 patients who did not respond sufficiently to UVB phototherapy alone, during either clearing or maintenance treatment. The treatment used for this purpose was UVB phototherapy plus Ro 10-9359 in a daily dose of 0.50 to 0.67 mg/kg body weight.

Materials and Methods

Patients: 14 patients (3 women and 11 men, aged between 16 and 64 years) with extensive psoriasis vulgaris who had failed to respond to UVB therapy alone, were selected for the combined treatment. Informed consent was obtained from each patient. Criteria for UVB failure were: 1. in the clearing treatment (CT), failure to achieve at least 80% clearance after maximally 40 irradiations, and 2. in the maintenance treatment (MT), failure to retain a clearance of at least 80% on at most one irradiation a week.

Retinoid Medication: Ro 10-9359 was given in 10 mg capsules according to the patient's body weight: patients weighing 40–60 kg, 60–80 kg or 80–100 kg received 3, 4, or 5 capsules per day, respec-

Abbreviations:
CT: Clearance treatment; MT: Maintenance treatment; CCT: Combined clearance treatment; CMT: Combined maintenance treatment

tively. For the 14 patients this gave a daily ranging from 0.50 to 0.67 mg/kg body weight for CT. In the course of MT the initial doses could generally be lowered, depending on the therapeutic response. Final maintenance doses ranged from 0.32 to 0.62 mg/kg body weight.

UVB: UVB irradiation was performed with a Waldmann UV-1000 cabin fitted with 28 Sylvania F75/85 watt UV-6 fluorescent lamps. The wave-length spectrum of these lamps extends from 280 nm into the visible region, with a broad peak at 313 nm. The spectral distribution is 280–320 nm: 51%, 320–400 nm: 31%, and >400 nm: 18%. The UVB spectral irradiation (280–320 nm) at a distance of 20 cm and a height of 75 cm was 0.75 mwatt/cm^2. The number of irradiations was four weekly during CT and one a week or less during MT. Further details of this treatment regimen have been reported elsewhere (1).

Combined Therapy (Ro 10-9359 and UVB): Where UVB alone failed during either CT or MT, Ro 10-9359 was added to treatment. A new combined clearing treatment (CCT) was then started (four irradiations a week). If the lesions did not show further improvement, the combined maintenance treatment (CMT) schedule was instituted (one irradiation a week or less).

The use of local treatment was recorded at each visit. All patients used white petrolatum with 2% salicylic acid throughout the study and only temporary use of some local corticosteroid preparations was frequent in the MT and CMT (because of the long-term nature of the trial).

Evaluation: Each week the per cent involvement was estimated relative to the original status of the lesions by evaluating the presence and degree of scaling, infiltration, and erythema. The therapeutic effect was then graded as follows: 0 = 0–24%, +1 = 25–49%, +2 = 50–79%, +3 = 80–94%, and +4 = >95% clearance of lesions.

Results

At the end of the CCT (═══), 12 of these 14 patients (86%) showed a grade 3 or 4 response, whereas at the end of the CT (UVB alone) (───) 9 of the 14 patients (64%) showed only a grade 3 response (Figs. 1 and 2). For the CMT (= = = =), 9 of the 14 patients (64%) showed a satisfactory response (grade 2, 3 or 4), 8 of the 9 (57% of the series) maintaining a grade 3 or 4 response on one irradiation a week or less (Figs. 1 and 2). The duration of follow-up for CMT ranged from 8 to 47 weeks (mean: 31.5 weeks).

Side Effects: The most common side effect was dryness of the lips, which was generally well tolerated. Further, there were four cases of palmo-plantar desquamation; two each of paronychia, conjunctivitis, transpiration and diffuse hair loss; and one patient complained of burning sensations of the skin. In one patient with a very good therapeutic response (grade 4) the retinoid therapy was terminated at the end of the CCT because of diffuse hair loss and conjunctivitis.

Discussion

Orfanos et al. (3) and Fritsch et al. (2) found Ro 10-9359 in a dosage of 1 mg/kg body weight combined with either SUP therapy (UVB) or PUVA to be superior to SUP or PUVA alone. We recommend starting with phototherapy alone. If the response is not satisfactory, combined therapy (in our study Ro 10-9359 and UVB) can be instituted. In this way the Ro 10-9359 medication can be restricted to a relatively small group of psoriasis patients. In the present study combined administration of UVB phototherapy and low-dosage Ro 10-9359 (0.50–0.67 mg/kg body weight) was successful in a majority of the patients with psoriasis who previously had not responded satisfactorily to UVB monotherapy. Even on CMT, 57% of our 14 patients maintained a clearance of 80–100% with one irradiation or less a week. We did not include a control group with Ro 10-9359 therapy alone, but in van der Rhee et al.'s study (5), Ro 10-9359 given alone according to the same low-dosage schedule as we used, had virtually no effect. Unlike their patients, ours were selected on the basis of failure to respond to UVB monotherapy.

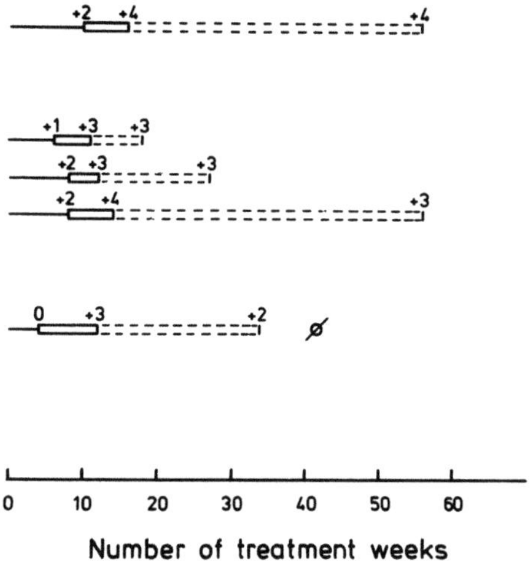

Fig. 1

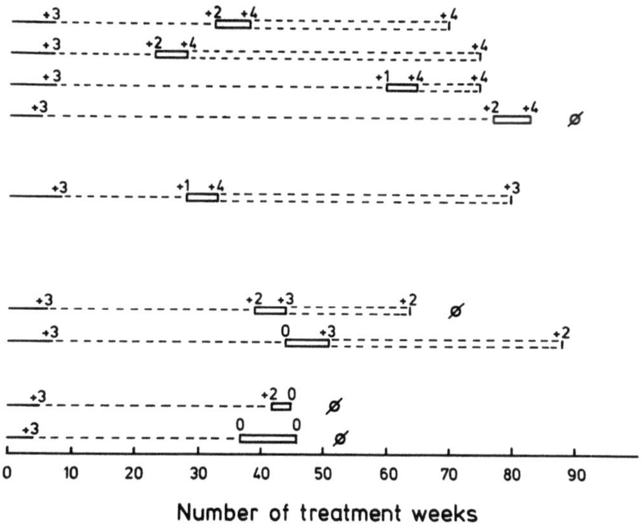

Fig. 2

Figs. 1 and 2. The duration in weeks of the different treatments in the clearing and maintenance failure group of UVB therapy, respectively. The patients are arranged according to the final degree of improvement obtained with a combined treatment.
(——) CT; (- - - -) MT; (══) CCT; (= = =) CMT.
0 to +4: improvement grade at the end of the different treatments.
Ø: drop outs

The combination we used caused relatively few side effects. Van der Rhee et al. (5) and Fritsch et al. (2) also found that lower Ro 10-9359 doses cause fewer side effects.

In sum, we consider it justified to conclude that the combination of UVB phototherapy and low-dosage oral retinoid (Ro 10-9359) offers a very useful therapy for psoriasis that responds inadequately to UVB alone.

Summary

Combined administration of UVB phototherapy and low-dosage Ro 10-9359 (0.50–0.67 mg/kg body weight) was successful in 14 patients with psoriasis who had not responded satisfactorily to UVB monotherapy. Twelve (86%) of these 14 patients showed a clearance of 80–100% on combined initial treatment (Ro 10-9359 and UVB), and 8 patients (57%) reached the same level on subsequent combined maintenance treatment consisting of one irradiation or less a week.

References

1. Boer J, Schothorst AA, Suurmond D (1980) UVB phototherapy of psoriasis. Dermatologica 161: 250–259
2. Fritsch PO, Hönigsmann H, Jaschke E, Wolff K (1978) Augmentation of oral methoxsalen-photochemotherapy with an oral retinoic acid derivative. J Invest Dermatol 70:178–182
3. Orfanos CE, Steigleder GK, Pullmann H, Bloch PH (1979) Oral retinoid and UVB radiation: a new, alternative treatment for psoriasis on an out patient basis. Acta Dermatol Venerol (Stockh) 59:241–244
4. Tronnier H, Heidbüchel H (1976) Zur Therapie der Psoriasis vulgaris mit UV-Strahlen. Z Haut Geschl Krankheiten 51:405–424
5. Van der Rhee HJ, Tijssen JGP, Herrmann WA, Waterman AH, Polano MK (1980) Combined treatment of psoriasis with a new aromatic retinoid (Tigason) in low dosage orally and triamcinolone acetonide cream topically: a double-blind trial. Br J Dermatol 102:203–212

C.E. Orfanos et al. (eds.)
Retinoids

Oral Retinoid Promotion of UV Light Action in Psoriasis. A Measure of UV Radiation Protection

W. Born, H. Wokalek and E. Schöpf

Preference of the lowest effective radiation exposure dose as a general principle of radiation protection in therapy requires measures to increase selectively the biological changes intended. This can be achieved by chemical or physical shielding of surrounding tissues, as well as by chemical and physical sensitization of the aim tissues.

The oral low-dose administration of an aromatic retinoid together with UVB radiation treatment has already shown to be much more effective against psoriasis than a similar radiation therapy without the drug, or as an even higher dose retinoid monotherapy (3).

Based on the convincing results obtained by that principle with a 4- to 6-day per week UVB treatment regimen, the intervals after each radiation were enlarged with the goal to reduce the total UVB dose, to increase biological recovery processes and, to make an outpatient treatment more convenient.

Methods

Within a total of 247 patients treated orally with the aromatic retinoid Ro 10-9359 for psoriasis (chronic, pustular, palmo-plantar, arthropathic), acne, ichthyosis, palmo-plantar hyperkeratosis, subcorneal pustulosis and surveyed by laboratory check as given below, a group of 16 patients (A-P in Fig. 1) with chronic psoriasis was treated by a modificated UV-retinoid regimen (3). A low-dose retinoid treatment was preferred in order to avoid adverse side effects.

Together with a daily administration of 25 mg aromatic retinoid Ro 10-9359, UVB irradiations were given every second day or only twice weekly with a METEC Helarium, producing no or only slightest visible solar erythema reactions. The course of clearing was followed and stated by a "+ better; 0 equal; - worse" classification (+++ almost or completely cleared; ++ almost or all scales and papules disappeared, stage of residual erythema; + substantially less papular lesions; - more lesions). The laboratory checks included blood count, GOT, GPT, LDH, creatinine.

Results

The therapeutical effect of UVB irradiations in psoriasis can be definitely increased by a low-dose oral administration of aromatic retinoid only if a certain interval time threshold is not exceeded. If the average interval time between two UVB exposures is longer than 2 days (for example 2.33 with 3-session weekly regimen), the UVB radiation treatment of psoriasis becomes little successful even if it is continued over long time periods and, in this case also

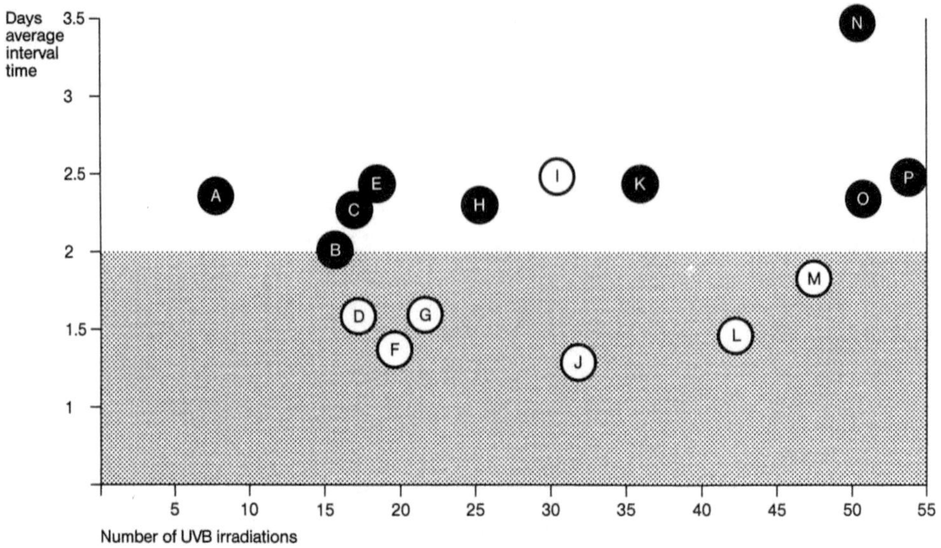

Fig. 1. Successful UVB treatment results in psoriasis were obtainable only within the range of 1–2 days average interval time between consecutive irradiations. Dark points indicate no sufficient therapy results (–, 0, +). Light points indicate a successful treatment (++, +++)

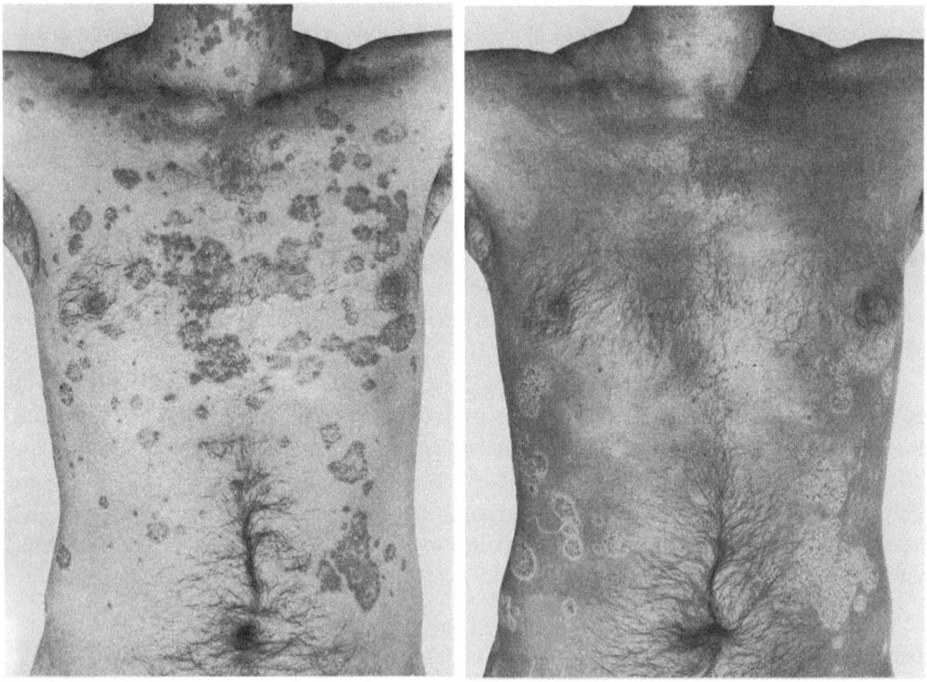

Fig. 2a, b. The typical results of regimens with 2 or more day average interval time between repeated therapeutical UVB irradiations in psoriasis is a lack of success even if the distribution and shape of lesions may change as shown **a** before treatment and **b** after a long time (4 months) continued combined UVB and low-dose oral retinoid therapy with average intervals of 2.39 days between a total of 55 irradiations no better results could be obtained with an additional low-dose retinoid administration than without (Fig. 2a, b).

Neither the clinical observation nor the laboratory controls showed adverse effects due to the low-dose retinoid treatment.

Conclusions

The daily oral low-dose administration of an aromatic retinoid Ro 10-9359 in psoriasis during UVB treatment periods allows to obtain a complete clearing with less radiation exposure than otherwise possible. This supporting principle can be used as an effective measure of UV radiation protection, but it turns into the opposite, if the recovery periods after each UVB application unto the next one exceed certain average values given.

The findings suggest to avoid UVB treatment regimens in psoriasis only every second day or less even if it is combined with additional antipsoriatic measures. The second and following UVB radiation hits are most effective if they are coincident with the reactive DNA synthesis increase periods after each single radiation exposure, as in UVB 1 day (2), in PUVA 3–7 days, in X-ray 1–2 weeks (1). From a radiobiological and also from a practical point of view, it may be an interesting question, whether UVB treatment regimens with continuous 3-day irradiation periods and following 4-day non-irradiation periods weekly lead to better and sufficient therapy results despite the same high average interval time of 2.33 days as in the non-sufficient every second work-day regimens.

References

1. Born W (1969) Die epidermale DNS-Synthese der Meerschweinchenflanke nach Röntgenbestrahlung. Strahlentherapie 138:749–753
2. Born W (1970) Zur Wirkung von Ultraviolettlicht auf die DNS-Synthese in der Epidermis. Arch klin exp Dermatol 237:466–471
3. Wokalek H, Roesch HW, Born W (1978) Erfolge mit UV-Retinoid bei therapieresistenter Psoriasis. Aktuel Dermatol 4:225–229

C.E. Orfanos et al. (eds.)
Retinoids

Treatment of Epidermodysplasia Verruciformis or Multiple Verrucae Planae by Oral Aromatic Retinoid (Ro 10-9359 - Tigason)

Y. Edelson, B. Berretti and Ch. Grupper

Authors discuss results observed in two patients affected with chronic epidermodysplasia verruciformis or generalized verrucae planae and treated by oral aromatic retinoid (AR) (Ro 10-9359, Tigason). HPV types 3 and 5 were isolated from the cutaneous lesions of one patient (Dr. Orth) and HLV type 3 in the other *Cell-mediated immune-response* (detected by delayed skin hypersensitivity tests) was depressed in the same patient and normal in the other one. Neither premalignant nor malignant cutaneous disorders were present at clinical examination or in the history of both patients.

Clearing of more than 80% of cutaneous lesions was obtained with an daily AR dose of 1 mg/kg during four to six weeks. Then, the treatment was continued with a decrease of AR dose to 0.5 mg/kg/day. In one patient, contemporaneously a *standard PUVA therapy* was combined with the AR. Side effects were mild. After four months' treatment, a new study on the immunological status of the two patients and a new viral investigation from the cutaneous lesions were performed. In spite of the clinical improvement, *histology, EM* and *virological studies* showed presence of virus.

The *oral AR seems a promising therapy* for these chronic viral cutaneous disorders, resistant to current treatments and whose prognosis is conditioned by a possible evolution to cutaneous cancers.

C.E. Orfanos et al. (eds.)
Retinoids

The Influence of Topical and Oral Retinoid Treatment on Photocarcinogenicity in Hairless Albino Mice

H.R. Hartmann and K. Teelmann

The etiological role of sunlight in human skin cancer is well established (3). The action spectrum of carcinogenic light irradiation lies between 280 and 320 nm (UV-B) (9, 10). Higher wave lengths of up to 400 nm (UV-A) increase the above-mentioned carcinogenic effect (12) as do chemicals which are known to be either photoactive, cancer initiating or cancer promoting agents (4, 5, 6). Epstein (7) has demonstrated that topical tretinoin in high concentrations can accelerate the tumorigenic process of UV-B light. Forbes et al. (8) have shown that topically applied tretinoin, even at very low concentrations, enhanced the carcinogenic effect of simulated sunlight in hairless albino mice. In a first investigation the influence on sunlight carcinogenesis by topical treatment with motretinid, an aromatic retinoid, was studied in comparison with tretinoin. The aim of a similar experiment was to study the influence of oral treatment with etretinate, another aromatic retinoid, on photocarcinogenesis. This is of particular importance since the combined clinical application of etretinate and UV-B irradiation induces a high percentage of complete remissions in severe psoriasis (11).

Materials and Methods

The following retinoids were applied in this study: tretinoin, all-trans-β-retinoic acid (Ro 1-5488); motretinid, all-trans-N-ethyl-9-(4-methoxy-2,3,6-trimethylphenyl)-3,7-dimethyl-2,4,6,8-nonatetraenamide (Ro 11-1430); etretinate, ethyl-all-trans-9-(4-methoxy-2,3,6-trimethylphenyl)-3,7-dimethyl-2,4,6,8-nonatetraenoate (Ro 10-9359).

Seven groups of 40 female hairless mice each (strain Fü-Alb hr/hr) were irradiated 3 times a week with simulated sunlight (Suntest apparatus, Original Hanau, Hanau/Main, FRG; equipped with a Xenon arc bulb and a Schott Suprax UV filter 1.7 mm). The irradiation applied per session was half an erythema dose (an average of 0.48 sunburn units, 11 min). The animals were exposed for 28 weeks and simultaneously treated topically with 0.1 ml of placebo, tretinoin or motretinid, evenly distributed on the back of the mice. 4 additional groups served as unirradiated controls, being topically treated with tretinoin or motretinid. A further group was neither irradiated nor treated topically.

In a second experiment, 3 groups of 40 mice were irradiated as described before and treated orally, 5 times a week, either with placebo or etretinate. The placebo, arachis oil, was dosed not exceeding 4 µl/g body weight. 2 groups served as etretinate treated unirradiated controls.

For arrangement of treatment groups and retinoid doses administered see Fig. 1.

Tumors were measured by means of a stencil, classified in diameter categories of >1 mm, >2 mm and >4 mm. Total tumor burden of an animal was expressed by the index T_i which was calculated as follows: $T_i = n_1 \times 1\,mm + n_2 \times 2\,mm + n_4 \times 4\,mm$. The mean tumor index $\bar{T}$ of a group was calculated as follows.

$$\bar{T}_j = \frac{1}{Z_j} \times \sum_{i=1}^{Z_j} T_i \quad (Z = \text{number of survivors})$$

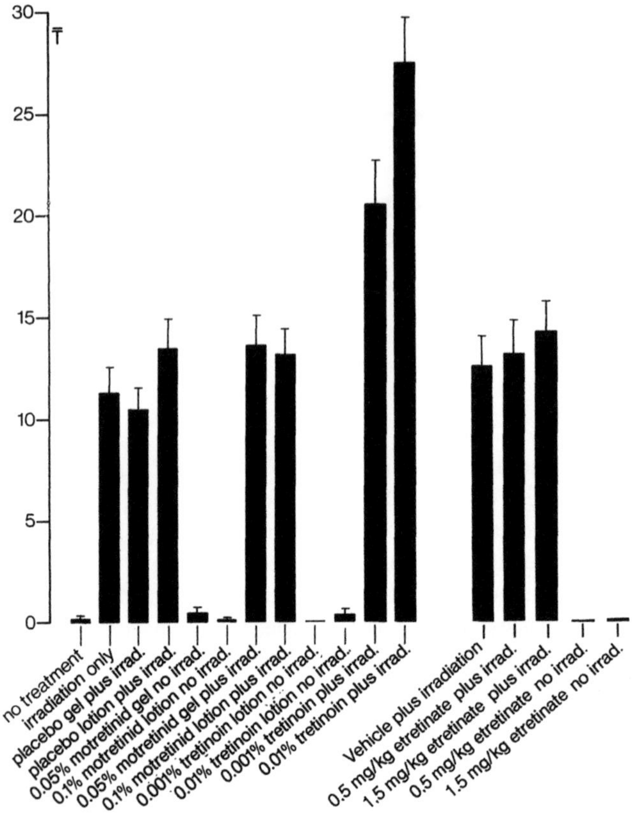

Fig. 1. Tumor indices after 28 weeks (end of treatment) with some retinoids

2 to 4 weeks after termination of treatment and irradiation all surviving mice were euthanized, dissected and macroscopically visible alterations were recorded. Representative samples of altered tissues, particularly skin samples, were fixed and processed for histological slide preparation, and H.E. stained sections were microscopically examined.

Results

Topical Retinoid Treatment

Topical treatment was well tolerated in all groups, no signs of local or systemic toxicity being observed. In treated and untreated unirradiated mice either no skin tumors or only a few papillomas developed.

At the end of the treatment period almost all irradiated animals carried multiple tumors on their backs. The first papillomas were observed in the 17th week. The mean tumor index of irradiated groups steadily increased during the treatment period and continued to grow after cessation of treatment and irradiation. Figure 1 shows the mean tumor index $\overline{T}$ of all groups after 28 weeks (end of treatment). The $\overline{T}$ of groups 3 and 4 (placebo gel and lotion, respectively) and groups 7 and 8 (0.05% and 0.1% motretinid gel and lotion, respectively) did not differ significantly from that of group 2 (irradiation only). In contrast to motretinid, tretinoin led to a dose dependent marked increase in tumors: the 0.001% lotion (group 11)

Table 1. Frequency distribution of skin lesions regarded at histopathologic examination

	no treatment	irradiation only	placebo gel plus irrad.	placebo lotion plus irrad.	0.05% motretinid gel no irrad.	0.1% motretinid lotion no irrad.	0.05% motretinid gel plus irrad.	0.1% motretinid lotion plus irrad.	0.001% tretinoin lotion no irrad.	0.01% tretinoin lotion no irrad.	0.001% tretinoin plus irrad.	0.01% tretinoin plus irrad.	Vehicle plus irradiation	0.5 mg/kg etretinate plus irrad.	1.5 mg/kg etretinate plus irrad.	0.5 mg/kg etretinate no irrad.	1.5 mg/kg etretinate no irrad.
No. of animals examined	40	34	37	33	38	40	37	39	37	38	37	32	34	38	39	36	37
Papilloma %	-	35	43	33	-	-	43	38	-	-	30	41	56	32	67	-	-
Focal squamous cell carcinoma %	-	50	49	33	-	-	24	50	-	-	41	16	56	58	59	-	-
Widespread squamous cell carcinoma %	-	41	38	58	-	-	73	38	-	-	84	76	24	18	28	-	-
Ratio of widespread to focal carcinoma	-	0.82	1.17		-	-	1.50		-	-	2.81		0.43	0.39		-	-

caused an increase of $\overline{T}$ of 53%, the 0.01% lotion (group 12) of 104% compared to the placebo group 4.

Histological observations revealed that local treatment with either motretinid or tretinoin without radiation caused a mild epidermal response with slight epithelial hyperplasia in approx. 5% of the mice treated with motretinid and in approx. 25% of those treated with tretinoin.

Macroscopically many tumors of the irradiated mice appeared to be small papilloma type proliferations, others were larger, sometimes involving ¼ or ⅓ of the back of the animals. Almost all irradiated mice had cicatrized skin areas.

Microscopically the skin of all mice exposed to simulated sunlight was markedly thickened with epithelial hyperplasia, enlargement of the follicular cysts and fat cells as well as some proliferation of the connective tissues. Tumors were primarily of epithelial origin and were diagnosed to be papillomas, focal or widespread squamous cell carcinomas. Most of the tumors seen were in a premalignant stage and nearly every mouse had benign tumor types as well.

Metastases of squamous cell carcinomas were seen only on two occasions. Keratoacanthomas, subepithelial tumors of mesenchymal origin like fibromas or fibrosarcomas, mixed tumors containing epithelial and fibrous cell types and hemangiomas usually located in the subcutaneous areas were noted only in a small number of irradiated mice.

In connection with treatment the spectrum of tumors remained basically similar and no shift to new tumor types became apparent. There appeared to be an increased frequency of carcinomas in the mice treated with tretinoin and furthermore the number of widespread squamous cell carcinomas in these mice was markedly enhanced in comparison to those mice only irradiated (Table 1).

Oral treatment was well tolerated in all groups; no signs of toxicity were observed. In unirradiated mice only 3 animals developed one skin papilloma each.

After termination of treatment all irradiated mice except one each in groups 13, 14 and 15 carried multiple tumors in their backs (see Fig. 1). The first tumors appeared in the 17th week and further development was similar as described in section a. No significant difference in mean tumor indices of the three irradiation groups (placebo, 0.5 and 1.5 mg/kg etretinate, respectively) was noted.

Histologically the skin of etretinate treated unirradiated mice appeared to be free of any cutaneous effect. Skin alterations in the irradiated mice were macroscopically and microscopically similar to that observed in section a., except that a distinct shift to more focal or circumscribed carcinomas became obvious in etretinate treated animals compared with all irradiated mice treated otherwise (Table 1).

Discussion

Exposure of hairless albino mice to simulated sunlight was followed by epithelial tumor formation, predominantly of malignant character. This finding is well in accordance with the results of Epstein and Epstein (3), Winkelmann et al. (15), and Stenbäck (14). Additional topical treatment with tretinoin enhances this tumor formation. These results confirm previous reports of Epstein (7) and Forbes et al. (8).

An important finding of this study is that neither topical motretinid nor oral etretinate administered in doses used in the clinic enhanced tumor formation. In contrast, topical tretinoin used in only one fiftieth and one fifth of clinical concentrations had a marked tumor enhancing effect.

The propagation of squamous cell carcinomas and the higher incidence of widespread tumors seen macroscopically in most of the tretinoin treated mice may be due to its ability to induce epithelial hyperplasia. This was found in this study in unirradiated mice and is due to its high stimulating effect on the proliferation of the epidermis, as was demonstrated by Zil (16), Plewig and Braun-Falco (13), and Cahn et al. (1). Christophers (2) reported that in contrast to tretinoin, motretinid failed to have such an effect in guinea pig and human skin.

Histopathologically the tumor types remained basically similar in all irradiated groups. A constant histopathologic finding in almost all irradiated mice were areas of cicatrized skin. These areas were, in most of the cases, involved in the formation of small or widespread squamous cell carcinomas. The intensity of light irradiation in future studies should be such that dermal necrosis and ulceration do not occur.

So far, the hairless albino mouse is the experimental animal most often used for photocarcinogenesis studies. It is not known whether this model system has any relevance to humans who are not albinos.

Summary

Hairless albino mice were irradiated with simulated sunlight and treated either topically with a placebo, tretinoin or motretinid, respectively, or orally with a placebo or etretinate. Almost all irradiated animals developed multiple skin tumors. Compared with the placebo group, the mice receiving tretinoin showed an increased number, a larger size and an earlier appearance of tumors. In contrast, topical motretinid had no enhancing effect on photocarcinogenicity. Oral treatment with etretinate also did not enhance tumor formation. Histologically the range of tumor types was similar in all irradiated mice. The number of large tumors was slightly increased in animals topically treated with tretinoin. In mice orally treated with etretinate a tendency to a decreased number of large tumors was noted.

References

1. Cahn J, Bordier Ph, Herold M, Meunier MT (1975) Pharmacological studies on retinoic acid in Wistar and Atrichos rats. Acta Derm Venerol (Stockh) (Suppl 74) 55:33–35
2. Christophers E Influence of retinoic acid and Ro 11-1430 on proliferation of epidermal cells in vitro and in vivo. 1979, in preparation
3. Epstein JH, Epstein WL (1963) A study of tumor types produced by ultraviolet light in hairless and hairy mice. J Invest Dermatol 41:463–473
4. Epstein JH, Roth HL (1968) Experimental ultraviolet light carcinogenesis: A study of croton oil promoting effects. J Invest Dermatol 50:387–389
5. Epstein JH (1970) Ultraviolet carcinogenesis, in: Photophysiology V. Academic Press, New York, pp 235–237
6. Epstein JH (1978) Photocarcinogenesis: a review. Natl Cancer Inst Monogr 50:13–25
7. Epstein JH (1977) Chemicals and Photocarcinogenesis. Aust J Dermatol 18:57–61
8. Forbes PD, Urbach F, Davies RE (1979) Enhancement of experimental photocarcinogenesis by topical retinoic acid. Cancer Lett 7:85–90
9. Freeman RG, Hudson HI, Carnes R (1970) Ultraviolet wavelength factors in solar radiation and skin cancer. Int J Dermatol 9:232–235
10. Freeman RG (1975) Data on the action spectrum for ultraviolet carcinogenesis. J Natl Cancer Inst 55:1119–1122
11. Orfanos CE, Steigleder GK, Pullmann H, Bloch PH (1979) Oral retinoid and UVB radiation: a new, alternative treatment for psoriasis on an out-patient basis. Acta Derm Venerol (Stockh) 59:241–244
12. Parrish JA, Anderson RR, Urbach F, Pitts D (1978) UV-A, biological effects of ultraviolet radiation with emphasis on human responses to longwave ultraviolet. Plenum Press, New York, pp 165–171
13. Plewig G, Braun-Falco O (1975) Kinetics of epidermis and adnexa following vitamin A acid in the human. Acta Derm Venerol (Stockh) (Suppl 74) 55:87–98
14. Stenbäck F (1978) Life history and histopathology of ultraviolet light-induced skin tumors. Natl Cancer Inst Monogr 50:57–70
15. Winkelmann RK, Zollman PE, Baldes EJ (1963) Squamous cell carcinoma produced by ultraviolet light in hairless mice. J Invest Dermatol 40:217–224
16. Zil JS (1972) Vitamin A acid effects on epidermal mitotic activity, thickness and cellularity in the hairless mouse. J Invest Dermatol 59:228–232

C.E. Orfanos et al. (eds.)
Retinoids

Richner-Hanhart Syndrome (RHS) - Tyrosinemia Type II and Oral Aromatic Retinoid (Ro 10-9359). Report of two Cases

N. Hunziker, R. Brun and J.-P. Jeanneret

Since the first observations of Richner (10) and Hanhart (6), cases of Richner-Hanhart syndrome (RHS) are not frequently observed. Most of the cases are described by Franceschetti et al. (3) (18 cases) and Goldsmith (4) (7 cases).

This syndrome is characterized by bilateral herpetiform keratitis, hyperkeratotic painful lesions on the palms and soles with hyperhidrosis and mental retardation (see 8 between others).

Since 1973 an association of this syndrome was described with tyrosinemia type II (1, 5, 11).

With a diet low in both tyrosine and phenylalanine, the eye and skin lesions of such patients improved and mental retardation even was prevented.

The case reports of our two cases of RHS have already been published with a third one (7). Histological findings were practically identical in the three cases: hyperkeratosis, splits in the granular layer, acanthosis, discrete perivascular infiltrate in the upper dermis contain-

Report of Cases

1. T. Jean-Jacques, born in 1942, had eye lesions described as "herpetoid epithelial corneal dystrophy" in early childhood. Lamellar keratoplasty was performed on the right eye. Thereafter the ocular lesions stabilized. Mental retardation was also observed during the first years of life; however, during the last recent years his intellectual development improved spontaneously.

In 1977 he was still complaining of painful hyperkeratotic lesions (2–3 cm in diameter) on the palms and soles with hyperhidrosis. The tyrosinemia was 1847 µmol/l (NV 33–82 µmol/l) and the tyrosinuria was 1906 µmol/l (NV $<$ 1 µmol/l).

After 3 weeks of low tyrosine and phenylalanine diet the level of serum tyrosine was reduced greater than 50% and tyrosine in the urine almost disappeared. At this time the lesions improved with hyperhidrosis ceasing and pain decreasing. However, the diet was very difficult to follow, and as the serum tyrosine level increased, the lesions relapsed.

2. *Cl. Rosa,* born in 1938, had no ocular lesions and only very mild mental retardation. Circumscribed hyperkeratotic lesions on palms and soles and band-like hyperkeratotic lesions along the toes appeared at about the age of 14 years. Her younger brother had similar lesions. Serum and urine tyrosine levels were more than ten fold the normal rate: serum tyrosine was 1160 µmol/l (NV 33–82 µmol/l) and urinary tyrosine was 3918 µmol/24 h (NV $<$ 1 µmol/l).

After 2–3 weeks of diet the lesions almost disappeared and the patient was able to work normally. The level of serum tyrosine was lowered and tyrosine in urine almost disappeared. However, the diet is a vegetarian diet without cereals and very difficult to follow with a normal family life; with dietary indiscretion, serum tyrosine level increased and the lesions relapsed.

Already in 1979, a case of rare familial keratoderma of the palms and soles, Mal of Meleda was treated with the 13-cis-retinoic acid, a retinoid, with dramatic improvement (9).

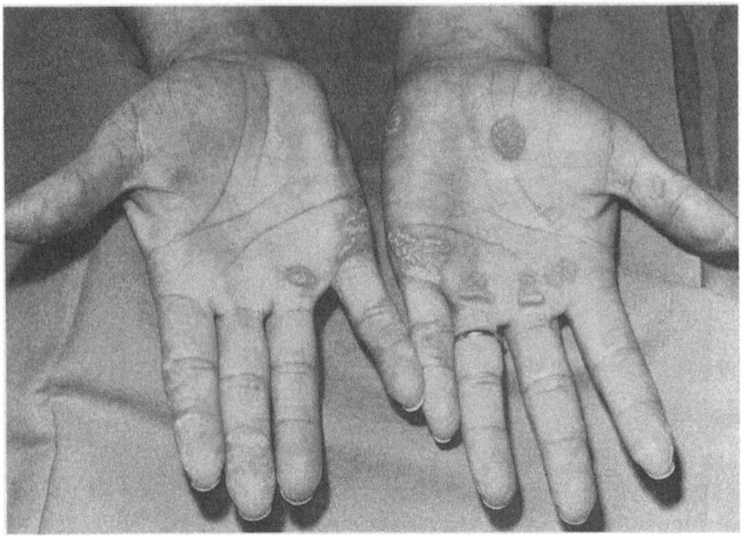

Fig. 1. Cl. Rosa, before treatment

ing many mast cells. In electron microscopic studies the most striking findings were in the dermis where we observed fibroblasts with different types of inclusions (2).

Knowing the effectiveness of oral retinoids in several disorders of keratinization, we treated our two cases orally with the retinoid, Ro 10-9359. Our two patients received orally a total of 1.0 mg/kg/day in three divided doses.

After 2 weeks of treatment the patients showed desquamation of the hyperkeratosis of hands and feet. Painful hyperkeratotic lesions and hyperhidrosis receded almost to normal by 8 weeks. The feet improved more slowly than the hands. Cl. Rosa stopped the treatment when she spent some weeks in Spain; the symptoms rapidly recurred. However after 4

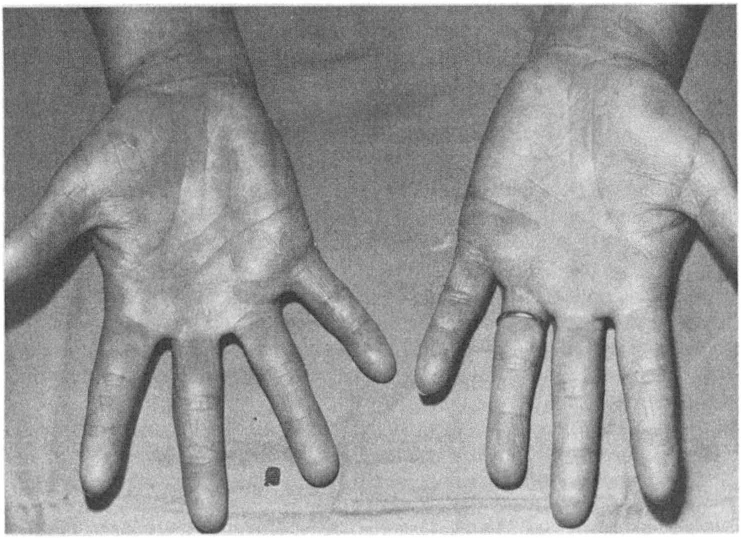

Fig. 2. Cl. Rosa, after 4 weeks' treatment with aromatic retinoid (Ro 10-9359)

weeks of treatment, a dramatic improvement was again observed (Fig. 1 and 2). The levels of tyrosine in serum and urine were never lowered.

T. Jean-Jacques has been treated with the aromatic retinoid now more than 2 years and Cl. Rosa for 18 months with an interruption of 6 weeks (it seems not possible to reduce the doses without some relapse). Even if some side effects are present, especially mild cheilitis and dryness of the skin, which did not force us to discontinue the treatment, our two patients are very happy and able to work and live normally.

In conclusion, treatment with oral aromatic retinoid (Ro 10-9359) improved the hyperkeratotic painful lesions on palms and soles associated with hyperhidrosis in the RHS - tyrosinemia type II, without influence on the inborn error of metabolism in this disorder.

References

1. Buist NRM, Kenneway NG, Fellman JH (1973) Eye and skin lesions in tyrosinemia. Lancet I: 620–621
2. Chavaz P, Hunziker N (1981) Richner-Hanhart Syndrome. Ultrastructure study of 3 cases. In press
3. Franceschetti AT, Schnyder UW, Felgenhauer WR (1971) Die Cornea beim Richner-Hanhart-Syndrom. Ber Dtsch Opththal Ges 71:109–112
4. Goldsmith LA (1978) Molecular biology and molecular pathology of a newly described molecular disease - tyrosinemia II (the Richner-Hanhart Syndrome). Exp Cell Biol 46:96–113
5. Goldsmith LA, Kang E, Bienfang DC, Jimbow K, Gerald P, Baden HP (1973) Tyrosinemia with plantar and palmar keratosis and keratitis. J Pediat 83:798–805
6. Hanhart E (1947) Neue Sonderformen von Keratosis palmo-plantaris, u.a. eine regelmäßig-dominante mit systematisierten Lipomen, ferner zwei einfach-rezessive mit Schwachsinn und z.T. mit Hornhautveränderungen des Auges (Ektodermalsyndrom). Dermatologica 94:286–308
7. Hunziker N (1980) Richner-Hanhart syndrome and tyrosinemia type II. Dermatologica 160:180–189
8. Jaeger W, Gallasch G, Schnyder UW, Lutz P, Schmidt H (1978) Tyrosinämie als Ursache einer doppelseitigen herpetiformen Hornhaut-Epithel-Dystrophie (Richner-Hanhart-Syndrom). Klin Mbl Augenheilk 173:506–515
9. Reed ML, Stanley J, Stengel F, Shupack JL, Benjamin DM (1979) Mal de Meleda treated with 13-cis-retinoic acid. Arch Dermatol 115:605–608
10. Richner H (1938) Hornhautaffektion bei Keratoma palmare et plantare hereditarium. Klin Mbl Augenheilk 100:580–588
11. Zaleski WA, Hill A, Kushniruk W (1973) Skin lesions in tyrosinosis: response to dietary treatment. Br J Derm 88:335–340

C.E. Orfanos et al. (eds.)
Retinoids

Light and Electron Microscopy Studies in Psoriasis Before and After Treatment with Retinoids (Ro 10-9359)

H. Kamino-Kamino, S. Gómez-Estrella, V. Tsutsumi, M.T. Hojyo-Tomoka and L. Domínguez-Soto

In two previous papers (6, 7) we presented the results obtained with the use of Ro 10-9359 in a group of patients with severe psoriasis; the first group was followed for a period of three months, the second of four months.

To summarize the outstanding points of our first observation, 20 patients were classified as excellent in 6, fair in 8, good in 4 and nil in 2 patients. The dosis used for this study was 50 mg a day for the first two weeks, reducing this to 25 mg a day for 6 weeks, and then to follow-up for another four weeks with placebo tablets. The side effects were quite consistent and they were mainly dryness of lips and other mucous membranes and a profuse desquamation of palms and soles.

In our second study with 10 patients the results were much better, as we achieved excellent results in 5, good results in 2, and fair results in 3 patients. The initial dose used was 100 mg daily for two weeks, then reduced to 50 mg for the following 6 weeks and to 25 mg for the

Table 1

Parameters	Number of cases			
	Before treatment	After treatment		
		Disappearence or normalization	Partial disappearance	Without changes
Number of mitosis per field (400 x)	8 (1 to 3)[a]	8 (0 to 1)[a]		
Parakeratosis	9	8	1	
Acanthosis	9	7	2	
Papillae edema	8	5	3	
Exocytosis	6	6		
Spongiosis	2	2		
Increased glycogen	5	5		
Munro microabscesses	4	4		
Dilated capillaries	8	2	4	2
Inflammatory infiltrate	9	2	6	1

[a] Number of mitosis

Table 2. Skin components studied by electron microscope

Layer	Component	Details
Basal layer	Epidermal-dermal junction	Basal lamina
		Hemidesmosomes
		Attachment filaments
	Melanocyte	
	Pigment in basal keratinocytes	
Spinous layer	Keratinocytes	Tonofibrils
		Junctional complex
		Intercellular space
	Langerhans' cells	
	Exocytosis (cell type)	
Stratum granulosum	Keratohyalin	
	Keratinosomes	
Stratum corneum: parakeratosis		
Vessels of dermal papillae		

next 4 weeks, and ending with a 4-week observation period with placebo. Side effects were the same, but more intense and they decreased as soon as the dose was reduced. No significant alterations were found in any of the laboratory tests.

Besides the clinical observation summarized in the previous paragraph, morphological studies with light- and electron microscopes were conducted in biopsies obtained from patients before and after treatment with Ro 10-9359.

Material and Methods

For the light- and electron microscopy studies, four skin samples were obtained from each of 9 patients: two before treatment, one of which was from a well-developed psoriatic plaque and the other from clinically healthy skin, one centimeter away from the rim of the same lesion. At the end of the treatment, two more samples were taken, a few millimeters away from the place where the first samples had been obtained. All these samples were obtained with a 3-mm punch.

For the light microscopy, 6 mm sections were obtained and stained with hematoxylin-eosin, PAS and the Feulgen techniques. The parameters studied are listed in Table 1. For electron microscopy, the samples were processed according to the routine procedure used in our laboratory: fixation in 3% glutaraldehyde (11), post-fixation in 1% osmium tetraoxide (9), and were observed in a Zeiss EM9A electron microscope. The parameters selected for the following study are listed in Table 2 (Figs. 6, 7 and 8).

Results

Histopathological Changes Observed Before Treatment

1. Clinically Healthy Skin. Under light microscopy, none of the 9 patients studied showed any epidermic changes (Fig. 1); except for the fact that a sparse lymphocytic infiltrate was seen in the papillary and subpapillary dermis in two of the cases (Fig. 1) and a capillary dilation and edema in one. In the observations made with the electron microscope, a great percentage of keratinocytes, mainly from the stratum spinosum, displayed a decrease in the density of the tonofilaments, and an increase in the number of mitochondria, which were localized mostly at the perinuclear region, a widened intercellular space with detachment of the cytoplasm of these cells, and the desmosomic junctions remaining intact (Fig. 9). The vessels seen both in the dermic papillae and in the subpapillary dermis, showed that the ca-

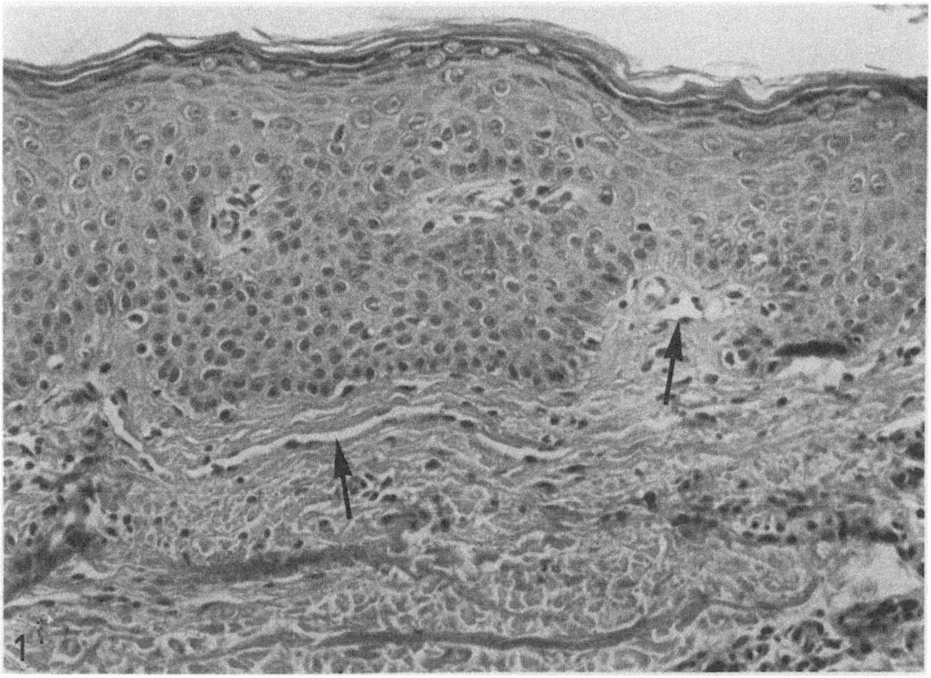

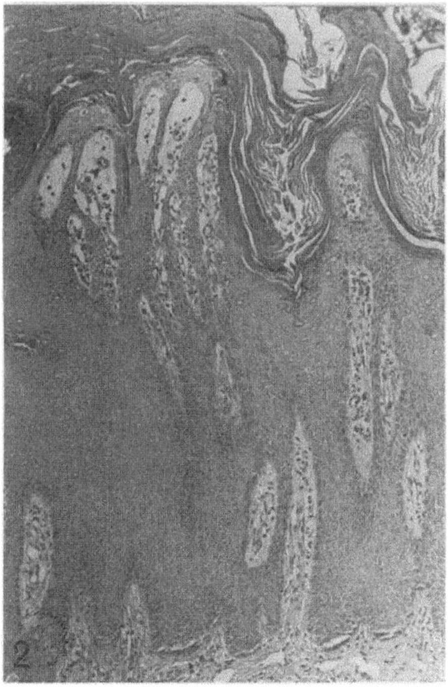

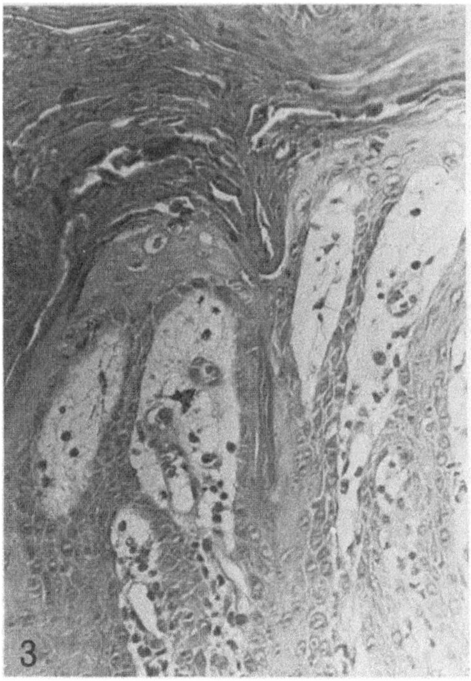

Fig. 1. Clinically healthy skin before treatment. Normal epidermis, capillary dilation (arrow) and sparse lymphocytic infiltrate

Fig. 2. Psoriatic skin before treatment: Hyperkeratosis with parakeratosis, acanthosis with rete ridge elongation, edematous papillae, capillary dilation and perivascular lymphocytic infiltrate

Fig. 3. Psoriatic skin before treatment: Parakeratosis, edematous papillae and capillary dilation

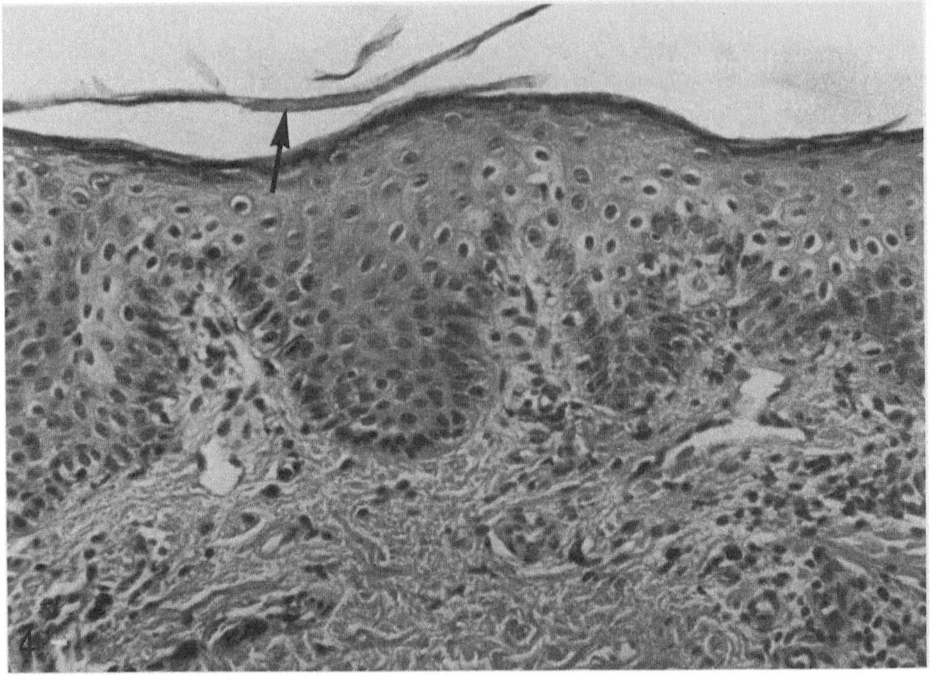

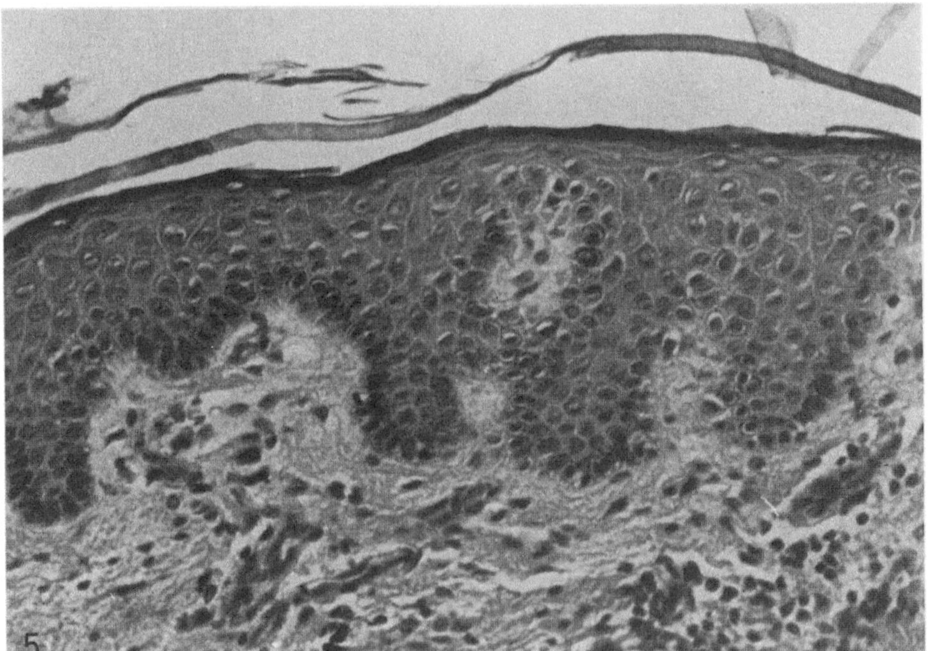

Fig. 4. Clinically healthy skin after treatment: Stratum corneum with tendency towards desquamation (arrow). The capillary dilation and inflammatory infiltrate persist

Fig. 5. Psoriatic skin after treatment: Desquamation of the stratum corneum. Normal malpighian layer, the perivascular lymphocytic infiltrate persist pillaries have a thinned endothelial wall in some areas and large vacuoles in other sites of the cytoplasm (1, 3, 4); the junction complexes between these cells were normal and pinocytic activity was observed at the cellular border (Fig. 10).

2. Skin from the psoriatic plaque. Under light microscopy, all the histological changes described by others (2, 5) for the diagnosis of psoriasis were observed (Figs. 2 and 3); 6 of them showed marked, 2 moderate and 1 slight changes, with a parallelism in the intensity of the dermic and epidermic changes (Fig. 2). In Table 1 we show the frequency with which these changes were observed.

Ultrastructurally, besides many mitosis, a definite decrease in the amount and density of the keratinocyte tonofilaments were observed with a significant increase in the amount of mitochondria in the previously mentioned location (Fig. 11). A well-developed rough endoplasmic reticulum and a Golgi apparatus (Fig. 12), and a large accumulation of glycogen in a rosette pattern were observed (Fig. 14). The intercellular space was very widened, even between the keratinocytes of the basal stratum, but without any alteration of the hemidesmosomic structures of the dermoepidermic junction (Fig. 13). In this intercellular space, a deposit of a flocculent granular material of a proteinaceous type was present (Fig. 13). The granular layer was observed in small areas and it was abnormal, the keratohyaline granules seen were scanty and small, tonofilaments were dispersed and only occasional keratinosomes were identified (Fig. 15). In the papillary dermis, capillary vessels were still observed with a thin wall and vacuoles in their cytoplasm.

Histopathological Changes Observed After Treatment

1. Clinically healthy skin. Under light microscopy, a looser stratum corneum with a tendency towards desquamation was detected in 6 of the cases (Fig. 4). The inflammatory infiltrate, edema and capillary dilation were similar to the cases presented before treatment. With the electron microscope a poorly organized fibrillar-type electrodense material was observed in the cytoplasm of the keratinocytes (Fig. 16), and also a decrease in the amount of mitochondria as compared to the samples of clinically healthy skin before treatment. Other epidermal layers were within normal limits (1).

2. Skin from the psoriatic plaque. The changes observed in affected skin after treatment (Fig. 5) are listed in Table 1. Summarizing, if we make an overall assessment of the degree of remission observed in every case, the results obtained in the 9 cases were as follows:
Total remission 1 case (11%)
Significant partial remission 7 cases (78%)
Moderate partial remission 1 case (11%)

Under electron microscopy, the reduction of the intercellular space between the keratinocytes was evident and also the restitution of a granular stratum of 2 to 3 layers (Fig. 17); in the keratinocytes of even the lower layers a considerable increase in the tonofilaments, with a significant decrease in the number of mitochondria, and other intracytoplasmic membranous organelles was observed (Fig. 17). Keratinocytes of the upper layer, the keratohyaline granules formed dense and abundant clumps with apparent aggregation of tonofilaments (Figs. 17 and 18). In the papillary dermis, the collagen fibers became compact and many blood vessels displayed a collapsed lumen with normal endothelial walls (Fig. 19); nevertheless, to a lesser degree, there were observed vessels with a wide lumen, thinned endothelial walls and the presence of vacuoles in the endothelial cytoplasm.

Although no morphological alterations were observed in melanocytes (Fig. 8), Langerhans' cells (Fig. 9) and pigment in the basal keratinocytes (Figs. 8 and 9), general quantitative differences were recorded. More melanocytes were seen in normal samples before and

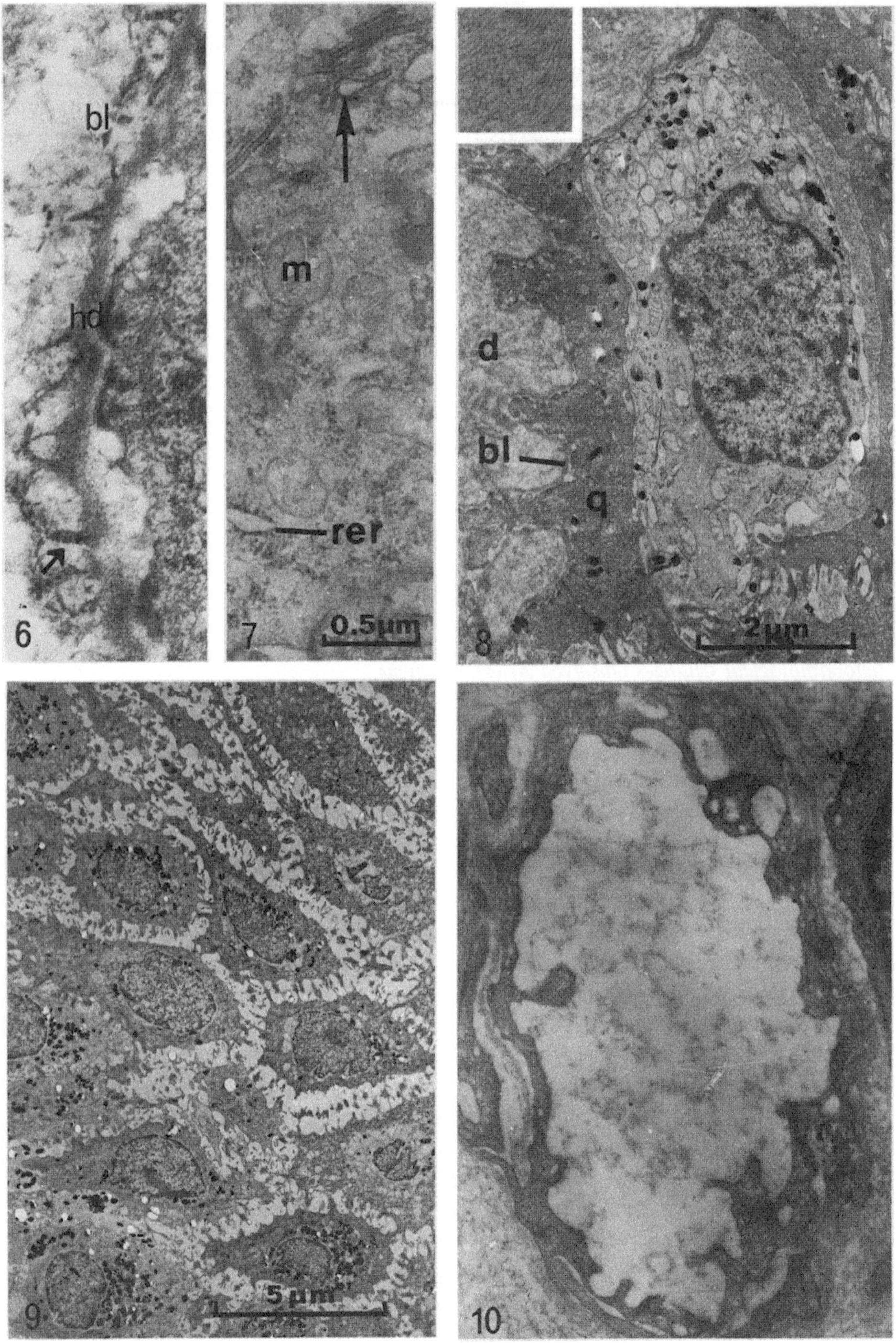

Figs. 6–10

after treatment as compared to the pathological samples before treatment, and their amount increased in the pathological samples after treatment. Less Langerhans' cells were seen in the pathological samples before treatment. The number of these cells increased in the pathological samples after treatment. The amount of pigment observed in basal keratinocytes in normal samples after and before treatment was abundant, practically absent in pathological samples before treatment and scarce in the pathological samples after treatment.

Comments

The observation of skin which was apparently normal both macroscopically and light-microscopically showed ultrastructural changes not only at the dermic level in various capillary vessels (3, 4), but also at the epidermic level, indicate that this is also an abnormal skin which has to be considered for further studies.

Based in the morphological changes observed after treatment with Ro 10-9359 which were more marked in the epidermis such as: a) the disappearance of epidermic inflammatory changes (spongiosis, exocytosis, Munro microabscesses); b) the trend towards maturation and restoration of an orderly keratinization pattern showed by light- and electronmicroscopy; and c) a tendency towards the regression of epidermic hyperplasia (remission of acanthosis and a decrease in the number of mitosis per field). We think that the inappropriate differentiation in keratinocytes in psoriasis could be one important factor that favours the considerable increase in the number of mitosis and the lack of an adequate production of keratinosomes which are essential for orthokeratinization (13); we also believe that the scarcity of these keratinosomes in affected skin is responsible for the abnormal exfoliation in corneal cells (14) and is one of the factors that explains the presence of hyperkeratosis. These keratinosomes are probably also involved in the production of a loose stratum corneum that was observed in those samples after treatment. On the other hand, we think that the lack of tonofilaments at the level of the desmosomic structures is probably an important factor that contributes to widening the intercellular space and makes it easier for the proteinaceous flocculent material to penetrate into these areas.

In contrast to the epidermis, the alterations in the dermis were changes to a lesser degree in damaged skin. Under electron microscopy the important observation was a compacting of the collagen fibers which indicates a remission of the edema. Most of the vessels showed a collapsed lumen and a normal endothelial wall; nevertheless vessels with the previously mentioned alterations were still sporadically identified.

The most marked regressive changes in the epidermis suggest that Ro 10-9359 act mainly in the epidermis, making a normal keratinization and reducing the proliferation of the keratinocytes. In this study we could not determine the exact mechanism for this. In previous study by Braun-Falco (2), were described the changes that occur in the lesions when psoria-

---

Fig. 6. Fine structure of the normal basal lamina (bl) in the epidermal-dermal junction. The attached anchoring fibrils with their typical periodicity (arrow) and normal hemidesmosomes (hd) are seen

Fig. 7. Detail of the cytoplasm of a Langerhans' cell which shows the characteristic granules (arrow), mitochondria (m), rough endoplasmic reticulum (rer)

Fig. 8. Electron micrograph of melanocyte with numerous melanosomes. d, dermis; q, keratinocyte; mb, basal lamina. Insert: Microfilaments within the cytoplasm of the same melanocyte

Fig. 9. Clinically healthy skin before treatment: Decrease on the number of tonofilaments and increase on the number of mitochondria within the cytoplasm of basal and spinous keratinocytes. Note the widened intercellular space

Fig. 10. Clinically healthy skin before treatment: capillary from papillar dermis shows a thin endothelial wall and gaps in the cytoplasm

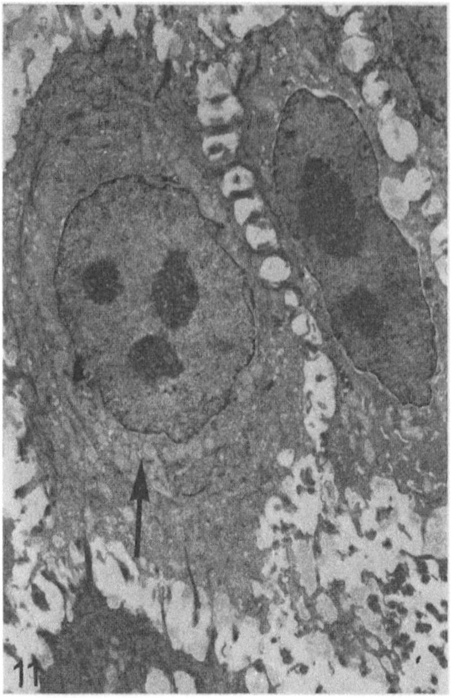

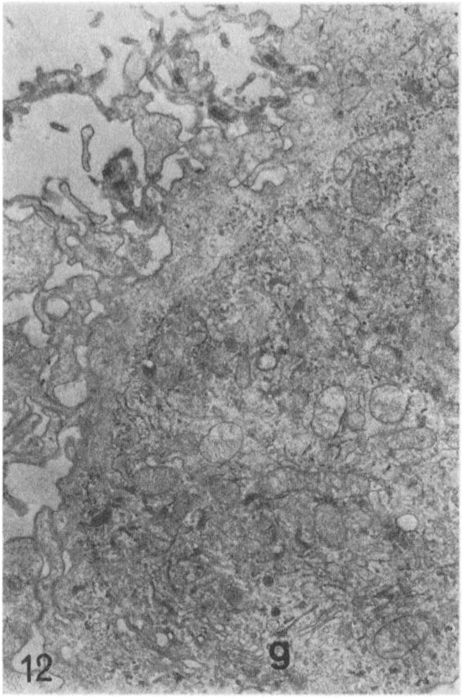

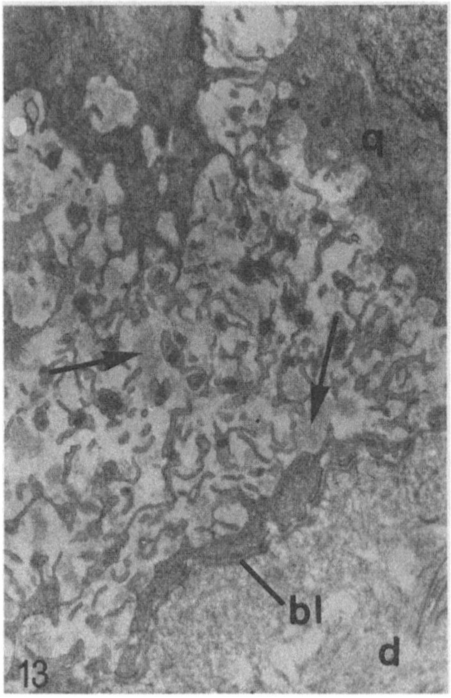

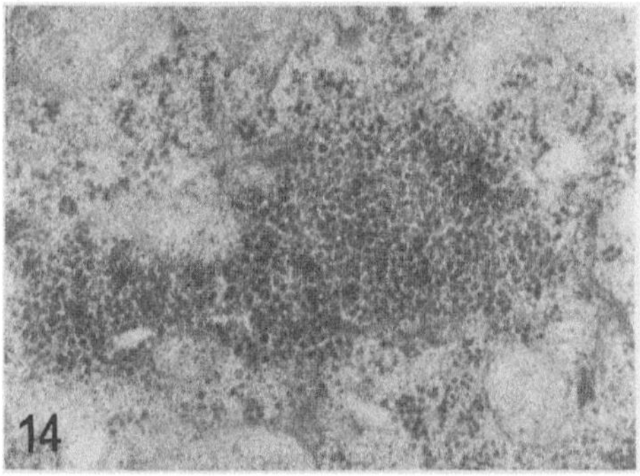

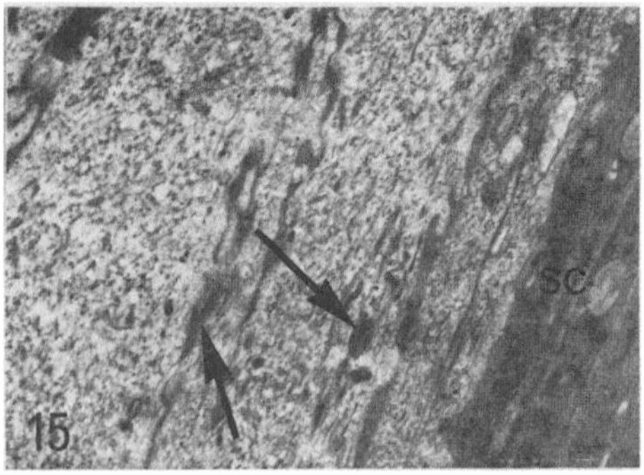

Fig. 11. Psoriatic skin before treatment: Detail of a basal keratinocyte with important decrease in the number and density of tonofilaments and increase of mitochondria (arrow)

Fig. 12. Psoriatic skin before treatment: Detail of well-developed membranous organelles in the keratinocyte cytoplasm

Fig. 13. Psoriatic skin before treatment: Within the widened intercellular space a proteineous granular material is present (arrows). (q) keratinocyte; (bl) basal lamina; (d) dermis

Fig. 14. Psoriatic skin before treatment: Large storage of glycogen in keratinocyte cytoplasm

Fig. 15. Psoriatic skin before treatment: Scarce and small keratohyaline granules (arrow) within the granular layer se = stratum corneum

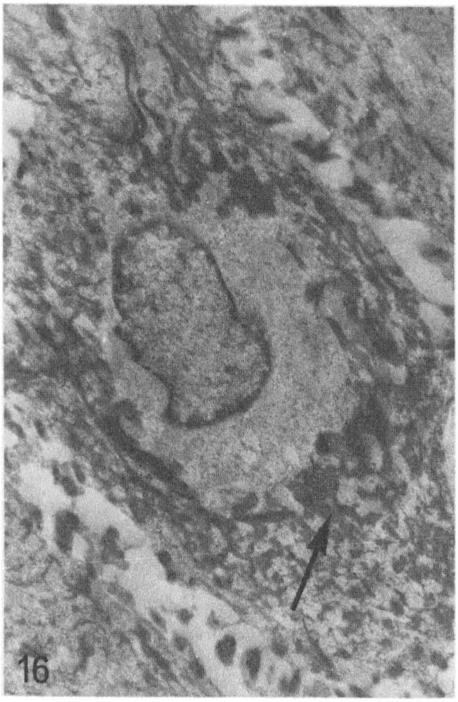

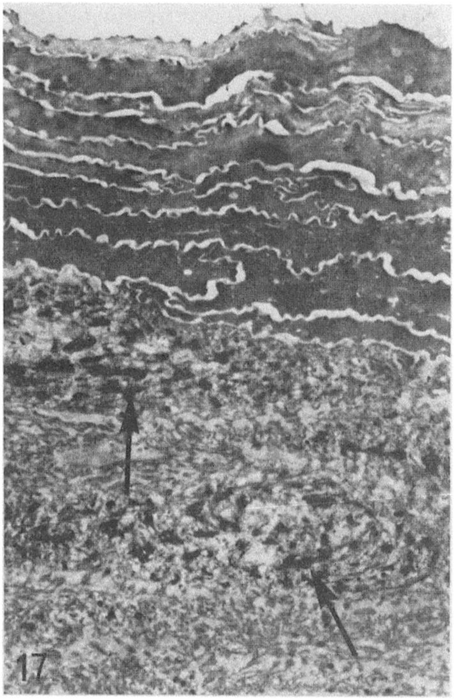

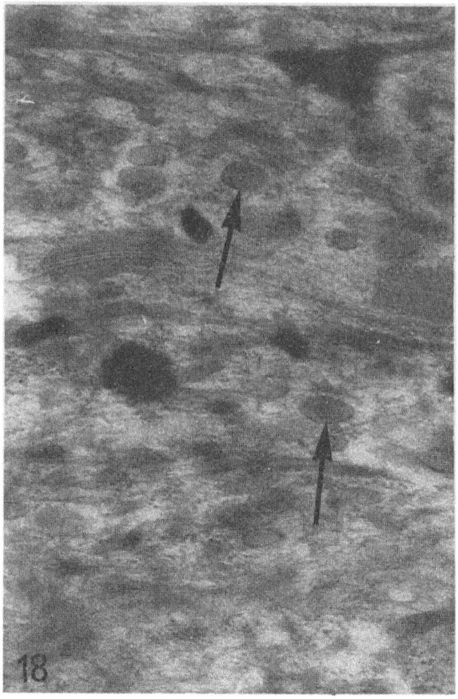

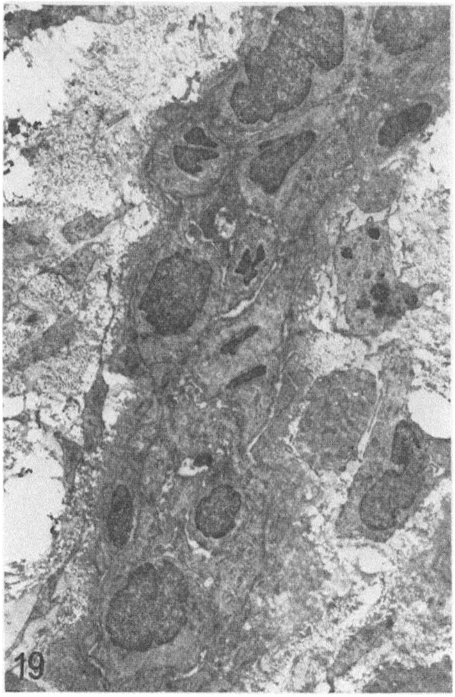

Fig. 16. Psoriatic skin after treatment: Detail of a keratinocyte of the spinous layer which shows within the cytoplasm an increase of loose fibrilar material (arrow). Important decrease in the number of mitochondria and reduced intercellular space are noted

Fig. 17. Psoriatic skin after treatment: A panoramic view which shows restitution of the granular layer with thick keratohyaline granules (arrows)

Fig. 18. Psoriatic skin after treatment: Detail of keratinosomes (arrows)

Fig. 19. Psoriatic skin after treatment: Vessel from dermis with collapsed lumen sis regresses with different treatments (methotrexate, ditranol, fluorcorticoids, etc.). The pharmacological action of these compounds is apparently different but, nevertheless, follows a sequence that is similar to the one described for this compound.

References

1. Breathnach AS (1971) In: A atlas of the ultrastructure of human skin. Churchill, London
2. Braun-Falco O (1971) Dynamics of growth and regression in psoriatic lesions: Alterations in the skin from normal into psoriatic lesion, and during regression of psoriatic lesion. In: Farber EM, Cox AJ (eds). Psoriasis: Proceedings of International Symposium, Stanford University, pp 215–317
3. Braverman IM, Cohen I, Keefe EO (1972) Metabolic and ultrastructural studies in a patient with pustular psoriasis. (Von Zumbusch) Arch Dermatol 105:189–196
4. Braverman IM, Yen A (1974) Microcirculation in psoriatic skin. J Invest Dermatol 62:493–502
5. Cox AJ, Watson W (1972) Histological variation in lesions of psoriasis. Arch Dermatol 106: 503–506
6. Domínguez-Soto L, Hojyo-Tomoka MT (1978) Aromatic retinoid (Ro 10-9359) in the treatment of psoriasis. Cutis 22:376–379
7. Domínguez-Soto L, Hojyo-Tomoka MT (1978) Ro 10-9359 in the treatment of psoriasis. Dermatologica 157 (Suppl 1):57–59
8. Luft JH (1961) Improvements in epoxy resin embedding methods. J Biophys Biochem Cytol 9:409–414
9. Milloning G (1961) Advantages of a phosphate buffer for osmium tetroxide solutions in fixation. J Appl Phys 32:1637
10. Reynolds ES (1963) The use of lead citrate at high pH as an electron opaque stain in electron microscopy. J Cell Biol 17:208–212
11. Sabatini DD, Bensch K, Barrnett RJ (1963) Cytochemistry and electron microscopy. The preservation of cellular ultrastructure and enzymatic activity by aldehyde fixation. J Cell Biol 17: 19–58
12. Watson ML (1958) Staining of tissue sections for electron microscopy with heavy metals. J Biophys Biochem Cytol 4:475–478
13. Weinstock M, Wilgram GF (1970) Fine structural observations on the formation and enzymatic activity of keratinosomes in mouse tongue filiform papillae. J Ultrastruct Res 30:262–274
14. Wolff K, Holubar K (1967) Odland-Körper (Membrane coating granules, Keratinosomen) als epidermale Lysosomen. Arch Klin Exp Dermatol 231:1–19

C.E. Orfanos et al. (eds.)
Retinoids

Electron Microscopic Characterization of the Mucus-like Material of the Epidermis Before and After Retinoid and Retinoid-PUVA (RePUVA) Treatment of Psoriasis

L. Kanerva, K.-M. Niemi, J. Lauharanta, T. Juvakoski and A. Lassus

Orfanos and Runne (9) were the first to report the fine-structural effects of an oral retinoid (Ro 10-9359) in psoriasis. They noted (a) enhanced inflammation with some cell degeneration in the malpighian layer, (b) extracellular accumulation of mucus-like material in the epidermis, (c) reappearance of keratohyaline granules and (d) normalization of other pathological changes both in the epidermis and the dermis.

In order to obtain more information about the effect of retinoid therapy in psoriasis, we extended the observation time to 14 weeks, during which time a clinical clearance of the psoriatic lesions occurred. We have also used the clinically highly effective therapy of retinoid followed by PUVA (RePUVA) (5, 8) and studied the biopsy samples electron-microscopically. In the present report special attention is paid to the intercellular area of the epidermis.

Material and Methods

Thirteen patients with severe psoriasis were studied. Four patients were treated with retinoid (Ro 10-9359), kindly donated by Hoffmann-La Roche Ltd.) for 14 weeks. The initial oral dose was 50–60 mg daily (0.5–1.0 mg/kg). This dose was gradually decreased to 0.3–0.5 mg/kg depending on the clinical response. Four patients were treated for 4 weeks with the same dose of retinoid and thereafter with conventional psoralen-UVA (PUVA) during the following 10 weeks. Biopsies were taken from a psoriatic lesion before treatment, and a biopsy from a corresponding area nearby was taken during treatment every 2 weeks.

Uninvolved skin from 5 psoriatics during PUVA therapy was also studied electron-microscopically.

Blocks, 1 mm^3 or smaller, were fixed for 2 hours or longer in 2.5% cacodylate buffered 0.1 M glutaraldehyde at 4 °C and postfixed with 1% osmium tetroxide, stained en bloc in uranyl acetate for 2 hours at room temperature, dehydrated in a graded series of alcohol and embedded in Epon 812. Ultrathin sections were cut with an LKB ultramicrotome, stained with lead citrate and examined with a Jeol 100S electron microscope operated at 80 kV.

Results and Discussion

The fine structure of the epidermis was studied carefully in untreated psoriasis, since it soon became evident that many features reported as being caused by retinoids (9), could be found in untreated psoriasis. Thus, the intercellular space, which was enlarged, contained a variety of finely granular or more coarsely granular material. This material was most abundant in the lower malpighian layer. Two main types of material could be distinguished: (a) A finely granular material, with granules about 80–150Å in diameter amongst an amorphic back-

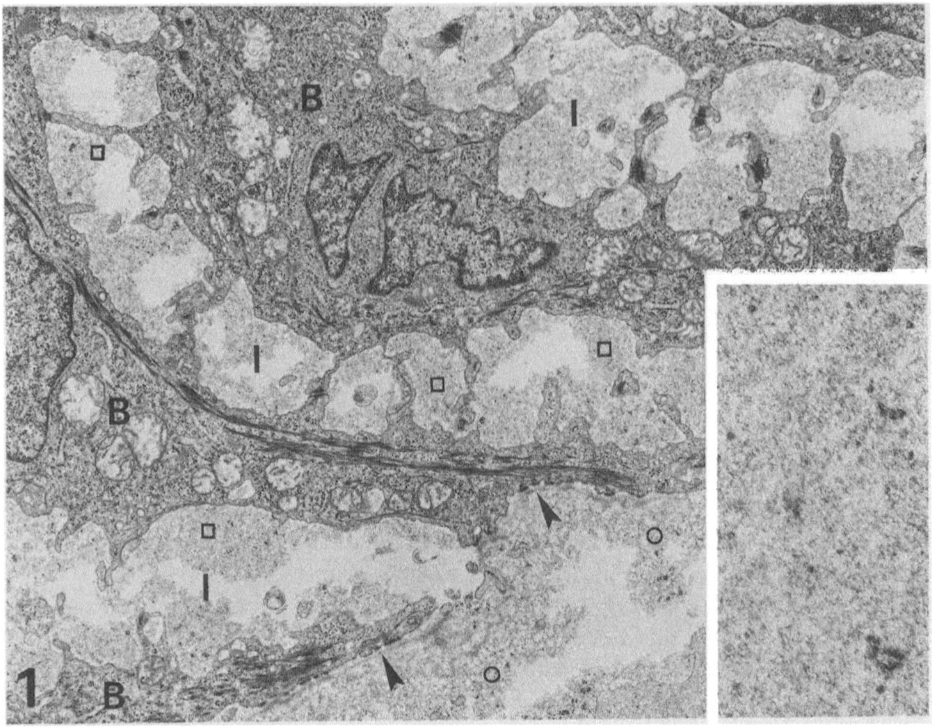

Fig. 1. Untreated psoriasis. Dermo-epidermal junction. Wide intercellular spaces (I) are found between the basal epidermal cells (B). The intercellular space is partly filled by a finely granular substance (□). A substance with the same fine structure (O) is found below the basal lamina (arrowhead) in the dermis. × 9300. Inset: Larger magnification of intercellular substance. × 39 200

ground substance (Fig. 1). This material was also found below the basal lamina, and we assume that it is a proteinous substance derived from the dermal vessels. It could also be derived from the epidermis and penetrate the basal lamina. (b) A substance with numerous coarser granules (Fig. 2), which were fine structurally identical to the abundant granules in the keratinocytes. The granules had a diameter of 120–150Å and their fine structure resembled that of ribosomes or beta particles of glycogen. This substance was not seen below the basal lamina and is probably formed in the keratinocytes. The granules were embedded in an amorphic ground substance. This substance was also found in the uninvolved skin of PUVA-treated psoriatics (Fig. 2). Probable mixtures of these two materials resulted in a sliding scale of intercellular substances with variable granularity. In the same specimen, the fine structural appearance varied in different adjacent areas.

After 2–6 weeks of retinoid treatment an increased amount of the intercellular substance could often be seen, though not always. No finely granular material was seen below the basal lamina, possibly indicating decreased leakage of proteinous substance through the dermal capillaries. The substance in the intercellular space could not be distinguished fine-structurally from the substances seen prior to treatment (Fig. 3). Thus, both coarse granular and fine granular substances were observed. The "mucous substance" in the epidermis after retinoid treatment has not previously been well described. Orfanos and Runne (9) described this substance as being a "fine granular material similar to mucus". However, so far cytochemical proof of the exact nature of the "mucous material" is lacking. No "threads with

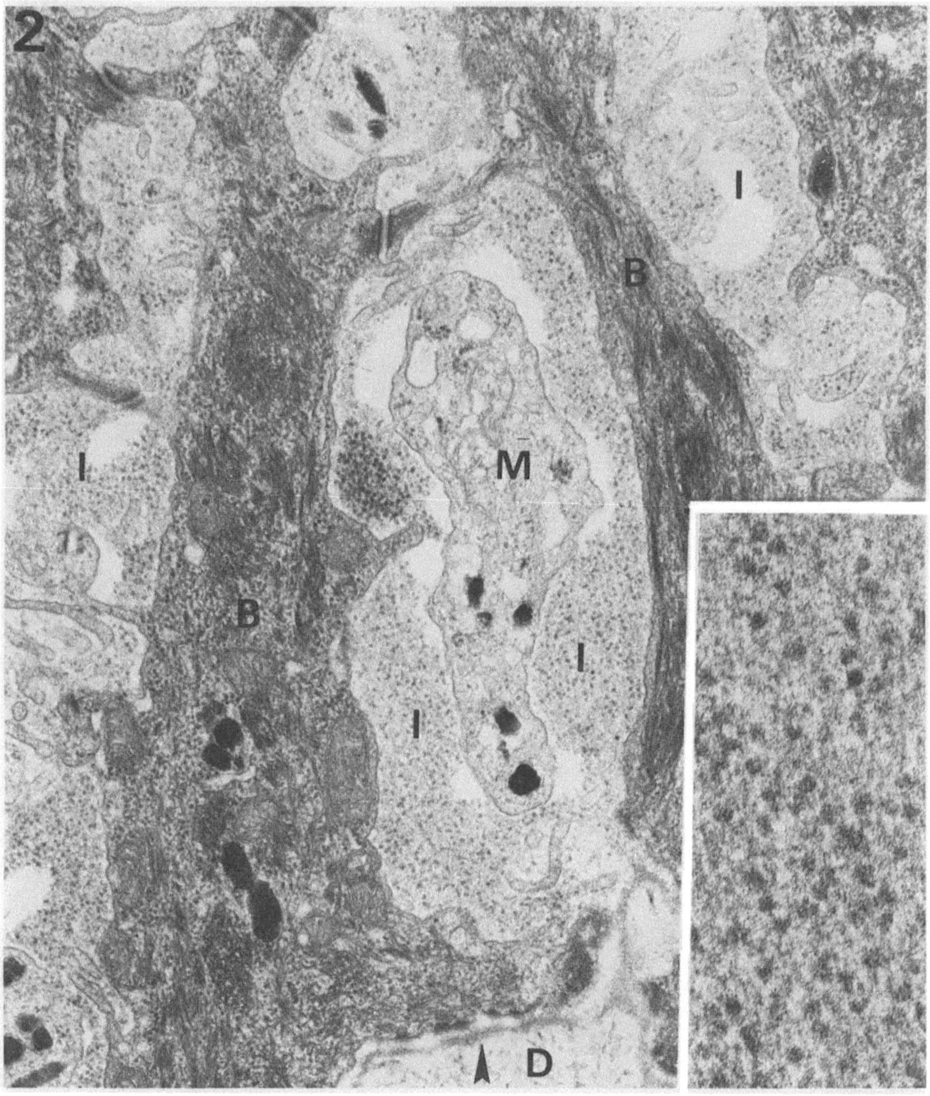

Fig. 2. PUVA-treated psoriasis, uninvolved skin. Dermo-epidermal junction. Widened intercellular spaces (I) with massive amounts of coarse granular substance. × 26,200. Inset: Larger magnification of intercellular substance. × 105 000 B, basal cell; M, melanocyte; D, dermis; arrowhead, basal lamina

knobs" or filaments reported as being characteristic of glycosaminoglycans (3, 4) were observed. Thus, there is no specific marker in the substance of the intercellular space that could prove this substance to be mucous, although biochemical evidence of stimulation of glycoprotein synthesis after retinoid administration has been presented (1).

In the intercellular space of the upper malpighian layers, a darker and more homogeneous material was occasionally observed in untreated psoriasis and somewhat more often after retinoid treatment (2–6 weeks) (Fig. 4). This substance seems fine structurally identical to that reported by Wolff et al. (10) to appear after topical vitamin A acid treatment of guinea pig epidermis. Wolff et al. (10) suspected that this substance would be the "mucous sub-

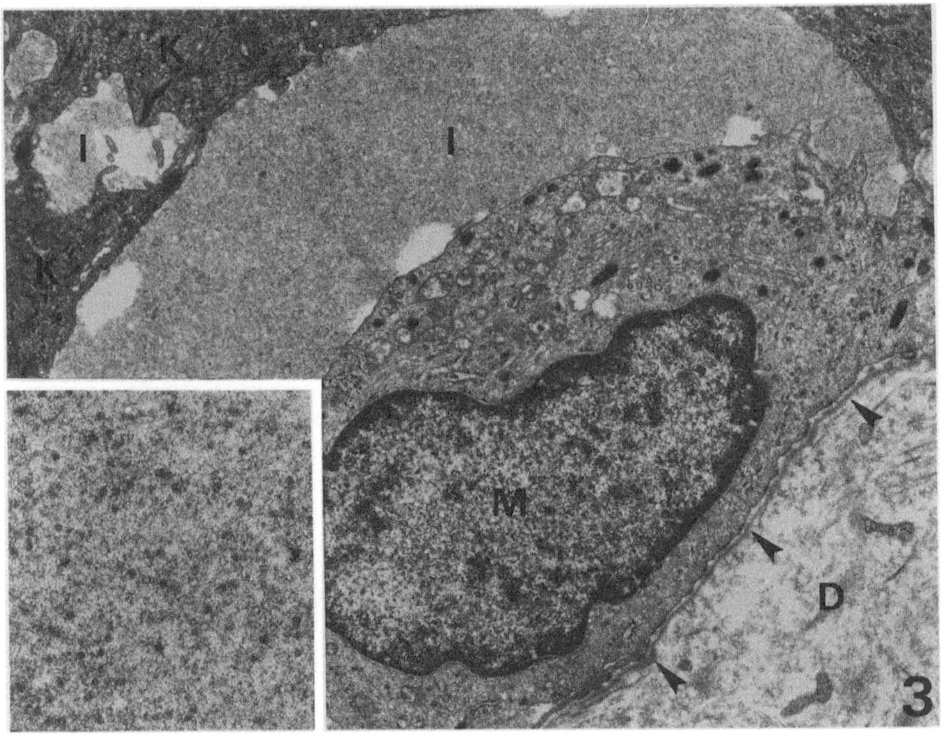

Fig. 3. 2 weeks of retinoid treatment. Dermo-epidermal junction. Enlarged intercellular space (I) with fine granular material. × 9,300. Inset: Larger magnification of intercellular substance. × 50,800. K, keratinocyte; M, melanocyte; D, dermis; arrowhead, basal lamina

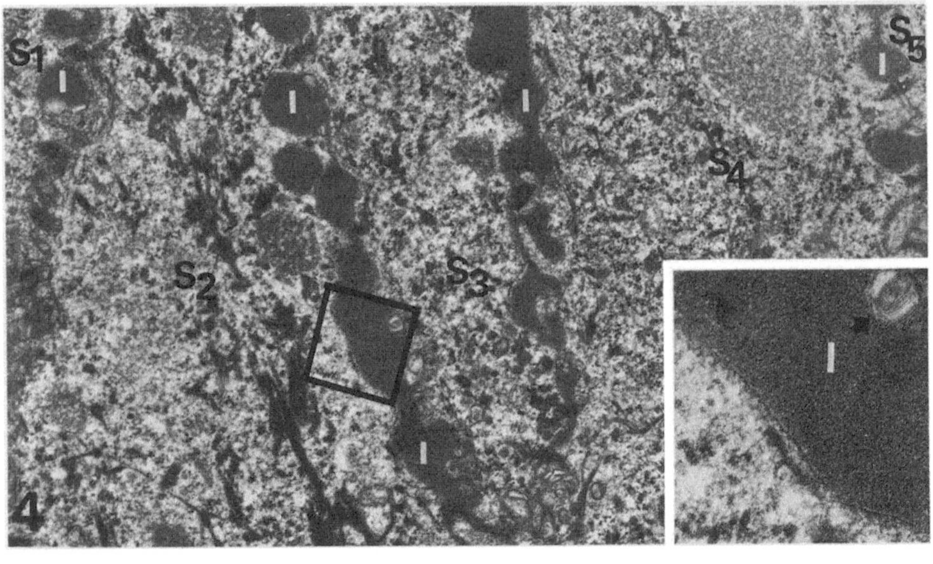

Fig. 4. 6 weeks of retinoid treatment. Spinous cell layer. Darker homogeneous substance in the intercellular space (I) between five spinous cells (S_1–S_5). × 16,400. Inset: Larger magnification of intercellular substance. A keratinosome is seen to protrude into the intercellular space (arrow). × 51,500

stance". Thus, also the nature of this material seems so far unknown, and cannot be attributed entirely to retinoid treatment, since it was sometimes seen before treatment as well. It could also be a condensed form of the fine granular substance seen in the lower malpighian layers.

Occasionally other cytoplasmic constituents, except the granular "mucous substance", were found in the intercellular space after retinoid treatment. Necrotic cells were only rarely encountered, and thus it is not probable that the bulk of the intercellular substance is derived from necrotic, dying cells, although Mayer et al. (7) have found increased amounts of necrotic cells during treatment of papillomas. Furthermore, organelles like mitochondria or myeloid bodies were only rarely observed intercellularly.

Vitamin A has previously been shown to alter the permeability and stability of the lipoprotein cell membranes (2, 6). This could explain the increased leakage of cytoplasmic constituents into the intercellular space, and also explain partly the increased amount of intercellular material after retinoid therapy.

During the following weeks of retinoid treatment or of RePUVA treatment (up to 14 weeks of total treatment), the biopsies regularly revealed some features of psoriasis, even though the skin appeared clinically cured. Compared to normal skin, the intercellular spaces were still widened and contained small amounts of fine or coarse granular substance. RePUVA treatment resulted in a strong melanocyte stimulation, but the intercellular space showed the same changes as described above.

In summary, the above findings, i.e. that finely to coarsely granular substance can be found before retinoid treatment, prove that the keratinocytes in psoriasis have the capacity to form such substances without retinoid treatment. On the other hand, retinoid seems to stimulate this synthesis. Fine-structural cytochemical techniques could clarify the nature of these substances.

Summary

Psoriatic epidermis was studied fine-structurally before and after retinoid or retinoid-PUVA (RePUVA) treatment for 14 weeks. Special attention was paid to the intercellular space. Before treatment, the intercellular space was widened and contained fine to coarse granular material embedded in an amorphous substance. After 2–6 weeks of retinoid treatment, the amount of this substance increased. The coarse granules resembled ribosomes or glycogen particles, the fine granules were less distinct in appearance. A darker more homogenous substance was produced in the upper malpighian intercellular spaces during treatment (2–6 weeks). The nature of the materials in the intercellular space is discussed.

Acknowledgments. We wish to express our gratitude for the support of Hoffmann-La Roche Ltd and for the excellent technical assistance given by Mrs. Liisa Erola.

References

1. Adamo S, DeLuca LM, Silverman-Jones CS, Yuspa ST (1979) Mode of action of retinol. Involvement in glycosylation of cultured mouse epidermal cells. J Biol Chem 254:3279–3287
2. Anderson OR, Roels OA, Dreher KD, Schulman JH (1967) The stability and structure of mixed lipid monolayers and bilayers. II. The effect of retinol and α-tocopherol on the structure and stability of lipid bilayers. J Ultrastruct Res 19:600–610
3. Kobayasi T, Asboe-Hansen G (1972) Ultrastructure of generalized scleroderma. Acta Derm Venerol (Stockh) 52:81–93
4. Kobayasi T, Danielsen L, Asboe-Hansen G (1971) Hyaluronate (?) microfibrils in human dermis. Acta Derm Venerol (Stockh) 51:27–34

5. Lauharanta J, Juvakoski T, Lassus A (1981) A clinical evaluation of the effects of an aromatic retinoid (Tigason), combination of retinoid and PUVA, and PUVA alone in severe psoriasis. Br J Dermatol, in press
6. Lucy JA, Dingle JT, Fell HB (1961) Studies on the mode of action of excess vitamin A. 2. A possible role of intracellular proteases in the degradation of cartilage matrix. Biochem J 79:500–508
7. Mayer H, Bollag W, Hänni R, Rüegg R (1978) Retinoids, a new class of compounds with prophylactic and therapeutic activities in oncology and dermatology. Experientia 34:1105–1119
8. Orfanos CE, Pullmann H, Sterry W, Künzig M (1978) Retinoid + PUVA (RePUVA): Systemische Kombinations-Behandlung bei Psoriasis. Z Hautkr 53:494–504
9. Orfanos CE, Runne U (1978) Tissue changes in psoriatic plaques after oral administration of retinoid. Dermatologica 157 (Suppl 1):19–25
10. Wolff HH, Christophers E, Braun-Falco O (1970) Beeinflussung der epidermalen Ausdifferenzierung durch Vitamin A-Säure. Eine elektronenmikroskopische Untersuchung. Arch Klin Exp Dermatol 237:774–795

C.E. Orfanos et al. (eds.)
Retinoids

Long-term Effects of All-trans-retinoic Acid on Epidermal Glycosaminoglycan, Glycoprotein and Protein Synthesis in vitro

I.A. King and A. Tabiowo

Studies on a number of cell types suggest that changes in the structure and composition of the cell surface may be involved in the biological effects of retinoids. Changes in morphology, adhesion, proliferation and density-dependent growth rate may be related to alterations in the synthesis of surface-associated components such as glycosaminoglycans (3, 10, 11), glycoproteins (2, 13) and glycolipids (8).

In a previous study we found increased synthesis of extracellular glycosaminoglycans (GAGs) in the epidermis when pig skin slices were cultured for 18 hours in the presence of all-trans-retinoic acid (6). The major GAG was identified as hyaluronic acid (5). The synthesis of plasma membrane glycoproteins (as measured by D-(^{3}H)glucosamine incorporation) was unaffected. In the work reported here we have extended these studies by examining the effect of all-trans-retinoic acid on glycoconjugate synthesis in the epidermis of longer-term cultures.

Methods

Organ culture of pig ear skin slices (1 cm^2, 0.2 mm thick) was as described previously (6). 10^{-5} M all-trans-retinoic acid in ethanol was included in the culture media which were changed every 2 days. After 0, 2, 4 or 8 day's culture in unlabelled medium skin slices were transferred to fresh medium containing the appropriate radioactive precursors (The Radiochemical Centre, Amersham, U.K.) for 18 hours.

Glycosaminoglycan Synthesis

D-(6-^{3}H)glucosamine hydrochloride (10 µCi/ml) and $^{35}SO_4^{2-}$ (50 µCi/ml) were used to label GAGs. After washing in phosphate-buffered saline (PBS) skin slices were separated with dispase, the epidermis was trypsinized and shaken, the stratum corneum was removed and the remaining cell suspension was centrifuged. Cellular and extracellular GAGs were isolated after papain digestion of the pellet and supernatant respectively and were analysed by cellulose acetate electrophoresis (5).

Particulate and Soluble Glycoprotein Synthesis

D-(6-^{3}H)glucosamine hydrochloride (25 µCi/ml), L-(1-^{3}H)fucose (40 µCi/ml) and L-U-^{14}C-labelled amino acid mixture (2 µCi/ml) were used to label glycoproteins. PBS-washed skin slices were mixed with 1 g of unlabelled pig skin, homogenized and fractionated by differential centrifugation to give a crude particulate epidermal fraction from which a vesicular plasma membrane fraction was isolated by sucrose density gradient centrifugation (4). Soluble glycoproteins were precipitated by treating the soluble fraction remaining after differential centrifugation with 10% trichloroacetic acid. Samples were dissolved in 2% sodium dodecyl sulphate (SDS), 10 mM mercaptoethanol and were analysed by polyacrylamide gel electrophoresis (4).

Protein Synthesis

Proteins were labelled using L-U-^{14}C-labelled amino acid mixture. PBS-washed skin slices were separated with 1 M $CaCl_2$, the epidermis was extracted with 8 M urea, 5% SDS, 10 mM mercaptoethanol at 100 °C, cooled and centrifuged (4). The protein (7) and radioactivity in the supernatant and pellet were measured and samples of the supernatant were analysed by polyacrylamide gel electrophoresis.

Results

The incorporation of D-(^{3}H)glucosamine into both cellular (Fig. 1a) and extracellular (Fig. 1b) GAGs was increased by exposure to retinoic acid for periods up to 8 days. Although D-(^{3}H)glucosamine incorporation decreased markedly with time, it continued to be stimulated 2- to 3-fold by retinoic acid. The major GAG labelled with D-(^{3}H)glucosamine was hyaluronic acid in both control and retinoic acid-treated epidermis. It accounted for 86% and 88% respectively of the total GAG at day 0 decreasing to 69% and 79% after 8 days. The synthesis of sulphated GAGs was stimulated to a lesser extent than hyaluronic acid by retinoic acid and

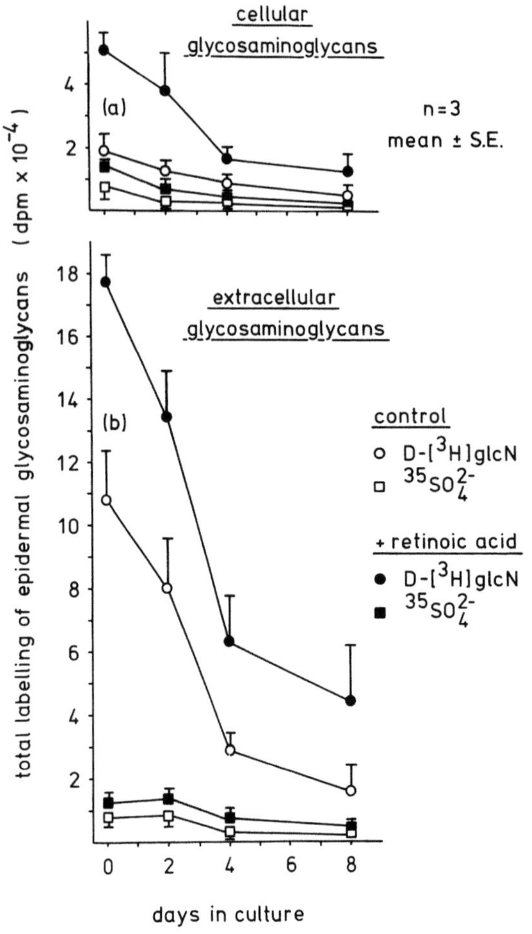

Fig. 1. Cellular and extracellular glycosaminoglycan synthesis in epidermis treated with all-trans-retinoic acid for up to 8 days

decreased less markedly with time. The major sulphated GAG in both control and retinoic acid-treated epidermis was heparan sulphate in all cases.

Compared to day 0 the incorporation of D-(^{3}H)glucosamine and L-(^{3}H)fucose into epidermal glycoproteins was increased after 2 to 4 days in culture (Fig. 2). This may be a consequence of the rapid decrease in GAG synthesis during this period (Fig. 1). However their incorporation into the glycoproteins of the particulate epidermal fraction (Fig. 2a) was not significantly affected by up to 8 days' treatment with retinoic acid. Similarly the labelling of a glycoprotein-enriched plasma membrane fraction from retinoic acid-treated epidermis was not consistently different to the controls (Fig. 2b). No significant changes could be detected in the (^{3}H)glycoprotein composition of the plasma membranes when they were subjected to polyacrylamide gel electrophoresis. The labelling of soluble glycoproteins with D-(^{3}H)glu-

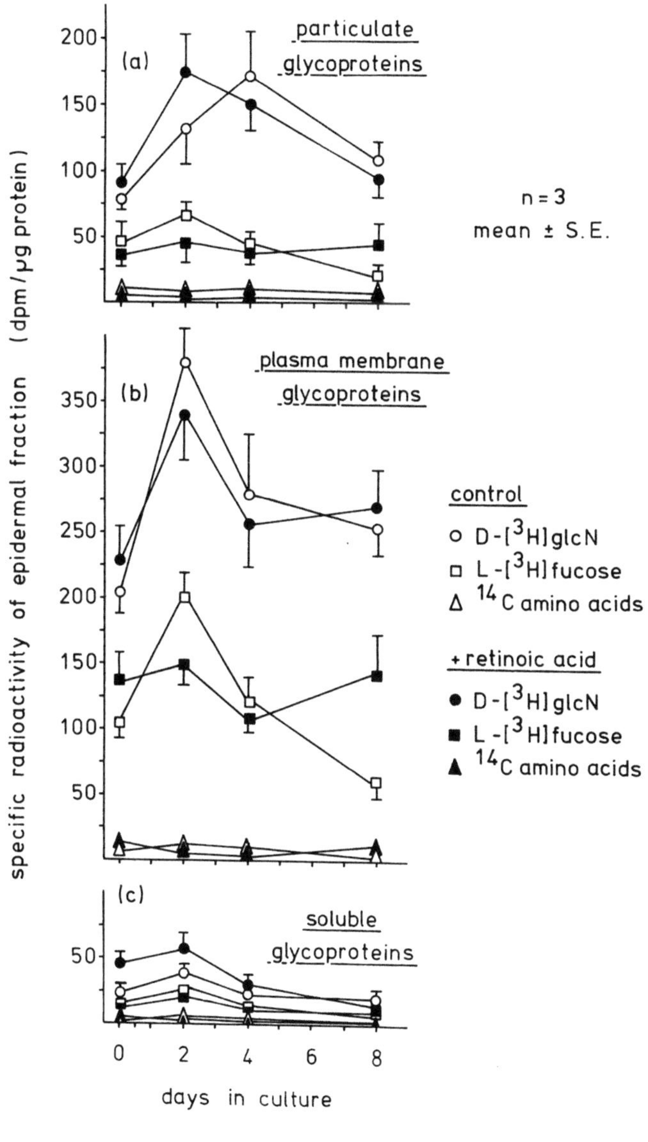

Fig. 2. Effect of up to 8 days' exposure to all-trans-retinoic acid on epidermal glycoprotein synthesis

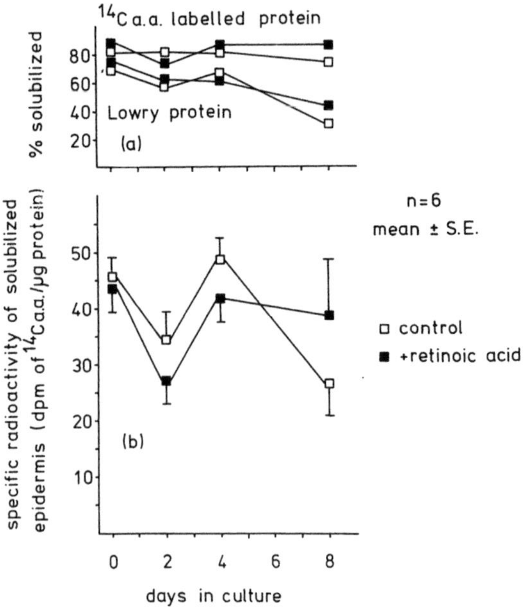

Fig. 3. Protein synthesis in epidermis treated with all-trans-retinoic acid for up to 8 days

cosamine but not with L-(^{3}H)fucose was increased during the first 4 days' exposure to retinoic acid.

The incorporation of ^{14}C amino acids into urea, SDS, mercaptoethanol-soluble epidermal proteins (mainly "keratin" polypeptides) was not significantly affected during 4 days' exposure to retinoic acid (Fig. 3). After this protein synthesis decreased in control cultures but appeared to be maintained in those treated with retinoic acid.

Discussion

The major epidermal cell surface changes induced by retinoids include a decrease in the number of desmosomes and an increase in the size of the extracellular spaces (1, 9, 12). The molecular basis for this apparent loss of cell adhesion is not known. However from the present and previous results (6) it is unlikely to be due to an alteration in the synthesis of plasma membrane glycoproteins. Changes in their degradation or their organization within the membrane cannot be ruled out. Decreased cell adhesion may simply be a result of the increased amounts of extracellular GAGs (mainly hyaluronic acid) synthesized by the epidermis in the presence of retinoids. However it is not yet possible to distinguish whether increased hyaluronic acid synthesis is a cause or a consequence of the changes in epidermal cell adhesion. The relevance of the increase in hyaluronic acid synthesis and the decrease in cell adhesion for the mechanism whereby retinoids "inhibit" keratinization remains to be established.

References

1. Barnett ML, Szabo G (1973) Effect of vitamin A on epithelial morphogenesis in vitro. Exp Cell Res 76:118–126
2. De Luca LM (1977) The direct involvement of vitamin A in glycosyl transfer reactions of mammalian membranes. Vitam Horm 35:1–57

3. Jetten AM, Jetten MER, Shapiro SS, Poon JP (1979) Characterization of the action of retinoids on mouse fibroblast cell lines. Exp Cell Res 119:289–299
4. King IA, Tabiowo A, Williams RH (1980) Incorporation of L-(^{3}H)fucose and D-(^{3}H)glucosamine into cell-surface-associated glycoconjugates in epidermis of cultured pig skin slices. Biochem J 190:65–77
5. King IA (1981) Characterization of epidermal glycosaminoglycans synthesized in organ culture. Biochim Biophys Acta 674. In press
6. King IA, Tabiowo A (1981) The effect of all-trans-retinoic acid on the synthesis of epidermal cell surface associated carbohydrates. Biochem J 194:341–350
7. Lowry OH, Rosebrough NJ, Farr AL, Randall RJ (1951) Protein measurement with the folin phenol reagent. J Biol Chem 193:265–275
8. Patt LM, Haya K, Hakomori S (1978) Retinol induces density-dependent growth inhibition and changes in glycolipids and LETS. Nature 273:379–381
9. Peck LP, Elias PM, Wetzel B In: Biochemistry of cutaneous epidermal differentiation (Seiji M & Bernstein IA, eds) pp 110–126, University Park Press, Baltimore
10. Shapiro SS, Poon JP (1978) Effect of retinyl acetate on sulfated glycosaminoglycan biosynthesis in dermal and epidermal cells in vitro. Connect Tissue Res 6:101–108
11. Shapiro SS, Poon JP (1979) Retinoic acid-induced alterations of growth and morphology in an established epithelial line. Exp Cell Res 119:349–357
12. Tsambaos D, Mahrle G, Orfanos CE (1980) Epidermal changes induced by oral excess of aromatic retinoid in guinea pigs. Arch Dermatol Res 267:141–152
13. Wolff G, Kiorpes TC, Masushige S, Schreiber JB, Smith MJ, Anderson RS (1979) Recent evidence for the participation of vitamin A in glycoprotein synthesis. Fed Proc 38:2540–2543

C.E. Orfanos et al. (eds.)
Retinoids

Clinical Aspects and Side Effects of Therapy by Oral Administration of Retinoids in Various Skin Diseases

S.V. Konstantinović

At the XVth International Congress of Dermatology in Mexico City in 1977 we have heard some preliminary reports on the successful treatment of various skin diseases with oral administration of retinoids.

We shall present here 23 patients treated in the period from April 1979 to July 1980 who suffered from the following skin diseases: keratosis follicularis (Darier's disease) - 5 cases; keratosis follicularis vegetans - 1 case; keratosis follicularis bullosa - 1 case; Hailey-Hailey disease - 1 cse; generalized psoriasis - 2 cases; erythrodermic psoriasis - 2 cases; generalized pustular psoriasis - 3 cases; palmo-plantar pustulosis - 2 cases; keratoderma climactericum - 1 case; ichthyosiform erythroderma - 3 cases; dominant ichthyosis vulgaris - 1 case, and acne conglobata - 1 case.

All these patients were treated before with various other topical and oral medicaments, but this treatment did not reveal any real result.

Before treatment the following laboratory analyses have been performed and controlled during therapy every two weeks: erythrocytes, hemoglobin, leukocytes, thrombocytes, blood sugar, urea, calcium, bilirubin, SGOT, SGPT, alkaline phosphatase, creatinine, blood sedimentation rate, and urine.

The *initial dose* at all patients was 1 mg/kg body weight (the maximum daily dose was 75 mg). Its efficacy was 10 days (1 patient), 3 weeks (10 patients), 4 weeks (9 patients), 5 weeks (1 patient), or 8 weeks (2 patients) respectively. The dose-dependency of doses given later was of different a degree.

The *reduced dose* was 0.75 mg/kg body weight. Its efficacy was 2 weeks (6 patients), 3 weeks (4 patients), 4 weeks (4 patients), 6 weeks (3 patients), 8 weeks (5 patients), or 11 weeks (1 patient), respectively.

The *maintenance dose* was 0.40–0.50 mg/kg body weight. In some cases the maintenance doses proved unsufficient (appearance of relapses), so that from time to time we had to increase it. No other therapy was applied.

Three cases were treated for *generalized pustular psoriasis*: 1) A 17-year-old girl at whom skin lesions had appeared at the age of 13. After 1 week's therapy there were no more pustules. After 8 weeks she was free of any skin lesions. Kept on maintenance doses (20 mg daily) during 15 months, she underwent no relapses. 2) An 18-year-old boy at whom skin lesions had appeared at the age of 3. After 2 weeks' therapy there were no more pustules. After 1 months' application of Tigason 0.50 mg/kg and PUVA he was free of any skin lesions. He was given PUVA therapy for 2 months with doses of 1 to 8 J/cm^2, and a maintenance dose (20 mg daily) for 7 months. After 3 months without treatment he underwent no relapses, except for a few typical small psoriatic plaques. 3) A 17-year-old girl at whom skin lesions had appeared 2 months ago. After 3 weeks' therapy there were no more pustules. After 9 weeks of treatment she was free of any skin lesions, but after 5 weeks without treatment, a relapse appeared. She received a new dose, and skin lesions regressed rapidly. To our opinion, the success of therapy at these patients was excellent.

Two cases were treated for *erythrodermic psoriasis*: 1) A 30-year-old woman at whom psoriatic skin lesions had appeared at the age of 20. After 4 months she was free of any skin lesions and after 13 months without treatment there was no relapse. 2) A 57-year-old woman at whom skin lesions had appeared at the age of 54. After 7 weeks the skin lesions regressed and the treatment lasted 13 months. The success of therapy was excellent.

Two cases of *generalized psoriasis*: 1) A 20-year-old woman. Almost all skin lesions disappeared after 2 months, and the treatment lasted 4 months. 2) A 20-year-old man, at whom almost all skin lesions disappeared after 3 weeks, and the treatment lasted 7 weeks. The success of therapy was very good.

Two cases of *palmo-plantar pustulosis*: 1) A 46-year-old woman. After 3 weeks she was free of any skin lesions, although the therapy is not yet finished. 2) A 29-year-old man. At reduced doses, a few new pustules appeared, thus the therapy is not yet finished. The success of therapy was excellent.

Five cases of *Darier's disease*: Two men, 18 and 23 years old, respectively, and three women, 30, 46 and 54 years old, respectively. The therapy lasted 12–14 months, and all patients were free of skin lesions. One patient was without therapy for 9 months without undergoing a relapse. The success of therapy was excellent.

One case of *keratosis follicularis vegetans* was a 36-year-old woman. The vegetating and verrucous lesions disappeared after 4 months, and the therapy lasted 16 months. The success of therapy was very good.

One case of *keratosis follicularis bullosa* was a 51-year-old woman. After 3 weeks there were no more bullous eruptions, but other skin lesions did not respond sufficiently. Success was moderate.

One case of *Hailey-Hailey disease* concerned a 57-year-old woman. After 3 weeks there were no more bullous eruptions, but complete clearing was not achieved. The success was moderate.

Three cases of *ichthyosiform erythroderma*: Three women, 43, 21 and 17 years old, respectively. After 3–4 months there remained only the lesions at palms and soles but the therapy had to be interrupted because of side effects (hair loss) and occurrence of relapses. The success was moderate.

One case of dominant *ichthyosis vulgaris* concerned a 27-year-old woman. After 10 days the skin became soft and rather moist, and after 8 months without therapy there remained only affections of arms and legs (dryness and roughness). The success was very good.

One case of *keratoderma climactericum* concerned a 54-year-old woman. After 6 weeks she was free of skin lesions, but the therapy is not yet finished. The success was excellent.

One case of *acne conglobata* concerned a 22-year-old girl the skin lesions of whom during therapy appeared continuous but in less intensity. The success was moderate.

The results of analyses at all patients during therapy were normal. Only in two cases of pustular psoriasis and one case of Darier's disease SGOT and SGPT were slightly increased. However, at some patients, values of SGOT and SGPT were slightly increased also during earlier corticosteroid therapy.

Like other authors we stated also many side effects at almost all patients: Cheilitis (9 patients), pruritus (8), paronychia (8), hair loss (7), onychodystrophia (5), peeling at the face (5), exfoliation at both palms and soles (3), mucosal dryness (3), conjunctivitis (3), dermatitis faciei (2), headache (2), dermatitis on the legs (2) and burning sensation (1). *Cheilitis* as a side effect appeared after 3 days (2 patients), 5 days (2), 7 days (3) or 14 days (2). *Pruritus* as a side effect appeared after 2 days (1), 1 week (2), 2 weeks (1), 3 weeks (3) or 3 months (1). *Paronychia* was observed after 3 weeks (1), 2 months (2), 3 months (2), 4 months (2) or 1 year (1 patient). *Hair loss* resulted after 3 weeks (4), 4 weeks (1) or 5 weeks (2). *Onychodystrophia* was observed after 4 months (2), 6 months (2) or 1 year (1). *Peeling at the face* occurred after 4 days (1), 6 days (1), 7 days (1), 10 days (1) or 1 month (1). *Exfoliation (at both palms and soles)* was stated after about 3 months. *Mucosal dryness* was seen after about 3 weeks. *Conjunctivitis* occurred after about 1 month. *Dermatitis faciei* and *dermatitis on legs* set in after 3 and 6 weeks and disappeared after 10 days. *Headache* occurred after 3 weeks, and *burning sensation* after 1 week. After several months' maintenance-dose therapy almost any side effects disappeared. Only in two cases from ichthyosiform erythroderma, therapy had to be interrupted because of hair loss.

Conclusions: The success of the treatment was evident, in all cases. It was excellent in cases of generalized pustular psoriasis, Darier's disease, erythrodermic psoriasis, keratoderma climacterium and palmo-plantar pustulosis; very good in cases of generalized psoriasis, keratosis follicularis vegetans and dominant ichthyosis vulgaris; and moderate in cases of ichthyosiform erythroderma, keratosis follicularis bullosa, Hailey-Hailey disease and acne conglobata.

C.E. Orfanos et al. (eds.)
Retinoids

Treatment of Severe Psoriasis by Ro 10-9359

J.J. Guilhou, B. Michel and J. Meynadier

In recent years several authors have reported the beneficial effect in psoriasis of the oral administration of an aromatic derivative of retinoic acid, Ro 10-9359 (7, 12, 13, 17, 18). The mechanisms of action of this compound are not fully understood but their analysis could be a useful tool in understanding mechanisms underlying psoriasis itself.

We have been using Ro 10-9359 for 5 years and in this paper we report on the remarkable action of this product on severe forms of the disease.

Material and Methods

We investigated 32 adult patients (25 males and 7 females) suffering from severe psoriasis, refractory to conventional therapy. Fourteen had generalized plaques (more than 60% of the body surface involved), 8 an erythroderma, 8 a pustular psoriasis (localized: 3, generalized: 5) and 2 had an invalidating palmo-plantar hyperkeratosis.

The aromatic retinoid (Ro 10-9359) was administered orally at initial doses of 0.75 to 1 mg/kg body weight/day for 4 to 6 weeks and then at maintenance doses of 0.50 mg/kg for several months (maximum duration: 3 years).

Clinical and laboratory tests (erythrocytes, hemoglobin, leukocytes, thrombocytes, urea, creatinine, alkalin phosphatase, bilirubin, SGOT and SGPT) were performed every 15 days for 4 to 6 months and then once a month.

Results (Table 1)

The clinical results were excellent (more than 75% improvement) in 20 patients, moderate in 9 patients and poor (no response) in 3 patients. The best response was obtained in pustular and in erythrodermic psoriasis. However, at maintenance doses, relapses occurred in several patients, leading to resumption of initial posology.

The side effects were essentially: cheilitis (27/32), thinning and/or palmo-plantar exfo-

Table 1. Results of treatment with Ro 10–9359

		Excellent	Moderate	Poor
Generalised plaques	14	7	5	2
Erythroderma	8	6	1	1
Pustular	8	6	2	0
Palmo-plantar keratoderma	2	1	1	0
Total	32	20	9	3

liation (22/32), hair loss (4/32), conjunctivitis (2/32) and moderate increase of transaminases (8/32). Usually these side effects were well tolerated but, in some patients, led to a discontinuation in the treatment.

Comments

This study confirms the effectiveness of Ro 10-9359 in psoriasis especially in severe forms of the disease. The Ro 10-9359 therapy is chiefly useful in erythrodermic and pustular psoriasis in which it could replace cytostatic drugs with more safety. The remarkable effectiveness in recalcitrant pustular psoriasis is to be emphasized since other treatments of this condition usually give poor results.

In disseminated psoriasis vulgaris Ro 10-9359 therapy could not be demonstrated better than PUVA of UVB therapies and seems to give more inconstant results. In follow-up studies with maintenance doses relapses seem to occur with the same frequency as with other therapies.

The mechanism by which Ro 10-9359 acts in psoriasis is not well understood. If we keep in mind that psoriasis is an epidermal proliferative disease with pharmacological imbalances (cyclic nucleotides – prostaglandins – polyamines), immunological disturbances (humoral and cellular) and with membrane abnormalities (review in 6) it is of interest to note that Ro 10-9359 could interact with each of these supposed pathogenic factors:

- *Modification of cell differenciation* and proliferation by Ro 10-9359 could be achieved in different ways:
- direct action on cell DNA since a cytosolic retinoic acid-binding protein has been demonstrated in nuclei of chick embryo skin (16),
- modulation of cyclic nucleotides (19), prostaglandins (20), and polyamines (1),
- labilization of lysosomal membranes (3) with subsequent release of hydrolases and proteases,
- modifications of basement membrane (14), cell membrane (11) and of gap junctions (15) leading to modified dermal-epidermal and cell-cell signals.

Stimulation of immune responses by Ro 10-9359 has been demonstrated (2, 4) and could result in restoration of deficient cellular immunity in psoriatic patients (5).

Finally *the action of Ro 10-9359 on a possible viral agent* of psoriasis (8) cannot be excluded since it seems effective in viral-induced proliferation of epidermodysplasia verruciformis (9, 10).

Summary

Ro 10-9359 has been demonstrated to be effective in 32 cases of severe psoriasis especially in erythrodermic and pustular forms. In these conditions it replaces cytostatic drugs with more safety. The possible mechanisms of action are discussed with regard to the pathogenetic factors of psoriasis.

References

1. Breeding J, Lowe N (1980) Vitamin A acid differentially modulates ultraviolet light-induced epidermal ornithine decarboxylase. J Invest Dermatol 74:246 (abstract)
2. Dennert G, Lotan R (1978) Effect of retinoic acid on the immune system: stimulation of T killer cell induction. Eur J Immunol 8:23–29
3. Fell HB, Dingle JT, Webb M (1962) Studies of the mode of action of excess vitamin A. Biochem J 83:63–69

4. Floersheim GL, Bollag W (1972) Accelerated rejection of skin homografts by vitamin A acid. Transplantation 15:564–567
5. Guilhou JJ, Clot J, Meynadier J (1976) Immunological aspects of psoriasis. II. Dissociated impairment of thymus-dependent lymphocytes. Br J Dermatol 95:295–301
6. Guilhou JJ, Clot J, Meynadier J (1978) New concepts in the pathogenesis of psoriasis. Br J Dermatol 98:585–592
7. Guilhou JJ, Malbos S, Meynadier J (1978) Traitement oral des psoriasis graves par un nouveau rétinoïde aromatique (Ro 10-9359). Ann Dermatol Vénéréol 105:813–818
8. Guilhou JJ T cell defect in psoriasis. Possible role of viruses E.S.D.R., Amsterdam, May 1980 (Workshop)
9. Guilhou JJ, Malbos S, Barneon G, Habib A, Baldet P, Meynadier J (1980) Epidermodysplasie verruciforme. Etude immunologique. Ann Dermatol Vénéréol 107:611–619
10. Lutzner M, Blanchet-Bardon (1980) Oral retinoid treatment of human papilloma virus type 5-induced epidermodysplasia verruciformis. N Engl J Med 302:1091
11. Nemanic MK, Elias PM (1980) Influence of retinoids on membrane glycosylation in epidermis. J Invest Dermatol 74:248 (abstract)
12. Orfanos CE, Goerz G (1978) Orale Retinoid-Therapie mit einem neuen aromatischen Retinoid (Ro 10-9359). Dtsch Med Wochenschr 5:195–199
13. Ott F, Bollag W (1975) Therapie der Psoriasis mit einem oral wirksamen neuen Vitamin A-Säure-Derivat. Schweiz Med Wochenschr 105:439–441
14. Peck GL, Elias PM, Wetzel B (1977) Effects of retinoic acid on embryonic chick skin. J Invest Dermatol 69:463–476
15. Prutkin L (1975) Vitamin A acid and keratoacanthomas. Acta Derm Venerol (Suppl 74):167–168
16. Sani BP (1977) Localisation of retinoic acid-binding protein in nuclei. Biochem Biophys Res Commun 75:7–12
17. Schimpf A (1976) Zur systemischen Anwendung eines aromatischen Vitamin A-Säure-Derivates (Ro 10-9359) bei Psoriasis und Keratosen. Z Hautkr 51:265–274
18. Viglioglia PA, Barclay A (1978) Oral retinoids and psoriasis. Dermatologica 157 (Suppl 1):32–37
19. Wilkinson DI, Orenberg EK (1980) Effect of vitamin A acid on cyclic nucleotides of cultured keratinocytes. Arch Dermatol Res 267:25–31
20. Ziboh VA (1975) Regulation of prostaglandin E2 biosynthesis in guinea-pig skin by retinoic acid. Acta Derm Venerol 55 (Suppl 74):56–60

C.E. Orfanos et al. (eds.)
Retinoids

Treatment of Psoriasis and Other Dermatoses with a New Aromatic Retinoid (Ro 10-9359)

J. Devaux, M. Pizzi, R. Gamby and Y. Privat

We have treated patients suffering from psoriasis and other dermatoses - such as keratotic and micaceous balanitis and porokeratosis of Mibelli - with an aromatic retinoid, Ro 10-9359 (Tigason).

1. Psoriasis

Our results merely concern the initial treatment of psoriasis. The results of further treatment will be the subject of another paper.

Material and Methods

1. Number of patients: 100. The patients had to comply with the following conditions:
- Age: more than 18 years;
- psoriasis having evoluted over five years and proving resistant to any classical treatment;
- as for women: having attained menopause age or being under anticonceptional treatment.
2. Type of study: A double-blind study could not be carried out due to persistent cheilitis at the inception of treatment.
3. Posology of Ro 10-9359:
   1–4 weeks: 1 mg/kg/day = 50–75 mg/day
   4–8 weeks: 0.66 mg/kg/day = 50 mg/day
   8–12 weeks: 0.33 mg/kg/day = 25 mg/day
4. Biological surveillance: Erythrocyte sedimentation rate, haemoglobin, erythrocyte, leukocyte and platelet count, alkaline phosphatase, transminase SGOT-SGPT, calcium, creatinine, serum electrolytes, cholesterol, triglycerides.
5. Codification of results:
   Very good: full clearance
   good: clearance of >75%
   moderate: clearance of 50–75%
   nil: clearance of < 50%

Results

The results are given in Tables 1–6.
The best percentage of "very good" and "good" results has been obtained in severe forms. Arthropathic forms have been improved in 8/39 patients (20.5%). The therapeutic result has been less satisfactory in very long-dating psoriasis.

Table 1. Total results (100 patients)

Very good	27 patients
Good	51 patients
Moderate	14 patients
Nil	8 patients

Table 2. Results in several clinical forms

Clinical form	Number of patients	Very good - good results	%
Erythrodermia	7	7	100
Pustular psoriasis	13	12	92.3
Inverse psoriasis	11	10	90.9
Psoriasis universalis	8	7	87.5
Psoriasis vulgaris	61	42	68.8
Total	100	78	78

Table 3. Results with reference to initial body involvement

Body involvement	Number of patients	Very good - good results	%
< 30%	13	8	61.5
30–50%	25	16	64
50–75%	28	24	85.7
75–100%	34	30	88.2
Total	100	78	78

The ‚very good‘ results have been observed in extensive forms

Table 4. Results with reference to duration of disease

Duration of disease	Number of patients	Very good - good results	%
5– 7 years	19	14	73.7
8–10 years	21	16	76.2
11–15 years	29	28	96.5
16–20 years	14	8	57.1
> 20 years	17	11	64.7
Total	100	77	77

Table 5. Results with reference to previously unsuccessful therapy

Unsuccessful therapy	Number of patients	Very good - good results	%
General cortico-therapy	11	10	90.9
Antimitotic therapy	2	2	100
Topical cortico-therapy	78	54	69.2
PUVA-therapy	26	21	80.8

Table 6. Side effects

Type	Number of patients
Cheilitis	89
Peeling	36
Mucosal dryness	22
Thinning of skin	14
Alopecia	12
Onychodystrophy	6
Transient elevation of transaminases	5

Ro 10–9359 therapy has been very efficient in psoriatic form proving resistant to other major therapy such as general cortico-therapy, antimitotics, PUVA.

No important side effect has been observed in this study, besides all the incidents disappeared when treatment was stopped.

Conclusion

Oral Ro 10-9359 therapy appeared to us not only as a new effective antipsoriatic agent, but also as an alternative to other treatments which prove dangerous (cytostatic drugs) or are associated with economic and practical problems (PUVA therapy).

2. Other Dermatoses

Keratotic and Micaceous Balanitis

a) *Case Report*

1. Clinical Aspect. A 57 year-old man has come to hospital for a keratotic tumor of the glans. An acquired and very serried phimosis has progressively become visible since 1977, with an anamnesis of inflammatory balanitis. The progressive spreading out of the glandular tumor since the second half-year 1977 calls for chirurgical circumcision. A wrong histologic diagnosis of acuminate condyloma requires an electro-coagulation of verrucous lesions.

In February 1979, a swift recurrence of lesions justifies hospitalisation.

Clinical data: Keratotic and painless tumors; micaceous aspect of the glans; normal systemic examination.

2. *Histological Finding*

Mucosa: Great parakeratotic hyperkeratosis; acanthosis; papillomatosis; no cellular atypia.
Corium: perivascular lymphocytic infiltrate.

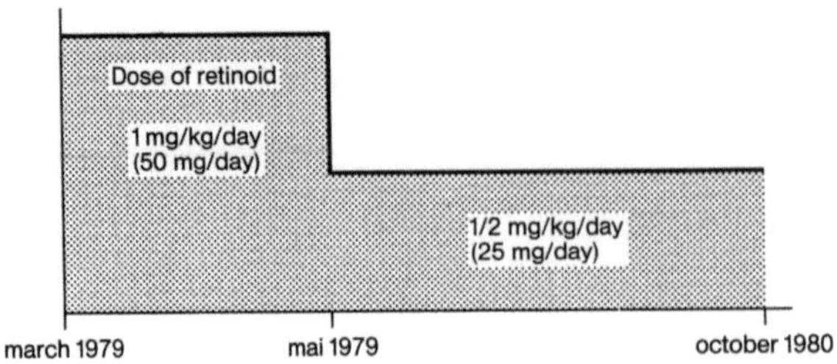

Fig. 1. Treatment with Ro 10-9359 in one case of micaceous balanitis

b) *Treatment*

Figure 1 visualized the posology of Ro 10-9359 from March 1979 to October 1980.

c) *Results*

1. *Clinical Results.* Very swift decrease of keratotic lesions and micaceous aspect of glans after 15 days of treatment.

Since sixteen months, in spite of the reduction of retinoid posology, absence of tumorous relapse, but persistence of scaly lesions on the glans. No side effect except cheilitis.

2. *Histological Findings.* One month after the beginning of treatment: Important decrease of hyperkeratosis and papillomatosis; keratotic maturation in the superficial layer of the mucosa; a lymphoplasmocytic infiltrate is still noticed.

d) *Discussion*

The aromatic retinoid Ro 10-9359 appears as a very good therapeutic for this type of balanitis, as the other therapies are ineffective in the cases referred to in literature.

Surgical treatment: Relapse of lesions in all of the four cases. Antimitotic agents: Relapse in one case and stabilisation in the remaining three cases.

The aromatic retinoid is likely to prevent the malignant transformation of both the keratosis and micaceous balanitis.

Porokeratosis of Mibelli

a) *Case Report*

A 46 year-old woman has been presenting for ten years a typical form of porokeratosis with linear lesions on the right forearm. Two years ago, the lesions extended to the right shoulder and both legs. Then, the patient was admitted to the Clinical Department of Dermatology (Prof. Y. Privat).

1. *Clinical Aspect.* A 10 cm long and 4 cm wide linear lesion was observed on the right forearm, presenting the typical aspect of porokeratosis. Ten lesions on both legs, presenting the same aspect. Two similar lesions on the right shoulder.

2. *Histological Findings before Treatment:* Typical aspects of the disease.

Ultrastructural study:

Basal membrane: There are replications.

Basal layer: Widening of the intercellular spaces by a great edema, autophagocytosed vacuoles and increasing tonofilaments in rare occasions.

Malpighian layer: Two types of pathological cells are intermingled with normal cells:

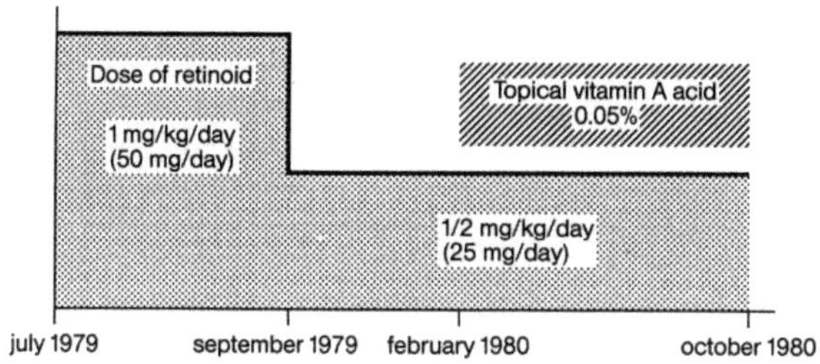

Fig. 2. Treatment with Ro 10-9359 in one case of porokeratosis of Mibelli

- Degenerative cells: Pycnotic nucleus, highly vacuolated cytoplasm with strands between nucleus and cell membrane.
- Dyskeratotic cells: Accumulation of perinuclear tonofilaments.

Intercellular oedema:

- Granular layer: Degenerative cells, dyskeratotic cells, some keratohyaline-granulated cells.
- Cornoid lamella: Globoid cells with pyknotic nuclei and autophagocytosed vacuoles; flattened cells with keratin filaments.

b) *Treatment*

Figure 2 visualizes the posology of Ro 10-9359 from July 1979 to October 1980.

c) *Results*

1. *Clinical Results.* Disappearance of lesions was observed after one month's treatment without inflammation; this result has been lasting for $1\frac{1}{2}$ years in spite of decreasing doses of retinoid and association to retinoic-acid topic treatment. Now we can only observe some scarce lesions. No side effects were noticed.

Table 7. Results of treatment with oral aromatic retinoid in porokeratosis of Mibelli (PM) (3 cases from literature)

Authors	Clinical forms	Posology of the retinoid	Results
Pehamberger and Konrad (6)	Linear PM of the arm Man, 15 years	1 mg/kg/day, 7 weeks	Reduction in thickness of the hyperkeratotic areas and thinning of elevated ridges. Pronounced inflammatory reduction.
		0.5 mg/kg/day	Disappearing of hyperkeratosis after 5 weeks' residual hyperpigmentation.
Bundino and Zina (1)	Case 1 Disseminated PM Man, 78 years	75 mg/day	First week: Inflammation and desquamation of lesions. Second week: Improvement of most lesions.
		50 mg/day, 3 weeks	Third week: Greatest improvement
Bundino and Zina (1)	Case 2 Disseminated PM Man, 62 years	25 mg/day, maintenance dose	The result acquired is being maintained, with relapse of a few lesions.

2. *Histological Findings After one Month of Treatment. Histological Study on a Cured Lesion:* Disappearance of the cornoid core. Restored granular layer. Spongiosis in malpighian layer. Lymphohistiocytic infiltrate in the superficial dermis.
Ultrastructural study: Normal basal membrane. Intense edema with disrupture of desmosomes in basal and malpighian layers.
Disappearance of pathological basal cells.
Disappearance of degenerative and dyskeratotic cells in the malpighian layer.
Rare spinous cells contain some vacuoles and pseudomyelinic figures. Restored granular layer with keratohyaline granules. Flattened cornoid lamella.

d) *Discussion*
The retinoid treatment has led to an almost complete disappearance of porokeratotic lesions, but this treatment is to be maintained. This treatment is likely to prevent the possible degenerative transformation of porokeratosis. We have collected 3 other cases quoted in literature as having been treated by retinoid (Table 7).

References

1. Bundino S, Zina AM (1980) Disseminated porokeratosis of Mibelli treated by oral retinoic acid. Dermatologica 160:328–336
2. Goerz G, Orfanos CE (1978) Systemic treatment of psoriasis with a new aromatic retinoid. Dermatologica 157 (Suppl 1):38–44
3. Guilhou JJ, Albos S, Meynadier J (1978) Traitement oral des psoriasis graves par un nouveau rétinoide aromatique (Ro 10-9359). Ann Dermatol 105:813–818
4. Lillie G, Guin JD (1961) Penil horn. Arch Dermatol 84:322–324
5. Lortat-Jacob, Civatte J (1966) Balanite pseudo-épithéliomateuse kératosique et micacée. Bull Soc Fr Dermatol Syph 73:931–935
6. Pehamberger H, Konrad K (1980) Treatment with an oral aromatic retinoid in linear porokeratosis. Dermatologica 160:270–274

C.E. Orfanos et al. (eds.)
Retinoids

Isoaccepting Serine t-RNAs Pattern as Marker of Epidermal Differentiation: its Alterations Under Retinoids

E. Schwarz and D. Tsambaos

Transfer RNAs (t-RNAs) act as carriers of specific individual amino acids during protein synthesis. Certain amino acids have more than one t-RNAs (isoaccepting). Changes in protein synthesis during cell differentiation are related to corresponding alterations in the relative amounts of isoaccepting t-RNAs.

Serine is an amino acid intimately involved in the differentiation processes of epidermal cells. Previous investigations (2) have shown that in normal guinea pig epidermis, certain isoaccepting serine t-RNAs occur, which are not detected in other tissues, being probably specific for keratinocytes.

Retinoids are of essential importance for the growth and differentiation of epithelial tissues. Therefore, we found it of interest to study their effects on the epidermal pattern of serine t-RNAs. This paper reports on the alterations of serine isoaccepting t-RNAs in the normal guinea pig epidermis under local treatment with retinoic acid and aromatic retinoid Ro 11-1430.

Material and Methods

20 male guinea pigs (300 g) were locally treated with 0.05% retinoic acid (10 animals) and 0.5% aromatic retinoid Ro 11-1430 (10 animals). Each drug was applied once daily for a period of one week.

Crude epidermal total t-RNA and aminoacyl t-RNA synthetases were prepared as described by Wittig et al. (3). Aminoacylation assay was performed using ^{3}H-serine (125 μCi/mmol) and ^{14}C-serine (50 μCi/mmol) according to Wittig et al. (3).

Reversed phase chromatography of ^{14}C- and ^{3}H-aminoacyl t-RNA was carried out using a 0.6 × 60 cm RPC-5 column as described by Pearson et al (1). Radioactivity measurements were done in a tricarb liquid scintillation counter; the plots of the figures were drawn by a graphometer after interactive correction.

Results

At least five peaks can be distinguished by RPC-5 chromatography of epidermal isoaccepting serine t-RNAs. They are numbered I through V according to the order of their appearance in the eluate from RPC-5 column and represent five chromatographically distinct serine t-RNA species.

Retinoic Acid (0.05%): Chromatographic analysis of ^{14}C-serine t-RNAs from the retinoic acid-treated epidermis reveals a decrease of the species I and V compared to the cochromatographed ^{3}H-serine t-RNAs from the normal untreated epidermis (Fig. 1).

Ro 11-1430 (0.5%): Chromatographic analysis of ^{14}C-serine t-RNAs from the retinoid-

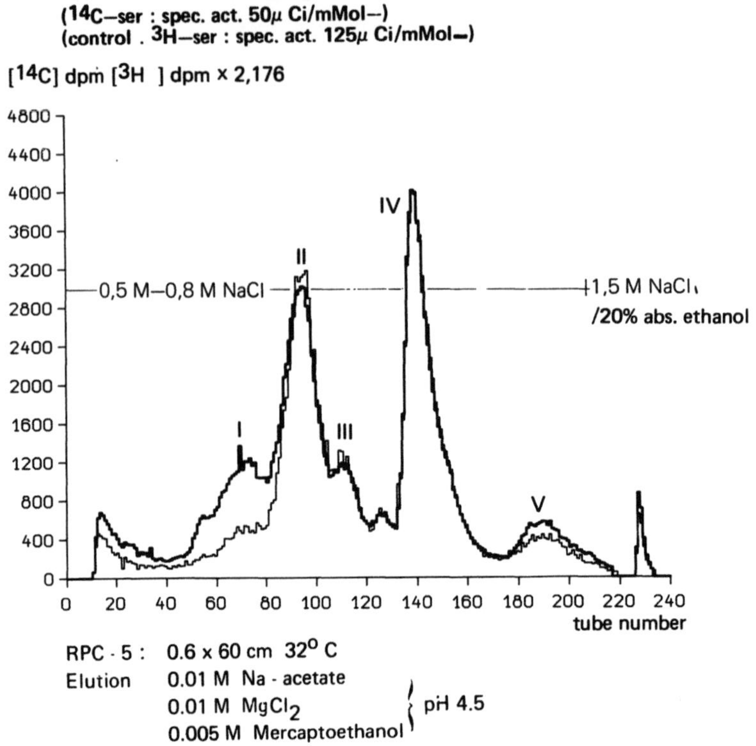

Fig. 1. Isoaccepting tRNA^{ser} from guinea pig epidermis after local treatment with retinoic acid (0.05%) daily over one week

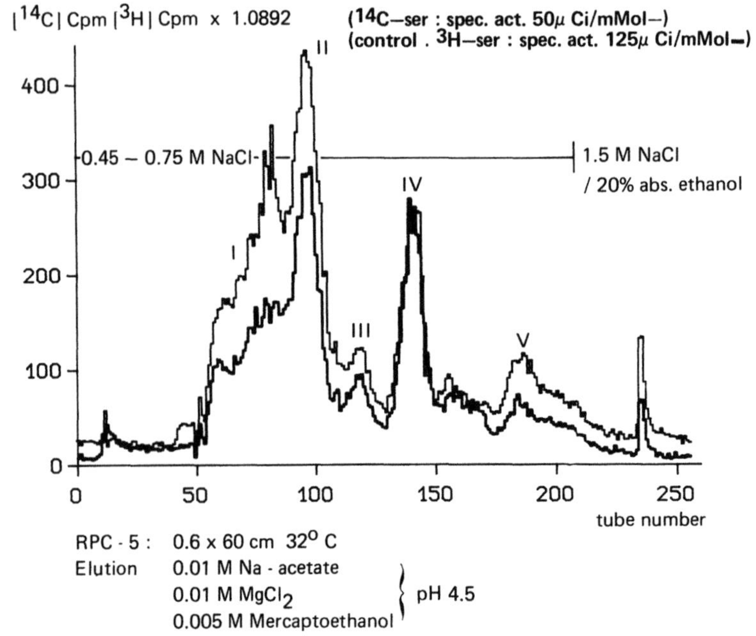

Fig. 2. Isoaccepting tRNA^{ser} from guinea pig epidermis after local treatment with Ro 11-1430 (0.5%) daily over one week

treated epidermis shows that all species but one (IV) are increased, as compared to the co-chromatographed ^{3}H-serine t-RNAs from the normal untreated epidermis (Fig. 2).

Conclusions

Retinoic acid and aromatic retinoid Ro 11-1430 exert a distinct influence on the isoaccepting serine t-RNAs from the locally treated guinea pig epidermis. Unter the present experimental conditions these retinoids seem to have some opposite effects on the epidermis-specific serine t-RNA species I and V, as assessed by their chromatographic behaviour.

Since the applied concentrations were not the same for both drugs, it must remain open to question, as to whether these effects are specific for each retinoid. It is possible, that they may represent qualitatively different expressions of a common dose-dependent pharmacological action.

There is growing evidence pointing towards a transcriptional and/or translational control of cell differentiation, involving shifts in protein synthesis. To change the type of protein to be synthesized, the t-RNA pool must be adapted to recognize the induced change in the m-RNA. It can be therefore assumed that the alterations in the epidermal isoaccepting serine t-RNAs found in this study, do reflect cell differentiation changes at the level of transcription and translation induced by the retinoids.

Summary

Changes of cell differentiation in mammalian tissues are related to certain alterations in the isoaccepting amino acid t-RNA species.

Serine is an amino acid intimately involved in the differentiation processes of epidermal cells. Reversed phase chromatographic analysis (RPC-5) of the serine specific t-RNA in normal guinea-pig epidermis revealed an elution pattern characterized by two fractions, which are not detected in other tissues, being probably specific for keratinocytes.

In the present study, alterations in the epidermal pattern of serine specific t-RNA under treatment with different retinoids are reported and their significance is discussed.

References

1. Pearson RL, Weiss JF, Kelmers AD (1971) Improved separation of transfer RNA's on polychlorotrifluoroethylene-supported reversed-phase chromatography columns. Biochim Biophys Acta 228:770–774
2. Schwarz E, Gottschling H (1980) J Biochem (in press)
3. Wittig B, Reuter S, Gottschling H (1973) Purification of the four lysine-specific transfer ribonucleic acids from chick embryos. Biochim Biophys Acta 331:221–230

C.E. Orfanos et al. (eds.)
Retinoids

Influence of Retinoic Acid[1] on Epidermal Wound Healing in Man

J.P. Ortonne, D. Schmitt, G. Bonnot and J. Thivolet

Topical retinoic acid is known to affect the epidermal homeostasy.

Using a new system (9, 10) allowing to measure epidermal wound-healing after pure epidermal wounding, the normal skin of ten controls and of ten subjects after topical treatment by retinoic acid solution of different concentration (1% and 2% in ethanol) was studied.

Material and Methods

Principle

Our system for evaluation of epidermal wound-healing combines the technique first reported by Kiistala and Mustakallio (6) to detache the epidermis from the dermis with suction, and the method of Eagelstein and Mertz (3) to quantitate the epidermal wound-healing after chemical separation of the epidermis and dermis.

Induction of the Blisters. Biopsies

Five suction blisters were induced on the abdominal skin of ten volunteers and of 10 subjects matched for sex and age after topical treatment with retinoic acid 1% in ethanol (3 subjects) and 2% in ethanol (7 subjects), twice a day, five days prior to the induction of the blisters[1].

When dermal-epidermal dissociation was obtained (time: 2 to 3 hours; 200 mm Hg), the roofs of the blisters were removed using a razor blade, then mounted on a glass slide for measurement. When the size of the blisters was irregular, they were not included in the study.

The wounds were covered with a dressing taped to the skin about 2 cm from the edges. Punch biopsies were undertaken at sequential periods of time from 18 to 90 hours after induction of the wounds. Each subject had three to four biopsies. The biopsied zone was randomly choosen. The excised skin contained the wound site and the surrounding normal skin.

Quantitative Evaluation

The specimen was then incubated in a 2 N sodium bromide solution at 37 °C for 2 hours allowing separation of the epidermis from the dermis. The separated epidermis was mounted on a glass slide, put in a photographic enlarger. The picture of the wounded site was cut out and weighed. This weight is proportional to the surface of the non-healed epidermis.

Statistical Analysis

For each subject, and for the whole group, the relationship between the surface of the wounded site and

[1] Retinoic acid (Cilag-Chimie)

the time after wounding was studied. Statistical analysis were performed in order to identify the best mathematical model for the interpretation of epidermal wound healing. Four models have been tested:
- linear model ($S = At + B$)
- second degree model ($S = At2 + Bt + C$)
- asymptotic model ($S = A + B \times R^t$)
- parabolic model ($S = T(Ro - Kt)^2$).
Two tests were performed:
- test of parallelism
- an algorithm for least squares estimation of nonlinear parameters (8).
The index of cicatrisation was also calculated (2, 5).

Results

Quantitative Results

The main quantitative results are summarized in Table 1. The other quantitative parameters and results will be published elsewhere.

Statistical Analysis

In the case of topical retinoic acid 1%, a linear model of regression can be used for the interpretation of epidermal repair. In these cases the linear regression equation is

$$S = 0.0033\ t + 0.2616$$

From this equation, the mean time of healing for a pure epidermal wound is 78 hours (extreme values were from 68 to 92 hours). For normal skin, the linear regression equation is

$$S = 0.0024\ t + 0.2376$$

(When the results are tested subject by subject, the different slopes of the linear regression are not statistically different as they are for normal skin).

In the case of topical retinoic acid 2%, a linear model of regression must be rejected and a second degree model of regression ($S = 0.0027\ t^2 + 0.34\ t + 0.97$) can be used. Although a linear model can not be used for the whole group, a linear regression can be applied to interprete the epidermal repair of each individual. This is probably a consequence of

1. slight differences in the blisters of each individual;
2. slight differences in the lag period before the initiation of keratinocytes migration. In this case, the different slopes are not statistically different.

If a second degree model of regression used to compare the epidermal repair of normal skin before and after treatment with topical retinoic acid it appears that for retinoic acid 1%, the three parameters of the second degree equation are significantly different from those of normal skin. Although, these differences are not statistically different in the case of the topical retinoic 2%, these values are much higher than for normal skin (Table 1).

Table 1. Values of the three parameters (A, B, C) in the second degree model of regression in normal skin before and after topical treatment by retinoic acid 1% and 2%

	A	$\hat{s}$ A	B	$\hat{s}$ B	C	$\hat{s}$ C
Normal skin	$1.16.10^{-5}$	$7.2.10^{-6}$	$-3.69.10^{-4}$	$7.96.10^{-4}$	0.264	0.019
Retinoic acid 1%	$5.71.10^{-6}$	$2.18.10^{-5}$	$-3.82.10^{-3}$	$2.13.10^{-3}$	0.272	0.002
Retinoic acid 2%	$2.81.10^{-5}$	$1.19.10^{-5}$	$-5.49.10^{-3}$	$1.23.10^{-3}$	0.27	0.025

In two patients treated with topical retinoic acid 0.1% in ethanol, the rate of epidermal repair was modified when compared to normal skin, although in one patient taking oral aromatic retinoid (1 mg per kg and per day during ten days prior to the experiment) normal values for epidermal repair were obtained.

The index of cicatrisation

$$\frac{\dfrac{S - S'}{S}}{t + \sqrt{T}} = i$$

has been calculated for normal skin before and after treatment (2) (S is the area of the wound S' is the area of the wound measured t days later, t is the time interval between the initial 2 measurements, and T is the total time between the formation of the wound and the first measurement S). A larger index indicates a wound that is closing faster. For normal skin, $i = 0.00125$ whereas for topical retinoic acid 1% $i = 0.0155$ and for topical retinoic acid 2% $i = 0.00160$.

Comments

These results show that topical retinoic acid increases the rate of epidermal repair in normal human skin. The reason accounting for stronger effect of topical retinoic acid 1% is unclear. It can be suggested that the concentration of 2% has a toxic effect which impairs the keratinocyte migration. It must be also pointed out that the number of subjects tested with topical retinoic acid 1% is low (three subjects). Topical 1% retinoic acid shows a lesser effect on the slope of the linear regression of the wound than 2% retinoic acid. On the other hand it seems likely that the lag period before the beginning of the keratinocyte migration is more increased by topical retinoic acid 2%.

This effect of topical retinoic acid on epidermal repair can be the result:

- of a non-specific effect partly due to ethanol. This possibility must be taken into account because numerous chemicals including inert vehicles are known to accelerate keratinocyte migration (4). Retinoic acid is also known to generate inflammation.

- of a specific effect. This hypothesis seems logical because retinoic acid is known to deeply modify the biology of epidermal keratinocytes. Furthermore retinoic acid has been shown to accelerate the rate of wound closure of dermal-epidermal wounds in rats (7).

Summary

A system allowing to measure epidermal wound-healing after pure epidermal wounding has been used on the normal skin of ten controls and of ten patients after topical treatment by retinoic acid solutions of different concentrations (1% and 2% in ethanol). The results show that the topical retinoic acid increases the rate of epidermal repair in normal human skin. The significance of this finding is discussed in relation to the known effects of retinoic acid on keratinocytes.

Acknowledgments. This work was supported by a grant from INSERM (CRL 79.5.517.2).

References

1. Christophers E, Wolff HH (1975) Effects of vitamin A acid in skin: in vivo and in vitro studies. Acta Dermato-vener (Stockh) 55 (Suppl 74):42–49
2. Du Nouy PL (1937) Biological time. New York: The MacMillan Company

3. Eagelstein WH, Mertz PM (1978) New method for assessing epidermal wound healing: the effects of triamcinolone acetonide and polyethylene film occlusion. J Invest Dermatol 71:382–384
4. Eagelstein WH, Mertz PM (1980) "Inert" vehicles do affect wound healing. J Invest Dermatol 74:90–91
5. Goodson WH, Hunt TK (1979) Wound healing and aging. J Invest Dermatol 73:88–91
6. Kiistala U, Mustakallio KK (1967) Dermoepidermal separation with suction: electron microscopic and histochemical study of initial events of blistering on human skin. J Invest Dermatol 48:466–477
7. Klein P (1975) Vitamin A acid and wound healing. Acta Dermatovener (Stockh) 55 (Suppl 74): 169-173
8. Marquardt DW (1963) An algorithm for least squares estimation of nonlinear parameters. J Soc Indust Appl Math 2:431–441
9. Ortonne JP, Schmitt D, Haftek M, Thivolet J (1980) Epidermal wound healing in man: quantitative evaluation immunofluorescence and ultrastructural study. J Invest Dermatol 74:448 (abstract)
10. Ortonne JP, Loning Th, Schmitt D, Thivolet J Immunomorphological and ultrastructural aspects of keratinocytes migration in epidermal wound healing. Virchows Archiv (in press)

C.E. Orfanos et al. (eds.)
Retinoids

Ro 10-9359 and Pregnancy

A.A. Cordero, M.A. Allevato and L. Donatti

Woman, aged 19, with erythrokeratodermia variabilis since age 6. She was under Tigason for 140 days (1.25 mg; 0.62 mg; and 0.25 mg/kg/day).

The skin was completely clear, the keratodermia was greatly improved. As this patient was living not in town (distant about 300 kilometers), we were forced to give her enough drug for two months. When she came for a periodical follow-up she was pregnant and had taken the drug during the first 55 days of pregnancy. Medication was stopped.

A child was born by cesarean section on the 36th week of gestation. Weight at birth: 3,200 g. Clinical examination: generalized lamellar scaling and dryness. Histopathology: moderate degree of hyperkeratosis, diminution of the granular layer, dermis normal. We have been following the baby for 2 years. He has no abnormalities. X-ray examination of the bones was normal. The mother received again Tigason and cleared perfectly as she did the first time.

The protocol on treatment with Ro 10-9359 closes:
1. The drug did not interfere with the course of pregnancy.
2. It did not produce any teratogenic effects.
3. It did not avoid the transmission of the ichthyotic process.

C.E. Orfanos et al. (eds.)
Retinoids

Elevated Levels of Triglycerides in Patients with Skin Disease Treated with Oral Aromatic Retinoid. The Significance of Risk Factors

H. Gollnick

The increasing significance of the use of synthetic retinoids for treatment of dermatological disorders and the broad spectrum of possible indications including other medical fields require and thorough investigations on the metabolic effects and side effects of this group of drugs.

Increased serum lipid levels have been reported, particularly of triglycerides, following administration of vitamin A acid ethylamide, all-trans vitamin A acid and 13-cis vitamin A acid (1–4) in humans and in animal experiments.

Can these observations be confirmed in patients with the skin diseases receiving treatment with the aromatic retinoid R 10-9359?

Patients. Serum triglyceride and cholesterol values were controlled repeatedly in 25 patients (14 women and 11 men aged between 18 and 88 years) receiving oral treatment with Ro 10-9359 in various dosages. Pretreatment values were available for 19 patients. Three patients had pretreatment lipid values at the upper limit of the normal range. The values of the other 6 patients were checked 6–8 months after beginning of therapy, in order to evaluate the effect of the drug after long-term treatment. No initial values have been recorded in these patients.

Dosage. 6 patients were on a decreasing dosage regime starting with 75 mg/day; 5 patients received increasing dosage starting with 35 mg/day and 9 were on a variable moderate dosage of about 50 mg/day.

Method. All patients were instructed to fast for at least 12 hours before the blood samples were taken. The laboratory investigation was carried out by means of the cholesteroloxidase-triglyceride kinase method in a centrifugal analyzer (Centrifichem Union Carbide).

Results

Triglycerides. In 5 patients (patients 1, 2, 3, 10 and 21) the triglyceride levels were found increased into the pathological range between 2 days and 12 weeks after beginning of treatment with Ro 10-9359. It seemed, moreover, that high initial dosages of retinoid may induce a rise of triglyceride levels rather and faster than lower dosage. In 2 cases the values improved after withdrawal of the drug or reduction of the daily dose, respectively (Fig. 1–3).
Cholesterol. In contrast, the cholesterol values varied, also extending into the pathological range, however, no positive relation was found either with the oral medication in general or with the dosage.

A striking observation in this study was the fact that the increases of blood lipid values occurred more readily in patients exhibiting risk factors. They were almost exclusively observed in this group. All patients with elevated lipid levels revealed one or more of such risk factors: *Obesity, alcohol abuse with alcoholic fatty liver, manifest or subclinical diabetes, and/or pre-existent disturbance of lipid metabolism* showing pretreatment lipid values at the upper normal range.

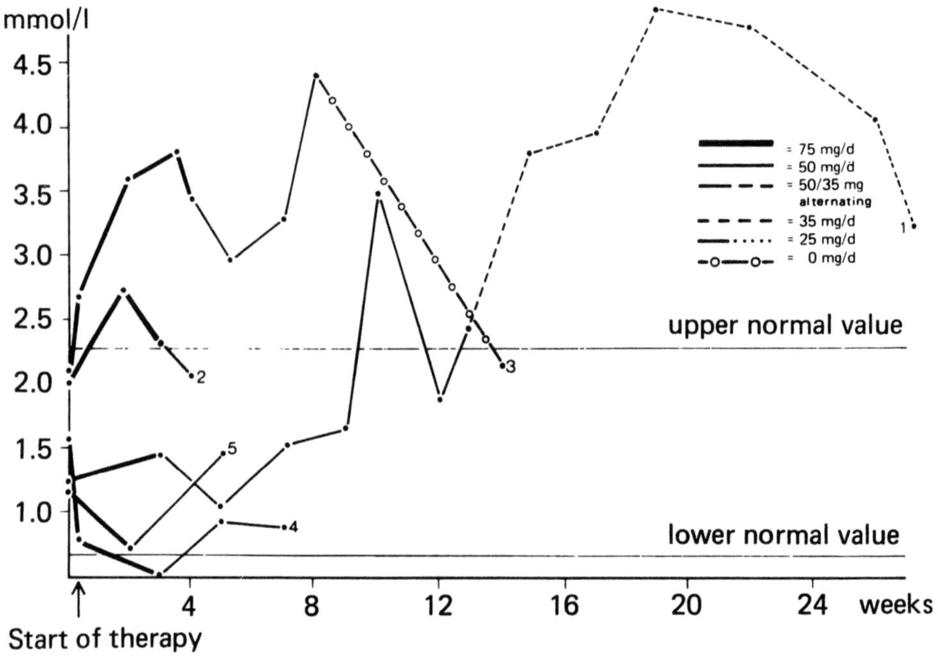

Fig. 1. Triglycerides during retinoid therapy in decreasing dosage (patients 1–5)

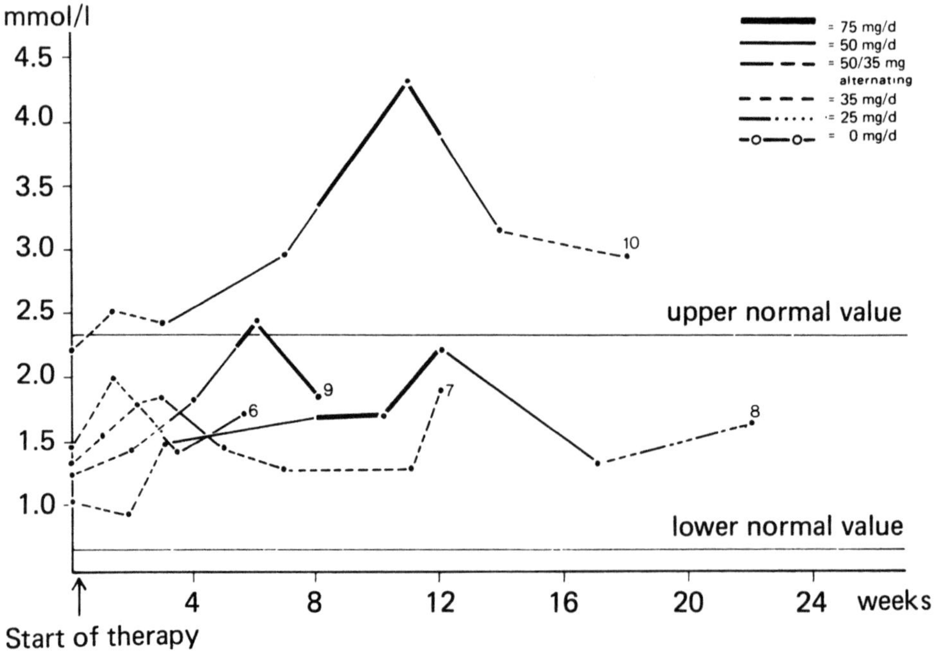

Fig. 2. Triglycerides during retinoid therapy in increasing dosage (patients 6–10)

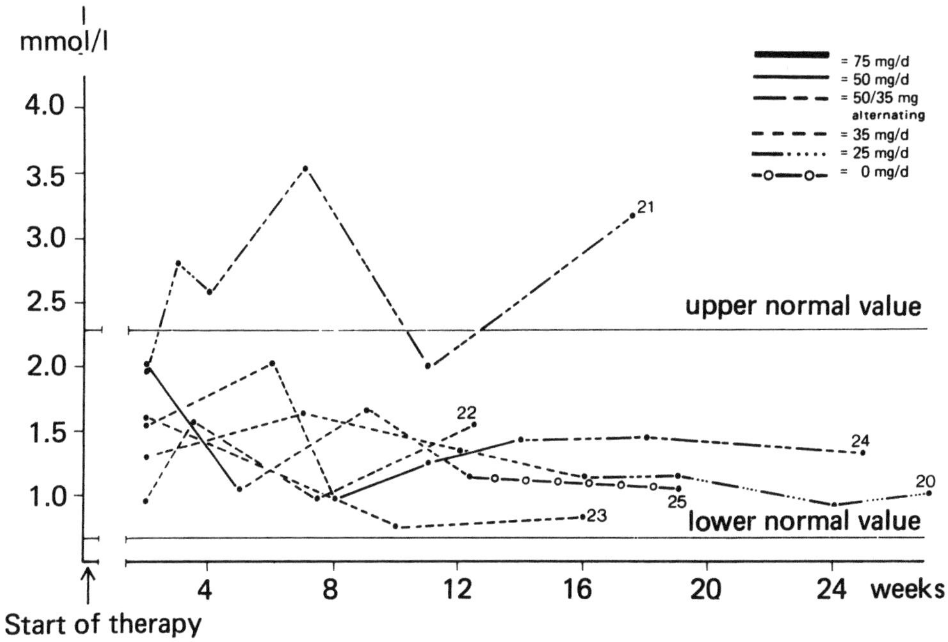

Fig. 3. Triglycerides during long-term (6–8 months) retinoid therapy (course control without initial values) (patients 20–25)

Discussion

The above results confirm that changes in serum triglycerides may occur after treatment with the aromatic retinoic Ro 10-9359. Therefore, regular controls must be carried out before, during and after oral retinoid treatment.

The presence of risk factors mentioned above must be taken into account when treatment with aromatic retinoids is considered, and lower dosage should be rather selected in such cases.

The assumption based on the results of animal studies conducted with vitamin A acid (all-trans and 13-cis) (1), that the effect of the retinoid is not mediated by chylomicrons but by VLDL-linked hypertriglyceridemia is subject for further investigation. Singh and Singh (5) have shown that the administration of vitamin A in rats leads to an increased mobilization of free fatty acids from adipose tissue and excessive deposits of neutral fats in hepatic tissue. Therefore, a more profound serum lipid analysis and investigations in a larger group of patients seem necessary.

References

1. Gerber LE, Erdman JW (1980) Comparative effects of all-trans and 13-cis-retinoic acid administration on serum and liver lipids in rats. J Nutr 110:343–351
2. Shuster S (1979) 13-cis retinoic acid. Lancet 2:8132
3. Peck GL (1980) Retinoids in dermatology. Arch Dermatol 116:283–284
4. Runne U, Orfanos CE, Gartmann H (1973) Perorale Applikation zweier Derivate der Vitamin A-Säure zur internen Psoriasis-Therapie: 13-cis-beta-Vitamin A-Säure und Vitamin A-Säure-aethylamid. Arch Dermatol Forsch 247:171–180
5. Singh M, Singh VN (1978) Fatty liver in hypervitaminosis. A: Synthesis and release of hepatic triglycerides. Am J Physiol 234:511–514

Present Status and Perspectives

C.E. Orfanos et al. (eds.)
Retinoids

Biological Effects of Retinoids

O. Braun-Falco

All those which did follow the fascinating and stimulating presentations during this symposion may agree, that this was a most successful meeting concerned to progress in dermatological treatment, induced by the development of retinoids. Without any doubt one can state that a new area in dermatotherapy has begun.

With vitamin A, various retinoic acids and the aromatic retinoids we know now a series of substances which, applicated locally or orally, have dramatic effects on skin diseases showing disturbances of epidermal and follicular keratinization, epidermal hyperproliferation and inflammatory dermal reactions. As we know, vitamin A regulates the growth and the differentiation of epithelial tissues; in cases of vitamin A deficiency the skin declines to develop hyperkeratosis and squamous metaplasia of mucous membranes. However, vitamin A has been a rather weak drug for treatment of keratotic conditions such as psoriasis or other dermatoses because, and it has only a small therapeutic range if given in effective doses.

The introduction of all-trans-retinoic acid was a further step for a better treatment of skin-diseases. However, for oral administration of this compound no indications exist today, because hypervitaminosis A syndromes could be seen rather frequently. Also after topical use, for example in acne vulgaris, skin irritation is regularly observed. Nevertheless, retinoic acid has still its place in the treatment of acne and similar conditions. Interesting effects were also seen in the treatment and prophylaxis of precancerous and cancerous skin conditions, as we have heard from Dr. Bollag (Switzerland). Even more interesting are new substances with a broader therapeutic range such as the aromatic retinoids etretinate and motretinid as well as the 13-cis-retinoic acid. Since these compounds may exert strong pharmacological effects it is important to know as much as possible about their pharmacology and toxicology; biological effects are indeed pharmacological effects.

The investigations of Dr. Paravicini (Switzerland) have shown that after a single dose of 100 mg etretinate given intravenously in animals, 75% of the dose is to be found in the faeces, 15% in the urine and 10% could not be discovered after 5 days. He also could show that plasma levels of both the unchanged drug and its metabolites corresponding to carboxylic acid may be detected up to 140 days after cessation of therapy. A half life of elimination of 80–100 days was calculated. The question as to where the drug may be stored in the human body is not yet clearly answered, p.e. in the liver or in the fatty tissue. It also could be shown, that there exists an intrahepatic circulation of retinoids. Due to biotransformation of retinoids metabolites may arise, characterized by a shortening of the polyene chain, by ring changes, by cis-trans-isomerization of the molecule or by glucuronidation; we know only little about the pharmacological effects of these metabolites. From these investigations it may be concluded that such substances which also have teratogenic effects should be applied in fertile woman only when contraceptive treatment is performed simultaneously longer than half a year after cessation of treatment.

The transport of retinoids has been also elucidated in the past years: Dr. Goodman (USA) reported, that there are two main *pathways for the transport of vitamin A and of retinoic esters.* It should be kept in mind that retinol is absorbed mainly via lymph chylomicrones, is metabolized into retinyl esters and is then stored in the liver. From the liver vitamin A is released into the plasma as a lipid soluble alcohol, bound to a specific transport protein: the retinol-binding-protein (RBP). Human RBP complexes with prealbumin in the same fashion are known for thyroxin. Since RBP may be decreased in liver diseases and increased in renal diseases, one should find disturbances of vitamin A delivery in these conditions. In contrast, retinoic acid and probably also other retinoids as well, are absorbed through the portal system and are transported in the plasma as carboxylate anions, bound to serum albumin, like free fatty acids. Recent observations seem to indicate that for the delivery of retinol to peripheral tissue specific surface RBP receptors are necessary; moreover, when retinol enters the target cell it may become associated to another intracellular binding protein (CRBP). This leads to the suggestion that in vitamin A toxicity clinical symptoms appear when excess of retinol begins to circulate in the plasma and is presented to the cell membranes in another form than bound to RBP. We do not know, however, how this relates to cutaneous tissues and how retinol is delivered to cutaneous cells. Because of this receptor regulating binding, vitamin A has a greater potential for toxicity. Also the experimental investigations of Dr. Vahlquist and others (Sweden) showed that there are no significant changes in physiological vitamin A transport in patients treated with etretinate, that means, that the two pathways for retinol and aromatic retinoids are rather unrelated one to the other. Since etretinate is mainly transported with lipoproteins, whereas the compound Ro 10-1670 migrates only with albumins, many different pathways may exist for every single substance.

According to our present knowledge all aromatic retinoids can induce more or less severe *side effects.* We are familiar with the clinical side effects. Dr. Teelmann (Switzerland) was able to show that under experimental conditions the side effects are dependent of the animal species (higher rate of side effects in rats than in mouse or dogs). In rats which received 0.5–3.0 mg/kg/day etretinate, he found reduction of body weight, bone deformations and enchondrial ossification as well as decrease of hemoglobin and increase of alkaline phosphatase; whereas, GOT/GPT did not show any significant changes. All these side effects in animal models were dose dependent and reversible after cessation in treatment. From those results we should conclude that especially in treating children with aromatic retinoids the indication should be choosen very carefully.

Of special practical importance are investigations on the *teratogenicity* and *mutagenicity* of aromatic retinoids. Dr. Hummler and Dr. Schüpbach (Switzerland) were able to show that the malformations and the teratogenic effects in animals treated with etretinate are rather similar to those found in hypervitaminosis A. They include eye abnormalities, cleft palate, craniofacial malformation and defects of the axial and appendicular sceleton. Interestingly enough, no mutagenic effects were observed. Dr. Happle and Dr. Niedworok (F.R. Germany) studied the chromosomal changes in 9 patients with psoriasis or other keratoses under treatment with etretinate. Their findings indicate that the retinoid etretinate given in usual oral doses (0.5–1.0 mg/kg/day) does not increase chromosomal instability in men. However, there are some preliminary results on sister chromatid exchanges under this type of treatment. Also the work of Dr. Obe and Dr. Tsambaos (F.R. Germany) on psoriatic patients under etretinate for 3–24 weeks did not reveal any changes in the frequency of exchange type aberrations in chromosomes of the peripheral lymphocytes compared to controls. From these investigations we can conclude, that aromatic retinoids have a definite teratogenic effect and that this effect is apparently not connected with mutagenic activities. This, however, does not tell us anything concerning carcinogenic effects of retinoids.

What are the *effects of retinoids on the skin?* We have heard so many, partly conflicting results in these few days that it is difficult to summarize the different observations made on different tissues using different substances in different concentrations and different application forms. It is without any doubt that these effects may be in relation to the different compounds available and dose dependent. However, the mode of action of aromatic retinoids and 13-cis-retinoic acid is not yet well understood. We have to realize that aromatic retinoids do effect ectodermal as well as mesodermal tissues and cells. The effects on ectodermal tissues comprise influences on proliferation and differentiation of epithelial tissues. The effects on mesodermal tissue seem to comprise influences on mesenchymal cells as well as immunological changes. Dr. Sporn (USA) reported that retinoids have hormone-like actions; they leed to inhibition of the proliferative action of prolactin on mammary epithelium. They also inhibit the proliferative paracrine effect of a polypeptide, the sarcoma growth factor on fibroblasts, and they block the autocrine effects of lymphokines or monokines on synovial cells.

It seems likely, that aromatic retinoids act as antiproliferative agents on proliferating epithelial tissues; however, there may also exert some proliferative action. The conflicting data which were reported during the symposion may be caused by technical problems.

As Dr. Bollag (Switzerland) said, chemically induced papillomas of the mouse skin are benign tumors, on which *antineoplastic activity* can be tested easily. Chemically induced skin papillomas regress under the influence of retinoic acids and aromatic retinoids. Together with the hypervitaminosis A syndrome-provoking activity of those substances he has come to an indicator for the therapeutic range of such compounds. Additional clinical observations have shown to us very clearly the antineoplastic effects of retinoids.

Dr. Verma (USA) studied the effects of retinoids on *tumor promotion* induced by carcinogenic chemical and biological alterations in the mouse epidermis. He found that retinoids do inhibit the skin tumor promotion induced by phorbolesters as well as, for example, by steroids. The inhibitory effect of retinoic acid on tumor promotion induced by phorbolesters seems to be reversible. Of particular interest is their finding that this inhibition is accompanied by rapid biochemical changes such as inhibition of the induction of ornithine decarboxylase activity (after 4 h) and elevation of putrescine (after 8 h). A clear parallelism between tumor induction and increasing levels of ornithine decarboxylase activity could be demonstrated. These experimental results seem to indicate, that the application of retinoids combined with steroids may result in a better inhibition of tumor promotion than by their separate application. The clinical consequences of these findings, however, cannot be discussed here.

The effects on *epithelial proliferation* induced by retinoic acid as well as of new synthetic aromatic retinoids were studied in epidermal cell cultures systems. Also here the results were not comparable. Dr. Pohl and Dr. Christophers (F.R. Germany) found that retinoic acid led to a remarkable increase of thymidin incorporation. This could be suggested, since we know the acanthogenic effect of retinoic acid. In higher doses, however, inhibition was observed – and this shows the dose-related problem! In contrast, etretinate as well as Ro 10-1670 did not show any significant stimulatory effect upon 3H-thymidin incorporation under these conditions. On the basis of experiments in combination with UVB they assume that retinoic acid probably may have a tumor promoting effect. The question however, as to where in the cell cycle retinoic acid and aromatic retinoids do attack, seems not to be clear at all. Dr. Mahrle, Dr. Wilkinson and Dr. Farber (USA) studied the effects of retinoic acid and of etretinate on cultured guinea pig epidermal cells growing on collagen gels. They showed that retinoic acid stimulates considerably the incorporation of 3H-thymidine and of 14C-leucine and increases the total epidermal cell number in the attached and detached fraction. However, an inhibitory effect could also be observed using higher concentrations. They also showed that etretinate increases the number of attached cells in early cell culture and decreases it in long term cell cultures. These effects are less understood. On the whole, however, these investigations seem to be good in vitro models for the understanding of the proliferative and shadding effects which can be seen in normal epidermis under oral retinoid treatment.

In general, we have to accept that under experimental conditions retinoic acid and aromatic retinoids may be able to induce epidermal hyperproliferation and may also act as antiproliferative agents. It is the antiproliferative effect which we use treating our patients with keratoacanthomas or praecanceroses in dermatology. In this relation the paper of Dr. Rusciani and his coworkers (Italy) is of interest. As they could show, there exist differences between the effect of etretinate on explants from psoriasis skin and from apparently healthy skin, taken from the same patients. Under experimental conditions they showed that etretinate decreases the mitotic activity of psoriasis cells, while it stimulates the cells of the apparently healthy skin. This seems to be a very important result. It shows that normal epidermis cells react in a different way compared to diseased and especially to acanthotic epidermal cells. We were able to observe similar results using tar under experimental conditions.

Most interesting are the effects of retinoic acid and aromatic retinoids on *epidermal differentiation.* From our clinical and dermatopathological experiences we know, that the normalisation of the horny layer in psoriasis preceeds the reduction of acanthosis. Dr. Marks (Great Britain) was able to show that there is perhaps in addition to the antiproliferative effect an specific effect on the process of keratinisation. He found, that under etretinate the indicative enzymes G6PDH is reduced quantitatively in the granular cell layer of the epidermis. The question, however, whether this is the consequence of reduced mitotic activity and epidermal cell turnover is not yet clear. Most significant are changes which perhaps may be interpreted as mucous metaplasia of human skin. Dr. Schultz-Ehrenburg and Dr. Orfanos (F.R. Germany) showed us excellent pictures on electron microscopical alterations of the diseased epidermis, especially in psoriasis, under treatment with oral retinoids. Most important seems the presence of a mucus-like material (MLM) intra- and extracellularly after one to three weeks in the lower layers of the stratum spinosum. Beside of this, vacuolar cytoplasmic degeneration, swelling of mitochondria and cell necrosis could be seen as signs of degeneration. This seems to indicate that there are dramatic effects on the epidermal differentiation under oral retinoid treatment; we showed the same to be true also under experimental conditions using retinoic acids. Interestingly enough MLM could also be found in clinically normal skin of psoriatic patients. Dr. Voorhees (USA) was able to show MLM with some granular components in the epidermis in all psoriatic patients he examined. However, he did not find any correlation between MLM and the course of the disease. Also the reduction of tonofibrils and desmosomes may be interpreted as a morphological sign of disturbed differentiation. The question about the synthesis and origin of the MLM (liver, surface glycoproteins, serum) is not yet answered. Certainly, the production of MLM is a sign of changed differentiation. One has to ask whether this is due to some interference of retinoids with the cellular DNA?

Dr. Madison and others (USA) could show that etretinate and its main metabolite TMMP, inhibit both proliferation and fibrous protein synthesis, namely the differentiation of isolated epidermal cells in culture. Interestingly enough, the retinoid effect on cell differentiation could be observed to occur earlier than the effect on epidermal proliferation. The question, therefore, arises whether these effects are independent one from another or not.

Also the effects of retinoids on *dermal cells* in psoriasis are rather dramatic. Dr. Schultz-Ehrenburg, Dr. Tsambaos, and Dr. Orfanos (F.R. Germany) showed us morphological changes indicating higher functional activity of Langerhans' cells; the intraepidermal migration of granulocytes seems to be inhibited, whereas Sézary-like stimulated lymphocytic cells do appear within the epidermis. In guinea pig skin as well as in psoriasis Dr. Tsambaos and Dr. Orfanos (F.R. Germany) found morphological alterations indicating activating effects of the drug on macrophages and fibroblasts, and also changes in the fibrous dermal tissue. The question whether these effects are drug-specific or a sign of cytotoxicity is not yet clear. It may be, that retinoids effect the cell surfaces. Dr. Bauer and Dr. Orfanos (F.R. Germany) found that under experimental conditions TMMP-retinoid may be bound to lectins and plasma cell membranes thus leading to interruption of lectin-cell interactions in vitro. Perhaps as a consequence of this reaction the response of human peripheral blood lymphocytes to mitogenic stimuli induced by lectins is inhibited. This is another paper with suggests effects of retinoids not only on the keratinizing epithelial tissue, but also on immunocompetent mesenchymal cells. On the basis of these results an *immunomodulatory action* of retinoid has been suggested.

We are just beginning to explore the effects of various retinoids on the cellular and humoral immune systems. In this respect the clinical observations of regression of lupus erythematosus and arthritis is of importance. Very interesting are the investigations of Dr. Hercend and coworkers (France) which showed that retinoids such as etretinate increase under experimental conditions the capacity of treated spleen cells to lyse antibody-coated chick erythrocytes and to activate peritoneal macrophages rendering them highly cytostatic for P815 mastocytoma cells in vitro. Similarly, the activation of T-cells and the induction of suppressor cells and natural killer cells is of particular interest. This may be in relation to the shortened transplantate reaction time which could be observed under experimental conditions. On the other hand, immunostimulatory effects on B-cells could not be observed. These data let us assume that retinoids may also stimulate antitumor immunity mechanisms. In my mind this is a very important observation which should stimulate us to continue in studying the effects of aromatic retinoids in immunologic skin disorders. Interesting are also special effects on leucocytes which could be found in acne patients by Dr. Plewig and others (Munich).

In conclusion, one can state that the new developments starting from retinoic acid and leading to new compounds such as the aromatic retinoids have opened new doors for treatment of skin diseases. We have a profound amount of basic information, which shows that these compounds are interfering with the normal growth and its steady state in epithelial tissues, with the differentiation of epithelial cells and also with the functional properties of dermal cells like fibroblasts, macrophages and inflammatory cells. With etretinate we know a drug which mainly effects the epithelial tissues and with 13-cis-retinoic acid a substance, which has stronger anti-inflammatory effects and effects on the sebaceous glands.

This allows us to assume that with the further development of such compounds we may receive substances, which exert normalizing effects mainly on epidermal disorders of keratinization, others which exert mainly antiproliferative effects, others with antiseborrhoic effects or again others with stronger anti-inflammatory effects. In some years from now we may have a new family of substances for oral treatment of skin diseases with disorders of keratinization, proliferative skin disorders and those, which are connected with inflammatory reactions. In this respect the further development of retinoids may reveal a gradual change of our treatment to a more internal type of treatment of dermatoses. Since all these substances exert only a morbostatic effects it is very important to take always into account the benefit-risk-ratio, when treating our patients. In this respect we are waiting for substances which have a broader therapeutic range as those available today. But beside of this, there is much to be done to elucidate the different pharmacological effects of this new series of highly reactive retinoids, which have led already now to such a great progress in dermatological treatment.

C.E. Orfanos et al. (eds.)
Retinoids

The Use of Oral Aromatic Retinoids in Psoriasis Therapy: an Overview of Past, Present, and Future Developments

E.M. Farber and L. Nall

Vitamin A research had its fundamental beginnings in 1909 when Steppe first described a fat-soluble principle, which proved essential for life (15). Now, more than seven decades later, a new therapeutic agent - the aromatic retinoid (Ro 10-9359) - has become available to provide dermatology with one of the most important drugs that has ever been introduced for the treatment of psoriasis. It is possible that Ro 10-9359 may replace many current agents in treating psoriasis and that the application of the retinoid as an adjuvant with anthralin or PUVA may be beneficial for the routine management of the disease in maintenance doses (16).

Psoriasis is a dynamic and variegated disease. There are periods of exacerbation as well as periods of decreased morbidity. It is a disease known to respond to an agent and subsequently become resistant to that same agent during various courses of treatment.

The following is a brief review of some of the papers and posters presented during this symposion set within a clinical frame of experience in many single and multicenter trials.

Early Investigations

Mayer, Bollag and others (15) have provided us with a comprehensive review of the retinoids as a new class of compounds with prophylactic activities in oncology and dermatology.

Vitamin A, vitamin A acid (retinoic acid), and their synthetic analogs or derivatives have been applied in the management of psoriasis with different therapeutic results. They influence the proliferation rate and the differentiation of human keratinizing epithelia and have beneficial effects on skin diseases with disturbances of keratinization.

Systemic application of vitamin A has been discontinued since high doses leading to clearing develop evident systemic toxicity, whereas the antipsoriatic effect of vitamin A acid is either moderate or restricted because of the hypervitaminosis A syndrome. In 1972–1973 Orfanos and his coworkers introduced for the first time new synthetic retinoids such as 13-cis-retinoid acid and retinoic acid ethylamide for oral treatment of psoriasis (25, 30). They tested their clinical efficacy and they described their side effects in humans, including elevations of triglycerides. In 1974 Bollag found in the animal experiment that the retinoic acid analog - aromatic retinoid "I" (later called Ro 10-9359) - possessed a therapeutic index which was 10 times more favorable than that of the retinoic acid (2, 3). With Ott (28) he tested the Ro 10-9359 in psoriasis patients and discovered that the therapeutic activity was good to excellent, and that the side effects of hypervitaminosis A were reversible upon cessation of treatment. The next year Orfanos and Runne (22) found that the combined regimen of oral retinoids with the topical application of anthralin increased the clinical response and shortened the duration of the traditional local treatment.

Current Investigations

Single and multicenter trials in many laboratories throughout the world have shown oral Ro 10-9359 to be effective in psoriasis as well as other skin diseases characterized by accelerated pathological keratinization (5, 7, 8, 10, 12, 18, 19, 20–26).

Although teratogenicity in humans has not been evaluated, the drug has proven to be so in animal studies; therefore, it is contraindicated in women in the child-bearing category; or in children unless the condition is so severe that the possible benefits outweigh the potential risks. The side effects from daily doses of Ro 10-9359 equal to or greater than 1 mg/kg/day almost invariably produce a dose-related appearance of a variety of symptoms characteristic of hypervitaminosis A: cheilitis, dryness of the nasal and buccal mucosa, desquamation of the palms and soles, hair loss along with varying side effects. These clinical manifestations are accompanied by possible elevations of the transaminases and the alkaline phosphatases; however, both clinical and laboratory side effects are reversible upon cessation of the treatment.

Symposion Papers

The Ro 10-9359 has not only been effective in treating generalized plaque psoriasis, but has been especially beneficial in erythroderma and pustular types as well as psoriasis with arthropathy as has been shown during this symposion where studies have been described in which a single therapy – the aromatic retinoid – was used (6, 9, 27), whereas other studies reported various combined therapies: such as the aromatic retinoid and PUVA (11, 14, 21), the retinoid and corticosteroid (32), and the retinoid and ultraviolet irradiation (1, 4, 26, 31).

Dominguez-Soto has presented the results of follow-up studies in which two dosage schedules with the Ro 10-9359 – continuous and intermittent – were carried out in 21 patients with psoriasis, that had been resistant to other forms of therapy. He reported on 18 of these patients in which the continuous treatment format utilized 1 mg/kg/day for one to two weeks, decreasing to 0.66 mg/kg/day by weeks 5 and 6, and down to 0.33 mg/kg/day in weeks 7 and 8. The next phase – intermittent – from weeks 9 to 52 employed 0.33 mg/kg/day alternating with placebo. Dominguez-Soto reported that the typical retinoid-associated side effects were evident at the beginning of the treatment and were dose related; however, a tapering off of the severity of these side effects was noted as treatment continued. His experience has shown that the continuous schedule was more effective than the intermittent regimen (6).

Jablonska (13) reported double-blind studies with Ro 10-9359 in which she and her coworkers observed good results in severe pustular psoriasis and psoriasis vulgaris, although only occasionally successful with the erythrodermic form. Orfanos (17) found that it was essential to employ different dosages of the aromatic retinoid for various forms of psoriasis. For example, he used minimal doses for the erythrodermic form and aggressive amounts for pustular psoriasis to achieve efficacy.

Results of long-term use of the aromatic retinoid was given by Ott (27) in patients suffering from psoriasis and various disorders of keratinization. Oral doses of 20 to 50 mg per day were administered for two years; of these, 42 had been treated for four years. In 11 patients with severe psoriasis, therapy with Ro 10-9359 has been administered for greater than six years. He has not observed any life threatening systemic problems or loss of efficacy from this long-term therapy.

It has been shown that a paradoxical reaction occasionally takes place in the use of the retinoids in that new areas of psoriasis appear in regions not previously involved. Rufli (29) reported that among the cutaneous side effects of the aromatic vitamin A acid derivative, Ro 10-9359, his group has seen a dermatitis, which shows characteristic primary lesions and distribution. A papulovesicular retinoid dermatitis appears first, which subsequently develops into psoriasis. It is possible that the retinoid dermatitis is a Koebner phenomenon due to increased skin fragility or increased thinness.

Lassus et al. (14) discussed another combination therapy: RePUVA (21). He employed the Ro 10-9359 and PUVA in four different groups:

1. Retinoid for 10 weeks
2. Retinoid for 4 weeks followed by PUVA for 6 weeks
3. Retinoid for 10 weeks simultaneously with PUVA during *last* 6 weeks
4. PUVA alone

Lassus found that Group 3 showed the greatest improvement: good to excellent in effectiveness in 75 to 100% of the patients; however, there was no significant difference between RePUVA and PUVA. Retinoid alone proved least effective. He pointed out that in addition to the high efficacy of RePUVA, there is a reduction of total UVA doses to about 40% as compared to PUVA, which is an important consideration for long-term treatment.

Grupper and Berretti (11) reported results observed in 126 patients affected with severe psoriasis who had been treated in accordance with five different schedules, three of them combining aromatic retinoid with PUVA therapy. The most effective results had been obtained with a schedule involving an initial treatment during a two-week period with the aromatic retinoid alone followed on the 15th day by the adjunction of the classical PUVA therapy, which in turn was followed by a progressive decrease in the retinoid daily dosage. There was therefore a reduction in the frequencies and lengths of PUVA treatments with a concomitant lessening in the amount of energy of irradiation required.

Another innovative approach to treating psoriasis with the aromatic retinoid was to combine it with topically applied corticosteroids, as investigated by van der Rhee and Polano (33). In a multicenter double-blind trial, the effect of three therapy regimes was studied in 90 psoriasis patients over a 6-week period.

1. Ro 10-9359 orally (0.5–0.66 mg/kg/body weight) and placebo cream topically
2. Ro 10-9359 (same dosage) with 0.1% triamcinolone acetonide and 5% salicylic acid in Lanette wax cream
3. Placebo capsules with the same corticosteroid dosage as in 2.

Their results indicated that according to regimen 2, good to excellent improvement was seen in 60% of the patients. In the first year after the start of the study, 31 patients interrupted treatment; 37 of the 59 remaining patients have been followed for two years and found to have had more or less constant remissions after two years; 43 patients are still under treatment. Thirty-one of this series have been in complete remission for two years on an average dose of 25 mg per day with neglible side effects. Some investigators voice a concern about sequelae stemming from long-term continuous corticosteroid application.

A number of studies reported clinical improvement with 1 mg/kg/body weight, using emolliation and UVB, reducing the dosage to 0.5 mg/kg/day as toxicity and side reactions appeared (26, 30). Boer and Suurmond (1) clearly confirmed that a 0.5 mg/kg/day of the Ro 10-9359 plus UVB irradiation was effective; more effective than 0.5 mg of the retinoid alone or the UVB alone. Born and his colleagues (4) also confirmed that lower doses of the retinoid are feasible when used concurrently with UVA-B.

Dr. Stöllenwerk (32), a rheumatologist, presented findings in using the Ro 10-9359 in 25 patients with psoriasis and arthropathy.

In spite of the drug-related side effects, she concluded that the Ro 10-9359 is effective in treating patients with both these diseases, and that the psoriatic lesions improved in more than 70% of the cases and that the "psoriatic arthritis" improved in 66%.

The relationship of psoriasis and arthritis is a highly controversial one, as pointed out by Dr. Grupper during the discussion period, since no satisfactory definition for "psoriatic arthritis" has been established by either the rheumatologists or dermatologists.

There is much to be done in the basic areas of determining the association of psoriasis and arthritis before we can fully evaluate the effectiveness of any regimen, including the aromatic retinoid.

Conclusions

In summarizing the findings in the literature and the symposion papers and posters, the following main points can be made with regard to the use of Ro 10-9359 in psoriasis.

As to the beneficial aspects:

Efficacy. The aromatic retinoid is the most effective treatment of pustular psoriasis to date. It is highly effective in palmar and plantar psoriasis, as well as erythrodermic psoriasis and psoriasis vulgaris.

Combination Therapy. When used in combination with other known effective modalities, lower retinoid dosage is possible with fewer retinoid-related side effects.

Toxicity. There is no bone marrow or renal toxicity in therapeutic doses. In man, there is transient elevation of transaminase, bilirubin, serum lipids, and alkaline phosphatase, but these are reversible.

Rebounds. There is no evidence of the occurrence of rebounds.

Cancers. The aromatic retinoid is not a carcinogen; in fact, it may act as a cancer chemopreventive agent. Immunologic patterns may be suppressed or stimulated; conflicting studies require continued work in this area.

As to the detrimental aspects:

Teratogenicity. Animal studies indicate the possibility of teratogenicity. Perhaps it would be wise to screen severely afflicted females of childbearing age by a committee including a dermatologist, psychologist, and a social worker – comparable to a Tumor Board.

Relapse. Like insulin, the oral retinoid is effective only as long as it is administered. It does not provide long-term remissions.

Side Effects. Muco-cutaneous side reactions are a burden to an otherwise satisfied patient.

Although the mode of action of the aromatic retinoid is not clear, it is reasonable to speculate that the drug is acting to modify the inflammatory response. The inflammatory responses include the invasion of the dermis and occasionally the epidermis by cellular elements such as neutrophils, plasma cells and lymphocytes. One could predict that the aromatic retinoid would be effective by initiating therapy with low dosage, e.g., 0.33 mg/kg/day along with emolliation, and after two to three months gradually increase the dosage up to 0.5 mg/kg/day with emolliation, and if necessary, ultraviolet light. On this regimen the clinician and the patient would have to be content to wait three to six months before noticeable improvement becomes apparent.

It is hoped that the future use of aromatic retinoids for psoriasis will be as judiciously and intelligently planned as the investigational studies reported at this congress. The practicing dermatologist has a grave responsibility to use the retinoid with an understanding of the natural history of psoriasis in the individual patient, and he should think of this drug in the context of the patient's need for total care.

References

1. Boer J, Suurmond D Combined UVB phototherapy and low dose oral retinoid Ro 10-9359 for psoriasis not sufficiently responding to UVB alone (poster). International Dermatology Symposion, Berlin, 1980
2. Bollag W (1972) Prophylaxis of chemically induced benign and malignant epithelial tumors by vitamin A acid (retinoic acid). Eur J Cancer 8:689–693
3. Bollag W (1974) Therapeutic effects of an aromatic retinoic acid analog on chemically induced skin papillomas and carcinomas of mice. Eur J Cancer 10:731–737
4. Born W, Wokalek H, Schöpf E Oral retinoid promotion of UV action in psoriasis - a measure of UV radiation protection (poster). International Dermatology Symposion, Berlin, 1980
5. Dahl B, Mollenbach K, Reymann F (1977) Treatment of psoriasis vulgaris with a new retinoic acid derivative Ro 10-9359. Dermatologica 154:261–267
6. Dominguez-Soto L, Hojyo-Tomoka MT Intermittent dose schedule of retinoids (Ro 10-9359) - long-term follow-up in psoriasis. International Dermatology Symposion, Berlin, 1980
7. Fredriksson T, Pettersson U (1978) Severe psoriasis - oral therapy with a new retinoid. Dermatologica 157:238–244
8. Fritsch P, Hönigsmann H, Jaschke E, Wolff K (1978) Augmentation of oral methoxypsoralen-photochemotherapy with an oral retinoic acid derivative. J Invest Dermatol 70:178–182
9. Gatti JC, Cardama JE, Gabrielli M, Cabrera H Treatment of severe forms of psoriasis with a retinoid acid derivative: Ro 10-9359. International Dermatology Symposion, Berlin, 1980
10. Goerz G, Orfanos C (1978) Systemic treatment of psoriasis with a new aromatic retinoid. Dermatologica 157 (Suppl 1):38–44
11. Grupper C, Berretti B Treatment of psoriasis by oral PUVA therapy combined with aromatic retinoid. International Dermatology Symposion, Berlin, 1980
12. Günther S (1973) The therapeutic value of retinoic acid in chronic discoid, acute guttate, and erythrodermic psoriasis: clinical observations on twenty-five patients. Br J Dermatol 89:515–517
13. Jablonska S, Wolska H, Dąbrowski J, Jarząbek-Chorzelska M, Kraińska T, Haftek M Aromatic retinoids in psoriasis: clinical, histological, histochemical, electron microscopical and immunological investigations. International Dermatology Symposion, Berlin, 1980
14. Lassus A, Lauharanta J, Juvakoski T Ro 10-9359, RePUVA and PUVA in the treatment of psoriasis. International Dermatology Symposion, Berlin, 1980
15. Mayer H, Bollag W, Hänni R, Rüegg R (1978) Retinoids, a new class of compounds with prophylactic and therapeutic activities in oncology and dermatology. Experientia 34:1105–1119
16. Orfanos CE (1978) Oral administration of retinoids. Dermatologica 157 (Suppl 1):2–4
17. Orfanos CE Retinoids: advances in basic research and therapy - introductory remarks. International Dermatology Symposion, Berlin, 1980
18. Orfanos C, Goerz G (1978) Orale Psoriasis-Therapie mit einem neuen aromatischen Retinoid (Ro 10-9359). Dtsch med Wochenschr 103:195–199
19. Orfanos C, Landes E, Bloch P (1978) Traitement du psoriasis pustuleux par un nouveau retinoide aromatique (Ro 10-9359). Ann Dermatol Venereol 105:807–811
20. Orfanos CE, Mahrle G, Goerz G, Happle R, Hofbauer M, Landes E, Schimpf A (1979) Laboratory investigations in patients with generalized psoriasis under oral retinoid treatment. A multicenter study of computerized data. Dermatologica 159:62–70
21. Orfanos CE, Pullmann H, Sterry W, Künzig M (1978) Retinoid PUVA (RePUVA): systemic combination therapy in psoriasis. Z Hautkr 53:494–504
22. Orfanos C, Runne U (1976) Systemic use of a new retinoid with and without local dithranol treatment in generalized psoriasis. Br J Dermatol 95:101–103
23. Orfanos C, Runne U (1978) Tissue changes in psoriatic plaques after oral administration of retinoid. Dermatologica 157 (Suppl 1):19–25
24. Orfanos CE, Schmidt HW, Mahrle G, Gartmann H, Lever WF (1973) Retinoic acid in psoriasis:

its value for topical therapy with and without corticosteroids. Br J Dermatol 88:167–181
25. Orfanos C, Schmidt H, Mahrle G, Runne U (1972) Die Wirksamkeit von Vitamin-A-Säure (VAS) bei Psoriasis. Örtliche Kombinationsbehandlung mit Corticoiden. Zwei neue VAS-Präparate zur peroralen Therapie. Arch Derm Forsch 244:424–428
26. Orfanos C, Steigleder G, Pullmann H, Bloch P (1979) Oral retinoid and UVB radiation: a new alternative treatment for psoriasis on an outpatient basis. Acta Derm Venerol (Stockh) 59: 241–244
27. Ott F Long-term experience with the retinoid Ro 10-9359 in the treatment of psoriasis and other keratinizing dermatoses. International Dermatology Symposion, Berlin, 1980
28. Ott F, Bollag W (1975) Therapie der Psoriasis mit einem oral wirksamen neuen Vitamin-A-Säure-Derivat. Schweiz med Wschr 105:439–441
29. Rufli T Psoriasis-like dermatitis in non-psoriatic patients as a side-effect of Ro 10-9359. International Dermatology Symposion, Berlin, 1980
30. Runne U, Orfanos CE, Gartmann H (1973) Perorale Applikation zweier Derivate der Vitamin A-Säure zur internen Psoriasis-Therapie. 13-cis-beta-Vitamin A-Säure und Vitamin A-Säure-aethylamid. Arch Derm Forsch 247:171–180
31. Steigleder GK, Orfanos CE, Pullmann H (1979) Retinoid-selective ultraviolet phototherapy (SUP) in psoriasis. Z Hautkr 54:19–23
32. Stollenwerk R, Fischer-Hoinkes H, Komenda K, Schilling F Clinical and scintigraphic studies in the treatment of psoriatic arthritis with the aromatic retinoid Ro 10-9359. International Dermatology Symposion, Berlin, 1980
33. van der Rhee HJ, Polano MK Treatment of psoriasis vulgaris with a combination of a low-dosage Ro 10-9359 orally and corticosteroids topically. International Dermatology Symposion, Berlin, 1980

C.E. Orfanos et al. (eds.)
Retinoids

Closing Remarks on Acne

J.S. Strauss

It is a pleasure for me to present the summation of the studies on acne. Most of the presentations have been given by investigators who have been identified with acne research for many years. However, I want to emphasize right from the beginning that Dr. Gary Peck of the National Cancer Institute in Bethesda deserves credit for first having alerted us to the effectiveness of 13-cis-retinoic acid in patients with severe acne. Had we not seen the photographs of his dramatic results, I doubt that the studies would have proceeded as far as they have by now.

There is no question that orally administered 13-cis-retinoic acid is an extremely effective drug for the treatment of severe nodulocystic acne. Placebo therapy was not part of any of the studies on acne reported in this conference. However, 1 mg/kg/day of 13-retinoic acid is much more active than the aromatic retinoid in producing a decrease in sebaceous gland activity and in causing clearing of cystic acne. This does demonstrate that 13-cis-retinoic acid is better than a placebo, if one considers the minimally effective aromatic retinoic to be the "placebo control". Furthermore, the patients treated with 13-cis-retinoic acid were taken from a treatment-resistant population. While investigators from Munich have shown us data that indicate that at a dosage level of 20 mg/kg the effect of 13-cis-retinoic acid and the aromatic derivative are comparable in decreasing sebaceous gland size in animals, this is an extremely large dose which is well beyond the dose range that is being used in man. The difference in effectiveness of the two drugs in acne is an indication of the specificity of the molecular structure of the retinoid in its follicular activity. It would appear that this difference does not exist in relation to the therapy of keratinizing disorders, where the aromatic compound is at least as effective as 13-cis-retinoic acid. The report by the Philadelphia group indicates that retinol also has sebum suppression and therapeutic activity when given orally, but it is not as efficacious as 13-cis-retinoic acid. The data seem to indicate that retinol and the aromatic compound are about equal in controlling acne, although they have not been compared side by side.

What are the characteristics of the response to 13-cis-retinoic acid? First of all, the dosage may be much smaller than that required for the keratinizing disorders. Clinical effectiveness with dosages as low as 0.1 mg/kg have been reported in this symposion. It has also been shown that sebum production is inhibited by this small dose although the level of inhibition is less than that observed with higher dosages. An outstanding characteristic of the response of 13-cis-retinoic acid and one that is extremely important is the production of long-term remissions. These remissions may or may not be related to prolonged inhibition of sebum production. Long-term inhibition of sebum production has been observed but it has not been a uniform finding. The response to therapy is rapid considering the degree of involvement, but it does lag approximately a month behind the inhibition of sebum production. It has been reported that the therapeutic response is more rapid in those patients who have more severe acne. Lesions of the face clear better than those on the back. Finally, one group of investigators has reported that clearing occurs faster in women.

How do the retinoids work in acne? The answers are by no means completely known, but if we consider the various mechanisms by which drugs work in acne, there are many promising leads. The aim of the modern approach to acne is to decrease sebaceous gland activity, to correct the altered pattern of keratinization within the follicle, to decrease the microbial flora and thereby the activity of microbial enzymes, and finally to produce an anti-inflammatory effect. There is definite evidence that sebaceous gland inhibition is produced by oral retinoids. The evidence is based on functional and histologic studies. Studies in humans have shown that the glands are smaller; sebum production is decreased; the labelling index is decreased; and that there are more undifferentiated cells than differentiated cells in the sebaceous lobules after treatment with the retinoids. Animal studies have been confirmatory and Dr. Gomez has proposed that since 13-cis-retinoic acid does not cause any change in the hair or the pigmentary system in hamster costovertebral glands, that the action on the sebaceous glands might be a post-hormonal effect. This remains to be determined.

Most of the reports given in this symposion relate to the use of retinoids in disorders of keratinization. Different dosages have been used, but it is my impression that with the aromatic retinoid, satisfactory results have been observed with dosages as low as 0.5 mg/kg/day. Data that I have seen from Dr. Peck's laboratory would indicate that higher dosages of 13-cis-retinoic acid are used in keratinizing diseases. An altered pattern of keratinization in the follicular duct is the initial finding in acne, and one might speculate that the oral retinoids are inhibiting or reversing this change in keratinization. This may not be true, however, for, as just mentioned, the dosage of 13-cis-retinoic acid used for keratinizing disorders probably exceeds the dose required for the treatment of acne.

We have heard that there is a decrease in the follicular microbial population in oral retinoid-treated patients, and this may be responsible for some of the clinical improvement. Along with this, it has been noted that the free fatty acids are decreased during retinoid therapy, indicating a decrease in the microbial enzymatic activity. Both of these effects may, however, be secondary to the decrease in sebaceous gland activity.

Finally, studies from the Munich group indicate that there is a decrease in the inflammatory response to potassium iodide patch tests in acne patients being treated with 13-cis-retinoic acid. This has been interpreted as an indication that the drug has anti-inflammatory activity, there are other studies that have been discussed in this symposion which also indicate that retinoids may influence immunologic events.

What are the questions for the future? First of all, it is extremely important that we continue investigative studies on the mechanism of action of the drug. We also need to continue to further define the optimal dose and duration of therapy. A third important question is what kind of acne should be treated with the oral retinoids. My own personal feeling is that at the present moment 13-cis-retinoic acid should be used primarily in severe inflammatory acne until we have more clinical and laboratory evidence on potential side effects. Finally, while 13-cis-retinoic acid is presently clearly the drug of choice for the treatment of acne, we should continue to search for other analogs which might be equally effective but have less potential for side effects. There is still considerable work to be done in spite of the fact that it would appear that a very effective agent has been developed.

Subject Index

MIX
Papier aus verantwortungsvollen Quellen
Paper from responsible sources
FSC® C105338

If you have any concerns about our products,
you can contact us on
ProductSafety@springernature.com

In case Publisher is established outside the EU,
the EU authorized representative is:
Springer Nature Customer Service Center GmbH
Europaplatz 3, 69115 Heidelberg, Germany

Printed by Libri Plureos GmbH
in Hamburg, Germany